D0787478

DSM-5® Made Easy

Also from James Morrison

Diagnosis Made Easier:
Principles and Techniques for Mental Health Clinicians, Second Edition

The First Interview, Fourth Edition

When Psychological Problems Mask Medical Disorders:
A Guide for Psychotherapists

For more information, see *www.guilford.com/morrison*

DSM-5® Made Easy

The Clinician's Guide to Diagnosis

James Morrison

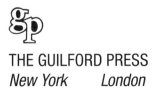

THE GUILFORD PRESS
New York   London

© 2014 The Guilford Press
A Division of Guilford Publications, Inc.
72 Spring Street, New York, NY 10012
www.guilford.com

All rights reserved

No part of this book may be reproduced, translated, stored in a retrieval system, or transmitted, in any form or by any means, electronic, mechanical, photocopying, microfilming, recording, or otherwise, without written permission from the publisher.

Printed in the United States of America

This book is printed on acid-free paper.

Last digit is print number: 9   8   7   6   5   4   3   2

The author has checked with sources believed to be reliable in his effort to provide information that is complete and generally in accord with the standards of practice that are accepted at the time of publication. However, in view of the possibility of human error or changes in behavioral, mental health, or medical sciences, neither the author, nor the editor and publisher, nor any other party who has been involved in the preparation or publication of this work warrants that the information contained herein is in every respect accurate or complete, and they are not responsible for any errors or omissions or the results obtained from the use of such information. Readers are encouraged to confirm the information contained in this book with other sources.

Library of Congress Cataloging-in-Publication Data

Morrison, James R., author.
    DSM-5 made easy : the clinician's guide to diagnosis / James Morrison.
        p. ;   cm.
    Includes bibliographical references and index.
    ISBN 978-1-4625-1442-7 (hardcover : alk. paper)
    I. Title.
    [DNLM: 1. Diagnostic and statistical manual of mental disorders. 5th ed
  2. Mental Disorders—diagnosis—Case Reports.   3. Mental Disorders—classification—Case Reports.   WM 141]
    RC469
    616.89′075—dc23
                                       2014001109

DSM-5 is a registered trademark of the American Psychiatric Association. The APA has not participated in the preparation of this book.

For Mary, still *my sine qua non*

About the Author

James Morrison, MD, is Affiliate Professor of Psychiatry at Oregon Health and Science University in Portland. He has extensive experience in both the private and public sectors. With his acclaimed practical books—including, most recently, *Diagnosis Made Easier, Second Edition,* and *The First Interview, Fourth Edition*—Dr. Morrison has guided hundreds of thousands of mental health professionals and students through the complexities of clinical evaluation and diagnosis. His website (*www.guilford.com/jm*) offers additional discussion and resources related to psychiatric diagnosis and DSM-5.

Acknowledgments

Many people helped in the creation of this book. I want especially to thank my wife, Mary, who has provided unfailingly excellent advice and continual support. Chris Fesler was unsparing with his assistance in organizing my web page.

Others who read portions of the earlier version of this book, *DSM-IV Made Easy*, in one stage or another included Richard Maddock, MD, Nicholas Rosenlicht, MD, James Picano, PhD, K. H. Blacker, MD, and Irwin Feinberg, MD. I am grateful to Molly Mullikin, the perfect secretary, who contributed hours of transcription and years of intelligent service in creating the earlier version of this book. I am also profoundly indebted to the anonymous reviewers who provided input; you know who you are, even if I don't.

My editor, Kitty Moore, a keen and wonderful critic, helped develop the concept originally, and has been a mainstay of the enterprise for this new edition. I also deeply appreciate the many other editors and production people at The Guilford Press, notably Editorial Project Manager Anna Brackett, who helped shape and speed this book into print. I would single out Marie Sprayberry, who went the last mile with her thoughtful, meticulous copyediting. David Mitchell did yeoman service in reading the manuscript from cover to cover to root out errors. I am indebted to Ashley Ortiz for her intelligent criticism of my web page, and to Kyala Shea, who helped get it web borne.

A number of clinicians and other professionals provided their helpful advice in the final revision process. They include Alison Beale, Ray Blanchard, PhD, Dan G. Blazer, MD, PhD, William T. Carpenter, MD, Thomas J. Crowley, MD, Darlene Elmore, Jan Fawcett, MD, Mary Ganguli, MD, Bob Krueger, PhD, Kristian E. Markon, PhD, William Narrow, MD, Peter Papallo, MSW, MS, Charles F. Reynolds, MD, Aidan Wright, PhD, and Kenneth J. Zucker, PhD. To each of these, and to the countless patients who have provided the clinical material for this book, I am profoundly grateful.

Contents

Frequently Needed Tables

Introduction

The summer after my first year in medical school, I visited a friend at his home near the mental institution where both of his parents worked. One afternoon, walking around the vast, open campus, we fell into conversation with a staff psychiatrist, who told us about his latest interesting patient.

She was a young woman who had been admitted a few days earlier. While attending college nearby, she had suddenly become agitated—speaking rapidly and rushing in a frenzy from one activity to another. After she impulsively sold her nearly new Corvette for $500, her friends had brought her for evaluation.

"Five hundred dollars!" exclaimed the psychiatrist. "That kind of thinking, that's schizophrenia!"

Now my friend and I had had just enough training in psychiatry to recognize that this young woman's symptoms and course of illness were far more consistent with an episode of mania than with schizophrenia. We were too young and callow to challenge the diagnosis of the experienced clinician, but as we went on our way, we each expressed the fervent hope that this patient's care would be less flawed than her assessment.

For decades, the memory of that blown diagnosis has haunted me, in part because it is by no means unique in the annals of mental health lore. Indeed, it wasn't until many years later that the first diagnostic manual to include specific criteria (DSM-III) was published. That book has since morphed into the enormous fifth edition of the *Diagnostic and Statistical Manual of Mental Disorders* (DSM-5), published by the American Psychiatric Association.

Everyone who evaluates and treats mental health patients must understand the latest edition of what has become the world standard for evaluation and diagnosis. But getting value from DSM-5 requires a great deal of concentration. Written by a committee with the goal of providing standards for research as well as clinical practice in a variety of disciplines, it covers nearly every conceivable subject related to mental health. But you could come away from it not knowing how the diagnostic criteria translate to a real live patient.

I wrote *DSM-5 Made Easy* to make mental health diagnosis more accessible to clinicians from all mental health professions. In these pages, you will find descriptions of every mental disorder, with emphasis on those that occur in adults. With it, you can learn how to diagnose each one of them. With its careful use, no one today would mistake that young college student's manic symptoms for schizophrenia.

What Have I Done to Make DSM-5 Easy?

Quick Guides. Opening each chapter is a summary of the diagnoses addressed therein—and other disorders that might afflict patients who complain about similar problems. It also provides a useful index to the material in that chapter.

Introductory material. The section on each disorder starts out with a brief description designed to orient you to the diagnosis. It includes a discussion of the major symptoms, perhaps a little historical information, and some of the demographics—who is likely to have this disorder, and in what circumstances. Here, I've tried to state that which I would want to know myself if I were starting out afresh as a student.

Essential Features. OK, that's the name I've given them in in *DSM-5 Made Easy*, but they're also known as *prototypes*. I've used them in an effort to make the DSM-5 criteria more accessible. For years, we working clinicians have known that when we evaluate a new patient, we don't grab a list of emotional and behavioral attributes and start ticking off boxes. Rather, we compare the data we've gathered to the picture we've formed of the various mental and behavioral disorders. When the data fit an image, we have an "aha!" experience and pop that diagnosis into our list of differential diagnoses. (From long experience and conversations with countless other experienced clinicians, I can assure you that this is exactly how it works.)

Very recently, a study of mood and anxiety disorders[*] has found that clinicians who make diagnoses by rating their patients against prototypes perform at least as well as, and sometimes better than, other clinicians who adhere to strict criteria. That is, it can be shown that prototypes have validity even greater than that of some DSM diagnostic criteria. Moreover, prototypes are reported to be usable by clinicians with a relatively modest level of training and experience; you don't have to be coming off 20 years of clinical work to have success with prototypes. And clinicians report that prototypes are less cumbersome and more clinically useful. (However—and I hasten to underscore this point—the prototypes used in the studies I have just mentioned were generated from the diagnostic criteria inherent in the DSM criteria.) The bottom line: Sure, we need criteria, but we can adapt them so they work better for us.

So once you've collected the data and read the prototypes, I recommend that you

---

[*]DeFife JA, Peart J, Bradley B, Ressler K, Drill R, Westen D: Validity of prototype diagnosis for mood and anxiety disorders. *JAMA Psychiatry* 2013; 70(2): 140–148.

assign a number to indicate how closely your patient fits the ideal of any diagnoses you are considering. Here's the accepted convention: 1 = little or no match; 2 = some match (the patient has a few features of the disorder); 3 = moderate match (there are significant, important features of the disorder); 4 = good match (the patient meets the standard—the diagnosis applies); 5 = excellent match (a classic case). Obviously, the vignettes I've provided will always match at the 4 or 5 level (if not, why would I use them as illustrative examples?), so I haven't bothered to grade them on the 5-point scale. But you should do just that with each new patient you interview.

Of course, there may be times you'll want to turn to the official DSM-5 criteria. One is when you're just starting out, so you can get a picture of the exact numbers of each type of criteria that officially count the patient as "in." Another would be when you are doing clinical research, where you must be able to report that participants were all selected according to scientifically studied, reproducible criteria. And even as an experienced clinician, I return to the actual criteria from time to time. Perhaps it's just to have in my mind the complete information that allows me to communicate with other clinicians; sometimes it is related to my writing. But mostly, whether I am with patients or talking with students, I stick to the prototype method—just like nearly every other working clinician.

The Fine Print. Most of the diagnostic material included in these sections is what I call *boilerplate*. I suppose that sounds pejorative, but each Fine Print section actually contains one or more important steps in the diagnostic process. Think of it this way: The prototype is useful for purposes of inclusion, whereas the boilerplate is useful largely for the also important exclusion of other disorders and delimitation from normal. The boilerplate verbiage includes several sorts of stereotyped phrases and warnings, which as an aid to memory I've dubbed *the D's*. (I started out by using "Don't disregard the D's" or similar phrases, but soon got tired of all the typing; so, I eventually adopted "the D's" as shorthand.)

Differential diagnosis. Here I list all the disorders to consider as alternatives when evaluating symptoms. In most cases, this list starts off with substance use disorders and general medical disorders, which despite their relative infrequency you should always place first on the list of disorders competing for your consideration. Next I put in those conditions that are most treatable, and hence should be addressed early. Only at the end do I include those that have a dismal prognosis, or that you can't do very much to treat. I call this the *safety principle* of differential diagnosis.

Distress or disability. Most DSM-5 diagnostic criteria sets require that the patient experience distress or some form of impairment (in work, social interactions, interpersonal relations, or something else). The purpose is to ensure that we discriminate people who are patients from those who, while normal, perhaps have lives with interesting aspects.

As best I can tell, *distress* receives one definition in all of DSM-5 (Campbell's *Psychiatric Dictionary* doesn't even list it). The DSM-5 sections on trichotillomania and excoriation (skin-picking) disorder both describe distress as including negative feelings such as embarrassment and forfeiture of control. It's unclear, however, whether the same definition is employed anywhere else, or what might be the dominant thinking throughout the manual. But for me, some combination of lost pride, shame, and control works pretty well as a definition. (DSM-IV didn't define *distress* anywhere.)

Duration. Many disorders require that symptoms be present for a certain minimum length of time before they can be diagnosed. Again, this is to ensure that we don't go around indiscriminately handing out diagnoses to everyone. For example, nearly everyone will feel blue or down at one time or another; to qualify for a diagnosis of a depressive disorder, it has to hang on for at least a couple of weeks.

Demographics. A few disorders are limited to certain age groups or genders.

Coding Notes. Many of the Essential Features listings conclude with these notes, which supply additional information about specifiers, subtypes, severity, and other subjects relevant to the disorder in question.

Here you'll find information about specifying subtypes and judging severity for different disorders. I've occasionally put in a signpost pointing to a discussion of principles you can use to determine that a disorder is caused by the use of substances.

Sidebars. To underscore or augment what you need to know, I have sprinkled sidebar information throughout the text (such as the one above). Some of these merely highlight information that will help you make a diagnosis quickly. Some contain historical information and other sidelights about diagnoses that I've found interesting. Many include editorial asides—my opinions about patients, the diagnostic process, and clinical matters in general.

Vignettes. I have based this book on that reliable device, the clinical vignette. As a student, I found that I often had trouble keeping in mind the features of diagnosis (such as it was back then). But once I had evaluated and treated a patient, I always had a mental image to help me remember important points about symptoms and differential diagnosis. I hope that the more than 130 patients I have described in *DSM-5 Made Easy* will do the same for you.

Evaluation. This section summarizes my thinking for every patient I've written about. I explain how the patient fits the diagnostic criteria and why I think other diagnoses are unlikely. Sometimes I suggest that additional history or medical or psychological testing should be obtained before a final diagnosis is given. The conclusions stated here allow you to match your thinking against mine. There are two ways you can do this. One is by picking out from the vignette the Essential Features I've listed for each diagnosis. But when you want to follow the thinking of the folks who wrote the actual DSM-5, I've also included references (in parentheses) to the individual criteria. If you disagree with any of my interpretations, I hope you'll e-mail me (*morrjame@ohsu.edu*). And for updated information, visit my website: *www.guilford.com/jm*.

Final diagnosis. Usually code numbers are assigned in the record room, and we don't have to worry too much about them. That's fortunate, for they are sometimes less than perfectly logical. But to tell the record room folks how to proceed, we need to put all the diagnostic material that seems relevant into verbiage that conforms to the approved format. My final diagnoses not only explain how I'd code each patient; they also provide models to use in writing up the diagnoses for your own patients.

Tables. I've included a number of tables to try to give you an overall picture of various topics—the variety of specifiers that apply across different diagnoses, a list of physical disorders that can produce emotional and behavioral symptoms. Those that are of principal use in a given chapter I've included in that chapter. A few, which apply more generally throughout the book, you'll find in the Appendix.

My writing. Throughout, I've tried to use language that is as simple as possible. My goal has been to make the material sound as though it was written by a clinician for use with patients, not by a lawyer for use in court. Wherever I've failed, I hope you will e-mail me to let me know. At some point, I'll try to put it right, either in a future edition or on my website (or both).

Structure of *DSM-5 Made Easy*

The first 18 chapters* of this book contain descriptions and criteria for the major mental diagnoses and personality disorders. Chapter 19 comprises information concerning other terms that you may find useful. Many of these are Z-codes (ICD-9 calls them V-codes), which are conditions that are not mental disorders but may require clinical attention anyway. Most noteworthy are the problems people with no actual mental disorder have in relating to one another. (Occasionally, you might even list a Z-code/V-code as the reason a patient was referred for evaluation.) Also described here are codes that indicate medications' effects, malingering, and the need for more diagnostic information.

---

*OK, I cheated a little. DSM-5 actually has 19, but for ease of description, I combined the two mood disorder chapters into one (which is how they were in DSM-IV). However, no confusion should result; DSM-5 doesn't number its chapters, anyway.

Chapter 20 contains a very brief description of diagnostic principles, followed by some additional case vignettes, which are generally more complicated than those presented earlier in the book. I've annotated these case histories to help you to review the diagnostic principles and criteria covered previously. Of course, I could include only a small fraction of all DSM-5 diagnoses in this section.

Throughout the book, I have tried to give you clinically relevant and accessible information, written in simple, declarative sentences that describe what you need to know in diagnosing a patient.

Quirks

Here are a few comments regarding some of my idiosyncrasies.

Abbreviations. I'll cop to using some nonstandard abbreviations, especially for the names of disorders. For example, BPsD (for brief psychotic disorder) isn't something you'll read elsewhere, certainly not in DSM-5. I've used it and others for the sake of shortening things up just a bit, and thus perhaps reducing ever so slightly the amount of time it takes to read all this stuff. I use these ad hoc abbreviations just in the sections about specific disorders, so don't worry about having to remember them longer than the time you're reading about these disorders. Indeed, I can think of two disorders that are sometimes abbreviated CD and four that are sometimes abbreviated SAD, so always watch for context.

My quest for shortening has also extended to the chapter titles. In the service of seeming inclusive, DSM-5 has sometimes overcomplicated these names, in my view. So you'll find that I've occasionally (not always—I've got *my* obsessive–compulsive disorder under control!) shortened them up a bit for convenience. You shouldn't have any problem knowing where to turn for sleep disorders (which DSM-5 calls *sleep–wake disorders*), mood disorders (*bipolar and related disorders* plus *depressive disorders*), psychotic (*schizophrenia spectrum and other psychotic*) disorders, cognitive (*neurocognitive*) disorders, substance (*substance-related and addictive*) disorders, eating (*feeding and eating*) disorders, and various other disorders from which I've simply dropped *and related* from the official titles. Similarly, I've sometimes dropped the */medication* from *substance/medication-induced* [just about anything].

{Curly braces}. I've used these in the Essential Features and in some tables to indicate when there are two mutually exclusive specifier choices, such as {with}{without} good prognostic features. Again, it just shortens things up a bit.

Severity specifiers. One of the issues with DSM-5 is its use of complicated severity specifiers that differ from one chapter to another, and sometimes from one disorder to the next. Some of these are easier to use than others.

For example, for the psychoses, we are offered the Clinician-Rated Dimensions of

Psychosis Symptom Severity (CRDPSS?), which asks us to rate on a 5-point scale, based on the past 7 days, each of eight symptoms (the five psychosis symptoms of schizophrenia [p. 58] plus impaired cognition, depression, and mania); there is no overall score, only the eight individual components, which we are encouraged to rate again every few days. My biggest complaint about this scale, apart from its complexity and the time required, is that it gives us no indication as to overall functioning—only the degree to which the patient experiences each of the eight symptoms. Helpfully, DSM-5 informs us that we are allowed to rate the patient "without using this severity specifier," an offer that many clinicians will surely rush to accept.

Evaluating functionality. Whatever happened to the Global Assessment of Functioning (GAF)? In use from DSM-III-R through DSM-IV-TR, the GAF was a 100-point scale that reflected the patient's overall occupational, psychological, and social functioning—but not physical limitations or environmental problems. The scale specified symptoms and behavioral guidelines to help us determine our patients' GAF scores. Perhaps because of the subjectivity inherent in this scale, its greatest usefulness lay in tracking changes in a patient's level of functioning across time. (Another problem: It was a mash-up of severity, disability, suicidality, and symptoms.)

However, the GAF is now G-O-N-E, eliminated for several reasons (as described in a 2013 talk by Dr. William Narrow, research director for the DSM-5 Task Force). Dr. Narrow (accurately) pointed out that the GAF mixed concepts (psychosis with suicidal ideas, for example) and that it had problems with interrater reliability. Furthermore, what's really wanted is a disability rating that helps us understand how well a patient can fulfill occupational and social responsibilities, as well as generally participate in society. For that, the Task Force recommends the World Health Organization Disability Assessment Schedule, Version 2.0 (WHODAS 2.0), which was developed for use with clinical as well as general populations and has been tested worldwide. DSM-5 gives it on page 747; it can also be accessed online (*www.who.int/classifications/icf/whodasii/en/*). It is scored as follows: 1 = none, 2 = mild, 3 = moderate, 4 = severe, and 5 = extreme. Note that scoring systems for the two measures are reciprocal; a high GAF score more or less equates with a low WHODAS 2.0 rating.

After quite a bit of experimentation, I decided that the WHODAS 2.0 is so heavily weighted toward physical abilities that it poorly reflects the qualities mental health clinicians are interested in. Some of the most severely ill mental patients received a only a moderate WHODAS 2.0 score; for example, Velma Dean (p. 90) scored 20 on the GAF but 1.6 on the WHODAS 2.0. In addition, calculation of the WHODAS 2.0 score rests on the answers given by the patient (or clinician) to 36 questions—a burden of data collection that many busy professionals will not be able to carry. And, because these answers cover conditions over the previous month, the score cannot accurately represent patients with rapidly evolving mental disorders. The GAF, on the other hand, is a fairly simple (if subjective) way to estimate severity.

So, after much thought, I've decided not to recommend the WHODAS 2.0 after all. (Anyone who is interested in further discussion can write to me; I'll be happy to send along a chart that compares the GAF with the WHODAS 2.0 for every patient mentioned in this book.) Rather, here's my fix as regards evaluating function and severity, and it's the final quirk I'll mention: Go ahead and use the GAF. Nothing says that we can't, and I find it sometimes useful for tracking a patient's progress through treatment. It's quick, easy (OK, it's also subjective), and free. You can specify the patient's current level of functioning, or the highest level in any past time frame. You'll find it in the Appendix of this book.

Using This Book

There are several ways in which you might use *DSM-5 Made Easy.*

Studying a diagnosis. Of course, you might go about this in several ways, but here's how I'd do it. Scan the introductory information for some background, then read the vignette. Next, compare the information in the vignette to the Essential Features, to assure yourself that you can pick out what's important diagnostically. If you want to see how well the vignettes fit the actual DSM-5 criteria, read through the vignette evaluations; there I've touched upon each of the important diagnostic points. In each evaluation section, you'll also find a discussion of the differential diagnosis, as well as some other conditions often found in association with the disorder in question.

Evaluating a patient whose diagnosis you think you know. Read through the Essential Features, then check the information you have on this patient against the prototype. Assign a 1–5 score, using the key given above (p. 3). Check through the D's to make sure you've considered all disqualifying information and relevant alternative diagnoses. If all's well and you've hit the mark, I'd also read through the evaluation section of the relevant vignette, just to make sure you've understood the criteria. Then you might want to read the introductory material for background.

Evaluating a new patient. Follow the sequence given just above, with one exception: After identifying one of several areas of clinical interest as a diagnostic possibility—let's say an anxiety disorder—you might want to start with the Quick Guide in the relevant chapter. There you will find capsule statements (too brief even to be called summaries) that might direct you to one or more disorders to consider further. Some patients will have problems in a number of areas, so you may have to explore several chapters to select all of the right diagnoses. Chapter 20 provides some additional pointers on diagnostic strategy.

Getting the broader view. Finally, there are a lot of disorders out there. Many will be familiar to you, but for others your information may be a little sketchy. So just reading through the book and hitting the high points (perhaps sampling the vignettes) may load your quiver with a few new diagnostic arrows. I hope that eventually you'll read the entire book. Besides introducing you to a lot of mental disorders, it should also give you a feel for how a diagnostician might approach an array of clinical problems.

Whatever course you take, I recommend that you confine your reading to relatively short segments. I have done my best to simplify the criteria and to explain the reasoning behind them. But if you consider more than a few diagnoses at a time, they'll probably begin to run together in your mind. I also recommend one other step to help you learn faster: After you have read through a vignette, go back and try to pick out each of the Essential Features before you look at my evaluation. You will retain the material better if you actively match the case history information with these features than if you just rely on passively absorbing what I have written.

Code Numbers

I'm afraid we've been played a rough trick as regards the code numbers we use. DSM-5 came out just as the 10th revision of the *International Classification of Diseases* (ICD-10) was about to be brought into full play in the United States. (For years, it has already been in use elsewhere in the world.) So at the time of DSM-5's publication, the old ICD-9* was still in use. The change-over is currently scheduled for October 1, 2014. DSM-5 has printed the ICD-10 code numbers for diagnoses in parentheses. I assume that readers will be using the book for many years, so I've given the ICD-10 versions pride of place, with the old numbers indicated in square brackets. Here's an example:

F40.10 [300.23]   Social anxiety disorder

However, we'll probably be translating back and forth between ICD-9 and ICD-10 for another decade or so.

One feature of ICD-10 codes is that they are much more complete than was true for ICD-9. That serves us well for accurate identification, retrieval of information for research, and other informational purposes. But it increases the number of, um, numbers we have to be familiar with. Mostly, I've tried to include what you need to know along with the diagnostic information associated with each disorder I discuss. Some of this information is so extensive and complex that I have condensed it into one or two tables. Most notable of these is Table 15.2 in Chapter 15, which gives the ICD-10 code numbers for substance-related mental disorders.

---

*Technically, both ICDs are a version called CM (for Clinical Modification)—hence ICD-9-CM and ICD-10-CM. I'll use the CM versions here, but I'm going to avoid the extra typing labor. So I refer just to ICD-10, period.

Using the DSM-5 Classification System

After decades of DSM advocacy for five axes on which to record the biopsychosocial assessment of our patients, DSM-5 has at last taken the ultimate step—and reversed course completely. Now all mental, personality, and physical disorders are recorded in the same place, with the principal diagnosis mentioned first. When you've made a "due to" diagnosis (such as catatonic disorder due to tuberous sclerosis), the ICD convention is to list first the physical disease process. The actual reason for the visit comes second, with the parenthetical statement *(reason for visit)* or *(principal diagnosis)* appended. I'm not sure just how often clinicians will adhere to this convention. Many will reason, I suspect, that this is a medical records issue and pay it no further mind. In any event, here is how you can write up the diagnosis.

Obviously, you need to record every mental diagnosis. Nearly every patient will have at least one of these, and many will have two or more. For example, imagine that you have a patient with two diagnoses: bipolar I disorder and alcohol use disorder. (Note, incidentally, that I've followed DSM-5's refreshing new style, which is to abandon the previous, somewhat Germanic practice of capitalizing the names of specific diagnoses.) Following the DSM-5 convention, first list the diagnosis most responsible for the current evaluation.

Suppose that, while evaluating the social anxiety disorder, you discovered that your patient also was drinking enough alcohol to qualify for a diagnosis of mild alcohol use disorder. Then the diagnosis should read:

F40.10 [300.23]   Social anxiety disorder
F10.10 [305.00]   Alcohol use disorder, mild

In this example, the first diagnosis would have to be social anxiety disorder (that's why the patient sought treatment). And of course, if the alcohol use was what had prompted the evaluation, you'd reverse the places for the two diagnoses.

DSM-IV required a separate location (the notorious Axis II) for the personality disorders and what was then called mental retardation. The purpose was to give special status to these lifelong attributes and to help ensure that they would not be ignored when we were dealing with our patients' often more pressing major pathology. But the logic of the division wasn't always impeccable—so, partly to coordinate its approach with how the rest of the world now views mental disorders, DSM-5 has done away with axes. In any event, personality disorders and mental retardation (or intellectual disability, as it now is) are included right along with all other diagnoses, mental and physical. I think that this is a good thing, though, like all change, it'll take a little while for us older clinicians to get used to it. It also means that material such as a patient's GAF score (or WHODAS 2.0 rating, should you opt to use it) will have to be placed in the body of your summary statement.

An Uncertain Diagnosis

When you're not sure whether a diagnosis is correct, consider using the DSM-5 qualifier *(provisional)*. This term may be appropriate if you believe that a certain diagnosis is correct, but you lack sufficient history to support your impression. Or perhaps it is still early in the course of your patient's illness, and you expect that more symptoms will develop shortly. Or you may be waiting for laboratory tests to confirm the presence of another medical condition that you suspect underlies your patient's illness. Any of these situations could warrant a provisional diagnosis. A couple of DSM-5 diagnoses— schizophreniform psychosis and brief psychotic disorder—require you to append *(provisional)* if the symptoms have not yet resolved. But you could use this term in just about any situation where it seems that safe diagnostic practice warrants it.

What about a patient who comes very close to meeting full criteria, who has been ill for a long time, who has responded to treatment appropriate for the diagnosis, and who has a family history of the same disorder? Such a patient deserves a definitive diagnosis, even though the criteria are not quite met. That's one reason I've gone over to the use of prototypes. After all, diagnoses are not decided by the criteria; diagnoses are decided by clinicians, who use criteria as guidelines. That's *guidelines*, as in "help you," not *shackles*, as in "restrain you."

Actually, DSM-5 has provided another way to list a diagnosis that seems uncertain: "other specified [name of] disorder." This allows you to put down the name of the category along with the specific reason you find the patient doesn't meet criteria for the diagnosis. For a patient who has a massive hoard of useless material in the house, but who has suffered no distress or disability, you could record "other specified hoarding disorder, lack of distress or impairment."

I'll bet we'd both be interested to learn just how often this option gets exercised.

Indicating Severity of a Disorder

DSM-5 includes specific severity specifiers for many diagnoses. They are generally pretty self-explanatory, and I've usually tried to boil them down just a bit, for the sake of your sanity and mine. DSM-IV provided the GAF as a generic way to indicate severity; I've already indicated above that I'd like to continue using it.

Other Specifiers

Many disorders include specifiers indicating a wide variety of information—with (or without) certain defined accompanying symptoms; current degrees of remission; and course features such as early (or late) onset or recovery, either partial or full. Some of these specifiers require additional code numbers; some are just a matter of added verbiage. Add as many of these as seem appropriate. Each one potentially helps the next clinician understand that patient just a little better.

Physical Conditions and Disorders

Physical illness may have a direct bearing on the patient's mental diagnoses; this is especially true of the cognitive disorders. In other cases, physical illness may affect (or be affected by) the management of a mental disorder. An example would be hypertension in a psychotic patient who believes that the medication has been poisoned. (Some of this stuff is formalized in the diagnosis of psychological factors affecting other mental conditions; see Chapter 8, p. 266.) In any event, whereas physical disorders used to have their own axis, that's no longer the case either. In fact, the ICD-10 recording scheme requires that when a mental disorder is due to a physical condition, the physical condition must be listed first.

Psychosocial and Environmental Problems

You can report certain environmental or other psychosocial events or conditions that might affect the diagnosis or management of your patient. These may have been caused by the mental disorder, or they may be independent events. They should have occurred within the year prior to your evaluation. If they occurred earlier, they must have contributed to the development of the mental disorder or must be a focus of treatment. DSM-5 requires that we use ICD-10 Z-codes (or ICD-9 V-codes) for the problems we identify. I've given a reasonably complete list of those available in Chapter 19. When stating them, be as specific as possible. You'll find plenty of examples scattered throughout the text.

Just What Is a Mental Disorder?

There are many definitions of *mental disorder*, none of which is both accurate and complete. Perhaps this is because nobody yet has adequately defined the term *abnormal*. (Does it mean that the patient is uncomfortable? Then many patients with manic episodes are not abnormal. Is abnormal that which is unusual? Then highly intelligent people are abnormal.)

The authors of DSM-5 provide the definition of mental disorder that they used to help them to decide whether to include a diagnosis in their book. Paraphrased, here it is:

> A *mental disorder* is a clinically important syndrome; that is, it's a collection of symptoms (these can be behavioral or psychological) that causes the person disability or distress in social, personal, or occupational functioning.

The symptoms of any disorder must be something more than an expected reaction to an everyday event, such as the death of a relative. Behaviors that primarily reflect a conflict between the individual and society (for example, fanatic religious or political ideology) are not usually considered mental disorders.

A number of additional points about the criteria for mental disorders bear emphasizing:

1. Mental disorders describe processes, not people. This point is made explicit to address the fears of some clinicians that by using the criteria, they are somehow "pigeonholing people." Patients with the same diagnosis may be quite different from one another in many important aspects, including symptoms, personality, other diagnoses they may have, and the many distinctive aspects of their personal lives that have nothing at all to do with their emotional or behavioral condition.

2. To a degree, some of what's abnormal, and of course far more that isn't, is determined by an individual's culture. Increasingly, we are learning to take culture into account when defining disorders and evaluating patients.

3. Don't assume that there are sharp boundaries between disorders, or between any disorder and so-called "normality." For example, the criteria for bipolar I and bipolar II disorders clearly set these two disorders off from one another (and from people who have neither). In reality, all bipolar conditions (and probably lots of others) are likely to fit somewhere along a continuum.

4. The essential difference between a physical condition such as pneumonia or diabetes, and mental disorders such as schizophrenia and bipolar I disorder, is that we know what causes pneumonia or diabetes. However, either mental disorder could turn out to have a physical basis; perhaps we just haven't yet found it. In operational terms, the difference between physical and mental disorders is that the former are not the subjects of DSM-5 or of *DSM-5 Made Easy.*

5. Basically, DSM-5 follows the medical model of illness. By this, I don't mean that it recommends the prescription of medication. I mean that it is a descriptive work derived (largely) from scientific studies of groups of patients who appear to have a great deal in common, including symptoms, signs, and life course of their disease. Inclusion is further justified by follow-up studies, which show that people belonging to these groups have a predictable course of illness months, or sometimes years, down the road.

6. With a few exceptions, DSM-5 makes no assumptions about the etiology of most of these disorders. This is the famous "atheoretical approach" that has been much praised and criticized. Of course, most clinicians would agree about the cause of some mental disorders (neurocognitive disorders, such as neurocognitive disorder due to Huntington's disease or with Lewy bodies, come to mind).

The descriptions of the majority of DSM-5 diagnoses will be well accepted by clinicians whose philosophical perspectives include social and learning theory, psychodynamics, and psychopharmacology.

Some Warnings

In defining mental health disorders, several warnings seem worth repeating:

1. The fact that the manual omits a disorder doesn't mean that it doesn't exist. Until now, with each new edition of the DSM, the number of listed mental disorders has increased. Depending on how you measure these things, DSM-5 appears to be an exception. On the one hand, it contains close to 600 codable conditions—nearly double the number included in its predecessor, DSM-IV-TR.[*] On the other hand, DSM-5 contains some 157 main diagnoses (by my count, 155), an overall reduction of about 9%. This feat was achieved through a fair amount of lumping conditions under one title (as occurred, for example, in the sleep–wake disorders chapter). However, there are probably still more conditions out there, waiting to be discovered. Prepare to invest in DSM-6 and *DSM-6 Made Easy.*

2. Diagnosis isn't for amateurs. Owning a set of prototypes is no substitute for professional training in interview techniques, diagnosis, and the many other skills that a mental health clinician needs. DSM-5 states—and I agree—that diagnosis consists of more than just checking off the boxes on a bunch of symptoms. It requires education, training, patience, and yes, patients (that is, the experience of evaluating many mental health patients).

3. DSM-5 may not be uniformly applicable to all cultures. These criteria are derived largely from studies of North American and European patients. Although the DSMs have been widely used with great success throughout the world, it is not assured that mental disorders largely described by North American and European clinicians will translate to other languages and other cultures. We should be wary of diagnosing pathology in patients who may express unusual beliefs that may be widely held in ethnic or other subcultures. An example would be a belief in witches once prevalent among certain Native Americans. Beginning on page 833 of DSM-5, you'll find a list of specific cultural syndromes.

4. DSM-5 isn't meant to have the force of law. Its authors recognize that the definitions used by the judicial system are often at odds with scientific require-

---

[*]To be fair, the vast bulk of the increase is due not to new disorders, but to ever-thinner slices of the original pie, served up with new numbers that reflect DSM-5's (and ICD-10's) finer diagnostic distinctions. Especially well represented are the now nearly 300 ways to say "substance/medication-induced this or that."

ments. Thus having a DSM-5 mental disorder may not exempt a patient from punishment or other legal restrictions on behavior.

5. Finally, the diagnostic manual is only as good as the people who use it. Late in his career, George Winokur, one of my favorite professors in medical school (and my first boss once I got out of training), co-wrote a brief paper[*] that investigated how well the DSM (at that time, it was DSM-III) assured consistency of diagnosis. Even among clinicians at the same institution with similar diagnostic approaches, it turned out, there were problems. Winokur et al. especially called attention to the amount of time expended on making a mental health diagnosis, to systematic misinterpretations of criteria, and to nonsystematic misreadings of the criteria. They concluded, "The Bible may tell us so, but the criteria don't. They are better than what we had, but they are still a long way from perfect." In DSM-5, those statements are still true.

The Patients

Many of the patients I've described in the vignettes are composites of several people I have known; some I've reported just as I knew them. In every instance, though (except the very few in which I have used actual well-known persons), I have tweaked the vital information to protect identities, to provide additional data, and sometimes just to add interest. Of course, the vignettes do not present all of the features of the diagnoses they are meant to illustrate, but then hardly any patient does. My intention has been, rather, to convey the flavor of each disorder.

Although I have provided over 130 vignettes to cover most of the major DSM-5 conditions, you'll notice some omissions. For one thing, there are just too many of them to illustrate every possible substance-related mood, psychotic, and anxiety disorder—that would occupy a book twice the length of this one. For disorders that begin in early life (Chapter 1), I have included vignettes and discussion only when a condition is also likely to be encountered in an adult. Specifically, these are intellectual disability, attention-deficit/hyperactivity disorder, autism spectrum disorder, and Tourette's disorder. However, you will find prototypes and brief introductory discussions for all disorders that begin during the neurodevelopmental period. *DSM-5 Made Easy* therefore contains diagnostic material pertinent to all DSM-5 mental disorders.

---

[*]Winokur G, Zimmerman M, Cadoret R: 'Cause the Bible tells me so. *Arch Gen Psychiatry* 1988; 45(7): 683–684.

CHAPTER 1

Neurodevelopmental Disorders

In earlier DSMs, the name of this chapter was even more of a mouthful: "Disorders Usually First Evident in Infancy, Childhood, or Adolescence." Now the focus is on the individual during the formative period, when the development of the nervous system takes place, hence, and logically enough, neurodevelopmental. However, *DSM-5 Made Easy* emphasizes the evaluation of older patients—later adolescence to maturity, and beyond. For that reason, I've taken some liberties in arranging the conditions discussed in this chapter—placing those that I discuss at length at the beginning, and listing later just the prototypes (with some discussion) for others.

Of course, many of the disorders considered in subsequent chapters can be first encountered in children or young adolescents; anorexia nervosa and schizophrenia are two examples that spring to mind. Conversely, many of the disorders discussed in this chapter can continue to cause problems for years after a child has grown up. But only a few commonly occupy clinicians who treat adults. For the remainder of the disorders DSM-5 includes in its first chapter, I provide introductions and Essential Features, but no illustrative case example.

Quick Guide to the Neurodevelopmental Disorders

In every Quick Guide, the page number following each item always refers to the point at which a discussion of it begins. Also mentioned below, just as in any other competent differential diagnosis, are various conditions arising in early life that are discussed in other chapters.

Autism and Intellectual Disability

Intellectual disability. This condition usually begins in infancy; people with it have low intelligence that causes them to need special help in coping with life (p. 20).

Borderline intellectual functioning. This term indicates persons nominally ranked in the IQ range of 71–84 who do not have the coping problems associated with intellectual disability (p. 598).

Autism spectrum disorder. From early childhood, the patient has impaired social interactions and communications, and shows stereotyped behaviors and interests (p. 26).

Global developmental delay. Use when a child under the age of 5 seems to be falling behind developmentally but you cannot reliably assess the degree (p. 26).

Unspecified intellectual disability. Use this category when a child 5 years old or older cannot be reliably assessed, perhaps due to physical or mental impairment (p. 26).

Communication and Learning Disorders

Language disorder. A child's delay in using spoken and written language is characterized by small vocabulary, grammatically incorrect sentences, and/or trouble understanding words or sentences (p. 46).

Social (pragmatic) communication disorder. Despite adequate vocabulary and the ability to create sentences, these patients have trouble with the practical use of language; their conversational interactions tend to be inappropriate (p. 49).

Speech sound disorder. Correct speech develops slowly for the patient's age or dialect (p. 47).

Childhood-onset fluency disorder (stuttering). The normal fluency of speech is frequently disrupted (p. 47).

Selective mutism. A child chooses not to talk, except when alone or with select intimates. DSM-5 lists this as an anxiety disorder (p. 187).

Specific learning disorder. This may involve problems with reading (p. 51), mathematics (p. 51), or written expression (p. 52).

Academic or educational problem. This Z-code is used when a scholastic problem (other than a learning disorder) is the focus of treatment (p. 591).

Unspecified communication disorder. Use for communication problems where you haven't enough information to make a specific diagnosis (p. 54).

Tic and Motor Disorders

Developmental coordination disorder. The patient is slow to develop motor coordination; some also have attention-deficit/hyperactivity disorder or learning disorders (p. 43).

Stereotypic movement disorder. Patients repeatedly rock, bang their heads, bite themselves, or pick at their own skin or body orifices (p. 44).

Tourette's disorder. Multiple vocal and motor tics occur frequently throughout the day in these patients (p. 39).

Persistent (chronic) motor or vocal tic disorder. A patient has either motor or vocal tics, but not both (p. 42).

Provisional tic disorder. Tics occur for no longer than 1 year (p. 42).

Other or unspecified tic disorder. Use one of these categories for tics that do not meet the criteria for any of the preceding (p. 43).

Attention-Deficit and Disruptive Behavior Disorders

Attention-deficit/hyperactivity disorder. In this common condition (usually abbreviated as ADHD), patients are hyperactive, impulsive, or inattentive, and often all three (p. 33).

Other specified (or unspecified) attention-deficit/hyperactivity disorder. Use these categories for symptoms of hyperactivity, impulsivity, or inattention that do not meet full criteria for ADHD (p. 38).

Oppositional defiant disorder. Multiple examples of negativistic behavior persist for at least 6 months (p. 380).

Conduct disorder. A child persistently violates rules or the rights of others (p. 381).

Disorders of Eating, Sleeping, and Elimination

Pica. The patient eats material that is not food (p. 288).

Rumination disorder. There is persistent regurgitation and chewing of food already eaten (p. 289).

Encopresis. At age 4 years or later, the patient repeatedly passes feces into clothing or onto the floor (p. 294).

Enuresis. At age 5 years or later, there is repeated voiding of urine (it can be voluntary or involuntary) into bedding or clothing (p. 293).

Non-rapid eye movement sleep arousal disorder, sleep terror type. During the first part of the night, these patients cry out in apparent fear. Often they don't really wake up at all. This behavior is considered pathological only in adults, not children (p. 333).

Other Disorders or Conditions That Begin in the Developmental Period

Parent–child relational problem. This Z-code is used when there is no mental disorder, but a child and parent have problems getting along (for example, overprotection or inconsistent discipline) (p. 589).

Sibling relational problem. This Z-code is used for difficulties between siblings (p. 590).

Problems related to abuse or neglect. A variety of Z-codes can be used to cover difficulties that arise from neglect or from physical or sexual abuse of children (p. 594).

Disruptive mood dysregulation disorder. A child's mood is persistently negative between severe temper outbursts (p. 149).

Separation anxiety disorder. The patient becomes anxious when apart from parent or home (p. 188).

Posttraumatic stress disorder in preschool children. Children repeatedly relive a severely traumatic event, such as car accidents, natural disasters, or war (p. 223).

Gender dysphoria in children. A boy or girl wants to be of the other gender (p. 374).

Factitious disorder imposed on another. A caregiver induces symptoms in someone else, usually a child, with no intention of material gain (p. 269).

Other specified (or unspecified) neurodevelopmental disorder. These categories serve for patients whose difficulties don't fulfill criteria for one of the above disorders (pp. 53–54).

Autism and Intellectual Disability

Intellectual Disability (Intellectual Developmental Disorder)

Individuals with intellectual disability (ID), formerly called mental retardation, have two sorts of problems, one resulting from the other. First, there's a fundamental deficit in their ability to think. This will be some combination of problems with abstract thinking, judgment, planning, problem solving, reasoning, and general learning (whether from academic study or from experience). Their overall intelligence level, as determined by a standard individual test (not one of the group tests, which tend to be less accurate), will be markedly below average. In practical terms, this generally means an IQ of less than 70. (For infants, you can only subjectively judge intellectual functioning.)

Most people with such a deficit need special help to cope. This need defines the other major requirement for diagnosis: The patient's ability to adapt to the demands of normal life—in school, at work, at home with family—must be impaired in some important way. We can break down adaptive functioning into three areas: (1) the conceptual, which depends on language, math, reading, writing, reasoning, and memory to solve problems; (2) the social, which includes deploying such abilities as empathy, communication, awareness of the experiences of other people, social judgment, and self-regulation; and (3) the practical, which includes regulating behavior, organizing tasks, managing finances, and managing personal care and recreation. How well these adaptations succeed depends on the patient's education, job training, motivation, personality, support from significant others, and of course intelligence level.

By definition, ID begins during the developmental years (childhood and adolescence). Of course, in most instances the onset is at the very beginning of this period—usually in infancy, often even before birth. If the behavior begins at age 18 or after, it is often called a major neurocognitive disorder (dementia); of course, dementia and ID can coexist. Diagnostic assessment must be done with caution, especially in younger children who may have other problems that interfere with accurate assessment. Some of these patients, once they have overcome, for example, sensory impairments of hearing or vision, will no longer appear intellectually challenged.

Various behavioral problems are commonly associated with ID, but they don't constitute criteria for diagnosis. Among them are aggression, dependency, impulsivity, passivity, self-injury, stubbornness, low self-esteem, and poor frustration tolerance. Gullibility and naïveté can lead to risk for exploitation by others. Some patients with ID also suffer from mood disorders (which often go undiagnosed), psychotic disorders, poor attention span, and hyperactivity. However, many others are placid, loving, pleasant people whom others find enjoyable to live and associate with.

Although many patients with ID appear normal, others have physical characteristics that seem obvious, even to the untrained observer. These include short stature, seizures, hemangiomas, and malformed eyes, ears, and other parts of the face. A diagnosis of ID is likely to be made earlier when there are associated physical abnormalities (such as those associated with Down syndrome). ID affects about 1% of the general population. Males outnumber females roughly 3:2.

The many causes of ID include genetic abnormalities, chemical effects, structural brain damage, inborn errors of metabolism, and childhood disease. An individual's ID may have biological or social causes, or both. Some of these etiologies (with the approximate percentages of all patients with ID they represent) are given below:

Genetic causes (about 5%). Chromosomal abnormalities, Tay–Sachs, tuberous sclerosis.

Early pregnancy factors (about 30%). Trisomy 21 (Down syndrome), maternal substance use, infections.

Later pregnancy and perinatal factors (about 10%). Prematurity, anoxia, birth trauma, fetal malnutrition.

Acquired childhood physical conditions (about 5%). Lead poisoning, infections, trauma.

Environmental influences and mental disorders (about 20%). Cultural deprivation, early-onset schizophrenia.

No identifiable cause (about 30%).

Though measurement of intelligence no longer figures in the official DSM-5 criteria, in the prototypes below I have included IQ ranges to provide some anchoring for the several severity specifiers. However, remember that adaptive functioning, not some number on a page, is what determines the actual diagnosis given to any individual.

Even individually administered IQ tests will have a few points of error. That's one reason why patients with measured IQs as high as 75 can sometimes be diagnosed as having ID: They still have problems with adaptive functioning that help define the condition. On the other hand, an occasional person with an IQ of less than 70 may function well enough not to qualify for this diagnosis. In addition, cultural differences, illness, and mental set can all affect the accuracy of IQ testing.

Interpretation of IQ scores also must consider the possibility of *scatter* (better performance on verbal tests than on performance tests, or vice versa), as well as physical, cultural, and emotional disabilities. These factors are not easy to judge; some test batteries may require the help of a skilled psychometrist. Such factors are among the reasons why definitions of ID have moved away from relying solely on the results of IQ testing.

Essential Features of **Intellectual Disability**

From their earliest years, people with ID are in cognitive trouble. Actually, it's trouble of two sorts. First, as assessed both clinically and with formal testing, they have difficulty with cognitive tasks such as reasoning, making plans, thinking in the abstract, making judgments, and learning from formal studies or from life's experiences. Both clinical judgment and the results of one-on-one intelligence tests are required to assess intellectual functioning. Second, their cognitive impairment leads to difficulty adapting their behavior so that they can become citizens who are independent and socially accountable. These problems occur in communication, social interaction, and practical living skills. To one degree or another, depending on severity, they affect the patient across multiple life areas—family, school, work, and social relations.

F70 [317] Mild. As children, these individuals learn slowly and lag behind schoolmates, though they can be expected to attain roughly sixth-grade academic skills by the time they are grown. As they mature, deficiencies in judgment and solving problems cause them to require extra help managing everyday situations—and personal relationships may suffer. They usually need help with such tasks as paying their bills, shopping for groceries, and finding appropriate accommodations. However, many work independently, though at jobs that require relatively little cognitive involvement. Though memory and the ability to use language can be quite good, these patients become lost when confronted with metaphor or other examples of abstract thinking. IQ typically ranges from 50 to 70. They constitute 85% of all patients with ID.

F71 [318.0] Moderate. When they are small children, these individuals' differences from nonaffected peers are marked and encompassing. Though they can learn to read, to do simple math, and to handle money, language use is slow to develop and relatively simple. Far more than mildly affected individuals do, in early life they need help in learning to provide their own self-care and engage in household tasks. Relationships with others (even romantic ones) are possible, though they often don't recognize the cues that govern ordinary personal interaction. Although they require assistance making decisions, they may be able to work (with help from supervisors and co-workers) at relatively undemanding jobs, typically at sheltered workshops. IQ will range from the high 30s to low 50s. They represent about 10% of all patients with ID.

F72 [318.1] Severe. Though these people may learn simple commands or instructions, communication skills are rudimentary (single words, some phrases). Under supervision, they may be able to perform simple jobs. They can maintain personal relationships with relatives, but require supervision for all activities; they even need help dressing and with personal hygiene. IQs are in the low 20s to high 30s. They make up roughly 5% of the total of all patients with ID.

F73 [318.2] Profound. With limited speech and only rudimentary capacity for social interaction, much of what these individuals communicate may be through gestures. They rely completely on other people for their needs, including activities of daily living, though they may help with simple chores. Profound ID usually results from a serious neurological disorder, which often carries with it sensory or motor disabilities. IQ ranges from the low 20s downward. About 1–2% of all patients with ID are so profoundly affected.

The Fine Print

Don't forget the D's: • Duration (from early childhood) • Differential diagnosis (autism spectrum disorder, cognitive disorders, borderline intellectual functioning, specific learning disorders)

Coding Notes

Specify level of severity (and code numbers) according to descriptions above.

Grover Peary

Grover Peary was born when his mother was only 15. She was an obese girl who hadn't even realized she was pregnant until she was 6 months along. Even then, she hadn't bothered to seek prenatal care. Born after 30 hours of hard labor, Grover hadn't breathed right away. After the delivery, his mother had lost interest in him; he had been reared alternately by his grandmother and an aunt.

Grover walked at 20 months; he spoke his first words at age 2½ years. A pediatrician pronounced him "somewhat slow," so his grandmother enrolled him in an infant school for children with developmental disabilities. At the age of 7, he had done well enough to be mainstreamed in his local elementary school. Throughout the remainder of his school career, he worked with a special education teacher for 2 hours each day; otherwise, he attended regular classes. Testing when he was in the 4th and 10th grades placed his IQ at 70 and 72, respectively.

Despite his disability, Grover loved school. He had learned to read by the time he was 8, and he spent much of his free time poring over books about geography and natural science. (He had a great deal of free time, especially at recess and lunch hour. He was clumsy and physically undersized, and the other children routinely excluded him from their games.) At one time he wanted to become a geologist, but he was steered toward a general curriculum. He lived in a county that provided special education and training for individuals with ID, so by the time he graduated, he had learned some manual skills and could navigate the complicated local public transportation. A job coach helped him to find work washing dishes at a restaurant in a downtown hotel and to learn the skills necessary to maintain the job. The restaurant manager got him a room in the hotel basement.

The waitresses at the restaurant often gave Grover a few quarters out of their tips. Living at the hotel, he didn't need much money—his room and food were covered, and the tiny dish room where he worked didn't require much of a wardrobe. He spent most of his money on expanding his CD collection and going to baseball games. His aunt, who saw him every week, helped him with grooming and reminded him to shave. She and her husband also took him to the ball park; otherwise, he would have spent nearly all of his free time in his room, listening to music and reading magazines.

When Grover was 28, an earthquake hit the city where he lived. The hotel was so badly damaged that it closed with no notice at all. Thrown out of work, all of Grover's fellow employees were too busy taking care of their own families to think about him. His aunt was out of town on vacation; he had nowhere to turn. It was summertime, so he placed the few possessions he had rescued in a heavy-duty lawn and leaf bag and walked the streets until he grew tired; he then rolled out some blankets in the park. He slept this way for nearly 2 weeks, eating what he could scrounge from other campers. Although federal emergency relief workers had been sent to help those hit by the earthquake, Grover did not request relief. Finally, a park ranger recognized his plight and referred him to the clinic.

During that first interview, Grover's shaggy hair and thin face gave him the appearance of someone much older. Dressed in a soiled shirt and baggy pants—they appeared to be someone's castoff—he sat still in his chair and gave poor eye contact. He spoke hesitantly at first, but he was clear and coherent, and eventually communicated quite well with the interviewer. (Much of the information given above, however, was obtained later from old school records and from his aunt upon her return from vacation.)

Grover's mood was surprisingly good, about medium in quality. He smiled when he talked about his aunt, but looked serious when he was asked where he was going to stay. He had no delusions, hallucinations, obsessions, compulsions, or phobias. He denied having any panic attacks, though he admitted he felt "sorta worried" when he had to sleep in the park.

Grover scored 25 out of 30 on the Mini-Mental State Exam. He was oriented except to day and month; he spent a great deal of effort subtracting sevens, and finally got two correct. He was able to recall three objects after 5 minutes, and managed a perfect score on the language section. He recognized that he had a problem with where to live, but, aside from asking his aunt when she returned, he hadn't the slightest idea how to go about solving the problem.

Evaluation of Grover Peary

Had Grover been evaluated before the hotel closed, he might not have fulfilled the criteria for ID. At that time he had a place to live, food to eat, and activities to occupy him. However, his aunt had to remind him about shaving and staying presentable. Despite low scores on at least two IQ tests (criterion A in DSM-5), he was functioning pretty well in a highly, if informally, structured environment.

Once his support system quite literally collapsed, Grover could not cope with change. He didn't make use of the resources available to others who had lost their homes. He was also unable to find work; only through the generosity of others did he manage even to eat—a pretty clear deficit of adaptive functioning (B). Of course, his condition had existed since early childhood (C). Therefore, despite the fact that his IQ had hovered in the low 70s, he seemed impaired enough to warrant a diagnosis of ID. (Note that, as an alternative, Grover would also comfortably match the prototype for mild ID.)

The differential diagnosis of ID includes a variety of learning and communication disorders, which are presented later in this chapter. **Dementia**, or **major neurocognitive disorder** in DSM-5, would have been diagnosed if Grover's problem with cognition had represented a marked decline from his previous level of functioning. (Dementia and ID sometimes coexist, though they can be difficult to discriminate.) At his IQ level, Grover might have been diagnosed as having **borderline intellectual functioning** had he not had such obvious difficulties in coping with life.

Youngsters and adults with ID often have associated mental disorders, which include **attention-deficit/hyperactivity disorder** and **autism spectrum disorder**; these conditions can be diagnosed concurrently. **Mood** and **anxiety disorders** are often present, though clinicians may not recognize them without adequate collateral information. Personality traits such as stubbornness are also sometimes concomitant. Patients with ID may have physical conditions such as **epilepsy** and **cerebral palsy**. Patients with Down syndrome may be at special risk for developing **major neurocognitive disorder due to Alzheimer's disease** as they approach their 40s. Adding in his homelessness (and a GAF score of 45, Grover's diagnosis would be as follows:

F70 [317]	Mild intellectual disability
Z59.0 [V60.0]	Homelessness
Z56.9 [V62.29]	Unemployed

Intellectual developmental disorder is the name for ID being proposed for use in—brace yourself!—ICD-11. The various editions of the DSM have recorded more than 200 changes in the names of mental disorders (a figure that doesn't even include new disorders added over the years). But the case of ID may be the only time that the name of a mental disorder was changed pursuant to an act of Congress.

During the 2009–2010 legislative session, Congress approved, and President Obama signed, a statute replacing in law the term *mental retardation* with *intellectual disability*. The inspiration was Rosa Marcellino, a 9-year-old girl with Down syndrome who, with her parents and siblings, worked to expunge the words *mentally retarded* from the health and education codes in Maryland, her home state.

Note further that the term *developmental disability* as it is used in law is not restricted to people with ID. The legal term applies to anyone who by age 22 has permanent problems functioning in at least three areas because of mental or physical impairment.

F88 [315.8] Global Developmental Delay

Use the category of global developmental delay for a patient under age 5 years who has not been adequately evaluated. Such a child may have delayed developmental milestones.

F79 [319] Unspecified Intellectual Disability

Use the category of unspecified ID for a patient 5 years of age or older who has additional disabilities (blindness, severe mental disorder) too severe to allow full evaluation of intellectual abilities.

F84.0 [299.00] Autism Spectrum Disorder

Autism spectrum disorder (ASD) is a heterogeneous neurodevelopmental disorder with widely varying degrees and manifestations that has both genetic and environmental causes. Usually recognized in early childhood, it continues through to adult life, though the form may be greatly modified by experience and education. The symptoms fall into three broad categories (DSM-5 lumps together the first two).

Communication. Despite normal hearing, the speech of patients with ASD may be delayed by as much as several years. Their deficits vary greatly in scope and severity, from what we used to call Asperger's disorder (these people can speak clearly and have normal, even superior, intelligence) to patients so severely affected that they can hardly communicate at all. Others may show unusual speech patterns and idiosyncratic use of phrases. They may speak too loudly or lack the prosody (lilt) that supplies the music of normal speech. They may also fail to use body language or other nonverbal behavior to communicate—for example, the smiles or head nods with which most of us express approval. They may not understand the basis of humor (the concept that the words people use can have multiple or abstract meanings, for instance). Autistic children often have trouble beginning or sustaining conversation; rather, they may talk to themselves or hold monologues on subjects that interest them, but not other people. They tend to ask questions over and again, even after they've obtained repeated answers.

Socialization. The social maturation of patients with ASD occurs more slowly than for normal children, and developmental phases may occur out of the expected sequence. Parents often become concerned in the second 6 months, when their child doesn't make eye contact, smile reciprocally, or cuddle; instead, the baby will arch away from a parent's embrace and stare into space. Toddlers don't point to objects or play with other children. They may not stretch out their arms to be picked up or show the normal anxiety at separation from parents. Perhaps as a result of frustration at the inability to communicate, ASD often results in tantrums and aggression in young children. With little apparent requirement for closeness, older children have few friends and seem not to share their joys or sorrows with other people. In adolescence and beyond, this can play out as a nearly absent need for sex.

Motor behavior. The motor milestones of patients with ASD usually arrive on time; it's the types of behavior they choose that mark them as different. These include compulsive or ritualistic actions (called *stereotypies*)—twirling, rocking, hand flapping, head banging, and maintaining odd body postures. They suck on toys or spin them rather than using them as symbols for imaginative play. Their restricted interests lead them to be preoccupied with parts of objects. They tend to resist change, preferring to adhere rigidly to routine. They may appear indifferent to pain or extremes of temperature; they may be preoccupied with smelling or touching things. Many such patients injure themselves by head banging, skin picking, or other repetitive motions.

Apart from the subtype formerly known as Asperger's disorder, ASD wasn't recognized at all until Leo Kanner introduced the term *early infantile autism* in 1943. Since then, the concept has expanded in scope and grown new subdivisions (DSM-IV listed four types plus the ubiquitous *not otherwise specified*), though it has now contracted again into the unified concept presented by DSM-5. Although the degree of disability varies widely, the effect upon the lives of most patients and their families is profound and enduring.

ASD is often associated with intellectual disability; discriminating these two disorders can be difficult. Sensory abnormalities occur in perhaps 90% of patients with ASD; some children hate bright lights or loud sounds, or even the prickly texture of certain fabrics or other surfaces. A small minority have cognitive "splinter" skills—special abilities in computation, music, or rote memory that occasionally rise to the level of savantism.

Physical conditions associated with ASD include phenylketonuria, fragile X syndrome, tuberous sclerosis, and a history of perinatal distress. Mental health comorbidity issues include anxiety disorders (especially prevalent) and depression (2–30%), obsessive–compulsive behavior (in about one-third), attention-deficit/hyperactivity disorder (over half), intellectual disability (about half), and seizures (25–50%). Some patients complain of initial insomnia or a reduced need for sleep; a few even sleep days and remain awake nights. Researchers have recently reported an association of a form of autism with a gene responsible for kidney, breast, colon, brain, and skin cancer.

Incorporating the former diagnoses of autistic, Rett's, Asperger's, and childhood disintegrative disorders, ASD's overall prevalence is about 6 per 1,000 children in the general population; some studies report even higher figures. And the numbers have increased in recent years, at least in part due to increased awareness of ASD. Autism affects all cultural and socioeconomic groups. Although boys are twice (perhaps up to four times) as often affected as girls, the latter are more likely to be severely affected. (The former Asperger's disorder, it should be said, is more heavily weighted toward girls.) Siblings of patients with ASD have a greatly elevated risk for the same disorder.

Note that ASD's impressive range of severity can be reflected in separate ratings for the social communication and behavioral components. Though the DSM-5 definitions for severity levels are a bit fussy, they boil down to *mild*, *moderate*, and *severe*. That's how I've listed them, but DSM-5 hasn't for a practical reason: Some members of the committee that wrote the criteria worried that a label of *mild* could give an insurance company leverage to deny services. Of course, that reasoning could cover just about any disorder in the book.

Essential Features of **Autism Spectrum Disorder**

From early childhood, contact with others affects to some extent nearly every aspect of how these patients function. Social relationships vary from mild impairment to almost complete lack of interaction. There may be just a reduced sharing of interests and experiences, though some patients fail utterly to initiate or respond to the approach of others. They tend to speak with few of the usual physical signals most people use—eye contact, hand gestures, smiles, and nods. Relationships with other people founder, so that patients with ASD have trouble adapting their behavior to different social situations; they may lack general interest in other people and make few, if any, friends.

Repetition and narrow focus characterize their activities and interests. They resist even small changes in their routines (perhaps demanding exactly the same menu every lunchtime or endlessly repeating already-answered questions). They may be fascinated with movement (such as spinning) or small parts of objects. The reaction to stimuli (pain, loud sounds, extremes of temperature) may be either feeble or excessive. Some are unusually preoccupied with sensory experiences: They are fascinated by visual movement or particular smells, or they sometimes fear or reject certain sounds or the feel of certain fabrics. They may use peculiar speech or show stereotypies of behavior such as hand flapping, body rocking, or echolalia.

The Fine Print

Note that there are varying degrees of ASD, some of which received separate diagnoses and codes in DSM-IV but no longer do. In particular, what was formerly called Asperger's disorder is relatively milder; many of these people communicate verbally quite well, yet still lack the other skills needed to form social bonds with others.

Deal with the D's: • Duration (from early childhood, though symptoms may appear only later, in response to the demands of socialization) • Distress or disability (work/ academic, social, or personal impairment) • Differential diagnosis (ordinary children may have strong preferences and enjoy repetition; consider also intellectual disability, stereotypic movement disorder, obsessive–compulsive disorder [OCD], social anxiety disorder, language disorder)

Coding Notes

Specify:

> {With}{Without} accompanying intellectual impairment
> {With}{Without} accompanying language impairment
> Associated with a known medical or genetic condition or environmental factor
> Associated with another neurodevelopmental, mental, or behavioral disorder
> With catatonia (see p. 100)

Specify severity (separate ratings are required for social communication and restricted, repetitive behavior).

Social communication

Level 1 (mild). The patient has trouble starting conversations or may seem less interested in them than most people. Code as "Requiring support."

Level 2 (moderate). There are pronounced deficits in both verbal and nonverbal communication. Code as "Requiring substantial support."

Level 3 (severe). Little response to the approach of others markedly limits functioning. Speech is limited, perhaps to just a few words. Code as "Requiring very substantial support."

Restricted, repetitive behaviors

Level 1 (mild). Change provokes some problems in at least one area of activity. Code as "Requiring support."

Level 2 (moderate). Problems in coping with change are readily apparent and interfere with functioning in various areas of activity. Code as "Requiring substantial support."

Level 3 (severe). Change is exceptionally hard; all areas of activity are influenced by behavioral rigidity. Causes severe distress. Code as "Requiring very substantial support."

Temple Grandin

Temple Grandin's career would have been noteworthy even had she not been born with ASD. Her life story serves as an inspiration for patients, for their families, and for all of us who would offer help. The following information, intended not to present a full picture of her life but to illustrate the features of ASD, has been abstracted from several of her own books.

Born in 1947, Temple began walking shortly after her first birthday. Even as a toddler, she didn't like to be picked up, and would stiffen when her mother tried to hold her. In her autobiographies, she recalls that she would sit and rock for long periods; rocking and spinning helped calm her when she felt overstimulated. Much later, she remembered that being touched by other people caused such sensory overload that she would struggle to escape; hugging was "too overwhelming." She couldn't even tolerate the feel of edges of clothing, such as seams of her underwear.

Temple was alert and well coordinated, and she had normal hearing; yet she didn't speak until after her fourth birthday. Later, she recalled her frustration at understanding what was said but being unable to respond. For many years thereafter, her voice was toneless and uninflected, without lilt or rhythm. Even as a college student, she would speak too loudly, unaware of the effect her voice was having on others.

As a small child, Temple was taken to a psychiatrist who diagnosed her as having "childhood schizophrenia"; her parents were advised that she might need institutionalization. Instead, she was given the benefit of private schooling, where her teachers taught the other students to accept her—and her eccentricities.

For example, she was unable to meet the gaze of others and lacked the sense of feelings attached to personal relationships. She would even hold a cat too tightly, not recognizing the signals of distress it was giving her. With no interest in playing with other children, she would instead sit and spin objects such as coins or the lids of cans or bottles. She had an intense interest in odors, and was fascinated by bright colors and the movement of sliding doors and other objects.

Sameness was balm for her. At school age, she resisted change in her routines and would repeatedly ask the same questions. She reacted badly to Christmas and Thanksgiving, because they entailed so much noise and confusion. As an older child, she became fixated on particular issues such as elections—the campaign buttons, bumper stickers, and posters for the governor of her state held special interest for Temple.

But emotional nuance escaped her. With no internal compass for navigating personal relationships, understanding normal social communication was, for her, like being "an anthropologist on Mars." Because she didn't have the feelings normal people attach to others, her social interactions had to be guided by intellect, not emotion. To communicate, she would use lines scripted in advance, because she didn't have the instinct to speak in a socially appropriate manner. What she has learned of empathy was attained by visualizing herself in the other person's place.

Although Temple had always rejected human contact, she nonetheless craved comfort. She found it one summer she spent on a farm, after observing that a device used to hold cattle so that they could be immunized appeared to calm them. As a result, she designed and built a squeezing machine that applied mechanical pressure to her own body; the result was tranquility she hadn't found by other means. Refined over the years, her invention led to her eventual career in creating devices used in animal husbandry.

As an adult, Temple still had trouble responding to unexpected social situations, and she would have severe panic attacks were they not controlled with a small dose of the antidepressant imipramine. But she became salutatorian of her college graduating class; eventually she earned a PhD and ran her own company. She is world-famous as a designer of machinery that helps calm animals on their road to slaughter. And she is a sought-after speaker on autism. But if someone's pager or cell phone goes off when she's giving a lecture, it still causes her to lose her train of thought.

Evaluation of Temple Grandin

Temple's books (and the HBO film named for her) provide a treasure trove of data bearing on the diagnosis of ASD. However, it would be better if we had had multiple sources of information—for her, as for any patient. I'll just touch on the basic material we'd use for diagnosis.

Working our way through the diagnostic criteria, I think we can agree, first of all, that she has had persistent problems in social interaction and communication (criterion A). They include social and emotional reciprocity (didn't want/need to be hugged—A1); use of nonverbal behaviors (poor eye contact—A2); and relationships (lacking interest in other children—A3). Although the DSM-5 criteria are not carefully worded, there must be deficits in each of these three areas for a person to be diagnosed as having ASD. That reading brings DSM-5 fully in line with the DSM-IV diagnostic criteria for autistic disorder.

Temple's restricted behavior and interests included examples of all four symptoms in the criterion B category (only two are required for diagnosis): stereotyped spinning of coins and other objects (she even twirled herself—B1); a rejection of change in routine (dislike of holiday festivities—B2); fixed, restricted interests in, for example, sliding doors and the paraphernalia of political campaigns (B3); and hyperreactivity to sounds and fascination with smells (B4). Temple's symptoms were present from early childhood (C); her biography and other books richly document the degree to which they dominated and impaired her everyday functioning (D). However, she eventually surmounted them brilliantly, thereby disposing of the final possible objection (E) that the symptoms must not be better accounted for by intellectual disability.

Patients with **stereotypic movement disorder** will exhibit motor behaviors that do not fulfill an obvious function, but the criteria for that diagnosis specifically exclude ASD. Temple spoke late and had difficulty communicating verbally, but the criteria for **social communication disorder** also exclude ASD. Her parents were supportive and sensitive to her needs, eliminating **severe psychosocial deprivation** as a possible etiology. We'd also need to consider general **medical problems** such as a **hearing deficit**, which Temple herself explicitly denies having.

She does have a history of severe anxiety, well controlled with medication, that would probably qualify for a comorbid diagnosis of **panic disorder**, though it cannot account for the vast majority of her past symptoms. (I'm leaving the details of that diagnosis as an exercise.) Although some aspects of her history are reminiscent of **obsessive–compulsive disorder**, she has many other symptoms that it cannot explain, either.

Besides panic and other anxiety disorders, ASD can be comorbid with intellectual disability, attention-deficit/hyperactivity disorder, developmental coordination disorder, specific learning disorders, and mood disorders. I'd judge Temple's childhood GAF score as about 55. Though today she may no longer meet DSM-5's diagnostic standards, she clearly did as a child, permitting us to list her diagnosis then as follows:

| F84.0 [299.00] | Autism spectrum disorder |
| F41.0 [300.01] | Panic disorder |

With the elimination of Asperger's disorder (and other specific autism diagnoses) from DSM-5, patient support groups have been up in arms. Asperger's disorder, used since 1944, has a history as extensive as autism. It seemed to define a group of people who, though clearly burdened by their symptoms, also possess a sometimes remarkable intelligence and range of capabilities that may even be superior. It's tempting to regard Asperger's as a sort of "autism lite." However, that would be a mistake, for patients with Asperger's have many of the same deficits as do other individuals with ASD. Perhaps desiring friends, but lacking the empathy necessary for normal social interaction, these solitary individuals might like to change but have no idea how to go about it.

So useful has the concept of Asperger's been, and so ingrained in the common usage of patients and professionals alike has it become, that it seems unlikely to disappear—even though it hasn't been blessed by the latest DSM. It is an irony that because of her language delay, DSM-IV criteria would have deemed Temple Grandin ineligible for a diagnosis of Asperger's, though she remains the poster person for that diagnosis. This is a great example in support of the prototype-matching method of diagnosis I have described in the Introduction (p. 2). Using it, I'd rate Temple (when she was a child) a 4 out of 5 for the diagnosis of Asperger's disorder. However, DSM-5, in a nod to vehement objections from the community of patients with Asperger's, does state that those who were formerly diagnosed as Asperger's can now be regarded as having ASD, whether or not they meet current criteria. That's the second irony in one paragraph.

Attention-Deficit/Hyperactivity Disorder

Attention-deficit/hyperactivity disorder (ADHD) has borne a long string of names since it was first described in 1902. Though it is one of the most common behavioral disorders of childhood, only recently—within a few decades, at most—have we recognized the persistence of ADHD symptoms into adult life.

Although this disorder usually isn't diagnosed until the age of 9, symptoms typically begin before a child starts school. (DSM-5 criteria require some symptoms before age 12.) Parents sometimes report that their children with ADHD cried more than their other babies, that they were colicky or irritable, or that they slept less. Some mothers will even swear that these children kicked more before they were born.

Developmental milestones may occur early; these children may be described as running almost before they could walk. "Motorically driven," they have trouble just sitting quietly. They may also be clumsy and have problems with coordination. At least one study found that they require more emergency care for injuries and accidental poisonings than children without ADHD do. They often cannot focus on schoolwork; therefore, though intelligence is usually normal, they may perform poorly in school. They tend to be impulsive, to say things that hurt the feelings of others, and to be unpopular. They may be so unhappy that they also fulfill criteria for persistent depressive disorder (dysthymia).

These behaviors usually decrease with adolescence, when many patients with ADHD settle down and become normally active and capable students. But some use substances or develop other forms of delinquent behavior. Adults may have continuing interpersonal problems, alcohol or drug use, or personality disorders. Adults may also complain of trouble with concentration, disorganization, impulsivity, mood lability, overactivity, quick temper, and intolerance of stress.

Until recently, ADHD was said to affect perhaps 6% of children in the United States, with a male preponderance ratio of 2:1 or greater. A (disputed) 2013 survey from the Centers for Disease Control and Prevention estimated the rate at closer to 11% of high school boys. The DSM-5 criteria identify perhaps 2.5% of adults age 17 and over, though the range reported in various studies is great. The male–female ratio is far less among adults, for reasons that are obscure.

The condition tends to run in families: Parents and siblings are more likely than average to be affected. Alcoholism and divorce, as well as other causes of family disruption, are common in the family backgrounds of these people. There may be a genetic association with antisocial personality disorder and somatic symptom disorder. Also associated with ADHD are learning disorders, especially problems with reading. In adults, look for substance use, mood, and anxiety disorders.

Several other disorders are likely to co-occur with ADHD. These include oppositional defiant disorder and conduct disorder, each of which will be present in a substantial minority of patients with ADHD. A newly devised condition, disruptive mood dysregulation disorder, may be even more strongly associated. Also look for specific learning disorders, obsessive–compulsive disorder, and tic disorders. Adults may have antisocial personality disorder or a substance use problem.

Essential Features of **Attention-Deficit/Hyperactivity Disorder**

Teachers often notice and refer for evaluation these children, who are forever in motion, disrupting class by their restlessness or fidgeting, jumping out of their seats, talking endlessly, interrupting others, seeming unable to take turns or to play quietly.

In fact, hyperactivity is only half the story. These children also have difficulty paying attention and maintaining focus on their work *or* play—the inattentive part of the story. Readily distracted (and therefore disliking and avoiding sustained mental effort such as homework), they neglect details and therefore make careless errors. Their poor organization skills result in lost assignments or other materials and an inability to follow through with chores or appointments.

These behaviors invade many aspects of their lives, including school, family relations, and social life away from home. Although the behaviors may be somewhat modified with increasing age, they may accompany these individuals through the teen years and beyond.

The Fine Print

Determine the D's: • Duration and demographics (6+ months; onset before age 12) • Disability (work/educational, social, or personal impairment) • Differential diagnosis (intellectual disability, anxiety and mood disorders, autism spectrum disorder, conduct disorder, oppositional defiant disorder, intermittent explosive disorder, specific learning disorders, disruptive mood dysregulation disorder, psychotic disorders, or other mental or personality disorders)

Coding Notes

Specify (for the past 6 months):

F90.0 [314.00] Predominantly inattentive presentation. Inattentive criteria met, but not hyperactive/impulsive criteria.

F90.1 [314.01] Predominantly hyperactive/impulsive presentation. The reverse.

F90.2 [314.01] Combined presentation. Both criteria sets are met.

Specify if:

In partial remission. When the condition persists (perhaps into adulthood), enough symptoms may be lost that the full criteria are no longer met but impairment persists.

Specify current severity:

Mild. Relatively few symptoms are found.

Moderate. Intermediate.

Severe. Many symptoms are experienced, far more than required for diagnosis.

If you read the actual DSM-5 criteria carefully, you'll encounter this anomaly: Criterion D specifies that the symptoms "interfere with, or reduce the quality of" the patient's functioning (p. 60), whereas nearly every other disorder in the book specifies "impairment" of functioning. The subcommittee that wrote the criteria apparently decided that "impairment" was too much influenced by culture. This, of course, prompts the question: Why should the diagnosis of ADHD pay more attention to cultural influences than does every other disorder in DSM-5?

The answer is, also of course, that it shouldn't, and neither should we. Stick with the Essential Features: They might just keep you sane.

Denis Tourney

"I think I've got what my son has."

Denis Tourney was a 37-year-old married man who worked as a research chemist. Throughout his life, Denis had had trouble focusing his attention on any task at hand. Because he was bright and personable, he had been able to overcome his handicap and succeed at his job for a major pharmaceutical manufacturer.

At home one evening the week before this appointment, Denis had been working on plans for a new chemical synthesis. His wife and children were in bed and it was quiet, but he had been having an unusually hard time keeping his mind on his work. Everything seemed to distract him—the ticking of the clock, the cat jumping up onto the table. Besides, his head was beginning to pound, so he grabbed what he thought were two aspirin tablets and washed them down with a glass of milk.

"What happened next seemed like magic," he told the clinician. "It was as if somebody had put my brain waves through a funnel and squirted them onto the paper I was working on. Within half an hour I had shut out everything but my work. In 2 hours I accomplished what would ordinarily take a day or more to get done. Then I got suspicious and looked at the pill bottle. I had taken two of the tablets that were prescribed last month for Randy."

Denis's son was 8, and until a month ago he had been considered the terror of the second grade. But after 4 weeks on Ritalin, he had seemed less driven; his grades had improved; and he had become "almost a pleasure to live with."

For years, Denis had suspected that he himself might have been hyperactive as a child. Like Randy, during the first few grades of elementary school he had been unable to sit still in his seat—bouncing up to use the pencil sharpener or to watch a passing ambulance. His teacher had once written a note home complaining that he talked constantly and that he "squirmed like a bug on a griddle." It was part of the family mythology that he had "crawled at 8 months, run at 10." On questioning, Denis admitted that as a kid he was always on the go and could hardly tolerate waiting his turn for anything ("I felt like I was going to climb right out of my skin").

He was almost stupifyingly forgetful. "Still am. I really can't recall much else about my attention span when I was a kid—it was too long ago," he said. "But I have the general impression that I didn't listen very well, just like I am today. Except when I took those two pills by mistake."

The remainder of Denis's evaluation was unremarkable. His physical health was excellent, and he had had no other mental health problems. Apart from some fidgeting in his chair, his appearance was unremarkable. His speech and affect were both completely normal, and he earned a perfect score on the Mini-Mental State Exam.

Denis had been born in Ceylon, where his parents were both stationed as career diplomats with the foreign service. His father drank himself into an early grave, but not before divorcing his mother when their only child was 7 or 8. Because it concerned him, Denis vividly remembered their last major argument. His mother had pleaded to have Denis's problems evaluated, but his father had banged his fist and sworn that no kid of his was "going to see some damn shrink." Not long afterwards, his parents split up.

Denis felt he had learned a lot from his father's example—he didn't drink, had never tried drugs, didn't argue with his wife, and had readily agreed when she suggested having Randy evaluated. "You always dream that your kids will have what you never did," he said. "In our case, it's Ritalin."

Evaluation of Denis Tourney

As a child, Denis undoubtedly had several symptoms of ADHD. It was easiest for him to remember the problems relating to his activity level (the A2 criteria). Those included the childhood symptoms of squirming (A2a), inability to remain seated (A2b) or wait his turn (A2h), always being on the go (A2e), excessive running (A2c), and excessive talking (A2f). (For children, DSM-5 requires six of these symptom—but, because they tend to be poorly remembered years later, only five for patients age 17 and above. The same numbers and rationale hold for symptoms of inattention.) Denis also thought that he had had problems with his attention span, though he was less clear about the exact symptoms.

These symptoms were present when Denis was a small child, certainly before age 12 (B); we have only anecdotal "clear evidence" that they interfered with the quality of his work, but at this remove, it would seem to be enough. His clinician should ascertain that he had had difficulties in more than one setting (such as school and at home;, C). But even three decades later, he remembered enough hyperactivity/impulsivity symptoms to justify the childhood diagnosis. As adults, many such patients recognize restlessness as their predominant symptom. It would be a good idea for the clinician to verify what Denis thought he remembered, perhaps by obtaining old school records.

In children, a number of other conditions make up the differential diagnosis. (Note that in a clinician's office, many children with ADHD are able to sit still and focus attention well; the diagnosis often hinges on the history.) Those with **intellectual disability** learn slowly and may be overly active and impulsive, but patients with ADHD, once their attention is captured, are able to learn normally. Unlike children with **autism spectrum disorder**, patients with ADHD communicate normally. **Depressed** patients may be agitated or have a poor attention span, but the duration is not usually lifelong. Many patients with **Tourette's disorder** are also hyperactive, but those who only have ADHD will not show motor and vocal tics.

Children reared in a **chaotic social environment** may also have difficulty with hyperactivity and inattention; although ADHD can be diagnosed in a child who lives in an unstable social environment, the process requires extra care and thought. Other **behavior disorders** (**oppositional defiant disorder**, **conduct disorder**) may involve behavior that runs afoul of adults or peers, but the behaviors appear purposeful and are not accompanied by the feelings of remorse typical of ADHD behavior. However, many children with ADHD have comorbid **conduct, oppositional defiant**, or **Tourette's disorder**.

The differential diagnosis in adults includes **antisocial personality disorder** and **mood disorders** (patients with mood disorders can have problems with concentration and agitation). The diagnosis should not be made if the symptoms are better explained by **schizophrenia**, an **anxiety disorder**, or a **personality disorder**.

As a child, Denis might have fulfilled criteria for ADHD, combined type; with the information currently available, however, this would be a tough sell to any hard-nosed coder. Although as an adult he continued to have severe problems concentrating, he overcame them by dint of raw intelligence. Until he compared his usual concentration to the kind of work he could do with medication, he never realized just how disabled he had been.

Although we have some specifics that would constitute a current DSM-5 diagnosis (he was distractible—A1b), even with more information we might not be able to dredge up enough detail to make a full adult diagnosis by contemporary standards. As a clinician, I feel more comfortable with the qualifier "in partial remission." A fuller examination, perhaps with added information from his wife (or boss), might justify a different final diagnosis. Oh, and I'd give him a GAF score of 70.

F90.2 [314.01]   Attention-deficit/hyperactivity disorder, combined presentation (in partial remission)

ADHD is probably underdiagnosed in adults. Although some writers have expressed skepticism about its validity, the evidence of its legitimacy in this age range is increasing. However, the fussiness of their language makes the specifier criteria seem ripe for neglect.

F90.8 [314.01] Other Specified Attention-Deficit/Hyperactivity Disorder

F90.9 [314.01] Unspecified Attention-Deficit/Hyperactivity Disorder

Use either other specified ADHD or unspecified ADHD for patients with prominent symptoms that do not fulfill the criteria for ADHD proper. Examples would include people whose symptoms begin after age 12 or whose symptoms are too few. Remember that, to qualify, those symptoms that are present should be associated with impairment. If you want to specify the reason why ADHD doesn't work for the patient, choose F90.8 and tack on something to the effect of "symptoms first identified at age 13." Otherwise, choose the second. See page 11 (sidebar).

Tic Disorders

A *tic* is a sudden vocalization or movement of the body that is repeated, rapid, and unrhythmic—so quick, in fact, that it can occur literally in (and sometimes is) the blink of an eye. Complex tics, which may include several simple tics in quick succession, naturally take longer. Tics are common; they can occur by themselves or as symptoms of Tourette's disorder.

Tics range from the occasional twitch to repetitive motor and vocal outbursts that can cluster into bouts and create utter (!) chaos in the classroom. Motor tics first appear in early childhood, sometimes as early as 2 years of age. Classically, they involve the upper part of the face (grimaces and twitching of the muscles around the eyes), though affected children can present with a wide range of symptoms that include abdominal tensing and jerking of shoulders, head, or extremities. Vocal tics tend to begin somewhat later. Simple vocal tics may include barks, coughs, throat clearing, sniffs, and single syllables that may be muttered or called out.

Tics cause children to feel out of control of their own bodies and mental processes, though as they get older, some patients do develop a "tension and release" buildup of the urge to tic that is relieved by the tic itself—not unlike what's encountered in kleptomania. Although tics are involuntary, patients can sometimes suppress them for a time; they usually disappear during sleep. Though tic disorders are described as persistent, they do change in intensity with time, perhaps disappearing entirely for weeks at a time. Frequency often increases when a person is sick, tired, or stressed.

Childhood tics are common, occurring in around 10% of boys and 5% of girls. Most of these are motor tics that disappear as the child matures; usually, they don't generate enough concern to warrant an evaluation. When they persist into adulthood, the prevalence is lower, though males still predominate. Adults rarely develop tics de novo; when it does happen, it is often in response to use of cocaine or other street drugs. The tics of adult patients tend to remain the same, varying in intensity though less severe than in childhood. Several factors contribute to a worse prognosis in an adult: comorbid mental conditions or chronic physical illness, lack of support at home, and psychoactive drug use.

Because tics look pretty much the same regardless of diagnosis, I've presented an example only in the context of Tourette's disorder.

F95.2 [307.23] Tourette's Disorder

Tourette's disorder (TD) was first described in 1895 by the French neurologist Georges Gilles de la Tourette. It entails many tics that affect various parts of the body. Motor tics of the head are usually present (eye blinking is often the first symptom to appear). Some patients have complex motor tics (for example, doing deep knee bends). The location and severity of motor tics in patients with TD typically change with time.

But the vocal tics are what make this disorder so distinctive and bring patients to the attention of professionals—often mental health clinicians rather than neurologists. Vocal tics can include an astonishing variety of barks, clicks, coughs, grunts, and understandable words. A sizeable minority (10–30%) of patients also have *coprolalia*, which means that they utter obscenities or other language that can render the condition intolerable by family and acquaintances. Mental coprolalia (intrusive dirty thoughts) can also occur.

Now acknowledged to be far from rare, TD affects up to 1% of young people, with males affected at two to three times the frequency of females. For unknown reasons, it is less common in African Americans than in other racial/ethnic groups. Associated symptoms include self-injury due to head banging and skin picking. TD is strongly familial, with concordance over 50% in monozygotic twins and 10% in dizygotic. There is often a family history of tics or obsessive–compulsive disorder (OCD), so that clinicians suspect a genetic linkage between Tourette's and early-onset OCD.

Typically, TD begins by age 6; most patients reach maximum severity by ages 10–12, after which improvement occurs in perhaps 75%. Under 25% will continue to have tics that are moderate or worse. Though there may be periods of remission, it usually lasts throughout life. Maturity, however, can bring reduced severity or even complete disappearance. Most patients have comorbid conditions, especially OCD and ADHD.

Essential Features of **Tourette's Disorder**

The first tics of patients with TD are often eye blinks that appear when the children are 6 or thereabouts. They are joined by vocal tics, which may initially be grunts or throat clearings. Eventually, patients with TD have multiple motor tics and at least one vocal tic. The best-known tic of all, coprolalia—swear words and other socially unacceptable speech—is relatively uncommon.

The Fine Print

Delve into the D's: • Duration and demographics (1+ years; beginning before age 18, though typically by age 4–6) • Differential diagnosis (OCD, other tic disorders, substance use disorders, and physical disorders)

Essential Features of **Tic Disorders (Compared)**

	Tourette's disorder	Persistent (chronic) motor or vocal tic disorder	Provisional tic disorder
Specific tic type	1+ vocal tics & 2+ motor tics (see The Fine Print)	Motor or vocal tics, but *not* both	Motor or vocal tics, or both, in any quantity
Duration	Longer than 1 year		Less than 1 year
Differential diagnosis	No other medical condition or substance use	No other medical condition or substance use; not TD	No other medical condition or substance use; not TD; not persistent (chronic) motor or vocal tic disorder
Demographics	Must begin by age 18		
Specify if	—	Motor tics only or vocal tics only	—
Tic definition	Abrupt, nonrhythmic, quick, repeated		

The Fine Print

In TD, motor and vocal tics need not occur in the same time frame

Gordon Whitmore

Gordon was a 20-year-old college student who came to the clinic with this chief complaint: "I stopped my medicine, and my Tourette's is back."

The product of a full-term pregnancy and uncomplicated delivery, Gordon had developed normally until he was 8½ years old. That was when his mother noticed his first tic. At the breakfast table, she was looking at him across the top of a box of Post Toasties. As he read what was written on the back, every few seconds he would blink his eyes, squeezing them shut and then opening them wide.

"She asked me what was wrong, said she wondered if I was having a convulsion," Gordon told the mental health clinician. He suddenly interrupted his story to yell, "Shit-fuck! Shit-fuck!" As he bellowed out each exclamation, he twisted his head sharply to the right and shook it so that his teeth actually rattled. "But I never lost consciousness or anything like that. It was only the beginning of my Tourette's."

Unperturbed by his sudden outburst, Gordon continued his story. Gradually throughout his childhood, he accumulated an assortment of facial twitches and other abrupt movements of his head and upper body. Each new motor tic earned renewed taunts from his classmates, but these were mild compared with the abuse he suffered once the vocal tics began.

Not long after he turned 13, Gordon noticed that a certain tension would seem to accumulate in the back of his throat. He couldn't describe it—it didn't tickle and it didn't have a taste. It wasn't something he could swallow down. Sometimes a cough would temporarily relieve it, but more often it seemed to require some form of vocalization to ease it. A bark or yelp usually worked just fine. But when it was most intense, only an obscenity would do.

"Shit-fuck! Shit-fuck!" he yelled again. Then "Cunt!" Gordon shook his head again and hooted twice.

Halfway through his junior year in high school, the vocal tics got so bad that Gordon was placed on "permanent suspension" until he could learn to sit in a classroom without creating pandemonium. The third clinician his parents took him to prescribed haloperidol. This relieved his symptoms completely, except for the tendency to blink when he was under stress.

He had remained on this drug until a month earlier, when he read an article about tardive dyskinesia and began to worry about his drug's side effects. Once he stopped taking the medication, the full spectrum of tics rapidly returned. He had recently been evaluated by his general physician, who had pronounced him healthy. He had never abused street drugs or alcohol.

Gordon was a neatly dressed, pleasant-appearing young man who sat quietly for most of the interview. He really seemed quite ordinary, aside from exaggerated blinking, which occurred several times a minute. He sometimes accompanied the blinks by opening his mouth and curling his lips around his teeth. But every few minutes there occurred a small explosion of hoots, grunts, yelps, or barks, along with a variety of tics that involved his face, head, and shoulders. Irregularly, but with some frequency, his outbursts would include the expletives mentioned above—uttered with more volume than conviction. Afterwards, he would placidly resume the conversation.

The remainder of Gordon's mental status was not remarkable. When he wasn't having tics, his speech was clear, coherent, relevant, and spontaneous, and he scored a perfect 30 on the Mini-Mental State Exam. He admitted that he was worried about his symptoms, but denied feeling depressed or especially anxious. He had never had hallucinations, delusions, or suicidal ideas. He also denied having obsessions and compulsions, adding, "You mean like Uncle George. He does rituals."

Evaluation of Gordon Whitmore

Gordon's symptoms had begun when he was a small child (criterion C) and included vocal as well as multiple motor tics (A), which had occurred frequently enough and long enough (B) to qualify him fully for a diagnosis of TD. He was otherwise healthy, so that **another medical condition** (especially a neurological disorder such as dystonia) would not appear to be a likely cause of his symptoms. Other mental disorders associated with abnormal movements include **schizophrenia** and **amphetamine intoxication**, but Gordon presented no evidence for either of these (D). The duration and full spectrum of vocal and multiple motor tics distinguished his condition from other tic disorders (persistent motor or vocal tic disorder, provisional tic disorder).

We should also inquire about conditions that may be associated with TD. These include OCD and ADHD of childhood. (Gordon's uncle may have had OCD.) Gordon's diagnosis would therefore be as follows (I'd assign him a GAF score of 55):

F95.2 [307.23]   Tourette's disorder

F95.0 [307.21] Provisional Tic Disorder

By definition, the tics in provisional tic disorder are transient. Usually, they are simple motor tics that begin at ages 3–10 and wax and wane over a period of weeks to months; vocal tics are less common than motor tics. A patient who has been diagnosed with persistent motor or vocal tic disorder can never receive the diagnosis of provisional tic disorder.

F95.1 [307.22] Persistent (Chronic) Motor or Vocal Tic Disorder

Once tics have been present for a year, they can no longer be considered provisional. Persistent motor tics also wax and wane over a range of severity. However, persistent vocal tics are rare. Even persistent motor tics usually disappear within a few years, though they may recur in adults when individuals are tired or stressed. Although persistent tics are probably related genetically to TD, patients with TD cannot receive this diagnosis.

F95.8 [307.20] Other Specified Tic Disorder

F95.9 [307.20] Unspecified Tic Disorder

Use unspecified tic disorder to code tics that don't fulfill criteria for one of the preceding tic disorders. Or you can specify the reason by using other specified tic disorder. One example would be tics that have apparently begun after age 18.

Motor Disorders

F82 [315.4] Developmental Coordination Disorder

Developmental coordination disorder (DCD) is perhaps better known by a pejorative label—"clumsy-child syndrome." More or less synonymous with *dyspraxia* (meaning difficulty in performing skilled movements despite normal strength and sensation), DCD remains a focus of some controversy. And it's a big one, inasmuch as it affects perhaps 6% of children ages 5–10; a third of these have severe symptoms. By a ratio of about 4:1, boys are affected more often than girls.

These young people have difficulty getting their bodies to perform as they might wish. Younger children experience delayed milestones, especially crawling, walking, speaking—even getting dressed. Older children, usually chosen last for team sports because they don't catch, run, jump, or kick well, may have trouble making friends. Some children even have trouble mastering classroom skills such as coloring, printing, cursive, and cutting with scissors.

Although the symptoms often stand on their own, for over half of patients DCD exists as part of a broader problem that includes attention deficits or learning problems such as dyslexia. Autism spectrum disorder has also been linked.

After years of study, the cause is still unknown. In the individual case, a variety of physical conditions must be ruled out: muscular dystrophy, congenital myasthenia, cerebral palsy, central nervous system tumors, epilepsy, Friedreich's ataxia, and Ehlers–Danlos disease. Obviously, late onset of motor incoordination after a normal start would weigh heavily against DCD.

Motor skill deficits can persist through adolescence and into adult life, though little is known about the course of DCD in mature patients.

Essential Features of **Developmental Coordination Disorder**

Motor skills are so much poorer than you'd expect, given a child's age, that they get in the way of progress in school, sports, or other activities. The specific motor behaviors involved include general awkwardness; problems with balance; delayed developmental milestones; and slow achievement of basic skills such as jumping, throwing or catching a ball, and handwriting.

The Fine Print

The D's: • Disability (work/educational, social, or personal impairment) • Differential diagnosis (physical conditions such as cerebral palsy; intellectual disability; autism spectrum disorder; ADHD)

F98.4 [307.3] Stereotypic Movement Disorder

Stereotypies are behaviors that people seem driven to perform over and again without any apparent goal—repetitive movement for the sake of motion. Such behavior is entirely normal in babies and young children, who will rock themselves, suck their thumbs, and put into their mouths just about anything that will fit. But when stereotypies persist until later childhood and beyond, they may come to clinical attention as stereotypic movement disorder (SMD).

The behaviors include rocking, hand flapping or waving, twiddling of fingers, picking at skin, and spinning of objects. Serious injury can result from biting, head banging, or striking fingers, mouth parts, or other body parts. You'll typically encounter these behaviors in patients with intellectual disability or autism spectrum disorder, though also in perhaps 3% of otherwise normal children with ADHD, tics, or OCD.

Just what percentage of adults may be affected is actually unknown, though, other than in individuals with intellectual disability, it's probably uncommon. Of 20 adults with SMD in one study, 14 were women; a lifetime history of mood and anxiety disorders was the rule in these patients.

Patients who abuse amphetamines may become fascinated with handling mechanical devices such as watches or radios, or picking at their own skin. Some will sort or rearrange small objects such as jewelry or even pebbles—*punding* (from a word popularized by amphetamine abusers), which may be related to excessive dopamine stimulation.

SMD behaviors are associated with blindness (especially when it's congenital), deafness, Lesch–Nyhan syndrome, temporal lobe epilepsy, and postencephalitic syndrome, as well as severe instances of schizophrenia and OCD. It has also been reported in individual patients with Wilson's disease and brainstem stroke, several with the genetic syndrome *cri du chat* ("cry of the cat," so called because of the characteristic sound the patients make as infants). You may also find SMD behavior in demented elderly patients. Perhaps 10% of people with intellectual disability who live in a facility have the self-injury type of SMD.

In 1995, *The New Yorker* reported that Bill Gates, then the CEO of Microsoft, rocks when he works. "[H]is upper body rocks down to an almost forty-five-degree angle, rocks back up, rocks down again. His elbows are often folded together, resting in his crotch. He rocks at different levels of intensity according to his mood. Sometimes people who are in the meetings begin to rock with him." Claiming it a holdover from "an extremely young age," Gates told the reporter, "I think it's just excess energy."

Essential Features of **Stereotypic Movement Disorder**

You can't find another physical or mental cause for the patient's pointless, repeated movements, such as head banging, swaying, biting (of self), or hand flapping.

The Fine Print

The D's: • Demographics (begins in early childhood) • Distress or disability (social, occupational, or personal impairment; self-injury can occur) • Differential diagnosis (OCD, autism spectrum disorder, trichotillomania, tic disorders, excoriation disorder, intellectual disability, substance use disorders, and physical disorders)

Coding Notes

Specify:

> {With}{Without} self-injurious behavior

Specify current severity:

> **Mild.** Symptoms are readily managed behaviorally.
> **Moderate.** Symptoms require behavior modification and specific protective measures.
> **Severe.** Symptoms require continuous watching to avert possible injury.

Specify if:

> **Associated with a known medical or genetic condition, neurodevelopmental disorder, or environmental factor** (such as intellectual disability or fetal alcohol syndrome)

Communication Disorders

Communication disorders are among the most frequent reasons why children are referred for special evaluation. For some children, problems with communication are symptomatic of broader developmental problems, such as autism spectrum disorder and intellectual disability. Many other children, however, have stand-alone disorders of speech and language.

Disorders of speech include lack of speech fluidity (for example, stuttering); inaccurately produced or appropriately used speech sounds (as in speech sound disorder); and developmental verbal dyspraxias, which result from impaired motor control and coordination of speech organs. Disorders of language comprise problems with formation of words (morphology) or sentences (syntax), language meaning (semantics), and the use of context (pragmatics). The old (DSM-IV) disorders of expressive and receptive language, as well as problems with reading and writing, have been subsumed within the latter category.

These disorders still are not well understood or (often) well recognized. While they are differentiable, they are also highly comorbid with one another.

F80.2 [315.32] Language Disorder

Language disorder (LD) is a new category intended to cover language-related problems including spoken and written language (and even sign language) that are manifested in receptive and expressive language ability—though these may be present to different degrees. Both vocabulary and grammar are usually affected. Patients with LD speak later and less than normal children, ultimately impairing academic progress. Later in life, occupational success may be impaired.

The diagnosis should be based on history, direct observation, and standardized testing, though no actual testing results are specified in the criteria. The condition tends to persist, so that affected teens and adults will likely continue to have difficulty expressing themselves. This disorder has strong genetic underpinnings.

Language impairments can also coexist with other developmental disorders, including intellectual disability, ADHD, and autism spectrum disorder.

Essential Features of **Language Disorder**

Beginning early in childhood, a patient's use of spoken and written language persistently lags behind age expectations. Compared to age-mates, patients will have small vocabularies, impaired use of words to form sentences, and reduced ability to employ sentences to express ideas.

The Fine Print

The D's: • Duration and demographics (begins in early childhood; tends to chronicity) • Disability (work/educational, social, or personal impairment) • Differential diagnosis (sensory impairment, autism spectrum disorder, intellectual disability, learning disorder—though each of these may coexist with LD)

F80.0 [315.39) Speech Sound Disorder

Substituting one sound for another or omitting certain sounds completely is the sort of error made by patients with speech sound disorder (SSD), formerly called phonological disorder. The difficulty can arise from inadequate knowledge of speech sounds or from motor problems that interfere with speech production. Consonants are affected most often, as in lisping. Other examples include errors in the order of sounds ("gaspetti" for *spaghetti*). The errors of speech found in those who learn English as a second language are *not* considered examples of SSD. When SSD is mild, the effects may appear quaint or even cute, but the disorder renders more severely affected individuals hard to understand, sometimes unintelligible.

Although SSD affects 2–3% of preschool children (it's more prevalent in boys), spontaneous improvement is the rule, reducing the prevalence to about 1 in 200 by late teens. The condition is familial and can occur with other language disorders, anxiety disorders (including selective mutism), and ADHD.

Essential Features of **Speech Sound Disorder**

The patient has problems producing the sounds of speech, compromising communication.

The Fine Print

The D's: • Duration (beginning in early childhood) • Disability (work/educational or social) • Differential diagnosis (physical disorders such as cleft palate or neurological disorders; sensory impairment such as hearing impairment; selective mutism)

F80.81 [315.35] Childhood-Onset Fluency Disorder

Although the loss of fluency and rhythm comprised by what used to be called simply *stuttering* (the title was changed to comply with ICD-10) is familiar to every layperson, the stutterer's agonized sense of dyscontrol is not. The momentary panic that ensues may cause these people to take extreme measures to avoid difficult sounds or situations—even such ordinary experiences as using a telephone. Typically, they report anxiety or frustration, even physical tension. You'll notice children clenching their fists or blinking their eyes in the effort to regain control, especially when there is extra pressure to succeed (as when speaking to a group).

Stuttering occurs especially with consonants; the initial sounds of words, the first word of a sentence; and words that are accented, long, or seldom used. It may be provoked by joke telling, saying one's own name, talking to strangers, or speaking to an authority figure. Stutterers often find that they are fluent when singing, swearing, or speaking to the rhythm of a metronome.

On average, stuttering starts at age 5, but it can begin as young as 2. Because young children often have dysfluencies of speech, early stuttering is often ignored. Sudden onset may correlate with greater severity. As many as 3% of young children stutter; the percentage is higher for children with brain injuries or intellectual disability. Boys outnumber girls at least 3:1. Although reports vary, the prevalence in adults is about 1 in 1,000, of whom 80% are male.

Stuttering runs in families, and there is some evidence of heritability. There are genetic (and some symptomatic) links to Tourette's disorder, which is a dopamine-related disorder; dopamine antagonists have been used to ameliorate the effects of stuttering.

Essential Features of
Childhood-Onset Fluency Disorder (Stuttering)

These patients have problems speaking smoothly, most notably with sounds that are drawn out or repeated; there may be pauses in the middle of words. They experience marked tension while speaking, and will repeat entire words or substitute easier words for those that are difficult to produce. The result: anxiety about the act of speaking.

The Fine Print

The D's: • Duration (beginning in early childhood) • Distress or disability (social, academic, or occupational) • Differential diagnosis (speech motor deficits; neurological conditions such as stroke; other mental disorders)

Coding Note

Stuttering that begins later in life should be recorded as adult-onset fluency disorder and coded F98.5 [307.0].

F80.89 [315.39] Social (Pragmatic) Communication Disorder

Social (pragmatic) communication disorder (SCD) describes patients who, despite adequate vocabulary and ability to form sentences, still have problems with the practical use of language. The world of communications calls this *pragmatics*, and it involves several principal skills:

- Using language to pursue different tasks, such as welcoming someone, communicating facts, making a demand, issuing a promise, or making a request.

- Adapting language in accord with the needs of a particular situation or individual, such as speaking differently to children than to adults or in class versus at home.

- Adhering to the conventions of conversation, such as taking turns, staying on topic, using nonverbal (eye contact, facial expressions) as well as verbal signals, allowing adequate space between speaker and listener, or restating something that's been misinterpreted.

- Understanding implied communications, such as metaphors, idioms, and humor.

Patients with SCD, whether children or adults, have difficulty understanding and using the pragmatic aspects of social communication, to the point that their conversations can be socially inappropriate. Yet they do not have the restricted interests and repetitive behaviors that would qualify them for a diagnosis of autism spectrum disorder. SCD can occur by itself or with other diagnoses, such as other communication disorders, specific learning disorders, or intellectual disability.

Essential Features of
Social (Pragmatic) Communication Disorder

From early childhood, the patient has difficulty with each of these features: using language for social reasons, adapting communication to fit the context, following the conventions (rules) of conversation, *and* understanding implied communications.

The Fine Print

The D's: • Disability (work/educational, social, or personal impairment) • Duration (usually first identified by age 4–5) • Differential diagnosis (physical or neurological conditions, autism spectrum disorder, intellectual disability, social anxiety disorder, ADHD)

F80.9 [307.9] Unspecified Communication Disorder

The usual drill applies: Diagnose unspecified communication disorder when a problem with communication doesn't fulfill criteria for one of the previously mentioned conditions, yet causes problems for the patient.

Specific Learning Disorder

Specific learning disorder (SLD) is a particular problem in acquiring information—a problem that isn't consistent with a child's age and native intelligence, and that can't be explained by external factors such as culture or lack of educational opportunity. SLD thus comprises a set of discrepancies (in reading, mathematics, and written expression, as well as some not yet specified) between the child's theoretical ability to learn and actual academic achievement.

Before a diagnosis can be affirmed, the criteria require evidence of significant deficit obtained from of an individually administered, standardized test that is psychometrically sound and culturally appropriate. Like the vast majority of DSM-5 disorders, SLD cannot be diagnosed unless it affects school, work, or social life. Of course, the child's intellectual level will affect the manifestation, prognosis, and remedy of the SLD.

Except for the descriptive specifier "with impairment in written expression," which can appear a year or two later than the others, SLD usually declares itself by the time the child reaches second grade. Two main groups of affected children have been identified. Most affected children have problems with language skills, including spelling and reading; these stem from a basic difficulty in processing sounds and symbols of language (in other words, they have a phonological processing disability). A smaller number have difficulties solving problems—visuospatial, motor, and/or tactile-perceptual problems that manifest as dyscalculia.

In one form or another, SLD affects 5–10% of Americans over the course of their lifetimes; boys are two to four times more often affected than girls. Of course, a child's behavioral and social consequences are proportional to the severity of the impairment and to the available educational remediation and social support. Overall, however, as many as 40% of children formally diagnosed with SLD leave school before completing high school, against a national average of about 6%. These disorders are likely to persist into adult life, where the prevalence is about half that for children. Of the types of SLD, problems with math are the most likely to have an influence on adult functioning.

Children with SLD are also more likely to have behavioral or emotional problems, specifically ADHD (which worsens the mental health prognosis), autism spectrum disorder, developmental coordination disorder, and communication disorders, as well as anxiety and mood disorders.

Specific Learning Disorder with Impairment in Reading (Dyslexia)

The best-studied disorder of this group, the reading type of SLD (aka dyslexia), occurs when a child (or adult, should it persist) cannot read at the level expected for age and intelligence. It can take several forms: difficulty with *comprehension* or *speed* when the person is reading silently; with *accuracy* when the person is reading aloud; with spelling when the person is, well, trying to spell. Normally distributed throughout the population (and occurring at every intelligence level), dyslexia affects about 4% of school-age children, most of them boys.

In the quest for causation, it is interesting to note that children are less likely to have reading problems when their native language has good correspondence between graphemes and phonemes (that is, the words sound generally the way they look). In that sense, English is relatively troublesome, Italian *facile*.

Dyslexia has been attributed to a variety of environmental factors (lead poisoning, fetal alcohol syndrome, low socioeconomic status) and familial causes (inheritance may account for as many as 30% of cases). Especially at risk are socially disadvantaged children, who are less likely to receive the early stimulation that is important to childhood development. Clinicians must rule out vision and hearing problems, behavioral disorders, and ADHD (which is often comorbid).

Prognosis for dyslexia depends on several factors, especially its severity in the individual patient: Reading at two standard deviations below the population mean signifies an especially poor outlook. Other factors include parents' educational levels and the child's overall intellectual capabilities.

Early identification of dyslexia improves outcome. One study showed that 40% of children treated when age 7 could read normally at age 14. However, some news isn't so good: Perhaps 40 million adult Americans are barely literate. Although reading accuracy tends to improve with time, fluency continues to be a problem into maturity. Adults may read slowly, confuse or mispronounce proper names and unfamiliar words, avoid reading aloud (due to embarrassment), or spell imaginatively (and choose words that are easier to spell). Frequently, reading is such a tiring chore that they choose not to read for pleasure.

Specific Learning Disorder with Impairment in Mathematics (Dyscalculia)

What do we know about the mathematics type of SLD? It's a little hard to figure. These people have difficulty performing mathematical operations—counting, understanding mathematical concepts and recognizing symbols, learning multiplication tables, performing operations as simple as addition or as complex as story problems—but we don't really know the cause. Perhaps it's part of a larger nonverbal learning disability, or a problem in making a connection between number sense and the representation of numbers.

Whatever the cause, about 5% of schoolchildren are affected. Of course, you won't find it in very young children. Although it's been shown that even babies have number sense, this condition cannot rear its head until the age at which children are expected to start doing math—sometimes in kindergarten, but more usually by the beginning of second grade.

Gerstmann's syndrome is a collection of symptoms that results from a stroke or other damage to the left parietal lobe of the brain in the region of the angular gyrus. It comprises four main disabilities: problems with writing clearly (*agraphia* or *dysgraphia*), understanding the rules for calculation (*dyscalculia*), telling left from right, and distinguishing fingers on the hand (*finger agnosia*). In addition, many adults have aphasia.

   The syndrome is sometimes reported in children, for whom the cause is unknown; some of these kids are otherwise quite bright. It is usually identified when a child starts school. Besides the four main symptoms, many children also have dyslexia and cannot copy simple drawings—a disability called *constructional apraxia*.

Specific Learning Disorder with Impairment in Written Expression

Patients with the written expression form of SLD have problems with grammar, punctuation, spelling, and developing their ideas in writing. Children have problems translating information from oral/auditory form to visual/written form; what they write may be too simple, too brief, or too hard to follow. Some have trouble generating new ideas. Note that though handwriting may be indecipherable, you wouldn't make this diagnosis when poor penmanship is the *only* problem.

   This problem usually doesn't appear until second grade or later—well after the usual onset of SLD in reading. Writing demands subsequently increase from third to sixth grade. It can be due to troubles with working memory (there's a problem with the organization of what the child is trying to say). The diagnosis is generally not appropriate if the patient is poorly coordinated, as in developmental coordination disorder.

Essential Features of **Specific Learning Disorder**

The patient has important problems with reading, writing, or arithmetic, *to wit*:

   Reading is slow or requires inordinate effort, or the patient has marked difficulty grasping the meaning.
   The patient has trouble with writing content (not the mechanics): There are

grammatical errors, ideas are expressed in an unclear manner or are poorly organized, or spelling is unusually "creative."

The patient experiences unusual difficulty with math facts, calculation, or mathematical reasoning.

Whichever skill is affected, standardized tests reveal scores markedly less than expected for age.

The Fine Print

School records of impairment can be used instead of testing for someone 17+ years of age.

The D's: • Demographics (beginning in early school years, though full manifestation may come only when demands exceed a patient's abilities) • Disability (social, academic, occupational) • Differential diagnosis (physical disorders such as vision, hearing, or motor performance; intellectual disability; ADHD)

Coding Notes

F81.0 [315.00] With impairment in reading. Specify word-reading accuracy, reading rate or fluency, or reading comprehension.

F81.81 [315.2] With impairment of written expression. Specify spelling accuracy, grammar and punctuation accuracy, legible or fluent handwriting, or clarity and organization of written expression.

F81.2 [315.1] With impairment of mathematics. Specify number sense, memorization of arithmetic facts, accurate or fluent calculations, or accurate math reasoning.

For each affected discipline (and subset), specify severity:

Mild. There are some problems, but (often with support) the patient can compensate well enough to succeed.

Moderate. There are marked difficulties, and these will require considerable remediation for proficiency. Some accommodation may be needed.

Severe. Critical problems will be difficult to overcome without intensive remediation. Even extensive support services may not promote adequate compensation.

F88 [315.8] Other Specified Neurodevelopmental Disorder

F89 [315.9] Unspecified Neurodevelopmental Disorder

Use these categories for those patients who have a disorder that appears to begin before adulthood and is not better defined elsewhere. For those in the first group, specify a reason, such as, "Neurodevelopmental disorder associated with ingestion of lead." The latter category is used especially when you lack adequate information.

CHAPTER 2

Schizophrenia Spectrum and Other Psychotic Disorders

Quick Guide to the Schizophrenia Spectrum and Psychotic Disorders

When psychosis is a prominent reason for a mental health evaluation, the diagnosis will be one of the disorders or categories listed below. The page number following each item indicates where a more detailed discussion begins. (To facilitate discussion, I have not adhered to the order in which DSM-5 presents these conditions.)

Schizophrenia and Schizophrenia-Like Disorders

Schizophrenia. For at least 6 months, these patients have had two or more of these five types of psychotic symptom: delusions, disorganized speech, hallucinations, negative symptoms, and catatonia or other markedly abnormal behavior. Ruled out as causes of the psychotic symptoms are significant mood disorders, substance use, and general medical conditions (p. 64).

Catatonia associated with another mental disorder (catatonia specifier). These patients have two or more of several behavioral characteristics (defined on p. 100). The specifier can be applied to disorders that include psychosis, mood disorders, autistic spectrum disorder, and other medical conditions (p. 100).

Schizophreniform disorder. This category is for patients who have the basic symptoms of schizophrenia but have been ill for only 1–6 months—less than the time specified for schizophrenia (p. 75).

Schizoaffective disorder. For at least 1 month, these patients have had basic schizophrenia symptoms; at the same time, they have prominent symptoms of mania or depression (p. 88).

Brief psychotic disorder. These patients will have had at least one of the basic psychotic symptoms for less than 1 month (p. 80).

Other Psychotic Disorders

Delusional disorder. These patients have delusions, but not the other symptoms of schizophrenia (p. 82).

Psychotic disorder due to another medical condition. A variety of medical and neurological conditions can produce psychotic symptoms that may not meet criteria for any of the conditions above (p. 97).

Substance/medication-induced psychotic disorder. Alcohol or other substances (intoxication or withdrawal) can cause psychotic symptoms that may not meet criteria for any of the conditions above (p. 93).

Other specified, or unspecified, schizophrenia spectrum and other psychotic disorder. Use one of these categories for patients with psychoses that don't seem to fit any of the categories above (p. 106).

Unspecified catatonia. Use when a patient has symptoms of catatonia but there isn't enough information to substantiate a more definitive diagnosis (p. 107).

Disorders with Psychosis as a Symptom

Some patients have psychosis as a symptom of mental disorders discussed in other chapters. These disorders include the following:

Mood disorder with psychosis. Patients with a severe major depressive episode (p. 112) or manic episode (p. 116) can have hallucinations and mood-congruent delusions.

Cognitive disorders with psychosis. Many patients with delirium (p. 477) or major neurocognitive disorder (p. 492) have hallucinations or delusions.

Personality disorders. Patients with borderline personality disorder may have transient periods (minutes or hours) when they appear delusional (p. 545). Patients with schizophrenia may have premorbid schizoid or (especially) schizotypal personality disorder (pp. 535, 538).

Disorders That Masquerade as Psychosis

The symptoms of some disorders appear to be psychotic, but are not. These disorders include the following:

Specific phobia. Some phobic avoidance behaviors can appear quite strange without being psychotic (p. 182).

Intellectual disability. Patients with intellectual disability may at times speak or act bizarrely (p. 20).

Somatic symptom disorder. Sometimes these patients will report pseudohallucinations or pseudodelusions (p. 251).

Factitious disorder imposed on self. These patients may feign delusions or hallucinations in order to obtain hospital or other medical care (p. 268).

Malingering. These persons may feign delusions or hallucinations in order to obtain money (insurance or disability payments), avoid work (such as in the military), or avoid *punishment* (p. 599).

Whatever happened to *folie à deux* ("madness of two")? For generations, this rarely encountered condition was a staple of mental health diagnostic schemes. It was termed shared psychotic disorder in recent DSMs, where it denoted patients who develop delusions similar to those held by a relative or other close associate. Often the second patient's delusions cleared up, once association with the first patient was severed. There are several reasons why this condition has been excluded from DSM-5.

Through the decades, there has been precious little research that would help us understand shared psychotic disorder. We have case reports, some describing multiple secondary patients dependent on one primary source (*folie à trois, à quatre, à famille*), but not much in the way of data.

Although most of these patients live with someone who has schizophrenia or delusional disorder, the phenomenon has also been linked to somatic symptom disorder, obsessive–compulsive disorder, and the dissociative disorders. In other words, *folie à deux* may be better conceptualized as a descriptive syndrome similar to the Capgras phenomenon (in which patients believe that close associates have been replaced by exact doubles).

Most patients who would formerly have been diagnosed as having *folie à deux* (shared psychotic disorder) will fulfill criteria for delusional disorder, which is how they should now be categorized. Otherwise, you'd have to diagnose them with other specified psychotic disorder and explain why.

Introduction

During the second half of the 20th century, one of the great leaps forward in mental health was to recognize that psychosis can have many causes. At least in part, this progress can be credited to DSM-III and its forebears and successors, which have established and popularized criteria for many forms of psychosis.

The existence of psychosis is usually not hard to determine. Delusions, hallucinations, and disorganized speech or behavior are generally obvious; they often represent a dramatic change from a person's normal behavior. But differentiating the various causes of psychosis can be difficult. Even experienced clinicians cannot definitively diagnose some patients, perhaps even after several interviews.

Symptoms of Psychosis

A psychotic patient is out of touch with reality. This state of mind can manifest in one or more of five basic types of symptom. These are DSM-5's criterion A inclusion requirements for schizophrenia.

Delusions

A *delusion* is a false belief that cannot be explained by the patient's culture or education; the patient cannot be persuaded that the belief is incorrect, despite evidence to the contrary or the weight of opinion of other people. Delusions can be of many types, including these:

Erotomanic. Someone (often of higher social station) is in love with a patient.

Grandeur. A patient is a person of exalted station, such as God or a movie star.

Guilt. A patient has committed an unpardonable sin or grave error.

Jealousy. A spouse or partner has been unfaithful.

Passivity. A patient is being controlled or manipulated by some outside influence, such as radio waves.

Persecution. A patient is being hounded, followed, or otherwise interfered with.

Poverty. Contrary to the evidence (a job and ample money in the bank), a patient faces destitution.

Reference. A patient is being talked about, perhaps in the press or on TV.

Somatic. Patients' body functions have altered, they smell bad, or they have a terrible disease.

Thought control. Others are putting ideas into patients' minds.

Delusions must be distinguished from *overvalued ideas*, which are beliefs that are not clearly false but continue to be held despite lack of proof that they are correct. Examples include belief in the superiority of one's own race or political party.

Hallucinations

A *hallucination* is a false sensory perception that occurs in the absence of a related sensory stimulus. Hallucinations are nearly always abnormal and can affect any of the five senses, though auditory and visual hallucinations are the most common. But they don't always mean that the person experiencing them is psychotic.

To count as psychotic symptoms, hallucinations must occur when a person is awake and fully alert. This means that hallucinations occurring only during delirium cannot be taken as evidence of one of the psychotic disorders discussed in this chapter. The same can be said for hallucinatory experiences that occur when someone is falling asleep (*hypnagogic*) or awakening (*hypnopompic*). These common experiences (which are not true hallucinations) are normal; they are better referred to as *imagery*.

Another requirement for a psychotic symptom is that a person must lack insight into its unreality. You might think that this would apply to pretty much everyone, but you'd be wrong. Consider, for example, the Charles Bonnet syndrome, in which people who have significant loss of vision see complex visual imagery—but with full realization that the experience is unreal.

Hallucinations must be discriminated from *illusions*, which are simply misinterpretations of actual sensory stimuli. They usually occur during conditions of decreased sensory input, such as at night. (For example, a person awakens to the impression that a burglar is bending over the bed; when the light comes on, the "burglar" is only a pile of clothes on a chair.) Illusions are common and usually normal.

Disorganized Speech

Even without delusions or hallucinations, a psychotic patient may have *disorganized speech* (sometimes also called *loose associations*), in which mental associations are governed not by logic but by rhymes, puns, and other rules not apparent to the observer, or by no evident rule at all.

Some disorganization of speech is quite common (try reading an exact transcript of a politician's off-the-cuff remarks, for example). But by and large, when those words were spoken, listeners understood perfectly well what was intended. To be regarded as psychotically disorganized, the speech must be so badly impaired that it interferes with communication.

Abnormal Behavior (Such as Catatonia)

Disorganized behavior, or physical actions that do not appear to be goal-directed—disrobing in public (without theatrical or, perhaps, political intent), repeatedly making the sign of the cross, assuming and maintaining peculiar and often uncomfortable postures—may indicate psychosis. Again, note how hard it can be to identify a given behavior as disorganized. There are plenty of people who do strange things; lots of these folks aren't psychotic. Most patients whose behavior qualifies as psychotic will have actual catatonic symptoms, each of which has been carefully defined (see p. 101).

Negative Symptoms

Negative symptoms include reduced range of expression of emotion (flat or blunted affect), markedly reduced amount or fluency of speech, and loss of the will to do things (*avolition*). They are called *negative* because they give the impression that something has been taken away from the patient—not added, as would be the case with hallucinations and delusions. Negative symptoms reduce the apparent textural richness of a patient's personality. However, they can be hard to differentiate from dullness due to depression, drug use, or ordinary lack of interest.

Distinguishing Schizophrenia from Other Disorders

DSM-5 uses four classes of information to distinguish among the various types of psychosis: type of psychotic symptom, course of illness, consequences of illness, and exclusions. Each of these categories (plus a few other features) can help you distinguish schizophrenia, the most common psychotic disorder, from other disorders that include psychosis among their symptoms. The reason for this emphasis is that the differential diagnosis of psychosis very often boils down to schizophrenia versus nonschizophrenia. In terms of the numbers of patients affected and the seriousness of implications for treatment and prognosis, it is the single most important cause of psychotic symptoms.

Psychotic Symptoms

Any form of psychosis must include at least one of the five types of psychotic symptoms described above, but to be diagnosed as having schizophrenia, a patient must have two or more. Therefore, the first task in diagnosing any psychosis is to determine the extent of the psychotic symptoms.

    When two or more of these types of psychotic symptoms have been present for at least 1 month, and at least one of them is hallucinations, delusions, or disorganized speech, criterion A for schizophrenia is said to be satisfied. DSM-5 specifies that these two or more psychotic symptom types must be present for a "significant portion of time" during that month. But what does *significant* mean in this context? It could be interpreted to mean that (1) these symptoms have been present on more than half the days in the month; (2) several persons independently may have observed on several days that the patient is having symptoms; or (3) the symptoms may have occurred at times when they are especially likely to affect the patient or the environment—as with, for example, a patient who has repeatedly interrupted a social gathering by screaming. Finally, note that a duration of less than 1 month is allowed if treatment has caused the symptoms to remit.

For behavior to be psychotic, it must be grossly abnormal, and the patient must lack insight into its nature. Examples of psychotic behavior would include symptoms of catatonia, such as mutism, negativism, mannerisms, or stereotypies—without apparent recognition that the behaviors in question are abnormal. (For definitions of these symptoms, see the p. 101 sidebar.) An example of bizarre behavior that is *not* psychotic would be obsessive–compulsive rituals, which patients usually recognize as excessive or unreasonable.

Delusions and hallucinations are the most commonplace symptoms of psychosis. As noted earlier, delusions must be discriminated from overvalued ideas, and hallucinations from illusions.

Disorganized speech means speech that goes beyond the merely circumstantial—it must show marked loosening of associations. Examples: "He tells me something in one morning and out the other," "Half a loaf is better than the whole enchilada." Or, in response to the question, "How long did you live in Wichita?": "Even anteaters like to Frenchkiss."

Negative symptoms can be hard to pinpoint, unless you ask an informant about changes in affective lability, volition, or amount of speech. Negative symptoms can also be mistaken for the stiffening of affect sometimes caused by neuroleptic medications.

For a diagnosis of schizophrenia, earlier DSM versions required only one type of psychotic symptom if it was either a bizarre delusion or hallucinated voices that talk to one another. We can feel pretty clear about the hallucinated voices, but what exactly does *bizarre* mean, anyway? Unhappily, the definition is neither exact nor constant across different studies. It isn't even consistent across different versions of the DSM, which refer to it with decreasing degrees of certitude: "with no possible basis in fact" (DSM-III), "totally implausible" (DSM-III-R), and "clearly implausible" (DSM-IV-TR). DSM-5 has nearly stepped away from the fray altogether, except as regards delusional disorder, where bizarre content is a specifier. There, *bizarre* is taken to mean not only "clearly implausible," but also neither understandable nor in accord with usual life experience.

So we might as well adopt the original sense that came to us several hundred years ago from French: *odd* or *fantastic*. Examples of delusions we could call bizarre include falling down a rabbit hole to Wonderland, being controlled (in thoughts or actions) by aliens from Halley's Comet, or having one's brain replaced by a computer chip. Examples of nonbizarre delusions include being spied upon by neighbors or betrayed by one's spouse. (The assessment of what is and is not bizarre may vary with our distance from those we seek to judge: "I am unique, you are odd, they are bizarre.")

The recent weight of opinion is that the quality of bizarreness has little importance when it comes to diagnosis or prognosis. Therefore, in DSM-5, all patients with schizophrenia must have two or more types of psychotic symptoms, no matter how fantastic any one of them might be.

Course of Illness

Cross-sectional symptoms are less important to the differential diagnosis of psychosis than is the course of illness. That is, the type of psychosis is largely determined by the longitudinal patterns and associated features of the disorder. Several of these factors are noted here:

Duration. How long has the patient been ill? A duration of at least 6 months is required for a DSM-5 diagnosis of schizophrenia. This rule was formulated decades ago, in response to the observation that psychotic patients who have been ill a long time tend at follow-up to have schizophrenia. Patients with a briefer duration of psychosis may turn out to have some other disorder. For years, we've operationally defined the time required as 6 months or longer.

Precipitating factors. Severe emotional stress sometimes precipitates a brief period of psychosis. For example, the stress of childbirth precipitates what we call a postpartum psychosis. A chronic course is less likely if there are precipitating factors, including this one.

Previous course of illness. A prior history of complete recovery (no residual symptoms) from a psychosis suggests a disorder other than schizophrenia.

Premorbid personality. Good social and job-related functioning before the onset of psychotic symptoms directs our diagnostic focus away from schizophrenia and toward another psychotic disorder, such as a psychotic depression or a psychosis due to another medical condition or substance use.

Residual symptoms. Once the acute psychotic symptoms have been treated (usually with medication), residual symptoms may persist. These are often milder manifestations of the person's earlier delusions or other active psychotic symptoms: odd beliefs, vague speech that wanders off the point, a reduced lack of interest in the company of others. They augur for the subsequent return of psychosis.

Consequences of Illness

Psychosis can seriously affect the functioning of both patient and family. The degree of this effect can help discriminate schizophrenia from other causes of psychosis. To be diagnosed as having schizophrenia, the patient must have materially impaired social or occupational functioning. For example, most patients with schizophrenia never marry and either don't work at all or hold jobs that require a lower level of functioning than is consistent with their education and training. The other psychotic disorders do not require this criterion for diagnosis. In fact, the criteria for delusional disorder even specify that functioning is not impaired in any important way except as it relates specifically to the delusions.

Exclusions

Once the fact of psychosis is established, can it be attributed to any mental disorder other than schizophrenia? We must consider at least three sets of possibilities.

First, the top place in any differential diagnosis belongs to disorders caused by physical conditions. History, physical examination, and laboratory testing must be scrutinized for evidence. See the table "Physical Disorders That Affect Mental Diagnosis" in the Appendix for a listing of some of these disorders.

Next, rule out substance-related disorders. Has the patient a history of abusing alcohol or street drugs? Some of these (cocaine, alcohol, psychostimulants, and the psychotomimetics) can cause psychotic symptoms that closely mimic schizophrenia. The use of prescription medications (such as adrenocorticosteroids) can also produce symptoms of psychosis. See the table "Classes (or Names) of Medications That Can Cause Mental Disorders" in the Appendix for more information.

Finally, consider mood disorders. Are there prominent symptoms of either mania or depression? The history of mental health treatment is awash in patients whose mood disorders have for years been diagnosed as schizophrenia. Mood disorders should be included early in the differential diagnosis of any patient with psychosis.

Other Features

You should also think about some features of psychosis that are not included in the DSM-5 criteria sets. Some of these can help predict outcome. They include the following:

Family history of illness. A close relative with schizophrenia increases your patient's chances of also having schizophrenia. Bipolar I disorder with psychotic features also runs in families. Always learn as much as you can about the family history, so you can form your own judgment; accepting another clinician's opinion about diagnosis can be risky.

Response to medication. Regardless of how psychotic the patient appears, previous recovery with, say, lithium treatment suggests a diagnosis of mood disorder.

Age at onset. Schizophrenia usually begins by a person's mid-20s. Onset of illness after the age of 40 suggests some other diagnosis. It could be delusional disorder, but you should consider a mood disorder. However, late onset does not completely rule out a schizophrenia diagnosis, especially of the type we used to call paranoid.

I have intentionally written up the material that follows in a different order from that adopted by DSM-5. The stated intention of that manual is to order its material along "a gradient of psychopathology" that clinicians should generally follow, so that they consider first conditions that don't attain full status as psychotic disorders or that affect relatively fewer aspects of a patient's life. Hence DSM-5 begins with schizotypal personality disorder and progresses next to delusional disorder and catatonia.

Here's the reasoning for my approach. As a general matter, I agree that we should evaluate our patients along a safety continuum, beginning with disorders that can be more readily treated (such as a substance-induced psychotic disorder) or those that have a relatively better prognosis (such as mood disorders with psychosis). However, from an educational point of view, it helps me to describe first a condition (schizophrenia) that includes all conceivable symptoms and then fiddle with variations. I believe that my approach is more likely to help you learn the basic features of psychosis.

The Schizophrenia Spectrum

F20.9 [295.90] Schizophrenia

In an effort to achieve precision, the DSM criteria for schizophrenia have become more complicated over the years. But the basic pattern of diagnosis remains so straightforward that it can be outlined briefly.

1. Before becoming ill, the patient may have a withdrawn or otherwise peculiar personality.

2. For some time (perhaps 3–6 years) before becoming clinically ill, the patient may have experiences that, while not actually psychotic, portend the later onset of psychosis. This *prodromal* period is characterized by abnormalities of thought, language, perception, and motor behavior.

3. The illness proper begins gradually, often imperceptibly. At least 6 months before a diagnosis is made, behavior begins to change. Right from the start, this may involve delusions or hallucinations; or it may be heralded by milder symptoms, such as beliefs that are peculiar but not psychotic.

4. The patient has been frankly psychotic during at least 1 month of those 6. There have been two or more of the five basic symptom types described at the start of this chapter; hallucinations, delusions, or disorganized speech must be one of the two.

5. The illness causes important problems with work and social functioning.

6. The clinician can exclude other medical disorders, substance use, and mood disorders as probable causes.

7. Although most patients improve with treatment, relatively few recover to such an extent that they return completely to their premorbid state.

There are several reasons why it is important to diagnose schizophrenia accurately:

Frequency. It is a common condition: Up to 1% of the general adult population will contract this disorder. For unknown reasons, males become symptomatic several years younger than do females.

Chronicity. Most patients who develop schizophrenia continue to have symptoms throughout their lives.

Severity. Although most patients do not require months or years of hospitalization, as was the case before neuroleptic medications were developed, incapacity for social and work functioning can be profound. Psychotic symptoms can vary in their degree of severity (see sidebar, p. 74).

Management. Adequate treatment almost always means using antipsychotic drugs, which, despite their risk of side effects, often must be taken lifelong.

Although nearly everyone does so, it is probably incorrect to speak of schizophrenia as if it were one disease. It is almost certainly a collection of several underlying etiologies, for which the same basic diagnostic criteria are used. It is also important to note that many symptoms in addition to the formal criteria are often found in patients with schizophrenia. Here are a few:

Cognitive dysfunction. Distractibility, disorientation, or other cognitive problems are often noted, though the symptoms of schizophrenia are classically described as occurring in a clear sensorium.

Dysphoria. Anger, anxiety, and depression are some of the common emotional reactions to ensuing psychosis. Other patients show inappropriate affect (such as giggling when nothing appears to be funny). Anxiety attacks and disorders are increasingly identified.

Absence of insight. Many patients refuse to take medicine in the mistaken belief that they are not ill.

Sleep disturbance. Some patients stay up late and arise late when they are attempting to deal with the onset of hallucinations or delusions.

Substance use. Especially common is tobacco use, which affects 80% of all patients with schizophrenia.

Suicide. Up to 10% of these patients (especially newly diagnosed young men) take their own lives.

Because schizophrenia can present in so many different ways, and because it is so important (to individuals, society, and the history of mental disorder), I will illustrate with the stories of four patients.

Essential Features of **Schizophrenia**

The classic picture of a patient with schizophrenia is of a young person (late teens or 20s) who has had (1) delusions (especially persecutory) and (2) hallucinations (especially auditory). However, some patients will have (3) speech that is incoherent or otherwise disorganized, (4) severely abnormal psychomotor behavior (catatonic symptoms), or (5) negative symptoms such as restricted affect or lack of volition (they don't feel motivated to do work, maintain family life). Diagnosis requires at least two of these five types of psychotic symptoms, at least one of which must be delusions, hallucinations, or disorganized speech (criterion A). The patient is likely to have some mood symptoms, but they will be relatively brief. Illness usually begins gradually, perhaps almost imperceptibly, and builds across at least 6 months in a crescendo of misery and chaos.

The Fine Print

Don't dismiss the D's: • Duration (6+ months, with criterion A symptoms for at least a month) • Distress or disability (social, occupational, or personal impairment) • Differential diagnosis (other psychotic disorders, mood or cognitive disorders, physical and substance-induced psychotic disorders, peculiar ideas—often political or religious—shared by a community)

Coding Notes

Specify:

> **With catatonia** (see p. 100)

If the disorder has lasted at least 1 year, specify course:

> **First episode, currently in acute episode**
> **First episode, currently in partial remission**
> **First episode, currently in full remission**
> **Multiple episodes, currently in acute episode**
> **Multiple episodes, currently in partial remission**
> **Multiple episodes, currently in full remission**
> **Continuous**
> **Unspecified**

You may specify severity, though you don't have to (see p. 74).

Whereas DSM-IV (and each of its predecessors) listed several subtypes of schizophrenia, DSM-5 has largely done away with them. Why is this? And why were they there in the first place?

Sadly, the venerable categories of hebephrenic (disorganized), catatonic, and paranoid types, each of which has roots deep in the 19th century, simply didn't predict much—not enough, at any rate, to justify their existence. Furthermore, they didn't necessarily hold true to type from one episode of psychosis to the next. Catatonia, always encountered more often in illnesses other than schizophrenia, has now been demoted to a specifier denoting behaviors that apply not just to schizophrenia but to mood disorders as well as to physical illnesses. And the other old categories, while interesting to discuss (at least by clinicians old enough to have been weaned on these concepts), have been relegated to history's dust bin, along with fever therapy and wet sheet packs.

Lyonel Childs

When he was young, Lyonel Childs had always been somewhat isolated, even from his two brothers and his sister. During the first few grades in school, he seemed almost suspicious if other children talked to him. He seldom seemed to feel at ease, even with those he had known since kindergarten. He never smiled or showed much emotion, so that by the time he was 10, even his siblings thought he was peculiar. Adults said he was "nervous." For a few months during his early teens, he was interested in magic and the occult; he read extensively about witchcraft and casting spells. Later he decided he would like to become a minister. He spent long hours in his room learning Bible passages by heart.

Lyonel had never been much interested in sex, but at age 24, still attending college, he was attracted to a girl in his poetry class. Mary had blonde hair and dark blue eyes, and he noticed that his heart skipped a beat when he first saw her. She always said "Hello" and smiled when they met. He didn't want to betray too great an interest, so he waited until an evening several weeks later to ask her to a New Year's Eve party. She refused him, politely but firmly.

As Lyonel mentioned to an interviewer months later, he thought that this seemed strange. During the day Mary was friendly and open with him, but when he ran into her at night, she was reserved. He knew there was a message in this that eluded him, and it made him feel shy and indecisive. He also noticed that his thoughts had speeded up so that he couldn't sort them out.

"I noticed that my mental energy had lessened," he told the interviewer, "so I went to see the doctor. I told him I had gas forming on my intestines, and I thought it was giving me erections. And my muscles seemed all flabby. He asked me if I used drugs or was feeling depressed. I told him neither one. He gave me a prescription for some tranquilizers, but I just threw it away."

Lyonel's skin was pasty white and he was abnormally thin, even for someone so slightly built. Casually dressed, he sat quietly without fidgeting during that interview. His speech was entirely ordinary; one thought flowed logically into the next, and there were no made-up words.

By summer, he had become convinced that Mary was thinking about him. He decided that something must be keeping them apart. Whenever he had this feeling, his thoughts seemed to become so loud that he felt sure other people must be able to hear. He neglected to look for a summer job that year and moved back into his parents' house, where he kept to his room, brooding. He wrote long letters to Mary, most of which he destroyed.

In the fall, Lyonel realized that his relatives were trying to help him. Although they would wink an eye or tap a finger to let him know when she was near, it did no good. She continued to elude him, sometimes only by minutes. At times there was a ringing in his right ear, which caused him to wonder whether he was becoming deaf. His suspicion seemed confirmed by what he privately called "a clear sign." One day while driving he noticed, as if for the first time, the control button for his rear window defroster. It was labeled "rear def," which to him meant "right-ear deafness."

When winter deepened and the holidays approached, Lyonel knew that he would have to take action. He drove off to Mary's house to have it out with her. As he crossed town, people he passed nodded and winked at him to signal that they understood and approved. A woman's voice, speaking clearly from just behind him in the back seat, said, "Turn right!" and "Atta boy!"

Evaluation of Lyonel Childs

Two of the five symptoms listed in DSM-5's criterion A must be present for a diagnosis of schizophrenia, and Lyonel did have two—delusions (criterion A1) and hallucinations (A2). Note this new feature in DSM-5: A diagnosis of schizophrenia requires that at least one of delusions, hallucinations, and disorganized speech be among the patient's psychotic symptoms.

As with Lyonel, the hallucinations of **schizophrenia** are usually auditory. Visual hallucinations often indicate a **substance-induced psychotic disorder** or **psychotic disorder due to another medical condition**; they can also occur in **major neurocognitive disorder (dementia)** and **delirium.** Hallucinations of sense or smell are more commonly experienced by a person whose psychosis is due to **another medical condition**, but their presence would not rule out schizophrenia.

As with Lyonel, auditory hallucinations are typically clear and loud; patients will often agree with the examiner who asks, "Is it as loud as my voice is right now?" Although the voices may seem to come from within a patient's head, the source may be located elsewhere—the hallway, a household appliance, the family's cat.

The special messages that Lyonel received (finger tapping, eye winking) are called **delusions of reference.** Patients with schizophrenia may also experience other sorts of delusions; I've listed these on page 58. Often delusions are to some extent **persecutory** (that is, the patient feels in some way pursued or interfered with). None of Lyonel's delusional ideas were so far from normal human experience that I'd call them *bizarre*.

Lyonel did not have disorganized speech, catatonic behavior, or negative symptoms, but others with schizophrenia may. His illness significantly interfered with his work (he didn't get a summer job) and his relationships with others (he stayed in his room and brooded). We can infer that in each of these areas he functioned much less well than before he became ill (B).

Although Lyonel had heard voices for only a short time, he had been delusional for several months. The prodromal symptoms (his concerns about intestinal gas and feeling of reduced mental energy) had begun a year or more earlier. As a result, he easily fulfilled the requirement of a total duration (prodrome, active symptoms, and residual period) of at least 6 months (C).

The doctor Lyonel consulted found no evidence of another medical condition (E). Auditory hallucinations that may exactly mimic those encountered in schizophrenia can occur in **alcohol-induced psychotic disorder.** People who are withdrawing from **amphetamines** may even harm themselves as they attempt to escape terrifying persecutory delusions. We might suspect either of these disorders if Lyonel had recently used substances.

Lyonel also denied feeling depressed. **Major depressive disorder with psychotic features** can produce delusions or hallucinations, but often these are mood-congruent (they center around feelings of guilt or deserved punishment). **Schizoaffective disorder** could be excluded because he had no prominent mood symptoms (depressive or manic, D). From the duration of his symptoms, we know not to diagnose **schizophreniform disorder.**

Many patients with schizophrenia also have an abnormal premorbid personality. Often this takes the form of **schizoid** or, especially, **schizotypal personality disorder.** As a child, Lyonel had at least five features of schizotypal personality disorder (see p. 538). These included constricted affect, no close friends, odd beliefs (interest in the occult), peculiar appearance (as judged by peers), and suspiciousness of other children. However, he had no history that would cause us to consider autism spectrum disorder (F).

With two psychotic symptoms and a duration of more than 6 months, Lyonel's illness easily matches the prototype for typical schizophrenia. Note that (as with most DSM-5 disorders) medical and substance use causes must be ruled out, and other, more treatable mental etiologies must be deemed less likely.

Throughout his current episode, Lyonel had had no change of symptoms that might suggest anything other than a continuous course. He had been ill for just about 1 year. I'd peg his current GAF score at 30, and his overall diagnosis would be as follows:

F20.9 [295.90]	Schizophrenia, first episode, currently in acute episode
F21 [301.22]	Schizotypal personality disorder (premorbid)
Z56.9 [V62.29]	Unemployed

In evaluating patients who have delusions or hallucinations, be sure to consider the cognitive disorders. This is especially true in an older patient whose psychosis has developed quite rapidly. And patients with schizophrenia who have active hallucinations or delusions should be asked about symptoms of dysphoria. They are likely to have depression or anxiety (or both) that could require additional treatment.

Bob Naples

As his sister told it, Bob Naples was always quiet when he was a kid, but not what you'd call peculiar or strange. Nothing like this had ever happened in their family before.

Bob sat in a tiny consulting room down the hall. His lips moved soundlessly, and one bare leg dangled across the arm of his chair. His sole article of clothing was a red-and-white-striped pajama top. An attendant tried to drape a green sheet across his lap, but he giggled and flung it to the floor.

It was hard for his sister, Sharon, to say when Bob first began to change. He was never very sociable, she said; "You might even call him a loner." He hardly ever laughed and always seemed rather distant, almost cold; he never appeared to enjoy anything he did very much. In the 5 years since he'd finished high school, he had lived at their house while he worked in her husband's machine shop, but he never really lived *with* them. He had never had a girlfriend—or a boyfriend, for that matter, though he sometimes used to talk with a couple of high school classmates if they dropped around. About a year and a half ago, Bob had completely stopped going out and wouldn't even return phone calls. When Sharon asked him why, he said he had better things to do. But all he did when he wasn't working was stay in his room.

Sharon's husband had told her that at work, Bob stayed at his lathe during breaks and talked even less than before. "Sometimes Dave would hear Bob giggling to himself. When he'd ask what was funny, Bob would kind of shrug and just turn away, back to his work."

For over a year, things didn't change much. Then, about 2 months earlier, Bob had started staying up at night. The family would hear him thumping around in his room, banging drawers, occasionally throwing things. Sometimes it sounded like he was talking to someone, but his bedroom was on the second floor and he had no phone.

He stopped going in to work. "Of course, Dave'd never fire him," Sharon continued. "But he was sleepy from being up all night, and he kept nodding off at the lathe. Sometimes he'd just leave it spinning and wander over to stare out the window. Dave was relieved when he stopped coming in."

In the last several weeks, all Bob would say was "Gilgamesh." Once Sharon asked him what it meant and he answered, "It's no red shoe on the backspace." This astonished her so much that she wrote it down. After that, she gave up trying to ask him for explanations.

Sharon could only speculate how Bob came to be in the hospital. When she'd come home from the grocery store a few hours earlier, he was gone. Then the phone rang and it was the police, saying that they were taking him in. A security guard down at the mall had taken him into custody. He was babbling something about Gilgamesh and wearing nothing but a pajama top. Sharon blotted the corner of her eye with the cuff of her sleeve. "They aren't even his pajamas—they belong to my daughter."

Evaluation of Bob Naples

Do take a few moments to review Bob's history for the elements of the typical schizophrenia prototype. This is the picture to carry around in your head, against which you'll match future patients.

With several psychotic symptoms, Bob fully met the basic criteria for schizophrenia. Besides his badly disorganized speech (criterion A3) and behavior (going out nude, A4), he had the negative symptoms of not speaking and lack of volition (he stopped going to work—A5). Although he had had active symptoms for perhaps only a few months, his decreased (even for him) sociability had begun well over a year before, extending the total duration of his illness (C) well beyond the 6-month threshold. The vignette makes clear the devastating effect of symptoms on his work and social life (B). However, even with these typical features, there are still several exclusions to be ruled out.

Bob would say only one word when he was admitted, so it could not be determined whether he had a cognitive deficit, as would be the case in a **delirium** or in an **amphetamine-** or **phencyclidine-induced psychotic disorder.** Only after treatment was begun might his cognitive status be known for sure. Other evidence of **gross brain disease** (E) could be sought with skull X-rays, MRI, and blood tests as appropriate.

Patients with **bipolar I disorder** can show gross defect of judgment by refusing to remain clothed, but Bob did not have any of the other typical features of mania, such as euphoric mood or hyperactivity—certainly not pressured speech. The absence of prominent mood symptoms would rule out **major depressive episode** and **schizoaffective disorder** (D). Over a year earlier, Bob had been found giggling to himself at his lathe, so the early manifestations of his illness had been present for far longer than the 6-month minimum for schizophrenia; we can therefore dismiss **schizophreniform disorder.**

Several of Bob's symptoms are typical for what used to be called disorganized schizophrenia. His affect was inappropriate (he laughed without apparent cause), although reduced lability (termed *flat* or *blunted*) would also qualify as a negative symptom. By the time of his evaluation, his speech had been reduced to a single word, but earlier it had been incoherent (and peculiar enough that his sister even wrote some of it down). Finally, there was loss of volition (the will to do things): He had stopped going to work and spent most of his time in his room, apparently accomplishing nothing.

From Sharon's information, a premorbid diagnosis of some form of personality disorder would also seem warranted. Bob's specific symptoms included the following: no close friends, not desiring relationships, choosing solitary activities, lack of pleasure in activities, and no sexual experiences. This is a pattern, often noted in patients with schizophrenia, called schizoid personality disorder (p. 535).

Although Bob's eventual diagnosis would seem evident, we should await the results of lab testing to rule out causes of psychosis other than schizophrenia. Therefore, we'll add the qualifier *(provisional)* to his diagnosis. I'd give him a GAF score of just 15.

F20.9 [295.90]	Schizophrenia, first episode, currently in acute episode (provisional)
F60.1 [301.20]	Schizoid personality disorder (premorbid)

Disorganized schizophrenia was first recognized nearly 150 years ago. It was originally termed *hebephrenia* because it began early in life (*hebe* is Greek for *youth*). Patients with disorganized schizophrenia can appear the most obviously psychotic of all. They often deteriorate rapidly, talk gibberish, and neglect hygiene and appearance. More recent research, however, has determined that the pattern of symptoms doesn't predict enough to make disorganized schizophrenia a useful diagnostic subcategory—other than as a description of current symptoms.

Natasha Oblamov

"She's nowhere near as bad as Ivan." Mr. Oblamov was talking about his two grown children. At 30 years of age, Ivan had such severe disorganized schizophrenia (as it was then known) that, despite neuroleptics and a trial of electroconvulsive therapy, he could not put 10 words together so they made sense. Now Natasha, 3 years younger than her brother, had been brought to the clinic with similar complaints.

Natasha was an artist. She specialized in oil-on-canvas copies of the photographs she took of the countryside near her home. Although she had had a one-woman exhibition in a local art gallery 2 years earlier, she had never yet earned a dollar from her artwork. She had a room in her father's apartment, where the two lived on his retirement income. Her brother lived on a back ward of the state mental hospital.

"I suppose it's been going on for quite a while now," said Mr. Oblamov. "I should have done something earlier, but I didn't want to believe it was happening to her, too."

The signs had first appeared about 10 months ago, when Natasha stopped attending class at the art institute and gave up her two or three drawing pupils. Mostly she stayed in her room, even at mealtimes; she spent much of her time sketching.

Her father finally brought Natasha for evaluation because she kept opening the door. Perhaps 6 weeks earlier she had begun emerging from her room several times each evening, standing uncertainly in the hallway for several moments, then opening the front door. After peering up and down the hallway, she would retreat to her own room. In the past week, she had reenacted this ritual a dozen times each evening. Once or twice, her father thought he heard her mutter something about "Jason." When he asked her who Jason was, she only looked blank and turned away.

Natasha was a slender woman with a round face and watery blue eyes that never seemed to focus. Although she volunteered almost nothing, she answered every question clearly and logically, if briefly. She was fully oriented and had no suicidal ideas or other problems with impulse control. Her affect was as flat as one of her canvases. She would describe her most frightening experiences with no more emotion than she would making a bed.

Jason was an instructor at the art institute. Some months earlier, one afternoon when her father was out, he had come to the apartment to help her with "some special stroking techniques," as she put it (referring to her brush). Although they had ended up naked together on the kitchen floor, she had spent most of that time explaining why she felt she should put her clothes back on. He left unrequited, and she never returned to the art institute.

Not long afterward, Natasha "realized" that Jason was hanging about, trying to see her again. She would sense his presence just outside her door, but each time she opened it, he had vanished. This puzzled her, but she couldn't say that she felt depressed, angry, or anxious. Within a few weeks she started to hear a voice quite a bit like Jason's, which seemed to be speaking to her from the photographic enlarger she had set up in the tiny second bathroom.

"It usually just said the 'C word,'" she explained in response to a question.

"The 'C word'?"

"You know, the place on a woman's body where you do the 'F word.'" Unblinking and calm, Natasha sat with her hands folded in her lap.

Several times in the past several weeks, Jason had slipped through her window at night and climbed into her bed while she slept. She had awakened to feel the pressure of his body on hers; it was especially intense in her groin area. By the time she had fully awakened, he would be gone. The previous week when she went in to use the bathroom, the head of an eel—or perhaps it was a large snake—emerged from the toilet bowl and lunged at her. She lowered the lid on the animal's neck and it disappeared. Since then, she had only used the toilet in the hall bathroom.

Evaluation of Natasha Oblamov

Natasha had a variety of psychotic symptoms. They included visual hallucinations (the eel in the toilet—criterion A2) and a nonbizarre delusion about Jason (A1). She also had the negative symptom of flat affect (she talked about eels and her private anatomy without a hint of emotion—A5). Although her active symptoms had been evident for only a few months, the prodromal symptom of staying in her room had been present for about 10 months (C). I can't identify anything in the vignette I'd call lack of volition, but her disorder obviously interfered with her ability to complete a canvas (B).

Nothing in Natasha's history would suggest **another medical condition** (E) that could explain her symptoms. However, a certain amount of routine lab testing might be ordered initially: complete blood count, routine blood chemistries, urinalysis. No evidence is given in the vignette to suggest that she had a **substance-induced psychotic disorder**, and her affect, though flat, was pleasant enough—nothing like the severely depressed mood of a **major depressive disorder with psychotic features** (D). Furthermore, she had never had suicidal ideas, and nothing suggested a **manic episode.** Duration of illness longer than 6 months rules out **schizophreniform disorder** and **brief psychotic disorder.** Finally, her brother had schizophrenia. About 10% of the first-degree relatives (parents, siblings, and children) of patients with schizophrenia also develop this condition. Of course, this is not a criterion for diagnosis, but it does help point the way.

Natasha fulfilled all elements of the prototype: psychotic symptoms, duration, and absence of other causes (especially medical and substance use disorders). Although age of onset isn't included in the DSM-5 criteria, I've mentioned it in the prototype. Anyone who becomes psychotic after, say, age 35 needs an evaluation even more careful than usual—for other, possibly treatable causes.

In an earlier time (DSM-IV), Natasha's symptoms would have earned her a diagnostic subtype of *undifferentiated*; now everyone's diagnosis is undifferentiated. Because she'd been ill less than a year (though well over the 6-month minimum), there would be no course specifier. I'd assign her a GAF score of 30. Her diagnosis would be simply this:

F20.9 [295.90]   Schizophrenia, first episode, acute

DSM-5 encourages us to rate each patient's psychotic symptoms on a 5-point scale. Each of the five criterion A symptoms is rated as 0 = absent, 1 = equivocal (not strong or long enough to be considered psychotic), 2 = mild, 3 = moderate, or 4 = severe. In addition, the manual notes that a similar rating scheme should be used for impaired cognition, depression, and mania, because each of these features is important in the differential diagnosis of psychotic patients. These ratings can be attached to several of the different psychotic disorders discussed in this chapter. But the use of this rating system for severity is (happily, in my judgment) optional.

Ramona Kelt

When she was 20 and had been married only a few months, Ramona Kelt was hospitalized for the first time with what was then described as "hebephrenic schizophrenia." According to records, her mood had been silly and inappropriate, her speech disjointed and hard to follow. She had been taken for evaluation after putting coffee grounds and orange peels on her head. She told the staff about television cameras in her closet that spied upon her whenever she had sex.

Since then, she had had several additional episodes, widely scattered across 25 years. Whenever she fell ill, her symptoms were the same. Each time she recovered enough to return home to her husband.

Every morning Ramona's husband had to prepare a list spelling out her day's activities, even including meal planning and cooking. Without it, he might arrive home to find that she had accomplished nothing that day. The couple had no children and few friends.

Ramona's most recent evaluation was prompted by a change in medical care plans. Her new clinician noted that she was still taking neuroleptics; each morning her husband carefully counted them out onto her plate and watched her swallow them. During the interview, she winked and smiled when it did not seem appropriate. She said it had been several years since television cameras bothered her, but she wondered whether her closet "might be haunted."

Evaluation of Ramona Kelt

Ramona had been ill for many years with symptoms that included disorganized behavior (criterion A4) and a delusion about television cameras (A1). The diagnosis of disorganized (hebephrenic) schizophrenia would at one time have been warranted, based on her inappropriate affect and bizarre speech (A3) and behavior. When acutely ill, she also met DSM-5 criteria for schizophrenia.

At this evaluation she was between acute episodes, but showed peculiarities of affect (winking) and ideation (the closet might be haunted) that suggested attenuated psychotic symptoms. She did have one serious, ongoing negative symptom (A5), avolition: If her husband didn't plan her day for her, she would accomplish pretty close to nothing (this would earn her a GAF score of 51). However, with only one current psychotic symptom, she appeared to be partly recovered from her last episode of schizophrenia.

Of course, to receive a diagnosis of schizophrenia, Ramona would have to have none of the exclusions (**general medical conditions, substance-induced psychotic disorder, mood disorders, schizoaffective disorder**). I think we would be pretty safe in assuming that this was still the case, so her current diagnosis would be as given below. Note, too, that even the sketchy information in the vignette nicely fulfilled our typical schizophrenia prototype. The course specifier equates essentially to the old diagnosis of schizophrenia, residual type.

F20.9 [295.90]   Schizophrenia, multiple episodes, currently in partial remission

Psychotic Disorders Other Than Schizophrenia

F20.81 [295.40] Schizophreniform Disorder

Its name sounds as if it must be related to schizophrenia, but the diagnosis of schizophreniform disorder (SphD) was devised in the late 1930s to deal with patients who may have something quite different. These people look as if they do have schizophrenia, but some of them later recover completely with no residual effects. The SphD diagnosis is valuable because it prevents closure: It alerts all clinicians that the underlying nature of the patient's psychosis has not yet been proven. (The *-form* suffix means this: The symptoms look like schizophrenia, which it may turn out to be. But with limited information, the careful clinician feels uncomfortable rushing into a diagnosis that implies lifelong disability and treatment.)

The symptoms and exclusions required for SphD are identical to those of basic schizophrenia; where the two diagnoses differ is in terms of duration and dysfunction. DSM-5 doesn't require evidence that SphD has interfered with the patient's life. However, when you think about it, most people who have had delusions and hallucinations for a month or more have probably suffered some inconvenience socially or in the workplace.

The real distinguishing point is the length of time the patient has been symptomatic: From 1 to 6 months is the period required. The practical importance of the interval is this: Numerous studies have shown that psychotic patients who have been briefly ill have a much better chance of full recovery than do those who have been ill for 6 months or longer. Still, over half of those who are initially diagnosed as having SphD are eventually found to have schizophrenia or schizoaffective disorder.

SphD isn't really a discrete disease at all; it's a place filler that's used about equally for males and females who are of about the age as patients with schizophrenia when they are first diagnosed. The diagnosis is made only about one-fifth as often as schizophrenia is, especially in the United States and other Western countries.

In the late 1930s, the Norwegian psychiatrist Gabriel Langfeldt coined the term *schizophreniform psychosis*. In the United States it was perhaps more relevant at that time, when the diagnosis of schizophrenia was so often made for patients who had psychotic symptoms but not the longitudinal course typical of schizophrenia. As Langfeldt made clear in a 1982 letter in the *American Journal of Psychiatry*, when he devised the concept he meant to include not only psychoses that look exactly like schizophrenia except for the duration of symptoms, but other presentations as well. These include what we would today call brief psychosis, schizoaffective disorders, and even some bipolar disorders. Time and custom have narrowed the meaning of his term, to the point where it is hardly ever used. I consider that to be a great pity; it's a useful device that helps keep clinicians on their toes and patients off chronic dosing with medication.

Essential Features of **Schizophreniform Disorder**

Relatively rapid onset and offset characterize SphD. The term usually indicates a young person (late teens or 20s) who for 30 days to 6 months has (1) delusions (especially persecutory) and (2) hallucinations (especially auditory). However, some patients will have (3) speech that is incoherent or otherwise disorganized, (4) severely abnormal psychomotor behavior (catatonic symptoms), or (5) negative symptoms such as restricted affect or lack of volition (they don't feel motivated to do work or maintain family life). Diagnosis requires at least two of these five types of psychotic symptoms, at least one of which must be delusions, hallucinations, or disorganized speech. The patient recovers fully within 6 months.

The Fine Print

The D's: • Duration (30 days to 6 months) • Differential diagnosis (physical and substance-induced psychotic disorders, schizophrenia, mood disorders, or cognitive disorders)

Coding Notes

Specify:

> **{With}{Without} good prognostic features,** which include: (1) Psychotic symptoms begin early (in first month of illness); (2) confusion or perplexity at peak of psychosis; (3) good premorbid functioning; (4) affect not blunted. Two to four of these = With good prognostic features; none or one = Without.
>
> **With catatonia** (see p. 100)

If it's within 6 months and the patient is still ill, use the specifier *(provisional)*. Once the patient has fully recovered, remove the specifier.

If the patient is still ill after 6 months, SphD can no longer apply. Change the diagnosis to schizophrenia or some other disorder.

You may specify severity, though you don't have to (see p. 74).

Arnold Wilson

When he was 3, Arnold Wilson's family had entered a witness protection program. At least that's what he told the mental health intake interviewer.

Arnold was slim, of medium height, and clean-shaven. He wore a name tag identifying him as a medical student. His eye contact was direct and steady, and he sat quietly as he described his experiences. "It was on account of my dad," he explained. "When we lived back East, he used to be in the Mob."

Arnold's father, the principal informant, later remarked, "OK, I'm an investment banker. You might think that's bad enough, but it isn't the Mob. Well, anyway, it's not *that* mob."

Arnold's ideas had come to him as a revelation 2 months earlier. He was at his desk, studying for a physiology test, when he heard a voice just behind him. "I jumped up, thinking I must have left my door open, but there was no one in the room but me. I checked the radio and my iPod, but everything was turned off. Then I heard it again."

The voice was one he recognized. "But I can't tell you whose. She told me not to." The woman's voice spoke very clearly to him and seemed to move around a lot. "Sometimes she seemed like she was just behind me. Other times, she stood outside whatever room I was in." He agrees that she spoke in complete sentences. "Sometimes full paragraphs. What a gabby person!" he remarked with a laugh.

At first, the voice told him he "needed to cover my tracks, whatever that meant." When he tried to ignore it, she became "really angry, told me to believe her, or . . . " Arnold didn't finish the sentence. The voice pointed out that his last name, before he was 3, was Italian. "You know, she was really beginning to make sense."

"The name change part's true," his father explained. "When I married his mother, Arnold was part of the deal. His biological father had died of cancer of the kidney. We both thought it would be best if I adopted him." That was 20 years ago.

Arnold had had difficulty in middle school. His attention wandered, and so did he. As a result, he spent a lot of time in the principal's office. Although several teachers despaired of him, in high school he'd hit his stride. There he'd made excellent grades, gotten into a good college, and then been accepted at a better medical school. That autumn, just before starting his freshman year, his physical exam (and a panel of blood tests) had been completely normal. He said his roommate would testify that he hadn't used any drugs or alcohol.

"It was pretty confusing, at first—the voice, I mean. I wondered if I was losing my mind. But then we talked it over, she and I. Now it seems pretty clear."

When Arnold talked about the voice, he became quite animated, using appropriate hand gestures and vocal inflections. Throughout, he gave full attention to the interviewer, except once when he turned his head, as though listening to something. Or someone.

Evaluation of Arnold Wilson

Arnold's two psychotic symptoms—delusions and auditory hallucinations—are enough to get us past the criterion A requirements, which are the same for SphD as for schizophrenia. The vignette doesn't describe the extent to which his social or school functioning had been compromised, but the SphD criteria set doesn't require this information.

The clinical features of Arnold's psychosis closely resembled those of **schizophrenia.** Of course, that's the whole point of SphD: At the time you make the diagnosis, you don't know whether the outcome will be full recovery or long-term illness. Arnold's symptoms had been present too long for **brief psychotic disorder**, which lasts less than 1 month, and too briefly for **schizophrenia.** He didn't use alcohol to excess, and on his roommate's evidence (OK, by proxy), he didn't use drugs at all; this would rule out a **substance-induced psychotic disorder.** The usual **general medical** causes of psychosis would have to be investigated, but his recent physical exam had been normal. With no symptoms of mania or depression, **bipolar I disorder** would seem vanishingly unlikely.

Whenever possible for patients with SphD, a statement of prognosis should be made. In Arnold's case, the treating clinician noted the following evidence of good prognosis: (1) As far as anyone could tell, his illness had begun abruptly with prominent psychotic symptoms (auditory hallucinations). (2) His premorbid functioning (both work and social life) had been good. (3) Lacking flattening or inappropriateness, his affect was intact during this evaluation. The fourth good-prognosis feature specified by DSM-5 is perplexity or confusion. Arnold did say that he was confused at first, but by the time of his evaluation, at the height of his illness, his cognitive processes seemed intact. Thus he had three of the features that favor a good prognosis; only two are needed.

The criteria require that a qualifier of *(provisional)* be appended if the diagnosis of SphD is made before the patient recovers, as was the case for Arnold. Assuming that he recovered completely within the 6-month limit, this qualifier could then be removed. However, if the illness lasted longer than 6 months and it interfered with Arnold's work or social life, the diagnosis might need to be changed—probably to schizophrenia.

Right now, Arnold's diagnosis should read as given below. And I'd give him a GAF score of 60: Though his psychotic symptoms were serious, his behavior hadn't been markedly affected. Yet.

F20.81 [295.40]   Schizophreniform disorder (provisional), with good prognostic features

---

Do you need a place to park your patient while you collect more evidence? Even in DSM-5, there persist a couple of diagnostic "sidings" that you can use to indicate that something is wrong, but you're waiting for more information before you commit to a diagnosis. Of course, there's always "other specified _____" or "unspecified _____," but even beyond those useful (and vague, and sometimes indiscriminately used) locutions, we have some other terms that gain much the same advantage.

SphD is one—it can go either way, to chronicity or to recovery. And then brief psychotic disorder was manufactured to cover the month of psychosis before you can diagnose SphD. In Chapter 6, we'll see that acute stress disorder was cobbled together to cover the month before posttraumatic stress disorder can be diagnosed. But that's about the sum of it. The problem is, we mental health clinicians are still dependent on our patients' *appearance* to inform how we view them. Other medical disciplines use lab tests, and so may avoid the diagnostic way station.

F23 [298.8] Brief Psychotic Disorder

Patients with brief psychotic disorder (BPsD) are psychotic for at least 1 day and return to normal within 1 month. It doesn't matter how many symptoms they have had or whether they have had trouble functioning socially or at work. (In parallel with schizophreniform disorder, any patient who remains symptomatic longer than 1 month must be given a different diagnosis.)

BPsD isn't an especially stable diagnosis; many patients will eventually be rediagnosed with another psychotic disorder. (This is hardly surprising for a diagnosis you can have for only 30 days.). As few as 7% of first-time patients with psychotic disorders have this as the initial diagnosis. Some patients who experience a psychosis around the time of giving birth may be given this diagnosis. Even then, it is a rare condition: The incidence of postpartum psychosis is only about 1 or 2 per 1,000 women who give birth. Indeed, BPsD is overall twice as common among women as men.

European clinicians are more likely to diagnose BPsD. (This doesn't mean that the condition occurs more frequently in Europe, just that European clinicians are apparently more alert to it—or more likely to overdiagnose it.) BPsD may be more common among young patients (teenagers and young adults) and among patients who are from lower socioeconomic strata or who have preexisting personality disorders. Patients with certain personality disorders (such as borderline) who have very brief psychotic symptoms precipitated by stress do not require a separate diagnosis of BPsD.

Over two decades ago, in DSM-III-R, this category was called *brief reactive psychosis*. That name and its criteria reflected the notion that it may occur in response to some overwhelmingly stressful event, such as death of a relative. In the DSM-5 criteria, this concept is retained only in the form of specifiers.

The decision about the diagnosis of BPsD is relatively straightforward. To compensate, we face decisions about specifiers that are fraught. We must determine whether a stressor could have caused the psychosis. Of course, anything could precede the onset, and to learn what it might be could require interviewing a spouse, relative, or friend. We'd want to learn about possible traumatic events, but also about the patient's premorbid adjustment, past history of similar reactions to stress, and the chronological relationship between stressor and the onset of symptoms. Even with all this, we're still stuck with deciding whether the event is likely to have caused psychosis. DSM-5 tells us only that the event(s) must be severe enough to cause stress for anyone of the patient's situation and culture. But it doesn't help us at all to decide whether psychosis is *in response* to stress. My solution: Ignore the words *in response*; if there's marked stress, say so, and move on.

Essential Features of **Brief Psychotic Disorder**

All within the course of a single month, the patient develops, then recovers *completely* from an episode of psychosis that includes delusions, hallucinations, or disorganized speech (disorganized behavior may also be present). The episode lasts at least 1 day but less than 1 month.

The Fine Print

The D's: • Duration (1 day to 1 month) • Differential diagnosis (mood or cognitive disorders, psychoses caused by medical conditions or substance use, schizophrenia)

Coding Notes

If you make the diagnosis without waiting for recovery, you'll have to append the term *(provisional)*.

You can specify:

> **With postpartum onset.** Symptoms begin within 4 weeks of giving birth.
> **{With}{Without} marked stressors.** The stressors must appear to cause the symptoms, must occur shortly before their onset, and must be severe enough that nearly anyone of that culture would feel markedly stressed.
> **With catatonia** (see p. 100)

You may specify severity, though you don't have to (see p. 74).

Melanie Grayson

This was Melanie Grayson's first pregnancy, and she had been quite apprehensive about it. She had gained 30 pounds, and her blood pressure had been slightly too high. But she had needed only a spinal block for anesthesia, and her husband was in the room with her when she delivered a healthy baby girl.

That night she slept fitfully; she was irritable the next day. But she breastfed her baby and seemed to listen attentively when the nurse practitioner came to instruct her on bathing and other postpartum care.

The next morning, while Melanie was having breakfast, her husband came to take her and the baby home. When she ordered him to turn off the radio, he looked around the room and said he didn't hear one. "You know very well what radio," she yelled, and threw a tea bag at him.

The mental health consultant noted that Melanie was alert, fully oriented, and cognitively intact. She was irritable but not depressed. She kept insisting that she heard a radio playing: "I think it's hidden in my pillow." She unzipped the pillowcase and felt around inside. "It's some sort of a news report. They're talking about what's happening in the hospital. I think I just heard my name mentioned."

Melanie's flow of speech was coherent and relevant. Apart from throwing the tea bag and looking for the radio, her behavior was unremarkable. She denied hallucinations involving any of the other senses. She insisted that the voices she heard could not be imaginary, and she didn't think someone was trying to play a trick on her. She had never used drugs or alcohol, and her obstetrician vouched for her excellent general health. After much discussion, she agreed to remain in the hospital a day or two longer to try to get to the bottom of the mystery.

Evaluation of Melanie Grayson

Despite her obvious psychosis (hallucinations and delusions), the brevity of her symptoms kept Melanie from meeting the criterion A requirements for **schizophrenia, schizophreniform disorder,** or **schizoaffective disorder.** What's left?

Although Melanie remained alert and cognitively intact, any patient with abrupt onset of psychotic symptoms should be carefully evaluated for a possible **delirium.** (They will often be confused, which may be the fact with patients who have BPsD, too. Be careful in your evaluation.) Many **general medical conditions** can also produce psychotic symptoms. Anyone who becomes psychotic soon after entering the hospital should be evaluated for a **substance-induced psychotic disorder with onset during withdrawal.** Melanie had no prominent mood symptoms; if she had had any, a diagnosis of a **mood disorder with psychotic features** might have been entertained.

It is worth noting that many patients who develop psychosis after delivery may have mixtures of symptoms that include euphoria, psychosis, and cognitive changes. Many of these patients have some form of mood disorder (often **bipolar I disorder**). Diagnosis should be made with extreme care in all cases of postpartum psychosis; the diagnosis of schizophrenia should never be made, except in the most obvious and certain of circumstances.

With a very brief duration of psychosis and none of the exclusions, Melanie would fulfill the somewhat undemanding criteria for BPsD. Until she recovered, the diagnosis would have to be made provisionally. I'd put her GAF score at 40. Her full diagnosis at this time would be as follows:

| F23 [298.8] | Brief psychotic disorder, with postpartum onset (provisional) |
| O80 [650] | Normal delivery |

F22 [297.1] Delusional Disorder

Persistent delusions are the chief characteristic of delusional disorder. Usually they can seem entirely believable; however, it is no longer necessary that they be nonbizarre, as DSM-IV required. Still, patients tend to appear pretty normal, as long as you don't touch on one of their delusions. There are half a dozen possible themes, which I've outlined in the Coding Notes.

Although the symptoms can seem similar to those of schizophrenia, there are several reasons to list delusional disorder separately:

- The age of onset is often later in life (mid- to late 30s) than that of schizophrenia.

- Family histories of the two illnesses are dissimilar.

- At follow-up, these patients are rarely rediagnosed as having schizophrenia.

- The infrequent hallucinations take a back seat to the delusions, and are understandable in the context of those delusions.

Most importantly, compared to that of schizophrenia, the course of delusional disorder is less fraught with intellectual and work-related deterioration. In fact, behavior won't be much altered, outside of responses to the delusions: for instance, phoning the police for protection, or letter-writing campaigns to complain of sundry imagined insults or infractions. As you might suppose, resulting domestic problems are frequent—and, depending on their subtype, these patients may be swept up in litigation or endless medical tests.

Delusional disorder is uncommon (by some estimates, schizophrenia is 30 times more frequent). Chronically reduced sensory input (being deaf or blind) may contribute to its development, as may social isolation (such as being an immigrant in a strange country). Delusional disorder may also be associated with family traits that include suspiciousness, jealousy, and secretiveness. The persecutory type is by far the most common of the subtypes; the jealous type ranks a distant second.

One problem that crops up frequently is the presence of mood symptoms in patients with delusional disorder. These may be quite unsurprisingly gloomy responses to the perception that others do not agree with closely held beliefs. Depressive mood can create difficult questions of differential diagnosis: Most notably, does the patient have a primary mood disorder? The DSM-5 criteria do not provide a bright line separating the two concepts; the time course of two sets of symptoms—mood and psychotic—may help in the differentiation. Of course, in the case of serious question, I'd consider first the more conservative mood disorder, though delusional disorder may look better and better as time passes.

Shared Delusions

Though such instances are extremely rare, cases in which one or more persons develop delusions as a result of close association with another delusional person are dramatic and inherently interesting. DSM-IV called this condition shared psychotic disorder; as long ago as 150 years it was known as *folie à deux*, which means "double insanity." Usually two people are involved, but three, four, or more can become caught up in the delusion. Shared delusions affect women more often than men, and they usually occur within families. Social isolation may play a role in the development of this strange condition.

One of the persons affected is independently psychotic; through a close (and often dependent) association, the other has come to believe in the delusions and other experiences of the first. Though occasionally bizarre, the content of the delusion is usually believable, if often unconvincing. Isolating the independently psychotic patient may cure the other(s), but this remedy doesn't always work. For one thing, the parties involved are often closely related and persist in reinforcing their mutual psychopathology.

A few patients whose delusions mirror those of people with whom they are intimately associated will, for one reason or another, not fully qualify for a diagnosis of delusional disorder. For them, you'll have to use the category of other specified (or unspecified) schizophrenia spectrum and other psychotic disorder, as described at the end of this chapter.

Essential Features of **Delusional Disorder**

For at least a month, the patient has had delusions but no other psychotic symptoms, and any mood symptoms are relatively brief. Other than consequences of the delusions, behavior isn't much affected.

The Fine Print

OK, there might be some hallucinations of touch or smell, but only as they relate to the delusions. And they won't be prominent.

The D's: • Duration (1+ months) • Distress and disability (none, except as related to the delusional content) • Differential diagnosis (physical and substance-induced psychotic disorders, mood or cognitive disorders, schizophrenia, obsessive–compulsive disorder)

Coding Notes

You can specify type of delusion: **erotomanic, grandiose, jealous, persecutory, somatic, mixed, or unspecified.**

Specify if:

> **With bizarre content.** This denotes obviously improbable delusions (see sidebar, p. 61).

If the delusional disorder has lasted at least 1 year, specify course:

> **First episode, currently in acute episode**
> **First episode, currently in partial remission**
> **First episode, currently in full remission**
> **Multiple episodes, currently in acute episode**

Multiple episodes, currently in partial remission
Multiple episodes, currently in full remission
Continuous
Unspecified

You may specify severity, though you don't have to (see p. 74).

Molly McConegal

Molly McConegal, a tiny sparrow of a woman, sat perched on the front of her waiting room chair. On her lap she tightly clutched a scuffed black handbag; her gray hair was caught up in a fierce little bun at the back of her head. Through spectacles as thick as highball glasses, she darted myopic, suspicious glances about the room. She had already spent 45 minutes with the consultant behind closed doors. Now she was waiting while her husband, Michael, had a turn.

Michael confirmed much of what Molly had already said. The couple had been married for over 40 years, had two children, and had lived in the same neighborhood (the same house, in fact) nearly all of their married life. Both were retired from the telephone company, and they shared an interest in gardening.

"That was where it all started, in the garden," said Michael. "It was last summer, when I was out trimming the rose bushes in the front yard. Molly said she caught me looking at the house across the street. The widow woman who lives there is younger than we are, maybe 50. We nod and say 'Hi,' but in 10 years, I've never even been inside her front door. But Molly said I was taking too long on those rose bushes, that I was waiting for our neighbor—her name is Mrs. Jessup—to come out of the house. Of course, I denied it, but she insisted. Kept talking about it for days."

In the following months, Molly pursued the idea of Michael's supposed extramarital relationship. At first she only suggested that he had been trying to lure Mrs. Jessup out for a meeting. Within a few weeks, she "knew" that they had been together. Soon this had become a sex orgy.

Molly had talked of little else and had begun to incorporate many commonplace observations into her suspicions. A button undone on Michael's shirt meant that he had just returned from a visit with "the woman." The adjustment of the living room Venetian blinds tipped her off that he had been trying to semaphore messages the night before. A private detective Molly hired for surveillance only stopped by to chat with Michael, submitted a bill for $500, and resigned.

Molly continued to do the cooking and washing for herself, but Michael now had to take care of his own meals and laundry. She slept normally, ate well, and—when she wasn't with him—seemed to be in good spirits. Michael, on the other hand, was becoming a nervous wreck. Molly listened in on his telephone calls and steamed open his mail. Once she told him that she would file for divorce, but she "didn't want the children to find out." Twice he had awakened at night to find her wrapped tightly in her bathrobe and standing beside his bed, glowering down at him. "Waiting for me to make my move," he said. Last week she had strewn the hallway outside his room with thumbtacks, so that he would cry out and awaken her when he sneaked away for his late-night sexual rendezvous.

Michael smiled and said sadly, "You know, I haven't had sex with anybody for nearly 15 years. Since I had my prostate operation, I just haven't had the ability."

Evaluation of Molly McConegal

If you compare the features of delusional disorder with those of schizophrenia, you will note many differences.

First, consider symptoms. Delusions are the only psychotic symptom found to any important degree in delusional disorder. The delusion could be any of the types listed in the Coding Notes. In Molly's case, they were of the jealous type, but the persecutory and grandiose types are also common. Note that with the exception of occasional olfactory or tactile hallucinations that support the content of delusions, patients with delusional disorder will never fulfill criterion A for schizophrenia (this nonfulfillment constitutes delusional disorder's criterion B).

The delusions need last only 1 month; however, by the time they come to professional attention, most patients, like Molly, have been ill much longer (A). The average age of patients may be around 55. The consequences are usually relatively mild for delusional disorder. Indeed, aside from the direct effects of the delusion (in Molly's case, her marital harmony), work and social life may not be affected much at all (C).

However, the exclusions are pretty much the same as for schizophrenia. Always rule out **another medical condition** or **cognitive disorder**, especially a **dementia with delusions**, when evaluating delusional patients (D). This is especially important in older patients, who can be quite crafty at disguising the fact that they are cognitively impaired. **Substance-induced psychotic disorders** can closely mimic delusional disorder. This is especially true for **amphetamine-induced psychotic disorder with onset during withdrawal**, in which fully oriented patients may describe how they are being attacked by gangs of pursuers (E).

Molly McConegal had neither history nor symptoms to support any of the foregoing disorders; however, laboratory and toxicology studies may be needed for many patients. Other than irritability in the company of her husband, she had no symptoms of a **mood disorder.** Even then, her affect was quite appropriate to her content of thought. However, many of these patients can develop mood syndromes secondary to the delusions. Then the diagnosis depends on the chronology and severity of mood symptoms. Information from relatives or other third parties is often required to determine which came first. Also, the mood symptoms must be relatively mild and brief to sustain a diagnosis of delusional disorder.

Although these patients may have associated conditions—including **body dysmorphic disorder**, **obsessive–compulsive disorder**, or **avoidant, paranoid, or schizoid personality disorder**—there was no evidence for any of these in Molly McConegal.

Molly had been ill a bit less than a full year, so no course of illness could be specified. Her GAF score would be 55 (highest level in the past year). Her diagnosis would be as follows:

F22 [297.1]   Delusional disorder, jealous type

Miriam Phillips

Miriam Phillips was 23 when she was hospitalized. She had spent nearly all her life in the Ozarks, where she sometimes attended class in a three-room school. Although she was bright enough, she had little interest in her studies and often volunteered to stay home to care for her mother, who was unwell. She dropped out of 12th grade to stay home full-time.

It was lonely living in the hills. Miriam's father, a long-distance trucker, was away most of the time. She had never learned to drive, and there were no close neighbors. Their television set received mostly snow; there was little in the way of mail; and there were no visitors at all. So she was surprised late on a Monday afternoon when two men paid a call.

After identifying themselves as FBI agents, they asked if she was the Miriam Phillips who 3 weeks earlier had written a letter to the president. When she asked how they had known, they showed her a faxed copy of her own letter:

> Dear Mr. President, what do you plan to do about the Cubans? They have been working on mother. Their up to no good. Ive seen the police, but they say Cubans are your job, and I guess their right. You have to do your job or Ill have a dirty job to do. Miriam Phillips.

When Miriam finally figured out that the FBI agents thought she had threatened the president, she relaxed. She hadn't meant that at all. She had meant that if no one else took action, she'd have to crawl under the house to get the gravity machines.

"Gravity machines?" The two agents looked at each other.

She explained. They had been installed under the house by Cuban agents of Fidel Castro after the Bay of Pigs invasion in the 1960s. The machines pulled your body fluids down toward your feet. They hadn't affected her yet, but they had bothered her mother for years. Miriam had seen the hideous swelling in her mother's ankles. Some days it extended almost to her knees.

The two agents listened to her politely, then left. As they passed through town on their way to the airport, they called at the local community mental health clinic. Within a few days, a mental health worker came to interview Miriam, who agreed to enter the hospital voluntarily for a "checkup."

On admission, Miriam appeared remarkably intact. She had a full range of appropriate affect and normal cognitive abilities and orientation. Her reasoning ability seemed good, aside from the story about the gravity machines. As far back as her teens, her mother had told her how the machines came to be installed in the crawlspace under their house. Mother had been a nurse, and Miriam had always accepted her word in medical matters. By some unspoken agreement, the two had never discussed the matter with Miriam's father.

After Miriam had been on the ward for 3 days, her clinician asked whether she thought any other explanation for her mother's edema was possible. Miriam considered. She had never felt the gravity effects herself. She had believed that her mother told her the truth, but she now supposed that even Mother could have been mistaken.

Though Miriam was given no medication, after a week she stopped talking about gravity machines and asked to be discharged. At the end of their shift that afternoon, two young attendants gave her a lift home. As they walked her to the front door, it was opened by a short woman, quite stout, with salt-and-pepper hair. Her lower legs were neatly wrapped in elastic bandages. Through the partly opened door she darted a glance at the two men.

"Hmmm!" she said. "You look like Cubans."

Evaluation of Miriam Phillips

Though we don't know exactly how long, Miriam had had delusions far longer than a month (criterion A) without hallucinations or negative symptoms, and with no disordered behavior or affect. Therefore, **schizophrenia** could be ruled out just on the basis of insufficient variety of symptoms (B). She wasn't depressed or manic (D), and there was no history or other evidence to support **substance-induced psychotic disorder** or **psychotic disorder due to another medical condition** (E). Her delusions hadn't caused any occupational or social dysfunction; her own isolation appeared to have begun at least 5 years earlier, before the onset of her shared delusion (C).

With an admission GAF score of 40, Miriam's delusions became less prominent after just a few days of separation from her mother. (If they had persisted for a long time, the diagnosis of a different, independent psychosis would have been considered.) In working further with her, a therapist would also want to consider the possibility of a personality disorder, such as **dependent personality disorder.** Her delusion, and that of her mother, was certainly bizarre, but I'm not confident she had been ill longer than a year, so I wouldn't give her any other specifiers.

F22 [297.1]   Delusional disorder, persecutory type, with bizarre content

Schizoaffective Disorder

Schizoaffective disorder (SaD) is just plain confusing. (William Carpenter, chairperson of the DSM-5 psychosis study group, stated during a 2013 presentation about his committee's work, "We don't even know if it exists in nature.") Over the years, it has meant many different things to clinicians. Partly because there were so many interpretations in use, DSM-III included no criteria at all in 1980. DSM-III-R first attempted to specify criteria in 1987. These endured for 7 years, until they were substantially rewritten for DSM-IV. Showing admirable restraint, DSM-5 has made relatively few changes to those criteria. Even with the (minimal) tweaking of criteria, in my opinion the value of this diagnosis remains pretty low.

Most interpretations suggest that SaD is some sort of cross between a mood disorder and schizophrenia. Some writers regard it as a form of bipolar disorder, because certain patients seem to respond well to lithium. Other commentators believe that it is closer to schizophrenia. Still others hold that it is an entirely separate type of psychosis, or simply a collection of confusing, sometimes contradictory symptoms.

With its various percentage and minimal time requirements, SaD could unfold in a variety of ways: mania first, depression first, psychosis first. Of course, there are the usual exclusions for substance use and general medical conditions. If you examine the various time requirements, you can determine that the entire illness must last at minimum for a bit longer than 1 month, though many patients will be ill much longer.

No one really knows much about the demographic features of SaD. It is probably less common than schizophrenia; its prognosis lies between that of schizophrenia and the mood disorders. Recent studies indicate that patients with SaD whose manic symptoms predominate (the bipolar type) may have a better prognosis than those with the depressive type of this condition.

I find it easier to remember the requirements for SaD if I think of them as follows:

The mood symptoms are important in that they must be present during half or more of the total duration of illness.

The psychosis symptoms are important in that they must be present *by themselves* for at least 2 weeks. (Note that the criteria are silent on whether to count psychosis symptoms that are present during the time that mood symptoms have disappeared under treatment.)

In this graphic representation of the minimum time requirements that are possible, given the criteria, the overall length of the box represents the totality of the individual's illness, not just an episode. Of course, it will be impossible for any clinician to know whether the criteria for a mood episode are met throughout the illness; we'll have to rely on prototypes for the overall gestalt.

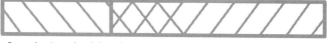

2 weeks (psychosis)　　2+ more weeks (mood episode)

Note that the "solo" psychotic episode (criterion A) could come at any point in the episode: the start, the end, somewhere in the middle. Unhappily, DSM-5 is silent on the question of whether, during the psychosis period, there can be mood symptoms that don't fully qualify as an episode of mania, hypomania, or depression. (DSM-IV was more forthright; it said "in the absence of prominent mood symptoms.") Start saving for DSM-6.

Essential Features of **Schizoaffective Disorder**

A patient has a period of illness during which a manic episode or a major depressive episode lasts half of more of the total time involved. For at least a fortnight during this same continuous period, the patient fulfills the criterion A requirements for schizophrenia *without* having a mood episode.

The Fine Print

If the patient has a major depression, one of the symptoms must be depressed mood; "mere" loss of interest doesn't cut it.

The D's: • Duration (a total of 1+ months) • Differential diagnosis (psychotic mood disorders, substance use, and physical disorders)

Coding Notes

Specify:

> **F25.0 [295.70] Bipolar type** (if during a manic episode)
> **F25.1 [295.70] Depressive type**

Specify:

> **With catatonia** (see p. 100)

If the disorder has lasted at least 1 year, specify course:

> **First episode, currently in acute episode**
> **First episode, currently in partial remission**
> **First episode, currently in full remission**
> **Multiple episodes, currently in acute episode**
> **Multiple episodes, currently in partial remission**
> **Multiple episodes, currently in full remission**
> **Continuous**
> **Unspecified**

You may specify severity, though you don't have to (see p. 74).

Velma Dean

Velma Dean's lips curled upwards, but the smile didn't touch her eyes. "I'm really sorry about this," she told her therapist, "but I guess—well, I don't know what." She reached into the large shopping bag she had carried into the office and pulled out a 6-inch kitchen knife. First she grasped it in her hand, with her thumb along the blade. Then she tried clutching it in her fist. The therapist reached for the alarm button under the desk top, ruefully aware of yet another change of course in this patient's multifaceted history.

A month before her 18th birthday, Velma Dean had joined the Army. Her father, a colonel of artillery, had wanted a son, but Velma was his only child. Over the feeble protests of her mother, Velma's upbringing had been strict and semimilitary. After working 3 years in the motor pool, Velma herself had just been promoted to sergeant when she became ill.

Her illness started with 2 days in the infirmary for what seemed like bronchitis, but as the penicillin took effect and her fever resolved, the voices began. At first they seemed to be located toward the back of her head. Within a few days they had moved to her bedside water glass. As nearly as she could tell, their pitch depended on the contents of her glass: If the glass was nearly empty, the voices were female; if it was full to the top, they spoke in a rich baritone. They were always quiet and mannerly. Often they gave her advice on how to behave, but at times she said they "nearly drove me crazy" by constantly commenting on what she was doing.

A psychiatrist diagnosed Velma's condition as schizophrenia and prescribed neuroleptics. The voices improved, but never quite disappeared. She concealed the fact that she had "figured out" that her illness had been caused by her first sergeant, who for months had tried unsuccessfully to get her into bed. She also hid the fact that for several weeks she had been drinking nearly a pint of Southern Comfort each evening. The Army retired her as medically unfit, 100% disabled. When she was well enough to travel, her father drove her the 600 miles back home.

For her treatment, Velma enrolled at her local Department of Veterans Affairs (VA) outpatient clinic. There, her new therapist verified (1) the continuing presence (now for nearly 8 months) of her barely audible hallucinations, and (2) her increasingly profound symptoms of depression. These included low self-esteem and hopelessness (much worse in the morning than in the evening); loss of appetite; a 10-pound weight loss over the past 8 weeks; insomnia that caused her to awaken early most mornings; and the guilty conviction that she had disappointed her father by "deserting" the Army before her hitch was up. She denied thoughts of injuring herself or other people.

Velma's VA clinician initially deferred making a diagnosis, noting that she had been ill too long for schizophreniform disorder and that her mood symptoms seemed to argue against schizophrenia. Physical exam and laboratory testing ruled out general medical conditions. Although Alcoholics Anonymous helped her stop drinking, her depressive and psychotic symptoms continued.

Because Velma's depressive symptoms might be secondary to a partly treated psychosis, her neuroleptic dose was increased. This completely eliminated the hallucinations and delusions, but the depressive symptoms continued virtually unabated. The antidepressant imipramine at 200 mg/day only produced side effects; after 4 weeks, lithium was added. Once a therapeutic blood level was reached, her depressive symptoms melted completely away. For 6 months she remained in a good mood and free of psychosis, though she never obtained a job or did very much with her time.

Now it seemed that Velma might actually be suffering from a major depressive disorder with psychotic features. At this point, her clinician became uneasy that the neuroleptic could produce side effects such as tardive dyskinesia. With Velma's consent, the neuroleptic was gradually reduced by about 20% per week. After 3 weeks, she began once again to hear voices commanding her to run away from home. During this time her mood remained good; with the exception of some difficulty getting to sleep at night, she developed none of the vegetative symptoms she had formerly had with depression. Her full former dose of neuroleptic medication was rapidly restored.

After several months of renewed stability, Velma and her therapist decided to try again. This time they began cautiously to reduce the imipramine, by 25 mg each week. Each week they met to evaluate her mood and check for symptoms of psychosis. By December she had been free of the antidepressant for 2 months, and had remained symptom-free (except for her habitual bland, smiling affect). Now her therapist took a deep breath and decreased her lithium by one tablet per day. The following week Velma returned to the office, hallucinating and wondering whether to hold a kitchen knife in her hand or in her fist.

Evaluation of Velma Dean

With Velma's story, we can illustrate the current thinking about SaD. Her condition really seemed to be a mixture of mood and psychotic symptoms, though the latter had clearly begun first. She had what appeared to be a single period of illness (her only "well" periods were when she was taking medication; even then, she had residual lack of initiative), with both psychotic symptoms (auditory hallucinations and a delusion that the sergeant had caused her illness) and a major depressive episode (criterion A). During this period her mood symptoms, which occurred both with and without psychotic symptoms, had lasted for more than half the duration of her total illness (C). Although she abused alcohol at one time during her illness, it appeared to be a consequence of her illness, not the cause; both her mood and psychotic symptoms continued long after she quit drinking (D). The psychosis had begun first and had lasted at least 2 weeks before the mood symptoms commenced (B). The prototype symptoms are also met at level 4, and say more or less the same thing.

Although we can rattle off these criteria with relative ease (and, to be honest, a crib sheet), Velma's history illustrates how difficult it can be to apply them. The therapist, whose thinking has already been described in the vignette, was smart initially to defer diagnosis; this should remind all clinicians to keep thinking about the diagnosis and to reject any label that might close their minds to further therapeutic plans. She could not be diagnosed as having **schizophrenia**, because it excludes prominent, lasting mood episodes. A **mood disorder with psychosis** could be eliminated because she had psychotic symptoms even when not depressed. After many months of care, she showed no evidence of **another medical condition**.

The relative duration of psychosis and mood symptoms is very important in SaD. DSM-5 states that the mood symptoms must be present for a majority of the overall duration of illness. Velma's depressive symptoms lasted for at least 2 months; there is every reason to suspect they would have gone on much longer had she not received effective treatment. Her criterion A symptoms for schizophrenia had been present for 2 weeks without mood symptoms. However carefully the criteria try to operationalize the duration of various symptoms, it remains to some degree a judgment call on the part of each clinician. (DSM-5 is silent on the issue of treated depression and SaD; I'm claiming clinician's prerogative and declaring that because antidepressant treatment seems to have made all the difference, SaD should be her diagnosis.)

Eventually, many patients with both mood and psychotic symptoms will comfortably fit the criteria for schizophrenia or a mood disorder. If they were followed long enough, perhaps the majority of patients with SaD could be rediagnosed. Given the highly restrictive nature of the current definition, it seems likely that this diagnosis will rarely be used. If you ever make the diagnosis, ask yourself, "Have I overlooked anything that is more reasonable?" SaD is a diagnosis best used for patients who have a long-standing history of both sets of symptoms. **Other specified (or unspecified) schizophrenia spectrum** and **other psychotic disorder** may prove to be much more useful to most clinicians. Velma's mood symptoms were depressive, which defined her subtype diagnosis. At the time she was wielding her knife, I felt that her GAF score was down around 20.

F25.1 [295.70]   Schizoaffective disorder, depressive type

Substance/Medication-Induced Psychotic Disorder

This category includes all psychoses caused by mind-altering substances. The predominant symptoms are usually hallucinations or delusions; depending on the substance, they can occur during withdrawal or acute intoxication. Usually the course is brief, though they can persist long enough to cause confusion with endogenous psychoses.

Although most of these psychoses are self-limiting, early recognition is crucial. Patients have died while experiencing a substance-induced psychotic disorder, several of which can closely mimic schizophrenia. Many diagnoses are possible, if we include all the possible combinations of different substances with the type and duration of psychosis and its relation to intoxication or withdrawal. The incidence is unknown, though a substantial minority of first-episode psychoses may belong to this class—enough that we should remain alert for them. See the "Classes (or Names) of Medications . . ." table in the Appendix for a list of medications associated with psychosis.

Essential Features of
Substance/Medication-Induced Psychotic Disorder

The use of some substance appears to have caused hallucinations or delusions (or both).

The Fine Print

For tips on identifying substance-related causation, see sidebar, page 95.

The D's: • Distress or disability (work/academic, social, or personal impairment) • Differential diagnosis (schizophrenia and its cousins, delusional disorder, ordinary substance intoxication or withdrawal, delirium)

You'd only make this diagnosis when the symptoms are serious enough to justify clinical attention *and* they are worse than you'd expect from ordinary intoxication or withdrawal.

Coding Notes

When writing down the diagnosis, use the name of the exact substance in the title: for example, methamphetamine-induced psychotic disorder.

ICD-9 kept coding simple: 291.9 for alcohol, 292.9 for all other substances. Coding in ICD-10 depends on the substance used and whether symptoms are met for an actual substance use disorder—and how severe the use disorder is. Refer to Table 15.2 in Chapter 15.

Specify if:

> **With onset during {intoxication}{withdrawal}.** This gets tacked on at the end of your string of words. It also affects the ICD-10 number.
> **With onset after medication use.** You can use this in addition to other specifiers (see the sidebar just below).

You may specify severity, though you don't have to (see p. 74).

Actually, DSM-5 mentions *with onset after medication use* as an optional specifier for substance/medication-induced anxiety disorder, obsessive–compulsive and related disorder, and sexual dysfunctions, but not for psychotic, mood, or sleep disorders. (This despite the fact that the titles of these disorders even begin, uniformly, "substance/medication-induced [this or that].")

I am told that there wasn't enough communication among the different subcommittees, so that inconsistencies such as this one crept into the final version. Inasmuch as prescribed medications can cause virtually any sort of emotional or behavioral problem, I plan to go right ahead and use the medication specifier any time it seems warranted. But that's easy for me to say—in my state, the governor has declared a moratorium on capital punishment.

Danny Finch

Danny Finch put up with the ear problem for 3 days before he finally called for an appointment. The doctor poked at this and that, and worried a little over his tremor.

"You don't drink, do you?"

"A little. But what about my ear?"

"It's perfectly normal."

"But I hear something. It's like someone chanting. I can almost make out what they're saying. You're sure no one's put something in there, a hearing aid?" He dug at the ear with his little finger.

"Nope, clean as a whistle. Here, don't do that!" The doctor scribbled a referral to the mental health clinic down the hall. That was late on a Friday afternoon, so of course the clinic was closed.

On Monday afternoon, when he finally got to his appointment, Danny could once again write his name legibly and eat solid food. But the voices were in full throat. As he talked with the interviewer, he could hardly concentrate for the shouting: "Don't tell about the drinking!" and "Why don't you just kill yourself?" He was so terrified that he accepted with relief a voluntary commitment to the mental health ward, where his admitting diagnosis was schizophrenia. Twice a day he was given a potent neuroleptic medication, which he tucked under his tongue and discarded in the tissue when he pretended to blow his nose.

Danny slept soundly at night and cleaned his plate at every meal while the voices shouted on. At the end of the week, he was visited by a consultant who learned that the voices came from about 2 feet behind him and talked in sentences. Reluctantly, he admitted that they told him not to talk about his drinking.

A rapid review of Danny's chart revealed no mention of alcohol use, but a little coaxing soon pried loose the whole story. Since his early 20s, there had been heavy drinking, loss of two jobs (he had a shaky hold on his present one), and a divorce, all related to his fondness for bourbon. Most recently he had been drinking more than a pint each evening, often a fifth on the weekends. Usually he managed to taper off; this time, he had quit suddenly after a bout of what he called "the stomach flu."

DSM-5 repeatedly refers to classes of symptoms that may appear to be caused by a substance. It is up to you to evaluate your patient for evidence that this might *not* be the case. Here are several findings, mostly based on chronology, that might constitute such evidence:

1. Your patient had a prior episode of the same, or very similar, symptoms that did *not* occur in the context of substance use.
2. The disorder continues long after the use of (or withdrawal from) the substance is over.
3. Rather obviously, a disorder that begins before substance use begins wouldn't be due to the substance use.
4. The symptoms are worse than you'd expect, considering the amount and duration of the substance misuse.

None of these is exactly iron-clad. For example, a prior history of major depressive disorder doesn't confer subsequent immunity to depression that originates in a bottle of Scotch. Still, the cues are there, for your thoughtful consideration.

And here are some of the reasons why you *should* consider a substance-use causation:

1. The symptoms begin soon after (or during) the use of a substance or its withdrawal.
2. They start after a patient has begun use of a medication.
3. The drug/medication is known to be capable of causing the symptoms in question.
4. Of course, if your patient has had a prior episode of the same symptoms that did follow the use of the same substance, that's perhaps the best evidence of all.

Evaluation of Danny Finch

Danny had auditory hallucinations (criterion A) that had been present far too briefly for **schizophrenia**, though he described them in similar terms (C). A **brief psychotic disorder** might be possible, except for the requirement that a **substance-induced psychotic disorder** does not better explain the symptoms. He had just been seen by a physician, who pronounced him fit; there was no evidence of any other **general medical condition.** The fact that he seemed fully oriented and maintained his attention would rule out **delirium** and other **cognitive disorders** (D). Though he appeared (appropriately) frightened by his experiences, he presented no evidence of **mood disorder.**

Danny's psychosis—in the distant past it was called *alcoholic auditory hallucinosis*—is a disorder of withdrawal that usually occurs only after weeks or months of heavy drinking (B). By about a 4:1 ratio, it occurs much more commonly in men than in women, approximating the sex ratio for alcohol use disorder itself. Auditory hallucinosis is sometimes misidentified as **alcohol withdrawal delirium**, though the problems with orientation and attention in the latter make the differences clear (see p. 483).

Withdrawal from other drugs can also produce psychosis. **Barbiturates**, which have many of the same effects as alcohol, are the most notorious of these. Some patients who use **phencyclidine** or **other hallucinogens** such as LSD experience prolonged psychosis, the risk for which may be greater in people who have **personality disorders.**

Danny's symptoms were clearly more serious than we'd expect in **alcohol withdrawal with perceptual disturbances** (which would be diagnosed had he retained insight that his experiences weren't "real"). His GAF score was only 35 on admission; his diagnosis (from Table 15.2 in Chapter 15) would be as follows:

F10.259 [291.9]   Severe alcohol use disorder with alcohol-induced psychotic disorder, with onset during withdrawal

Psychotic Disorder Due to Another Medical Condition

A psychosis arising in a patient who has another medical condition shouldn't be especially rare. Many diseases can produce psychosis, and a number of them are relatively common. But few, if any, studies bear on questions of epidemiology. When such patients do appear, they are too often misdiagnosed as having schizophrenia or some other psychosis. This can lead to real tragedy: A patient who is not appropriately treated early enough may go on to experience (or cause) serious harm. Prevalence rates are not known exactly, but they're probably low; as you might imagine, frequency increases with age.

Note that a patient with mainly disorganized behavior would instead be diagnosed as having catatonic disorder due to another medical condition.

It's often a struggle to determine that a physical illness or medical condition has caused any mental disorder. Here are a few straws in the wind that can help out.

- Timing of onset: Mental or behavioral symptoms that begin shortly after the start of the physical illness offer a pretty obvious etiological clue.
- Remission follows treatment for the physical issue.
- Proportionality of symptoms: As the physical disorder worsens, so do the behavioral or emotional symptoms.
- Above all, there must be a known physiological connection between the physical condition and the symptom in question. That is, the physical disorder must be known to be capable of producing the symptom (for example, through production of chemicals, by impinging on brain structures). It cannot simply be that the prospect of having a serious illness evokes psychosis, depression, anxiety, and so forth.

OK, so these pointers aren't exactly iron-clad. Remember, they're straws, not steel.

Essential Features of
Psychotic Disorder Due to Another Medical Condition

A physical condition causes hallucinations or delusions.

The Fine Print

For pointers on deciding when a physical condition may have caused a mental disorder, see the sidebar just above.

The D's: • Distress or disability (work/academic, social, or personal impairment) • Differential diagnosis (delirium, substance-induced psychotic disorder, schizophrenia and its cousins, delusional disorder)

Coding Notes

In recording the diagnosis, use the name of the responsible medical condition, and list *first* the medical condition, with its code number.

Code, based on the predominant symptoms:

F06.2 [293.81] With delusions
F06.0 [293.82] With hallucinations

You may specify severity, though you don't have to (see p. 74).

Rodrigo Chavez

After he retired from teaching at age 65, Rodrigo Chavez spent most of his time sitting alone in his room. Sometimes he played the acoustic guitar; once or twice he shot targets at the rifle range. True to his lifelong habit, he never drank. Other than his immediate family, he had few social contacts. "My cigarettes are my best friends," he put it during the forensic examination.

When Rodrigo was nearly 70, an inoperable carcinoma of the lung was diagnosed. After a course of palliative radiotherapy, he declined further treatment and settled down in his apartment to die. Four months later, he first noticed right-sided headaches that would sometimes awaken him in the middle of the night. Because the doctors had told him he was terminally ill, he didn't seek further medical attention. Then he began to associate the headaches with natural gas, which he smelled coming out of the ventilator duct in his bathroom. When he called to report the problem to Mrs. Riordan, his landlady, she sent around the building's handyman, who could find nothing wrong.

When his headaches and the odors increased, Rodrigo recalled that, weeks before, Mrs. Riordan had gone out several times to watch while repairmen from the power company dug up the street outside the apartment building. The logical conclusion fairly burst upon him: His landlady was trying to poison him.

His anger mounted as the odor worsened. It had begun to affect his voice, which had become raspy and high-pitched. He had several shouted arguments with Mrs. Riordan. One of these they carried on through her apartment door at 2 A.M., several weeks after he first noticed the gas. He threatened to report her to the housing authority; she called him "a crazy old coot." After he threatened her ("If I'm not safe, your life isn't worth 15 cents!"), they both made 911 telephone calls. The police could find nothing to charge anyone with and admonished them both to behave.

The night he was arrested, Rodrigo had sat just inside his open doorway, yelling insults at Mrs. Riordan. When she lumbered to the top of the stairs to investigate, he shot her once, just behind her left ear. The arresting officers noted that he seemed "strangely detached" from the murder of his landlady. One of them wrote down this statement: "It wouldn't matter, just for me. But I couldn't stand her gassing all those other people in the house."

The forensic examiner noted that Rodrigo Chavez was an elderly, slightly built man who was clean-shaven and neatly groomed. He was gaunt, looking as if he had lost considerable weight. His speech was clear, coherent, relevant, and spontaneous, but his voice was high-pitched and gravelly. He appeared calm, and he described his mood as "medium," but he became angry when describing his landlady's attempts to poison him. He was oriented to person, place, and time, and he earned a perfect score on the Mini-Mental State Exam. He was fully aware that he had lung cancer. Insight for the fact of his psychosis was nil, and his judgment by recent history had been extremely poor.

An X-ray of his chest showed a right lung full of tumor; compared with a previous series, skull films suggested a metastatic lesion located in the right frontal lobe.

Evaluation of Rodrigo Chavez

Rodrigo Chavez was clearly psychotic: He had prominent olfactory hallucinations and an elaborate delusion about being poisoned. These had been present for several months (criterion A). (If insight is retained that the hallucinations and delusions are a product of the patient's own mind, one would generally not diagnose a psychotic disorder. Also note that, though Rodrigo's symptoms clearly met the criterion A inclusion requirements for schizophrenia, they didn't have to: A person can qualify for this diagnosis with just one of either hallucinations or delusions.)

Aside from his psychosis, Rodrigo's thinking was clear. He was oriented and he scored well on the Mini-Mental State Exam, so he had no evidence of a **delirium** or **dementia** (D). He had had no history of drinking or taking drugs, ruling out a **substance-induced psychotic disorder.** His mood had been at times angry, but appropriately so, given the content of his delusion and hallucination, so a **mood disorder with psychotic features** would also seem unlikely. There was no previous history of behavior or personality change that would qualify him for a diagnosis of **schizophrenia** (C). Other features atypical for schizophrenia included the late age of onset and relatively brief duration. **Schizophreniform disorder** could be ruled out because another diagnosis was more likely. Mrs. Riordan's unhappy end provides mute testimony to the clinical importance of his illness (E).

Rodrigo had a history of a cancer that is known to metastasize to the brain; his headaches suggested that it had already done so. The findings on chest X-ray and MRI confirmed the diagnosis (B). His gravelly, high-pitched voice could be due to extension of the growth or to another metastasis within his chest or neck. (Other **medical conditions** that can cause psychosis include temporal lobe epilepsy, primary [that is, not metastatic] brain tumors, endocrine disorders such as thyroid and adrenal disease, vitamin deficiency states, central nervous system syphilis, multiple sclerosis, systemic lupus erythematosus, Wilson's disease, and head trauma.)

Although Rodrigo had *both* hallucinations and delusions, the olfactory hallucinations appeared first and seemed to predominate, resulting in the diagnosis as recorded. My assessment of his GAF score was 15.

C79.31 [198.3]	Cancer of the lung, metastatic to the brain
F06.0 [293.82]	Psychotic disorder due to metastatic carcinoma, with hallucinations
Z65.3 [V62.5]	Arrested for murder

F06.1 [293.89] Catatonia Associated with Another Mental Disorder (Catatonia Specifier)

Catatonia, which we've always thought of as a classic schizophrenia subtype, was first described by Karl Kahlbaum in 1874; in 1896, Emil Kraepelin included it with the disorganized (it was called hebephrenic then) and paranoid types as a major subgroup of what he termed *dementia praecox*. During the early part of the 20th century, each of these subtypes constituted about a third of all U.S. hospital admissions for schizophrenia. Since that time, the prevalence of the catatonic type has declined markedly, so that it is now unusual to encounter such a patient on an acute care inpatient service. When it does occur, we would now call it catatonia associated with schizophrenia.

F06.1 [293.89] Catatonic Disorder Due to Another Medical Condition

In recent decades, we've come to realize that catatonia is more often found in association with various medical disorders. Most published accounts tend to describe only a handful of patients, but the responsible illnesses include viral encephalitis, subarachnoid hemorrhage, ruptured berry aneurysm in the brain, subdural hematoma, hyperparathyroidism, arteriovenous malformation, temporal lobe tumors, akinetic mutism, and penetrating head wounds. There has even been a description of one patient who had a reaction to fluorides. A neurologist or mental health clinician who does a lot of consulting in a busy medical center may occasionally encounter a case.

Catatonic symptoms (see sidebar below) are essentially the same, whether they occur in patients with a mood disorder, with schizophrenia, or with a physical disorder. A patient with another medical condition is more likely to have the characteristic symptoms of what is called *retarded* catatonia. These include posturing, catalepsy, and waxy flexibility. Such patients may also drool, stop eating, or become mute. The catatonic features usually associated with mania include hyperactivity, impulsivity, and combativeness. These patients may also refuse to keep their clothes on. Depressed patients may show markedly reduced mobility (even to the point of stupor), mutism, negativism, mannerisms, and stereotypies.

Partly to save space, I've omitted definitions of catatonic symptoms from my Essential Features for these two disorders and gathered them all into one convenient place: right here. Each of these behaviors tends to be a repeated rather than a one-off occurrence.

Agitation. Excessive motor activity that appears to have neither a purpose nor an external cause. **Stupor** would be more or less the polar opposite.

Catalepsy. Maintaining an uncomfortable posture, even when told it is not necessary.

Echolalia. Verbatim repetition of someone else's words when another response is indicated.

Echopraxia. Imitating another person's physical behavior, even when asked not to do so.

Exaggerated compliance. At the slightest touch, moving in the direction indicated by another person (the old German term is *mitgehen*).

Grimace. Facial contortions not made in response to a noxious stimulus.

Mannerisms. Repeated movements that seem to have a goal, but are excessive for the purpose.

Mutism. Absence of speech despite apparent physical ability to speak.

Negativism. Without apparent motive, the patient offers resistance to passive movement or repeatedly turns away from the examiner.

Posturing. Voluntarily assuming an unnatural or uncomfortable pose.

Stereotypy. Repeated movement that is a nonessential part of goal-directed behavior.

Waxy flexibility. Maintaining a position, even if uncomfortable, for several minutes or more, even if asked to change it.

Essential Features of **Catatonia Associated with Another Mental Disorder (Catatonia Specifier)**

The patient has prominent symptoms of catatonia, such as catalepsy, negativism, posturing, stupor, stereotypy, grimacing, echolalia, and others (see the sidebar above for definitions).

The Fine Print

Relax, it's only a specifier. No Fine Print.

Coding Notes

You can apply the catatonia specifier to manic, hypomanic, or major depressive episodes; to schizophrenia; and to schizophreniform, schizoaffective, brief psychotic, and substance-induced psychotic disorders. It can even be used for autism spectrum disorder.

List first the other mental disorder, then **F06.1 [293.89]**, then **catatonia associated with [the other mental disorder].**

Edward Clapham

Edward Clapham, a 43-year-old single man, was admitted to the university hospital's mental health service. He gave no chief complaint; he was entirely mute. He had been transferred from the state psychiatric hospital, where his diagnosis had been schizophrenia, catatonic type. For the past 8 years, he had not communicated by speech or writing.

According to the transfer note, Edward had been intensively treated with neuroleptics during his entire hospitalization, though none of these medications had relieved his basic symptoms. He reportedly spent the entire day every day lying on his back, toes pointing towards the foot of his bed, fists clenched and turned inward. From years of maintaining this position, he had developed severe muscle contractures at both ankles and both wrists. Most of the time he could be spoon-fed, but occasionally he refused to swallow and had to be fed by nasogastric tube. This had often been the case during the past 6 months; despite the tube feedings, he had lost about 30 pounds.

Ten days earlier Edward had developed a high fever (104.6°F) and had been transferred to the medical service, where the staff treated a *Klebsiella* pneumonia with tetracycline. Subsequently he was moved to the mental health service, where this evaluation took place.

Very little was known about Edward's background. He had been reared in the Midwest, the second child of a farm family. He may have attended some college, and he had worked for approximately 10 years as a tractor salesman. On admission, his mental status examination read as follows:

Mr. Clapham lies flat on his back in bed. He is totally mute, so nothing can be learned of his thought content or flow of thought. Similarly, his cognitive processes, insight, and judgment cannot be assessed. His toes point down and his fists are rotated inward. There is a noticeable tremor of his feet and his hands; he contracts the muscles of his arms and legs so strongly that they actually shake.

Besides being mute, he shows other signs of catatonia. *Negativism:* When he is approached from one side, he gradually turns his head so that he gazes in the opposite direction. *Catalepsy:* When a limb is placed in any position (for instance, raised high above his head), he will maintain that position for several minutes, even if told that he can drop his hand. *Waxy flexibility:* Any attempt to bend his arm at the elbow, where there are no contractures, is met with resistance. It is evident that the biceps and triceps muscles are contracting together, causing motion at the joint to feel as if one were bending a rod made of wax or some other stiff substance. *Grimacing:* Every four or five minutes, he wrinkles his nose and purses his lips. This expression lasts for 10 or 15 seconds, then relaxes. There is no apparent purpose to these motions, and they are not accompanied by any motions of the tongue or other indications of tardive dyskinesia.

Evaluation of Edward Clapham

Counting his negative symptoms (lack of speech and affect) and his grossly abnormal motor behavior, Edward fulfilled the criterion A requirements for **schizophrenia.** His illness had lasted far longer than the minimum 6 months (schizophrenia criterion C); it is hard to imagine how it could have had a greater effect on every aspect of his life (B). Nonetheless, on admission to the mental health unit, he was given a diagnosis of unspecified schizophrenia spectrum and other psychotic disorder. This provisional diagnosis was given because the clinician could not be sure from the initial presentation whether the symptoms were due to the effects of his dehydration and loss of weight (another medical condition), schizophrenia, or another cause such as a mood disorder, which is perhaps the most frequent cause of catatonic symptoms.

The list of **medical conditions** that can produce catatonic behavior includes liver disease, strokes, epilepsy, and uncommon disorders such as Wilson's disease (a defect of copper metabolism) and the inherited disorder (autosomal dominant), tuberous sclerosis. These possibilities should be vigorously pursued with neurological and medical consultation and with the appropriate laboratory and X-ray studies. Urine or blood screens for toxic substances or drugs of abuse should be considered a part of every such patient's workup. Any patient who presents with a first episode of catatonia should probably have an MRI. When Edward Clapham was diagnosed, there was no MRI; we'll have to take criterion E on faith.

Many patients who have been diagnosed as having schizophrenia, catatonic type, really have a manic phase of **bipolar I disorder** (D). On the other hand, a patient with severe psychomotor slowing should be considered for a diagnosis of **major depressive disorder with melancholic features.** Although patients with **somatic symptom disorder** are occasionally mute or have abnormal motor activity, such episodes are usually short-lived, lasting only a few hours or days, not years. Edward had been ill for years; a chronic, psychotic, catatonic mood disorder seems unlikely.

Edward's symptoms were classic for catatonia associated with schizophrenia. He demonstrated grimacing (catatonia specifier criterion A10), muteness (A4), waxy flexibility (A3), and catalepsy (A2). He could not be called stuporous because he was alert enough to turn away from an approaching stimulus (negativism—A5). His behavior range was insufficient to demonstrate other typical catatonic behaviors.

Because he had already been extensively (and unsuccessfully) treated with neuroleptics, Edward was given a course of electroconvulsive therapy. Although the first three bilateral treatments produced no noticeable effect, after the fourth he asked for a glass of water. After a total of 10 treatments, he was conversing with others on the ward, feeding himself, and walking—always on tiptoe because of the severe contractures at his ankles. Although he continued to show residual symptoms of his disease, his catatonic symptoms disappeared. He eventually left the hospital, whereupon he was lost to follow-up.

Edward's 8-year course of illness had been continuous; I scored his GAF at discharge at 60 (on admission, it would have been pretty close to 1). After appropriate medical investigations and additional history ruled out other possible causes of his abnormal behavior, his revised diagnosis was as given below.

By the way, without reference to the official DSM-5 severity criteria for psychosis (p. 74), on admission I'd give Edward a rating of *severe*. I anticipate no backlash from outraged coding mavens, though I still feel that the overall global evaluation of the GAF does a better job. At discharge:

F20.9 [295.90]	Schizophrenia, first episode, currently in partial remission
F06.1 [293.89]	Catatonia associated with schizophrenia
M24.573 [718.47]	Contractures of ankles
M24.539 [718.43]	Contractures of wrists

Essential Features of **Catatonic Disorder Due to Another Medical Condition**

A physical illness appears to have caused symptoms of catatonia, such as catalepsy, negativism, posturing, stupor, stereotypy, grimacing, echolalia, and others (see sidebar just above) for definitions).

The Fine Print

For pointers on deciding when a physical condition may have caused a mental disorder, see sidebar, page 97.

The D's: • Differential diagnosis (delirium or other cognitive disorder, schizophrenia and its cousins, psychotic mood disorder, obsessive–compulsive disorder)

Coding Notes

Using the name of the responsible medical condition, record this diagnosis after you've coded the actual medical condition.

Marion Wright

Since graduating from high school 12 years earlier, Marion Wright had worked as a sign painter. In school he had shown some aptitude for art, though not enough that he saw himself as the next Pablo Picasso. Nor did he like school enough to study for a career in commercial art. But painting signs on buildings and billboards was undemanding, well-paying, immediately available, and largely open-air. Within a few years he was married, had two kids and a small house in a subdivision, and was still painting signs. He thought he was set for life.

One afternoon not long after his 30th birthday, his foreman drove by to inspect the billboard Marion had just finished. "You've painted the logo in script. The blueprint calls for block letters," the foreman pointed out. Marion said that he thought the script looked better, but without much grumbling he changed it. A week later he completed an ad for a local premium beer; the female model holding the bottle was naked from the waist up. The following day he was out of work.

Marion made a few efforts to find a new job, but within a week he was staying at home and watching daytime TV. His wife noted that he seemed to be talking less and less, but he ignored her suggestion to seek clinical evaluation. Although he continued to eat and sleep normally, his interest in sex had vanished. By the fourth week after losing his job, he had no spontaneous speech at all and would only answer a question if it was directly put to him. With the added persuasion of Marion's brother, his wife finally got him to the clinic. He was immediately hospitalized.

On admission Marion would answer questions appropriately, if briefly. Fully oriented, he denied feeling depressed or suicidal. He had no delusions, hallucinations, obsessions or compulsions. He earned a perfect score on the MMSE, though the examiner noted that he was slow to carry out instructions.

The following morning he deliberately turned away from the nurse who approached his bedside. Although he willingly accompanied the nurse to a table in the dining room, he refused to eat and was completely mute. In fact, the clinician who examined him later that morning found that Marion would readily move in any direction at the slightest touch of an examiner's hand. In the evening he seemed improved and even spoke a few words.

But the next day, he lay on his back in bed, again silently refusing to cooperate. When his pillow was removed, his head remained elevated about two inches above the mattress. This position appeared to cause him no discomfort; he seemed willing to maintain it all day. Later, an examiner noted that when Marion's arm was twisted into an awkward position (elevated at an angle over the bed), he maintained that position even when he was told that he could relax.

Marion's clinicians considered the diagnosis of schizophrenia, but they noted that he had been only briefly ill and had no family history of psychosis. His wife assured them that he had never abused drugs or alcohol. Despite the fact that his neurological exam remained normal, an MRI of his head was obtained. It revealed a tumor the size of a golf ball sitting on the convexity of his right frontal lobe. Once this was surgically removed, he quickly regained full consciousness. Two months later he was back on his ladder painting billboards, following instructions to the letter.

Evaluation of Marion Wright

Marion had several symptoms (three are required) that are classical for catatonia (criterion A). His included negativism and muteness (A5, A4), exaggerated compliance (though this is not one of the criteria DSM-5 mentions), a "psychological pillow" (a form of posturing in which he held his head unsupported above the mattress—A6), and catalepsy (A2).

Marion did not have the wandering attention found in **delirium** (D). Catatonic behavior can be found in **schizophrenia**, which his clinicians correctly rejected because he had been ill too briefly (C). Too few symptoms (and better choices) ruled out **schizophreniform disorder.** Muteness and marked motor slowing, even to the point of immobility, can be encountered in **major depressive episode**, but Marion specifically denied mood symptoms. Muteness may occasionally be encountered in **somatic symptom disorder** and in **malingering** and **factitious disorder**, but it would be unusual to encounter a full, persisting catatonic syndrome in one of these conditions.

Note that catatonic behavior can include excessive or even frenzied motor activity. Then the differential diagnosis would include **manic episode** and **substance use intoxication.** Of course, neither of these applies to Marion's case.

On laboratory examination of the surgical specimen, Marion was found to have a (benign) brain tumor, which can directly result in catatonic symptoms (B) and which caused manifest impairment (E). On admission, I'd put his GAF score at 21; his GAF score was 90 on discharge.

D32.9 [225.2]	Cerebral meningioma, benign
F06.1 [293.89]	Catatonic disorder due to cerebral meningioma

F28 [298.8] Other Specified Schizophrenia Spectrum and Other Psychotic Disorder

Use this category when you want to write down the specific reason your patient cannot receive a more definite psychotic disorder diagnosis. Here's an example: "other specified schizophrenia spectrum and other psychotic disorder, persistent auditory hallucinations."

Charles Bonnet syndrome. In this disorder (not specifically mentioned in DSM-5, but first described in 1790!), elderly people report complex visual hallucinations (scenes, people) but no other hallucinations or delusions. They also have insight that what they "see" is unreal. As such, they aren't truly psychotic, but one can argue that the condition belongs somewhere along the spectrum of psychotic disorders.

Attenuated psychosis syndrome. A patient has psychotic symptoms that do not meet the full criteria for any psychotic disorder (less disabling symptoms, relatively good insight, etc.).

Persistent auditory hallucinations. The patient experiences repeated auditory hallucinations without other symptoms.

Delusional symptoms in partner of individual with delusional disorder. Most people who develop delusions in response to close association with someone who is independently psychotic can be diagnosed as having a delusional disorder. However, those who don't fulfill criteria for delusional disorder can be classified here.

Other. The patient appears to have a psychotic disorder, but the information is conflicting or too inadequate to permit a more specific diagnosis.

F29 [298.9] Unspecified Schizophrenia Spectrum and Other Psychotic Disorder

This category is for symptoms or syndromes that don't meet guidelines for any of the disorders described earlier, and you do not wish to specify a reason.

Unspecified Catatonia

DSM-5 mentions unspecified catatonia as a possibility when the context is unclear or there is insufficient detail for a more precise diagnosis. But the coding itself is clear: First code **R29.818 [781.99] other symptoms involving nervous and musculoskeletal systems**; then code **F06.1 [293.89] unspecified catatonia.**

CHAPTER 3

Mood Disorders

DSM-5 notes that issues related to genetics and symptoms locate bipolar disorders as a sort of bridge between mood disorders and schizophrenia. That's why DSM-5 separated the deeply intertwined chapters on bipolar and depressive disorders. However, to explain mood disorders as clearly and concisely as possible, I've reunited them.

Quick Guide to the Mood Disorders

DSM-5 uses three groups of criteria sets to diagnose mental problems related to mood: (1) mood episodes, (2) mood disorders, and (3) specifiers describing most recent episode and recurrent course. I'll cover each of them in this Quick Guide. As usual, the page number following each item below refers to the point where a more detailed discussion begins.

Mood Episodes

Simply expressed, a *mood episode* refers to any period of time when a patient feels abnormally happy or sad. Mood episodes are the building blocks from which many of the codable mood disorders are constructed. Most patients with mood disorders (though *not* the majority of mood disorder types) will have one or more of these three episodes: major depressive, manic, and hypomanic. Without additional information, none of these mood episodes is a codable diagnosis.

Major depressive episode. For at least 2 weeks, the patient feels depressed (or cannot enjoy life) and has problems with eating and sleeping, guilt feelings, low energy, trouble concentrating, and thoughts about death (p. 112).

Manic episode. For at least 1 week, the patient feels elated (or sometimes only irritable) and may be grandiose, talkative, hyperactive, and distractible. Bad judgment leads to marked social or work impairment; often patients must be hospitalized (p. 116).

Hypomanic episode. This is much like a manic episode, but it is briefer and less severe. Hospitalization is not required (p. 120).

Mood Disorders

A mood disorder is a pattern of illness due to an abnormal mood. Nearly every patient who has a mood disorder experiences depression at some time, but some also have highs of mood. Many, but not all, mood disorders are diagnosed on the basis of a mood episode. Most patients with mood disorders will fit into one of the codable categories listed below.

DEPRESSIVE DISORDERS

Major depressive disorder. These patients have had no manic or hypomanic episodes, but have had one or more major depressive episodes. Major depressive disorder will be either recurrent or single episode (p. 122).

Persistent depressive disorder (dysthymia). There are no high phases, and it lasts much longer than typical major depressive disorder. This type of depression is not usually severe enough to be called an episode of major depression (though chronic major depression is now included here). (p. 138).

Disruptive mood dysregulation disorder. A child's mood is persistently negative between frequent, severe explosions of temper (p. 149).

Premenstrual dysphoric disorder. A few days before her menses, a woman experiences symptoms of depression and anxiety (p. 146).

Depressive disorder due to another medical condition. A variety of medical and neurological conditions can produce depressive symptoms; these need not meet criteria for any of the conditions above (p. 153).

Substance/medication-induced depressive disorder. Alcohol or other substances (intoxication or withdrawal) can cause depressive symptoms; these need not meet criteria for any of the conditions above (p. 151).

Other specified, or unspecified, depressive disorder. Use one of these categories when a patient has depressive symptoms that do not meet the criteria for the depressive diagnoses above or for any other diagnosis in which depression is a feature (pp. 169, 170).

BIPOLAR AND RELATED DISORDERS

Approximately 25% of patients with mood disorders experience manic or hypomanic episodes. Nearly all of these patients will also have episodes of depression. The severity and duration of the highs and lows determine the specific bipolar disorder.

Bipolar I disorder. There must be at least one manic episode; most patients with bipolar I have also had a major depressive episode (p. 129).

Bipolar II disorder. This diagnosis requires at least one hypomanic episode plus at least one major depressive episode (p. 135).

Cyclothymic disorder. These patients have had repeated mood swings, but none that are severe enough to be called major depressive episodes or manic episodes (p. 143).

Substance/medication-induced bipolar disorder. Alcohol or other substances (intoxication or withdrawal) can cause manic or hypomanic symptoms; these need not meet criteria for any of the conditions above (p. 151).

Bipolar disorder due to another medical condition. A variety of medical and neurological conditions can produce manic or hypomanic symptoms; these need not meet criteria for any of the conditions above (p. 153).

Other specified, or unspecified, bipolar disorder. Use one of these categories when a patient has bipolar symptoms that do not meet the criteria for the bipolar diagnoses above (pp. 167, 169).

Other Causes of Depressive and Manic Symptoms

Schizoaffective disorder. In these patients, symptoms suggestive of schizophrenia coexist with a major depressive or a manic episode (p. 88).

Major and mild neurocognitive disorders with behavioral disturbance. The qualifier *with behavioral disturbance* can be coded into the diagnosis of major or mild neurocognitive disorder (p. 492). OK, so mood symptoms don't sound all that behavioral, but that's how DSM-5 elects to indicate the cognitive disorders with depression.

Adjustment disorder with depressed mood. This term codes one way of adapting to a life stress (p. 228).

Personality disorders. Dysphoric mood is specifically mentioned in the criteria for borderline personality disorder (p. 545), but depressed mood commonly accompanies avoidant, dependent, and histrionic personality disorders.

Uncomplicated bereavement. Sadness at the death of a relative or friend is a common experience. Because *uncomplicated* bereavement is a normal reaction to a particular type of stressor, it is recorded not as a disorder, but as a Z-code [V-code]. See page 590.

Other disorders. Depression can accompany many other mental disorders, including schizophrenia, the eating disorders, somatic symptom disorder, sexual dysfunctions, and gender dysphorias. Mood symptoms are likely in patients with an anxiety disorder (especially panic disorder and the phobic disorders), obsessive–compulsive disorder, and posttraumatic stress disorder.

Specifiers

Two special sets of descriptions can be applied to a number of the mood episodes and mood disorders.

SPECIFIERS DESCRIBING CURRENT OR MOST RECENT EPISODE

These descriptors help characterize the most recent major depressive episode; all but the first two can also apply to a manic episode. (Note that the specifiers for severity and remission are described on p. 158.)

With atypical features. These depressed patients eat a lot and gain weight, sleep excessively, and have a feeling of being sluggish or paralyzed. They are often excessively sensitive to rejection (p. 160).

With melancholic features. This term applies to major depressive episodes characterized by some of the "classic" symptoms of severe depression. These patients awaken early, feeling worse than they do later in the day. They lose appetite and weight, feel guilty, are either slowed down or agitated, and do not feel better when something happens that they would normally like (p. 161).

With anxious distress. A patient has symptoms of anxiety, tension, restlessness, worry, or fear that accompanies a mood episode (p. 159).

With catatonic features. There are features of either motor hyperactivity or inactivity. Catatonic features can apply to major depressive episodes and to manic episodes (p. 100).

With mixed features. Manic, hypomanic, and major depressive episodes may have mixtures of manic and depressive symptoms (p. 161).

With peripartum onset. A manic, hypomanic, or major depressive episode (or a brief psychotic disorder) can occur in a woman during pregnancy or within a month of having a baby (p. 163).

With psychotic features. Manic and major depressive episodes can be accompanied by delusions, which can be mood-congruent or -incongruent (p. 164).

SPECIFIERS DESCRIBING COURSE OF RECURRING EPISODES

These specifiers describe the overall course of a mood disorder, not just the form of an individual episode.

With rapid cycling. Within 1 year, the patient has had at least four episodes (in any combination) fulfilling criteria for major depressive, manic, or hypomanic episodes (p. 165).

With seasonal pattern. These patients regularly become ill at a certain time of the year, such as fall or winter (p. 165).

Introduction to Mood Episodes

Mood refers to a sustained emotion that colors the way we view life. Recognizing when mood is disordered is extremely important, because as many as 20% of adult women and 10% of adult men may have the experience at some time during their lives. The prevalence of mood disorders seems to be increasing in both sexes, accounting for half or more of a mental health practice. Mood disorders can occur in people of any race or socioeconomic status, but they are more common among those who are single and who have no "significant other." A mood disorder is also more likely in someone who has relatives with similar problems.

The mood disorders encompass many diagnoses, qualifiers, and levels of severity. Although they may seem complicated, they can be reduced to a few main principles.

Years ago, the mood disorders were called *affective disorders*; many clinicians still use the older term, which is also entrenched in the name *seasonal affective disorder*. Note, by the way, that the term *affect* covers more than just a patient's statement of emotion. It also encompasses how the patient appears to be feeling, as shown by physical clues such as facial expression, posture, eye contact, and tearfulness. Emphasis on the actual mood experience of the patient, rather than the sometimes fuzzy concept of *affect*, dictates the current use of *mood*.

In this section, I'll describe three types of mood episodes. You will find case vignettes illustrating each one in the sections on the mood disorders themselves, which follow.

Major Depressive Episode

Major depressive episode is one of the building blocks of the mood disorders, but it's not a codable diagnosis. You will use it often—it is one of the most common problems for which patients seek help. Apply it carefully after considering a patient's full history and mental status exam. (Of course, we should be careful in using every label and every diagnosis.) I mention this caution here because some clinicians tend to use the major depressive episode label almost as a reflex, without really considering the evidence. Once it gets applied, too often there is a reflexive reaching for the prescription pad.

A major depressive episode must meet five major requirements. There must be (1) a quality of depressed mood (or loss of interest or pleasure) that (2) has existed for a minimum period of time, (3) is accompanied by a required number of symptoms, (4) has resulted in distress or disability, and (5) violates none of the listed exclusions.

Quality of Mood

Depression is usually experienced as a mood lower than normal; patients may describe it as feeling "unhappy," "downhearted," "bummed," "blue," or many other terms expressing sadness. Several issues can interfere with the recognition of depression:

- Not all patients can recognize or accurately describe how they feel.

- Clinicians and patients who come from different cultural backgrounds may have difficulty agreeing that the problem is depression.

- The presenting symptoms of depression can vary greatly from one patient to another. One patient may be slowed down and crying; another will smile and deny that anything is wrong. Some sleep and eat too much; others complain of insomnia and anorexia.

- Some patients don't really feel depressed; rather, they experience depression as a loss of pleasure or reduced interest in their usual activities, including sex.

- Crucial to diagnosis is that the episode must represent a noticeable change from the patient's usual level of functioning. If the patient does not notice it (some are too ill to pay attention or too apathetic to care), family or friends may report that there has been such a change.

Duration

The patient must have felt bad most of the day, almost every day, for at least 2 weeks. This requirement is included to ensure that major depressive episodes are differentiated from the transient "down" spells that most of us sometimes feel.

Symptoms

During the 2 weeks just mentioned, the patient must have at least five of the *italicized* symptoms below. Those five must include either depressed mood or loss of pleasure, and the symptoms must overall indicate that the person is performing at a lower level than before. *Depressed mood* is self-explanatory; *loss of pleasure* is nearly universal among depressed patients. These symptoms can be counted either if the patient reports them or if others observe that they occur.

Many patients lose *appetite and weight*. More than three-fourths report trouble with *sleep*. Typically, they awaken early in the morning, long before it is time to arise. However, some patients eat and sleep more than usual; most of these patients will qualify for the atypical features specifier (p. 160).

Depressed patients will usually complain of *fatigue*, which they may express as tiredness or low energy. Their speech or physical movements may be slowed; sometimes there is a marked pause before answering a question or initiating an action. This is called *psychomotor retardation*. Speech may be very quiet, sometimes inaudible. Some patients simply stop talking completely, except in response to a direct question. At the extreme, complete muteness may occur.

At the other extreme, some depressed patients feel so anxious that they become *agitated*. Agitation may be expressed as hand wringing, pacing, or an inability to sit still. The ability of depressed patients to evaluate themselves objectively plummets; this shows up as *low self-esteem or guilt*. Some patients develop trouble with *concentration* (real or perceived) so severe that sometimes a misdiagnosis of dementia may be made. Thoughts of death, *death wishes*, and *suicidal ideas* are the most serious depressive symptoms of all, because there is a real risk that the patient will successfully act upon them.

To count as a DSM-5 symptom for major depressive episode, the behaviors listed above must occur nearly every day. However, thoughts about death or suicide need only be "recurrent." A single suicide attempt or a specific suicide plan will also qualify.

In general, the more closely a patient resembles this outline, the more reliable will be the diagnosis of major depressive episode. We should note, however, that depressed patients can have many symptoms besides those listed in the DSM-5 criteria. They can include crying spells, phobias, obsessions, and compulsions. Patients may admit to feeling hopeless, helpless, or worthless. Anxiety symptoms, especially panic attacks (see p. 173), can be so prominent that they blind clinicians to the underlying depression.

Many patients drink more (occasionally, less) alcohol when they become depressed. This can lead to difficulty in sorting out the differential diagnosis: Which should be treated first, the depression or the drinking? (Hint: Usually, both at once.)

A small minority of patients lose contact with reality and develop delusions or hallucinations. These psychotic features can be either *mood-congruent* (for example, a depressed man feels so guilty that he imagines he has committed some awful sin) or *mood-incongruent* (a depressed person who imagines persecution by the FBI is not experiencing a typical theme of depression). Psychotic symptoms are indicated in the severity indicator (it's verbiage you add to the diagnosis, *and* the final number in either the ICD-9 or ICD-10 code, as discussed later in this chapter). The case vignette of Brian Murphy (p. 124) includes an example.

There are three situations in which you should not count a symptom toward a diagnosis of major depressive episode:

1. A symptom is fully explained by another medical condition. For example, you wouldn't count fatigue in a patient who is recovering from major surgery; in that situation, you expect fatigue.
2. A symptom results from mood-incongruent delusions or hallucinations. For

example, don't count insomnia that is a response to hallucinated voices that keep the patient awake throughout the night.

3. Feelings of guilt or worthlessness that occur because the patient is too depressed to fulfill responsibilities. Such feelings are too common in depression to carry any diagnostic weight. Rather, look for guilt feelings that are way outside the boundaries of what's reasonable. An extreme example: A woman believes that her wickedness caused the tragedies of 9/11.

Impairment

The episode must be serious enough to cause material distress or to impair the patient's work (or school) performance, social life (withdrawal or discord), or some other area of functioning, including sex. Of the various consequences of mental illness, the effect on work may the hardest to detect. Perhaps this is because earning a livelihood is so important that most people will go to great lengths to hide symptoms that could threaten their employment.

Exclusions

Regardless of the severity or duration of symptoms, major depressive episode usually should not be diagnosed in the face of clinically important substance use or a general medical disorder that could cause the symptoms.

Essential Features of **Major Depressive Episode**

These people are miserable. Most feel sad, down, depressed, or some equivalent; however, some few will instead insist that they've only lost interest in nearly all their once-loved activities. All will admit to varying numbers of other symptoms—such as fatigue, inability to concentrate, feeling worthless or guilty, and wishes for death or thoughts of suicide. In addition, three symptom areas may show either an increase or a decrease from normal: sleep, appetite/weight, and psychomotor activity. (For each of these, the classic picture is a decrease from normal—in appetite, for example—but some "atypical" patients will report an increase.)

The Fine Print

Also, children or adolescents may only feel or seem irritable, not depressed.

Don't disregard the D's: • Duration (most of nearly every day, 2+ weeks) • Distress or disability (work/educational, social, or personal impairment) • Differential diagnosis (substance use and physical disorders)

Coding Notes

No code alert: Major depressive episode is not a diagnosable illness; it is a building block of major depressive, bipolar I, and bipolar II disorders. It may also be found in persistent depressive disorder (dysthymia). However, certain specifier codes apply to major depressive episodes—though you tack them on only after you've decided on the actual mood disorder diagnosis. Relax; this will all become clear as we proceed.

The bereavement exclusion that was used through DSM-IV is not to be found in DSM-5, because recent research has determined that depressions closely preceded by the death or loss of a loved one do not differ substantially from depressions preceded by other stressors (or possibly by none at all). There's been a lot of breast beating over this move, or rather removal. Some claim that it places patients at risk for diagnosis of a mood disorder when context renders symptoms understandable; a substantial expansion in the number of people we regard as mentally ill could result.

I see the situation a little differently: We clinicians now have one fewer artificial barriers to diagnosis and treatment. However, as with any other freedom, we must use it responsibly. Evaluate the whole situation, especially the severity of symptoms, any previous history of mood disorder, the timing and severity of putative precipitant (bereavement plus other forms of loss), and the trajectory of the syndrome (is it getting worse or better?). And reevaluate frequently.

I've included examples of major depressive episode in the following vignettes: Brian Murphy (p. 124), Elizabeth Jacks (p. 131), Winona Fisk (p. 133), Iris McMaster (p. 136), Noah Sanders (p. 141), Sal Camozzi (p. 304), and Aileen Parmeter (p. 127). In addition, there may be some examples in Chapter 20, "Patients and Diagnoses"—but you'll have to find them for yourself.

Manic Episode

The second "building block" of the mood disorders, manic episode, has been recognized for at least 150 years. The classic triad of manic symptoms consists of heightened self-esteem, increased motor activity, and pressured speech. These symptoms are obvious and often outrageous, so manic episode is not often overdiagnosed. However, the psychotic symptoms that sometimes attend manic episode can be so florid that clinicians instead diagnose schizophrenia. This tendency to misdiagnosis may have decreased since 1980, when the DSM-III criteria increased clinicians' awareness of bipolar illness. The introduction of lithium treatment for bipolar disorders in 1970 also helped promote the diagnosis.

Manic episode is much less common than major depressive episode, perhaps affecting 1% of all adults. Men and women are about equally likely to have mania.

The features that must be present in order to diagnose manic episode are identical to those for major depressive episode: (1) A mood quality that (2) has existed for a required period of time, (3) is attended by a required number of symptoms, (4) has resulted in a considerable degree of disability, and (5) violates none of the listed exclusions.

Quality of Mood

Some patients with relatively mild symptoms just feel jolly; this bumptious good humor can be quite infectious and may make others feel like laughing with them. But as mania worsens, this humor becomes less cheerful as it takes on a "driven," unfunny quality that creates discomfort in patients and listeners alike. A few patients will have mood that is only irritable; euphoria and irritability sometimes occur together.

Duration

The patient must have had symptoms for a minimum of 1 week. This time requirement helps to differentiate manic episode from hypomanic episode.

Symptoms

In addition to the change in mood (euphoria or irritability), the patient must also have an increase in energy or activity level during a 1-week period. With these changes, at least three of the *italicized* symptoms listed below must also be present to an important degree during the same time period. (Note that if the patient's *abnormal mood* is only irritable—that is, without any component of euphoria—four symptoms are required in addition to the increased activity level.)

Heightened self-esteem, found in most patients, can become grandiose to the point that it is delusional. Then patients believe that they can advise presidents and solve the problem of world hunger, in addition to more mundane tasks such as conducting psychotherapy and running the very medical facilities that currently house them. Because such delusions are in keeping with the euphoric mood, they are called *mood-congruent*.

Manic patients typically report feeling *rested on little sleep*. Time spent sleeping seems wasted; they prefer to pursue their many projects. In its milder forms, this *heightened activity* may be goal-directed and useful; patients who are only moderately ill can accomplish quite a lot in a 20-hour day. But as they become more and more active, agitation ensues, and they may begin many projects they never complete. At this point they have *lost judgment* for what is reasonable and attainable. They may become involved in risky business ventures, indiscreet sexual liaisons, and questionable religious or political activities.

Manic patients are eager to tell anyone who will listen about their ideas, plans, and work, and they do so in speech that is loud and difficult to interrupt. Manic *speech* is often *rapid and pressured*, as if there were too many dammed-up words trying to escape through a tiny nozzle. The resulting speech may exhibit what is called *flight of ideas*, in which one thought triggers another to which it bears only a marginally logical association. As a result, a patient may wander far afield from where the conversation (or monologue) started. Manic patients may also be *easily distracted* by irrelevant sounds or movements that other people would ignore.

Some manic patients retain insight and seek treatment, but many will deny that anything is wrong. They rationalize that no one who feels this well or is so productive could possibly be ill. Manic behavior therefore continues until it ends spontaneously or the patient is hospitalized or jailed. I consider manic episodes to be acute emergencies, and I don't expect many clinicians will argue.

Some symptoms not specifically mentioned in the DSM-5 criteria are also worth noting here.

1. Even during an acute manic episode, many patients have brief periods of depression. These "microdepressions" are relatively common; depending on the symptoms associated with them, they may suggest that the specifier *with mixed features* is appropriate (p. 161).

2. Patients may use substances (especially alcohol) in an attempt to relieve the uncomfortable, driven feeling that accompanies a severe manic episode. Less often, the substance use temporarily obscures the symptoms of the mood episode. When clinicians become confused about whether the substance use or the mania came first, the question can usually be sorted out with the help of informants.

3. Catatonic symptoms occasionally occur during a manic episode, sometimes causing the episode to resemble schizophrenia. But a history (obtained from informants) of acute onset and previous episodes with recovery can help clarify the diagnosis. Then the specifier *with catatonic features* may be indicated (p. 100).

What about episodes that don't start until the patient undergoes treatment for a depression? Should they count as fully as evidence of spontaneous mania or hypomania? To count as evidence for either manic or hypomanic episode, DSM-5 requires that the *full* criteria (not just a couple of symptoms, such as agitation or irritability) be present, and that the symptoms last longer than the expected physiological effects of the treatment. This declaration nicely rounds out the list of possibilities: DSM-IV stated flatly that manic episodes caused by treatment could not count toward a diagnosis of bipolar I disorder, whereas DSM-III-R implied that they could. And DSM-III kept silent on the whole matter.

The authors of the successive DSMs may have been thinking of Emerson's famous epigram: A foolish consistency is the hobgoblin of little minds.

Impairment

Manic episodes typically wreak havoc on the lives of patients and their associates. Although increasing energy and effort may at first actually improve productivity at work (or school), as mania worsens a patient becomes less and less able to focus attention. Friendships are strained by arguments. Sexual entanglements can result in disease, divorce, and unwanted pregnancy. Even when the episode has resolved, guilt and recriminations remain behind.

Exclusions

The exclusions for manic episode are the same as for major depressive episode. General medical conditions such as hyperthyroidism can produce hyperactive behavior; patients who misuse certain psychoactive substances (especially amphetamines) will appear speeded up and may report feeling strong, powerful, and euphoric.

Essential Features of **Manic Episode**

Patients in the throes of mania are almost unmistakable. These people feel euphoric (though sometimes they're only irritable), and there's no way you can ignore their energy and frenetic activity. They are full of plans, few of which they carry through (they are so distractible). They talk and laugh, and talk some more, often very fast, often with flight of ideas. They sleep less than usual ("a waste of time, when there's so much to do"), but feel great anyway. Grandiosity is sometimes so exaggerated that they become psychotic, believing that they are exalted personages (monarchs, rock stars) or that they have superhuman powers. With deteriorating judgment (they spend money unwisely, engage in ill-conceived sexual adventures), functioning becomes impaired, often to the point they must be hospitalized to force treatment or for their own protection or that of other people.

The Fine Print

The D's: • Duration (most of nearly every day, 1+ weeks) • Distress or disability (work/educational, social, or personal impairment) • Differential diagnosis (substance use and physical disorders, schizoaffective disorder, neurocognitive disorders, hypomanic episodes, cyclothymia)

Coding Notes

Manic episode is not a diagnosable illness; it is a building block of bipolar I disorder.

Elisabeth Jacks had a manic episode; you can read her history beginning on page 131. Another example is that of Winona Fisk (p. 133). Look for other cases in the patient histories given in Chapter 20.

Hypomanic Episode

Hypomanic episode is the final mood disorder "building block." Comprising most of the same symptoms as manic episode, it is "manic episode writ small." Left without treatment, some patients with hypomanic episode may become manic later on. But many, especially those who have bipolar II disorder, have repeated hypomanic episodes. Hypomanic episode isn't codable as a diagnosis; it forms the basis for bipolar II disorder, and it can be encountered in bipolar I disorder, after the patient has already experienced an episode of actual mania. Hypomanic episode requires (1) a mood quality that (2) has existed for a required period of time, (3) is attended by a required number of symptoms, (4) has resulted in a considerable degree of disability, and (5) violates none of the listed exclusions. Table 3.1 compares the features of manic and hypomanic episodes.

Quality of Mood

The quality of mood in hypomanic episode tends to be euphoric without the driven quality present in manic episode, though mood can instead be irritable. However described, it is clearly different from the patient's usual nondepressed mood.

TABLE 3.1. Comparing Manic and Hypomanic Episodes

	Manic episode	Hypomanic episode
Duration	1 week or more	4 days or more
Mood	Abnormally and persistently high, irritable, or expansive	
Activity/energy	Persistently increased	
Symptoms that are changes from usual behavior	Three or more[a] of grandiosity, ↓ need for sleep, ↑ talkativeness, flight of ideas or racing thoughts, distractibility (self-report or that of others), agitation or ↑ goal-directed activity, poor judgment	
Severity	Results in psychotic features, hospitalization, or impairment of work, social, or personal functioning	Clear change from usual functioning *and* Others notice this change *and* No psychosis, hospitalization, or impairment
Other	Rule out substance/medication-induced symptoms With mixed features if appropriate[b]	

[a]Four or more if the only abnormality of mood is irritability.

[b]Both manic and hypomanic episodes can have the specifier *with mixed features.*

Duration

The patient must have had symptoms for a minimum of 4 days—a marginally shorter time requirement than that for manic episode.

Symptoms

As with manic episode, in addition to the change in mood (euphoria or irritability), the patient must also have an increase in energy or activity level—but again, only for 4 days. Then at least three symptoms from the same list must be present to an important degree (and represent a noticeable change) during this 4 days. If the patient's *abnormal mood* is irritable and *not* elevated, four symptoms are required. Note that hypomanic episode precipitated by treatment can be adduced as evidence for, say, bipolar II disorder—if it persists longer than the expected physiological effects of the treatment.

The *sleep* of hypomanic patients may be brief, and *activity level* may be increased, sometimes to the point of agitation. Although the degree of agitation is less than in a manic episode, hypomanic patients can also feel driven and uncomfortable. *Judgment* deteriorates, and may lead to untoward consequences for finances or for work or social life. *Speech* may become rapid and pressured; *racing thoughts* or *flight of ideas* may be noticeable. *Easily becoming distracted* can be a feature of hypomanic episode. Heightened *self-esteem* is never so grandiose that it becomes delusional, and hypomanic patients are never psychotic.

In addition to the DSM-5 criteria, note that in hypomanic episode, as in manic episode, substance use is common.

Impairment

How severe can the impairment be without qualifying as a manic episode? This is to some extent a judgment call for the practitioner. Lapses of judgment, such as spending sprees and sexual indiscretions, can occur in both manic and hypomanic episodes—but, by definition, only the patient who is truly manic will be seriously impaired. If behavior becomes so extreme that hospitalization is needed or psychosis is evident, the patient can no longer be considered hypomanic, and the label must be changed.

Exclusions

The exclusions are the same as those for manic episode. General medical conditions such as hyperthyroidism can produce hyperactive behavior; patients who misuse certain substances (especially amphetamines) will appear speeded up and may also report feeling strong, powerful, and euphoric.

Essential Features of **Hypomanic Episode**

Hypomania is "mania lite"—many of the same symptoms, but never to the same outrageous degree. These people feel euphoric or irritable and they experience high energy or activity. They are full of plans, which, despite some distractibility, they sometimes actually implement. They talk a lot, reflecting their racing thoughts, and may have flight of ideas. Judgment (sex and spending) may be impaired, but not to the point of requiring hospitalization for their own protection or that of others. Though the patients are sometimes grandiose and self-important, these features never reach the point of delusion. You would notice the change in such a person, but it doesn't impair functioning; indeed, sometimes these folks get quite a lot done!

The Fine Print

The D's: • Duration (most of nearly every day, 4+ days) • Disability (work/educational, social, and personal functioning are *not* especially impaired) • Differential diagnosis (substance use and physical disorders, other bipolar disorders)

Coding Notes

Specify if: **With mixed features.**

There is no severity code.

Hypomanic episode is not a diagnosable illness; it is a building block of bipolar II disorder and bipolar I disorder.

Mood Disorders Based on the Mood Episodes

From this point, the format of my presentation differs somewhat from both that of the DSM-5 and that of the Quick Guide at the beginning of the chapter. First, I'll discuss the mood disorders that use the mood episode "building blocks"—major depressive disorder and bipolar I and II disorders. Afterwards, I'll cover the disorders that do *not* crucially involve these episodes.

Major Depressive Disorder

A patient who has one or more major depressive episodes, and no manic or hypomanic symptoms, is said to have major depressive disorder (MDD). It is a common condition, affecting about 7% of the general population, with a female preponderance of roughly 2:1. MDD usually begins in the middle to late 20s, but it can occur at any time of life, from childhood to old age. The onset may be sudden or gradual. Although episodes last on average from 6 to 9 months, the range is enormous, from a few weeks to many years. Recovery usually begins within a few months of onset, though that too can vary enormously. A full recovery is less likely for a person who has a personality disorder or symptoms that are more severe (especially psychotic features). MDD is strongly hereditary; first-degree relatives have a risk several times that of the general population.

Some patients have only a single episode during an entire lifetime; then they are diagnosed with (no surprise) MDD, single episode. However, roughly half the patients who have one major depressive episode will have another. At the point they develop a second episode (to count, it must be separated from the first by at least 2 months), we must change the diagnosis to MDD, recurrent type.

For any given patient, symptoms of depression remain pretty much the same from one episode to the next. These patients will have an episode roughly every 4 years; there is some evidence that the frequency of episodes increases with age. Multiple episodes of depression greatly increase the likelihood of suicide attempts and completed suicide. Unsurprisingly, patients with recurrent episodes are also much more likely than those with a single episode to be impaired by their symptoms. One of the most severe consequences is suicide, which is the fate of about 4% of patients with MDD.

Perhaps 25% of patients with MDD will eventually experience a manic or hypomanic episode, thereby requiring yet another change in diagnosis—this time to bipolar (I or II) disorder. We'll talk more about them later.

Essential Features of **Major Depressive Disorder, {Single Episode}{Recurrent}**

The patient has {one}{or more} major depressive episodes and no spontaneous episodes of mania or hypomania.

The Fine Print

Two months or more without symptoms must intervene for episodes to be counted as separate.

Decide on the D's: • Differential diagnosis (substance use and physical disorders, other mood disorders, ordinary grief and sadness, schizoaffective disorder)

Coding Notes

From type of episode and severity, find code numbers in Table 3.2. If applicable, choose specifiers from Table 3.3. Both tables are located and discussed near the end of this chapter (pp. 167 and 168).

Brian Murphy

Brian Murphy had inherited a small business from his father and built it into a large one. When he sold out a few years later, he invested most of his money; with the rest, he bought a small almond farm in northern California. With his tractor, he handled most of the farm chores himself. Most years the farm earned a few hundred dollars, but as Brian was fond of pointing out, it really didn't make much difference. If he never made a dime, he felt he got "full value from keeping busy and fit."

When Brian was 55, his mood, which had always been normal, slid into depression. Farm chores seemed increasingly to be a burden; his tractor sat idle in its shed.

As his mood blackened, Brian's body functioning seemed to deteriorate. Although he was constantly fatigued, often falling into bed by 9 P.M., he would invariably awaken at 2 or 3 A.M. Then obsessive worrying kept him awake until sunrise. Mornings were worst for him. The prospect of "another damn day to get through" seemed overwhelming. In the evenings he usually felt somewhat better, though he'd sit around working out sums on a magazine cover to see how much money they'd have if he "couldn't work the farm" and they had to live on their savings. His appetite deserted him. Although he never weighed himself, he had to buckle his belt two notches smaller than he had several months before.

"Brian just seemed to lose interest," his wife, Rachel, reported the day he was admitted to the hospital. "He doesn't enjoy anything any more. He spends all his time sitting around and worrying about being in debt. We owe a few hundred dollars on our credit card, but we pay it off every month!"

During the previous week or two, Brian had begun to ruminate about his health. "At first it was his blood pressure," Rachel said. "He'd ask me to take it several times a day. I still work part-time as a nurse. Several times he thought he was having a stroke. Then yesterday he became convinced that his heart was going to stop. He'd get up, feel his pulse, pace around the room, lie down, put his feet above his head, do everything he could to 'keep it going.' That's when I decided to bring him here."

"We'll have to sell the farm." That was the first thing Brian said to the mental health clinician when they met. Brian was casually dressed and rather rumpled. He had prominent worry lines on his forehead, and he kept feeling for his pulse. Several times during the interview, he seemed unable to sit still; he would get up from the bed where he was sitting and pace over to the window. His speech was slow but coherent. He talked mostly about his feelings of being poverty-stricken and his fears that the farm would have to go on the block. He denied having hallucinations, but admitted to feeling tired and "all washed up—not good for anything any more." He was fully oriented, had a full fund of information, and scored a perfect 30 on the MMSE. He admitted that he was depressed, but he denied having thoughts about death. Somewhat reluctantly, he agreed that he might need treatment.

Rachel pointed out that with his generous disability policy, his investments, and his pension from his former company, they had more money coming in than when he was healthy.

"But still we have to sell the farm," Brian replied.

Evaluation of Brian Murphy

Unfortunately, clinicians (including some mental health specialists) commonly make two sorts of mistakes when evaluating patients with depression.

First, we sometimes focus too intently on a patient's anxiety, alcohol use, or psychotic symptoms and ignore underlying symptoms of depression or dysthymia. Here's my lifelong rule, formulated from bitter experience (not all mine) as far back as when I was a resident: Always look for a mood disorder in any new patient, even if the chief complaint is something else.

Second, the presenting depressive or manic symptoms can be quite noticeable, even dramatic—to the point that clinicians may fail to notice, lurking underneath, the presence of alcohol use disorder or another disorder (good examples are neurocognitive and somatic symptom disorders). And that suggests another, equally important rule, almost the mirror image of the first rule: Never assume that a mood disorder is your patient's only problem.

First, let's try to identify the current (and any previous) mood episodes. Brian Murphy had been ill much longer than 2 weeks (criterion A). Of the major depressive episode symptoms listed (five are required by DSM-5), he had at least six: low mood (A1), loss of interest (A2), fatigue (A6), sleeplessness (A4), low self-esteem (A7), loss of appetite (A3), and agitation (A5). (Note that either low mood or loss of interest is required for diagnosis; Brian had both.) He was so seriously impaired (B) that he required hospitalization. Although we do not have the results of his physical exam and laboratory testing, the vignette provides no history that would suggest **another medical condition** (for example, pancreatic carcinoma) or **substance use** (C). However, his clinician would definitely need to ask both Brian and his wife about this—depressed people often increase their drinking. He was clearly severely depressed and different from his usual self. He easily fulfilled the criteria for **major depressive episode.**

Next, what type of mood disorder did Brian have? There had been no manic or hypomanic episodes (E), ruling out **bipolar I or II disorder.** His delusions of poverty could suggest a psychotic disorder (such as **schizoaffective disorder**), but he had too few psychotic symptoms, and the timing of mood symptoms versus delusions was wrong (D). He was deluded but had no additional A criteria for schizophrenia. His mood symptoms ruled out **brief psychotic disorder** and **delusional disorder.** He therefore fulfilled the requirements for MDD.

There are just two subtypes of MDD: single episode and recurrent. Although Brian Murphy might subsequently have other episodes of depression, this was the only one so far.

For the further description and coding of Brian Murphy's depression, let's turn ahead to Table 3.2. His single episode dictates the column to highlight under MDD. And he was delusional, so we'd code him as *with psychotic features.*

But wait: Suppose he hadn't been psychotic? What severity would we assign him then? Despite the fact that he wasn't suicidal (he didn't want death; rather, he feared it), he did have most of the required symptoms, and he was seriously impaired by his depressive illness. That's why I'd rate him as severely depressed (but remember, the code number has already been determined).

Now we'll turn to the panoply of other specifiers, which I'll discuss toward the end of this chapter (p. 159). Brian had no manic symptoms; that rules out *with mixed features*. His delusion that he was poor and would have to sell the farm was *mood-congruent*—that is, in keeping with the usual cognitive themes of depression. (However, the thought that his heart would stop and the pulse checking were probably not delusional. I'd regard them as signifying the overwhelming anxiety he felt about the state of his health.) The words we'd attach to his diagnosis (so far) would be MDD, single episode, severe with mood-congruent psychotic features.

But wait; there's more. There were no abnormalities of movement suggestive of catatonic features, nor did his depression have any atypical features (for example, he didn't have increased appetite or sleep too much). Of course, he would not qualify for peripartum onset. But his wife complained that he didn't "enjoy anything any more," suggesting that he might qualify for melancholic features. He was agitated when interviewed (marked psychomotor slowing would have also qualified for this criterion), and he had lost considerable weight. He reported awakening early on many mornings (terminal insomnia). The interviewer did not ask him whether this episode of depression differed qualitatively from how he felt when his parents died, but I'd bet that it did. So, we'll add *with melancholic features* to the mix.

I wrote this vignette before a new specifier, *with anxious distress*, was a gleam in anyone's eye, but I think Brian Murphy qualifies for it as well. He appeared edgy and tense, and he was markedly restless. Furthermore, he seemed to be expressing the fear that something horrible—possibly a catastrophic health event—would occur. Even though nothing was said about poor concentration, he had at least three of the symptoms required for the *with anxious distress* specifier, at a moderate severity rating. The evidence is that this specifier has real prognostic importance, suggesting, in the absence of treatment, the possibility of a poor outcome—even suicide.

Some patients with severe depression also report many of the symptoms typical of **panic disorder, generalized anxiety disorder**, or some other **anxiety disorder.** In such a case, two diagnoses could be made. Usually the mood disorder is listed first as the primary diagnosis. Anxiety symptoms that do not fulfill criteria for one of the disorders described in Chapter 4 may be further evaluated as evidence for the anxious distress specifier.

Of course, Brian wouldn't qualify for rapid cycling or seasonal pattern; with only one episode, there could be no pattern. I'd give him a GAF score of 51, and his final diagnosis would be as given below.

Let me just say that the prospect of using so many different criteria sets to code one patient may seem daunting, but taking it one step at a time reveals a process that is really quite logical and (once you get the hang of it) fairly quick. The same basic methods should be applied to all examples of depression. (Of course, you could argue—I certainly would—that using the prototypical descriptions of depression and mania and their respective disorders simplifies things still further. But again, remember always to consider the possibility of substance use and physical causes of any given symptom set.)

F32.3 [296.24]   Major depressive disorder, single episode, severe with mood-congruent psychotic features, with melancholic features, with moderate anxious distress

---

There's a situation in which I like to be extra careful about diagnosing MDD. That's when a patient also has somatic symptom disorder (see p. 251). The problem is that many people who seem to have too many physical symptoms can also have mood symptoms that closely resemble major depressive episodes (and sometimes manic episodes). Over the years, I've found that these people tend to get treatment with medication, electroconvulsive therapy (ECT), and other physical therapies that don't seem to help them much—certainly not for long. I'm not saying that drugs never work; I maintain only that if you encounter a patient with somatic symptom disorder who is depressed, other treatments (such as cognitive-behavioral therapy or other forms of behavior modification) may be more effective and less fraught with complications.

Aileen Parmeter

"I just know it was a terrible mistake to come here." For the third time, Aileen Parmeter got out of her chair and walked to the window. A wiry 5 feet 2 inches, this former Marine master sergeant (she had supervised a steno pool) weighed a scant 100 pounds. Through the slats of the Venetian blinds, she peered longingly at freedom in the parking lot below. "I just don't know whatever made me come."

"You came because I asked you to," her clinician explained. "Your nephew called and said you were getting depressed again. It's just like last time."

"No, I don't think so. I was just upset," she explained patiently. "I had a little cold for a few days and couldn't play my tennis. I'll be fine if I just get back to my little apartment."

"Have you been hearing voices or seeing things this time?"

"Well, of course not." She seemed rather offended. "You might as well ask if I've been drinking."

After her last hospitalization, Aileen had been well for about 10 months. Although she had taken her medicine for only a few weeks, she had remained active until 3 weeks ago. Then she stopped seeing her friends and wouldn't play tennis because she "just didn't enjoy it." She worried constantly about her health and had been unable to sleep. Although she didn't complain of decreased appetite, she had lost about 10 pounds.

"Well, who wouldn't have trouble? I've just been too tired to get my regular exercise." She tried to smile, but it came off crooked and forced.

"Miss Parmeter, what about the suicidal thoughts?"

"I don't know what you mean."

"I mean, each time you've been here—last year, and 2 years before that—you were admitted because you tried to kill yourself."

"I'm going to be fine now. Just let me go home."

But her therapist, whose memory was long, had ordered Aileen held for her own protection in a private room where she could be observed one-on-one.

Sleepless still at 3 A.M., Aileen got up, smiled wanly at the attendant, and went in to use the bathroom. Looping a strip she had torn from her sweatsuit over the top of the door, she tried to hang herself. As the silence lengthened, the attendant called out softly, then tapped on the door, then opened it and sounded the alarm. The code team responded with no time to spare.

The following morning, the therapist was back at her bedside. "Why did you try to do that, Miss Parmeter?"

"I didn't try to do anything. I must have been confused." She gingerly touched the purple bruises that ringed her neck. "This sure hurts. I know I'd feel better if you'd just let me go home."

Aileen remained hospitalized for 10 days. Once her sore neck would allow, she began to take her antidepressant medication again. Soon she was sleeping and eating normally, and she made a perfect score on the MMSE. She was released to go home to her apartment and her tennis, still uncertain why everyone had made such a fuss about her.

Evaluation of Aileen Parmeter

Aileen never acknowledged feeling depressed, but she had lost interest in her usual activities. This change had lasted longer than 2 weeks, and—as in previous episodes— her other symptoms included fatigue, insomnia, loss of weight, and suicidal behavior (criterion A). (Although she reproached herself for entering the hospital, these feelings referred exclusively to her being ill and would not be scored as guilt.) She was sick enough to require hospitalization, fulfilling the impairment criterion (B).

Aileen could have a **mood disorder due to another medical condition**, and this would have to be pursued by her clinician, but the history of recurrence makes this seem unlikely (C). Symptoms of apathy and poor memory raise the question of **mild neurocognitive disorder**, but her MMSE showed no evidence of memory impairment. She denied alcohol consumption, so a **substance-induced mood disorder** would also appear unlikely (her clinician had known her for so long that further pursuit of the possibility would be wasted effort).

There was no evidence that Aileen had ever had mania or hypomania, ruling out **bipolar I** or **II disorder** (E), and absence of any psychotic symptoms rules out **psychotic disorders** (D). She therefore fulfills the criteria for MDD. She'd had more than one episode separated by substantially longer than 2 months, which would satisfy the requirement for the term *recurrent*. Turning ahead to Table 3.2, we can reject the rows there describing psychotic features (she emphatically denied having delusions or hallucinations) and remission.

Now we must consider the severity of her depression (p. 158). It is always a problem how best to score someone with so little insight. Even with the suicide attempt, Aileen appeared barely to meet the five symptoms needed for major depressive episode. According to the rules, she should receive a severity coding of no greater than moderate. However, for a patient who has just nearly killed herself, this would be inaccurate and possibly dangerous; one of her symptoms, suicidal behavior, was very serious indeed. As I've said before, the coding instructions are meant to be guides, not shackles: I'd call Aileen's depression severe.

She wouldn't qualify for any of the specifiers for the most recent episode—perhaps because her lack of insight prevented her from providing full information. (I suppose that longer observation might reveal criteria adequate for *with melancholic features*.)

Other diagnoses are sometimes found in patients with MDD. These include several of the **anxiety disorders, obsessive–compulsive disorder**, and the **substance-related disorders** (especially **alcohol use disorder**). There is no evidence for any of these. I'd give her a GAF score of only 15 on admission. Her GAF had improved to 60 by the time she was released. Her complete diagnosis would be as follows:

F33.2 [296.33]   Major depressive disorder, recurrent, severe

Bipolar I Disorder

Bipolar I disorder is shorthand for any cyclic mood disorder that includes at least one manic episode. Although this nomenclature has only been adopted within the past several decades, bipolar I disorder has been recognized for over a century. Formerly, it was called *manic–depressive illness*; older clinicians may still refer to it this way. Men and women are about equally affected, for a total of approximately 1% of the general adult population. Bipolar I disorder is strongly hereditary.

There are two technical points to consider in evaluating episodes of bipolar I disorder. First, for an episode to count as a new one, it must either represent a change of polarity (for example, from major depressive to manic or hypomanic episode), or it must be separated from the previous episode by a normal mood that lasts at least 2 months.

Second, a manic or hypomanic episode will occasionally seem to be precipitated by the treatment of a depression. Antidepressant drugs, ECT, or bright light (used to treat seasonal depression) may cause a patient to move rapidly from depression into a full-blown manic episode. Bipolar I disorder is defined by the occurrence of *spontaneous* depressions, manias, and hypomanias; therefore, any treatment-induced manic or hypomanic episode can only be used to make the diagnosis of a bipolar I (or, for that matter, bipolar II) condition if the symptoms persist beyond the physiological effect of that treatment. Even then, DSM-5 urges caution: Demand the *full* number of manic or hypomanic symptoms, not just edginess or agitation that some patients experience following treatment of depression.

In addition, note the warning that the mood episodes must not be superimposed on a psychotic disorder—specifically schizophrenia, schizophreniform disorder, delusional disorder, or unspecified psychotic disorder. Because the longitudinal course of bipolar I disorder differs strikingly from those of the psychotic disorders, this should only rarely cause diagnostic problems.

Usually a manic episode will be current, and the patient will have been admitted to a hospital. Occasionally, you might use the category *current or most recent episode manic* for a newly diagnosed patient who is on a mood-stabilizing regimen. Most will have had at least one previous manic, major depressive, or hypomanic episode. However, a single manic episode is hardly rare, especially early in the course of bipolar I disorder. Of course, the vast majority of such patients will later have subsequent major depressive episodes, as well as additional manic ones. Males are more likely than females to have a first episode that is manic.

Current episode depressed (I'm intentionally shorthanding the long and unwieldy official phrase) will be one of the most frequently used of the bipolar I subtypes; nearly all patients with this disorder will receive this diagnosis at some point during their lifetimes. The depressive symptoms will be very much like those in the major depressive disorders of Brian Murphy (p. 124) and Aileen Parmeter (p. 127). Elisabeth Jacks (p. 131), whose current episode was manic, had been depressed a few weeks before her current evaluation.

In a given patient, symptoms of mood disorder tend to remain the same from one episode to the next. However, it is possible that after an earlier manic episode, a subsequent mood upswing may be less severe, and therefore only hypomanic. (The first episode of a bipolar I disorder couldn't be hypomanic; otherwise, you'd have to diagnose bipolar II.) Although I have provided no vignette for bipolar I, most recent episode hypomanic, I have described a hypomanic episode in the case of Iris McMaster, a patient with bipolar II disorder (see p. 136).

Researchers who have followed bipolar patients for many years report that some have only manias. The concept of *unipolar mania* has been debated off and on for a long time. There are probably some patients who will never have a depression, but most will, given enough time. I have known of patients who had as many as seven episodes of mania over a 20-year period before finally having a first episode of depression. What's important here is that all patients with bipolar I (and II) disorder—and their families—should be warned to watch out for depressive symptoms. Bipolar I patients have a high likelihood of completing suicide; some reports suggest that these people account for up to a quarter of all suicides.

Essential Features of **Bipolar I Disorder**

The patient has had at least one manic episode, plus any number (including zero) of hypomanic and major depressive episodes.

The Fine Print

A manic episode that was precipitated by treatment (medication, ECT, light therapy) can be counted toward a diagnosis of bipolar I disorder *if* the manic symptoms last beyond the expected physiological treatment effects.

The D's: • Differential diagnosis (substance use and physical disorders, other bipolar disorders, psychotic disorder)

Coding Notes

From type of episode and severity, find code numbers in Table 3.2. Finally, choose from a whole lot of specifiers in Table 3.3.

Older patients who develop a mania for the first time may have a comorbid neurological disorder. They may also have a higher mortality. First-episode mania in the elderly may be quite a different illness from recurrent mania in the elderly, and should probably be given a different diagnosis, such as unspecified bipolar disorder.

Elisabeth Jacks

Elisabeth Jacks ran a catering service with her second husband, Donald, who was the main informant.

At age 38, Elisabeth already had two grown children, so Donald could understand why this pregnancy might have upset her. Even so, she had seemed unnaturally sad. From about her fourth month, she spent much of each day in bed, not arising until afternoon, when she began to feel a little less tired. Her appetite, voracious during her first trimester, fell off, so that by the time of delivery she was several pounds lighter than usual for a full-term pregnancy. She had to give up keeping the household and business accounts, because she couldn't focus her attention long enough to add a column of figures. Still, the only time Donald became really alarmed was one evening at the beginning of Elisabeth's ninth month, when she told him that she had been thinking for days that she wouldn't survive childbirth and he would have to rear the baby without her. "You'll both be better off without me, anyway," she had said.

After their son was born, Elisabeth's mood brightened almost at once. The crying spells and the hours of rumination disappeared; briefly, she seemed almost her normal self. Late one Friday night, however, when the baby was 3 weeks old, Donald returned from catering a banquet to find Elisabeth wearing only bra and panties and icing a cake. Two other just-iced cakes were lined up on the counter, and the kitchen was littered with dirty pots and pans.

"She said she'd made one for each of us, and she wanted to party," Donald told the clinician. "I started to change the baby—he was howling in his basket—but she wanted to drag me off to the bedroom. She said 'Please, sweetie, it's been a long time.' I mean, even if I hadn't been dead tired, who could concentrate with the baby crying like that?"

All the next day, Elisabeth was out with girlfriends, leaving Donald home with the baby. On Sunday she spent nearly $300 for Christmas presents at an April garage sale. She seemed to have boundless energy, sleeping only 2 or 3 hours a night before arising, rested and ready to go. On Monday she decided to open a bakery; by telephone, she tried to charge over $1,600 worth of kitchen supplies to their Visa card. She'd have done the same the next day, but she talked so fast that the person she called couldn't understand her. In frustration, she slammed the phone down.

Elisabeth's behavior became so erratic that for the next two evenings Donald stayed off work to care for the baby, but his presence only seemed to provoke her sexual demands. Then there was the marijuana. Before Elisabeth became pregnant, she would have an occasional toke (she called it her "herbs"). During the past week, not all the smells in the house had been fresh-baked cake, so Donald thought she might be at it again.

Yesterday Elisabeth had shaken him awake at 5 A.M. and announced, "I am becoming God." That was when he had made the appointment to bring her for an evaluation.

Elisabeth herself could hardly sit still during the interview. In a burst of speech, she described her renewed energy and plans for the bakery. She volunteered that she had never felt better in her life. In rapid succession she then described her mood (ecstatic), how it made her feel when she put on her best silk dress (sexy), where she had purchased the dress, how old she had been when she bought it, and to whom she was married at the time.

Patients who may have bipolar I disorder need a careful interview for symptoms of addiction to alcohol; alcohol use disorder is diagnosed as a comorbid disorder in as many as 30%. Often the alcohol-related symptoms appear first.

Evaluation of Elisabeth Jacks

This vignette provides a fairly typical picture of manic excitement. Elisabeth Jacks's mood was definitely elevated. Aside from the issue of marijuana smoking (which appeared to be a symptom, not a cause), her relatively late age of onset was the only atypical feature.

For at least a week Elisabeth had had this high mood (manic episode criterion A), accompanied by most of the other typical symptoms (B): reduced need for sleep (B2), talkativeness (B3), flight of ideas (a sample run is given at the end of the vignette, B4), and poor judgment (buying Christmas gifts at the April garage sale—B7). Her disorder caused considerable distress, for her family if not for her (C); this is usual for patients with manic episode. The severity of the symptoms (not their number or type) and the degree of impairment were what would differentiate her full-blown **manic episode** from a **hypomanic episode.**

The issue of another medical condition (D) is not addressed in the vignette. Medical problems such as hyperthyroidism, multiple sclerosis, and brain tumors would have to be ruled out by the admitting clinician before a definitive diagnosis could be made. **Delirium** must be ruled out for any postpartum patient, but she was able to focus her attention well. Although Elisabeth may have been smoking **marijuana**, misuse of this substance should never be confused with mania; neither cannabis intoxication nor withdrawal presents the combination of symptoms typical of mania. Although the depression that occurred early in her pregnancy would have met the criteria for **major depressive episode**, her current manic episode would obviate **major depressive disorder.** Because the current episode was too severe for hypomanic symptoms, she could not have **cyclothymic disorder.** Therefore, the diagnosis would have to be **bipolar I disorder** (because she was hospitalized, it could not be **bipolar II**). The course of her illness was not compatible with any psychotic disorder other than brief psychotic disorder, and that diagnosis specifically excludes a bipolar disorder (B).

The bipolar I subtypes, as described earlier, are based upon the nature of the most recent episode. Elisabeth's, of course, would be current episode manic.

Next we'll score the severity of Elisabeth's mania (see the footnotes to Table 3.2). These severity codes are satisfactorily self-explanatory, though there's one problem: Whether Elisabeth was actually psychotic is not made clear in the vignette. If we take her words literally, she thought she was becoming God, in which case she would qualify for *severe with psychotic features.* These would be judged *mood-congruent* because grandiosity was in keeping with her exalted mood.

The only possible episode specifier (Table 3.3) would be *with peripartum onset*: She developed her manic episode within a few days of delivery. With a GAF score of 25, the full diagnosis would be as follows:

F31.2 [296.44]   Bipolar I disorder, currently manic, severe with mood-congruent psychotic features, with peripartum onset

Winona Fisk

By the time she was 21, Winona Fisk had already had two lengthy mental health hospitalizations, one each for mania and depression. Then she remained well for a year on maintenance lithium, which in the spring of her junior year in college she abruptly discontinued because she "felt so well." When two of her brothers brought her to the hospital 10 days later, she had been suspended for repeatedly disrupting classes with her boisterous behavior.

On the ward, Winona's behavior was mostly a picture of manic excitement. She spoke nonstop and was constantly on the move, often rummaging through other patients' purses and lockers. But many of the thoughts flooding her mind were so sad that for 8 or 10 days she often spontaneously wept for several minutes at a time. She said she felt depressed and guilty—not for her behavior in class, but for being such a burden to her family. During these brief episodes, she claimed to hear the heart of her father beating from his grave, and she would express the wish to join him in death. She ate little and lost 15 pounds; she often awakened weeping at night and was unable to get back to sleep.

Nearly a month's treatment with lithium, carbamazepine, and neuroleptics was largely futile. Her mood disorder eventually yielded to six sessions of bilateral ECT.

Evaluation of Winona Fisk

Winona's two previous episodes of bipolar I disorder make that diagnosis crystal clear. Our only remaining task is to decide about the type and severity of the most recent episode.

In a typical manner, Winona's manic episode began with feeling "too good" to be ill; that got her into trouble with her lithium. Her symptoms, which included poor judgment (she was suspended from class for her behavior), talkativeness, and increased psychomotor activity fulfilled criteria A and B for manic episode; hospitalization (C) ruled out hypomanic episode. (Her clinician would have to make sure she had no other medical or substance use disorder—criterion D.)

But at times throughout the day, she also had "microdepressions" during which she experienced at least three depressive symptoms, which would fulfill the criterion A requirements for the specifier *with mixed features* (manic episode): She felt depressed (A1), she expressed feelings of (inappropriate) guilt (A5), and she ruminated about death (A6). We cannot include her problems with sleep and appetite/weight; because they are found in both manic and depressive episodes, they don't make the mixed features list. She didn't meet full major depressive criteria, so there's no need to fuss about whether to call her episode manic with mixed features, or major depressive with mixed features (C). And she didn't drink or use drugs (D).

The severity of Winona's episode should be judged on the basis of both the symptom count and the degree to which her illness affected her (and others). All things considered, her clinician felt that she was seriously ill, and coded her accordingly.

With a GAF score of 25, here's Winona's diagnosis:

F31.2 [296.44]	Bipolar I disorder, current episode manic, severe with mood-congruent psychotic features, with mixed features
Z55.9 [V62.3]	Academic or educational problem (suspended from school)

F31.81 [296.89] Bipolar II Disorder

The symptoms of bipolar II and bipolar I disorders have important similarities. The principal distinction, however, is the degree of disability and discomfort conferred by the high phase, which in bipolar II never involves psychosis and never requires hospitalization.* Bipolar II disorder consists of recurrent major depressive episodes interspersed with hypomanic episodes.

Like bipolar I disorder, bipolar II may be diagnosed on the basis of mood episodes that arise spontaneously or that are precipitated by antidepressants, ECT, or bright light therapy—if the induced symptoms subsequently last past the expected duration of the physiological treatment effects. (Be sure to ask the patient and informants whether there has been another hypomanic episode that was not precipitated by treatment; many patients will have had one.) Bipolar II is also associated with an especially high rate of rapid cycling, which carries added risk for a difficult course of illness.

Women may be more prone than men to develop bipolar II disorder (the sexes are about equally represented in bipolar I disorder); fewer than 1% of the general adult population are affected, though the prevalence among adolescents may be higher. The peripartum period may be especially likely to precipitate an episode of hypomania.

Comorbidity is a way of life for patients with bipolar II. Mostly they will have anxiety and substance use disorders, though eating disorders will also be in the mix, especially for female patients.

It is important to note that although I have earlier described hypomanic episode as "mania lite," we shouldn't imagine that the disorder is innocuous. Indeed, some studies suggest that patients with bipolar II are ill longer and spend more time in the depressive phase than is the case for patients with bipolar I. They may also be especially likely to make impulsive suicide attempts. And not a few (in the 10% range) will eventually experience a full-blown manic episode.

Sal Camozzi was another patient with bipolar II disorder; his history is given in Chapter 11 (p. 304).

Essential Features of **Bipolar II Disorder**

The patient has had at least one each of a major depressive episode *and* a hypomanic episode, but *no* manic episodes ever.

The Fine Print

The D's: • Distress or disability (work/educational, social, or personal impairment, but only for depressive episodes or for switches between episodes) • Differential diag-

---

*I suppose it's possible that a patient with bipolar II disorder might end up hospitalized without really needing it. In that case, I'd go with the predominant symptoms and call it bipolar II.

nosis (substance use and physical disorders, other bipolar disorders, major depressive disorder)

Coding Notes

Specify current or most recent episode as {hypomanic}{depressed}.

Choose any relevant specifiers, summarized in Table 3.3. For most recent episode, you can mention severity (free choice: mild, moderate, severe).

Iris McMaster

"I'm a writer," said Iris McMaster. It was her first visit to the interviewer's office, and she wanted to smoke. She fiddled with a cigarette but didn't seem to know what to do with it. "It's what I do for a living. I should be home doing it now—it's my life. Maybe I'm the finest creative writer since Dostoevsky. But my friend Charlene said I should come in, so I've taken time away from working on my play and my comic novel, and here I am." She finally put the cigarette back into the pack.

"Why did Charlene think you should come?"

"She thinks I'm high. Of course I'm high. I'm always high when I'm in my creative phase. Only she thinks I'm too nervous." Iris was slender and of average height; she wore a bright pink spring outfit. She looked longingly at her pack of cigarettes. "God, I need one of those."

Her speech could always be interrupted, but it was salted with bon mots, neat turns of phrase, and original similes. But Iris was also able to give a coherent history. At 45, she was married to an engineer and had a daughter who was nearly 18. And she really was a writer, who over the last several years had sold (mainly to women's magazines) articles about a variety of subjects.

For 3 or 4 months Iris had been in one of her high phases, cranking out an enormous volume of essays on wide-ranging topics. Her "wired" feeling was uncomfortable in a way, but it hadn't troubled her because she felt so productive. Whenever she was creating, she didn't need much sleep. A 2-hour nap would leave her rested and ready for another 10 hours at her computer. At those times, her husband would fix his own meals and kid her about having "a one-track mind."

Iris never ate much during her high phases, so she lost weight. But she didn't get herself into trouble: no sexual indiscretions, no excessive spending ("I'm always too busy to shop"). And she volunteered that she had never "seen visions, heard voices, or had funny ideas about people following me around." She had never spent time "in the funny farm."

As Iris paused to gather her thoughts, her fingers clutched the cigarette package. She shook her head almost imperceptibly. Without uttering another word, she grabbed her purse, arose from the chair, and swooped out the door. It was the last the interviewer saw of her for a year and a half.

In November of the following year, a person announcing herself as Iris McMaster dropped into that same office chair. She seemed like an impostor. She'd gained 30 or 40 pounds, which she had stuffed into polyester slacks and a bulky knit sweater. "As I was saying," were the first words she uttered. Just for a second, the corners of her mouth twitched up. But for the rest of the hour she soberly talked about her latest problem: writer's block.

About a year ago, she had finished her play and was well into her comic novel when the muse deserted her. For months now, she had been arising around lunchtime and spending long afternoons staring at her computer. "Sometimes I don't even turn it on!" she said. She couldn't focus her thinking to create anything that seemed worth clicking on "save." Most nights she tumbled into bed at 9. She felt tired and heavy, as though her legs were made of bricks.

"It's cheesecake, actually," was how Iris described her weight gain. "I have it delivered. For months I haven't been interested enough to cook for myself." She hadn't been suicidal, but the only time she felt much better was when Charlene took her out to lunch. Then she ate and made conversation pretty much as she used to. "I've done that quite a lot recently, as anyone can see." Once she returned home, the depression flooded back.

Finally, Iris apologized for walking out a year and a half earlier. "I didn't think I was the least bit sick," she said, "and all I really wanted to do was get back to my computer and get your character on paper!"

Evaluation of Iris McMaster

This discussion will focus on the episode of elevated mood Iris had during her first visit. There are two possibilities for such an episode: manic and hypomanic. As far as the time requirement was concerned, either type was possible—hypomanic requires 4 days (hypomanic episode criterion A), manic 1 week. She admitted that she felt "wired," and this feeling had apparently been sustained for several months. It was also abnormal for her. During her high phase, she had at least four symptoms (three required, B): high self-esteem, decreased need for sleep, talkativeness, and increased goal-directed activity (writing).

The mood of either a manic or hypomanic episode is excessively high or irritable, and it is accompanied by increased energy and activity. The real distinction between hypomania and mania consists in the *effects* of the mood elevation on patient and surroundings. The patient's functioning during a manic episode is markedly impaired, whereas in a hypomanic episode it is only a clear change from normal for the individual (C) that others can notice (D). During her high spells, Iris's writing productivity actually increased, and her social relationships (those with her husband and friends, though perhaps not with her hapless clinician) did not appear to suffer (E). Note that the collective effect of criteria C, D, and E is to allow some impairment of functioning, just not very much.

Assuming that Iris had no other **medical conditions** or **substance-induced mood disorder** (F), she could have one of these three: **bipolar I, bipolar II,** or **cyclothymic**

disorder. Judging from her lack of psychosis and hospitalizations, Iris had never had a true mania, ruling out bipolar I disorder. Her mood swings weren't nearly numerous enough to qualify for a diagnosis of cyclothymic disorder.

That leaves **bipolar II disorder.** But to qualify for that diagnosis, there must be at least one major depressive episode (bipolar II criterion A). On Iris's second visit to the clinician, her depressive symptoms included feeling depressed most of the time, weight gain, hypersomnia, fatigue, and poor concentration (her "writer's block"), which fulfill the criterion A requirements for major depressive episode. If her depression had not met the criteria for major depressive episode, her diagnosis would have been **unspecified** (or **other specified**) **bipolar disorder.** That's the same conclusion you'd reach for a patient who has never had a depression and only hypomanic episodes—or, for Iris McMaster, if she'd stayed the course for her first office visit.

In coding bipolar II disorder, clinicians are asked to specify the most recent episode. Iris's was a depression. Although bipolar II disorder provides no severity code for a hypomanic episode, we can rate her depression by the same criteria we'd use for any other major depressive episode. Though she had only the minimum number of symptoms needed for major depressive episode, her work had been seriously impaired. For that reason, moderate severity seems appropriate, and is mirrored in her GAF score of 60. If further interview revealed additional (or more serious) symptoms, I'd consider boosting her to *severe* level. These specifiers leave leeway for the clinician's judgment.

During her depression Iris had a number of symptoms of an episode specifier: *with atypical features.* That is, her mood seemed to brighten when she was having lunch with her friend; she also gained weight, slept excessively, and had a sensation of heaviness (bricks) in her limbs. With a total of four of these symptoms (only three are required), at the time of the second interview her full diagnosis would read as follows:

F31.81 [296.89]   Bipolar II disorder, depressed, moderate, with atypical features

Additional Mood Disorders

As we've discussed so far, many of the mood disorders seen in a mental health practice can be diagnosed by referring to manic, hypomanic, and major depressive episodes. These three mood episodes must be considered for any patient with mood symptoms. Next we'll consider several other conditions that do not depend on these episodes for their definition.

F34.1 [300.4] Persistent Depressive Disorder (Dysthymia)

The condition discussed here goes by several names—*dysthymic disorder, dysthymia, chronic depression,* and now *persistent depressive disorder.* Whatever you call it

(I'll generally stick with *dysthymia*), these patients are indeed chronically depressed. For years at a time, they have many of the same symptoms found in major depressive episodes, including low mood, fatigue, hopelessness, trouble concentrating, and problems with appetite and sleep. But notice what's absent from this list of symptoms (and from the criteria): inappropriate guilt feelings and thoughts of death or suicidal ideas. In short, most of these patients have an illness that's enduring, but also relatively mild.

In the course of a lifetime, perhaps 6% of adults have dysthymia, with women about twice as often affected as men. Although it can begin at any age, late onset is uncommon, and the classic case starts so quietly and so early in life that some patients regard their habitual low mood as, well, normal. In the distant past, clinicians regarded these patients as having *depressive personality* or *depressive neurosis*.

Dysthymic patients suffer quietly, and their disability can be subtle: they tend to put much of their energy into work, with less left over for social aspects of life. Because they don't appear severely disabled, such individuals may go without treatment until their symptoms worsen into a more readily diagnosed major depressive episode. This is the fate of many, probably most, dysthymic patients. In 1993 this phenomenon was recounted in a book that made *The New York Times* best-seller list: *Listening to Prozac*. However, the astonishing response to medication that book reported is by no means limited to one drug.

DSM-IV differentiated between dysthymic disorder and chronic major depressive disorder, but research has not borne out the distinction. So what DSM-5 now calls persistent depressive disorder is a combination of the two separate DSM-IV conditions. The current criteria supply some specifiers to indicate the difference. Here's what's clear: Patients who have depression that goes on and on (whatever we choose to call it) tend to respond poorly to treatment, are highly likely to have relatives with either bipolar disorders or some form of depression, and continue to be ill at follow-up.

There's one other feature that results from the lumping together of dysthymia and chronic major depression. Because some major depression symptoms do not occur in the dysthymia criteria set, it is possible (as DSM-5 notes) that a few patients with chronic major depression won't meet criteria for dysthymia: The combination of psychomotor slowing, suicidal ideas, and low mood/energy/interest would fit that picture (of those symptoms, only low energy appears among the B criteria for dysthymia). Improbable, I know, but there you are. We are advised that such patients should be given a diagnosis of major depressive disorder if their symptoms meet criteria during the current episode; if not, we'll have to retreat to other specified (or unspecified) depressive disorder.

Essential Features of **Persistent Depressive Disorder (Dysthymia)**

"Low-grade depression" is how these symptoms are often described, and they occur most of the time for 2 years (they are never absent for longer than 2 months running). Some patients aren't even aware that they are depressed, though others can see it. They will acknowledge such symptoms as fatigue, problems with concentration or decision making, poor self-image, and feeling hopeless. Sleep and appetite can be either increased or decreased. They may meet full requirements for a major depressive episode, but the concept of mania is foreign to them.

The Fine Print

For children, mood may be irritable rather than depressed, and the time requirement is 1 year rather than 2.

The D's: • Duration (more days than not, 2+ years) • Distress or disability (work/educational, social, or personal impairment) • Differential diagnosis (substance use and physical disorders, ordinary grief and sadness, adjustment to a long-standing stressor, bipolar disorders, major depressive disorder)

Coding Notes

Specify severity.

Specify onset:

> **Early onset**, if it begins by age 20.
> **Late onset**, if it begins at age 21 or later.

Specify if:

> **With pure dysthymic syndrome.** Doesn't meet criteria for major depressive episode.
> **With persistent major depressive episode.** Does meet criteria throughout preceding 2 years.
> **With intermittent major depressive episodes, with current episode.** Meets major depressive criteria now, but at times hasn't.
> **With intermittent major depressive episodes, without current episode.** Has met major depressive criteria in the past, though doesn't currently.

Choose other specifiers from Table 3.3.

Noah Sanders

For Noah Sanders, life had never seemed much fun. He was 18 when he first noticed that most of the time he "just felt down." Although he was bright and studied hard, throughout college he was often distracted by thoughts that he didn't measure up to his classmates. He landed a job with a leading electronics firm, but turned down several promotions because he felt that he could not cope with added responsibility. It took dogged determination and long hours of work to compensate for this "inherent second-rateness." The effort left him chronically tired. Even his marriage and the birth of his two daughters only relieved his gloom for a few weeks at a time, at best. His self-confidence was so low that, by common consent, his wife always made most of their family's decisions.

"It's the way I've always been. I am a professional pessimist," Noah told his family doctor one day when he was in his early 30s. The doctor replied that he had a depressive personality.

For many years, that description seemed to fit. Then, when Noah was in his early 40s, his younger daughter left home for college; after this, he began to feel increasingly that life had passed him by. Over a period of several months, his depression deepened. He had worsened to the point that he now felt he had never really been depressed before. Even visits from his daughters, which had always cheered him up, failed to improve his outlook.

Usually a sound sleeper, Noah began awakening at about 4 A.M. and ruminating over his mistakes. His appetite fell off, and he lost weight. When for the third time in a week his wife found him weeping in their bedroom, he confessed that he had felt so guilty about his failures that he thought they'd all be better off without him. She decided that he needed treatment.

Noah was started on an antidepressant medication. Within 2 weeks, his mood had brightened and he was sleeping soundly; at 1 month, he had "never felt better" in his life. Whereas he had once avoided oral presentations at work, he began to look forward to them as "a chance to show what I could do." His chronic fatigue faded, and he began jogging to use up some of his excess energy. In his spare time, he started his own small business to develop and promote some of his engineering innovations.

Noah remained on his medication thereafter. On the two or three occasions when he and his therapist tried to reduce it, he found himself relapsing into his old, depressive frame of mind. He continued to operate his small business as a sideline.

Evaluation of Noah Sanders

For most of his adult life, Noah's mood symptoms were chronic, rather than acute or recurring. He was never without these symptoms for longer than a few weeks at a time (criterion C for dysthymia), and they were present most of the day, most days (A). They included general pessimism, poor self-image, and chronic tiredness, though only two symptoms are required by criterion B. His indecisiveness encouraged his wife to assume the role of family decision maker, which suggests social impairment (H). The way he felt was not different from his usual self; in fact, he said it was the way he had always been. (The extended duration is one of two main features that differentiate dysthymia from **major depressive disorder.** The other is that the required dysthymia symptoms are neither as plentiful nor as severe as for major depression.) Noah had had no manic or psychotic symptoms that might have us considering bipolar or psychotic disorders (E, F).

The differential diagnosis of dysthymia is essentially the same as that for major depressive disorder. **Mood disorder due to another medical condition** and **substance-induced mood disorder** must be ruled out (G). The remarkable chronicity and poor self-image invite speculation that Noah's difficulties might be explained by a personality disorder, such as **avoidant** or **dependent personality disorder.** The vignette does not address all the criteria that would be necessary to make those diagnoses. However, an important diagnostic principle holds that the more treatable conditions should be diagnosed (and treated) first. If, despite relief of the mood disorder, Noah continued to be shy and awkward and to have a negative self-image, only then should we consider a personality diagnosis.

Now to the specifiers (Table 3.3). Though lacking psychotic symptoms, Noah had quite a number of depressive symptoms (including thoughts about death), which would suggest that he was severely ill. His dysthymia symptoms began when he was young (he first noticed them when he was just 18), so we'd say that his onset was early. Noah's recent symptoms would also qualify for a **major depressive episode**, which had begun fairly recently and precipitated his evaluation; DSM-5 notes that a dysthymic patient can have symptoms that fulfill criteria for such an episode (D). We would therefore give him the specifier *with intermittent major depressive episodes, with current episode.* None of the course specifiers would apply to Noah's dysthymia, but the following symptoms would meet the criteria for an episode specifier for the major depression— *with melancholic features*: He no longer reacted positively to pleasurable stimuli (being with his daughters); he described his mood as a definite change from normal; and he reported guilt feelings, early morning awakening, and loss of appetite.

Once treated, Noah seemed to undergo a personality change. His mood lightened and his behavior changed to the point that, by contrast, he seemed almost hypomanic. However, these symptoms don't rise to the level required for a hypomanic episode; had that been the case, criterion E would exclude the diagnosis of dysthymia. (Also, remember that a hypomanic episode precipitated by treatment that does not extend past the physiological effects of treatment does not count *toward* a diagnosis of bipolar II disorder. It should not count against the diagnosis of dysthymia, either.) I thought his GAF score would be about 50 on first evaluation; his GAF would be a robust 90 at follow-up. In the summary, I'd note the possibility of avoidant personality traits.

My full diagnosis for Noah Sanders would be as follows:

F34.1 [300.4]   Persistent mood disorder, severe, early onset, with
                       intermittent major depressive episode, with current
                       episode, with melancholic features (whew!)

F34.0 [301.13] Cyclothymic Disorder

Patients with cyclothymic disorder (CD) are chronically either elated or depressed, but *for the first couple of years*, they do not fulfill criteria for a manic, hypomanic, or major depressive episode. Note that there's a phrase back there dripping with italics. I'll explain in the sidebar below.

Cyclothymic disorder was at one time regarded as a personality disorder. This may have been partly due to the fact that it begins so gradually and lasts such a long time. Articles in the literature still refer to *cyclothymic temperament*, which may be a precursor to bipolar disorders.

The clinical appearance can be very variable. Some patients are nearly always dysphoric, occasionally shifting into hypomania for a day or so. Others can shift several times in a single day. Often the presentation is mixed.

Typically beginning gradually in adolescence or young adulthood, CD affects under 1% of the general population. However, clinicians diagnose it even less often than you'd expect. The sex distribution is about equal, though women are more likely to come for treatment. Not surprisingly, patients usually only come to clinical attention when they are depressed. Once begun, it tends toward chronicity.

What if your cyclothymic patient later develops a manic, hypomanic, or major depressive episode? In that case, you'll have to change the diagnosis to something different. Once a major mood episode rears its head, that patient can never revert to CD. If the new episode is major depressive, then you'll probably fall back on an unspecified (or other specified) bipolar disorder, inasmuch as, by definition, the "up" periods of CD will *not* qualify as a hypomanic episode. Note that this is a change from DSM-IV, which allowed a diagnosis of a bipolar disorder along with CD.

Essential Features of **Cyclothymic Disorder**

The patient has had many ups and downs of mood that *don't* meet criteria for any of the mood episodes (major depressive, hypomanic, manic). Although symptoms occur most of the time, as much as a couple of months of level mood can go by.

The Fine Print

The D's: • Duration (2+ years; 1+ year in children and adolescents) • Distress or disability (work/educational, social, or personal impairment) • Differential diagnosis (substance use and physical disorders, other bipolar disorders)

Coding Notes

Specify if: **With anxious distress.**

Honey Bare

"I'm a yo-yo!"

Without her feathers and sequins, Honey Bare looked anything but provocative. She had begun life as Melissa Schwartz, but she loved using her stage name. The stage in question was Hoofer's, one of the bump-and-grind joints that thrived near the waterfront. The billboard proclaimed that it was "Only a Heartthrob Away" from the Navy recruiting station. Since she'd dropped out of college 4 years earlier, Honey had been a front-liner in the four-girl show at Hoofer's. Every afternoon on her way to work she passed right by the mental health clinic, but this was her first visit inside.

"In our current gig, I play the Statue of Liberty. I receive the tired, the poor, and the huddled masses. Then I take off my robes."

"Is that a problem?" the interviewer wanted to know.

Most of the time, it wasn't. Honey liked her little corner of show biz. When the fleet was in, she played to thunderous applause. "In fact, I enjoy just about everything I do. I don't drink much, and I never do drugs, but I go to parties. I sing in our church choir, go to movies—I enjoy art films quite a bit." When she felt well, she slept little, talked a lot, started a hundred projects, and even finished some of them. "I'm really a happy person—when I'm feeling up."

But every couple of months, there'd be a week or two when Honey didn't enjoy much of anything. She'd paste a smile on her face and go to work, but when the curtain rang down, the smile came off with her makeup. She was never suicidal, and her sleep and appetite didn't suffer; her energy and concentration were normal. But it was as if all the fizz had gone out of her ginger ale. She could see no obvious cause for her mood swings, which had been going on for years. She could count on the fingers of both hands the number of weeks she had been "just normal."

Lately, Honey had acquired a boyfriend—a chief petty officer who wanted to marry her. He said he loved her because she was so vivacious and enthusiastic, but he had only seen her when she was bubbly. Always before, when she was depressed, he had been out to sea. Now he had written that he was being transferred to shore duty, and she feared it would be the end of their relationship. As she said it, two large tears trickled through the mascara and down her cheeks.

Four months and several visits later, Honey was back, wearing a smile. The lithium carbonate, she reported, seemed to be working well. The peaks and valleys of her moods had smoothed out to rolling hills. She was still playing the Statue of Liberty down at Hoofer's.

"My sailor's been back for nearly 3 months," she said, "and he's still carrying the torch for me."

As far back as the mid-19th century, Karl Kahlbaum—the German psychiatrist who first described catatonia—noted that some people experience frequent alterations between highs and lows so mild as not to require any treatment. His observations were confirmed and extended by his student and colleague, Ewald Hecker (who was best known for his description of hebephrenic schizophrenia).

But by the mid-20th century, the first DSM described cyclothymia as a cardinal personality type (along with schizoid, paranoid, and inadequate personalities). The description actually sounds pretty wonderful: "an extratensive and outgoing adjustment to life situations, an apparent personal warmth, friendliness and superficial generosity, an emotional reaching out to the environment, and a ready enthusiasm for competition." (I'll leave the looking-up of *extratensive* as an extra-credit exercise.) Anyway, thus was born cyclothymia as a temperament or personality style.

DSM-II kept cyclothymic personality with the other personality disorders, but in 1980 it was moved to the mood disorders and rechristened with its current name. However, its relationship to other mood disorders is fraught; experts argue about it even today. Many hold that it can be prodromal to a more severe bipolar disorder. Some point out the similarities between cyclothymia and borderline personality disorder (labile, irritable moods leading to interpersonal conflict), even suggesting that the latter disorder belongs on the bipolar spectrum—a speculation extreme enough to invite resistance.

All of this suggests that we still have work to do in determining cyclothymic disorder's exact place in the diagnostic firmament. Though the DSM-5 criteria are a step along the road to differentiation of this venerable diagnosis, they may not signify any real progress.

Evaluation of Honey Bare

The first and most obvious question is this: Had Honey ever fulfilled criteria for a manic, hypomanic, or major depressive episode (cyclothymic disorder criterion C)? When feeling down, she had no vegetative symptoms (problems with sleep or appetite) of **major depressive episode.** She had normal concentration, had never been suicidal, and did not complain of feeling worthless. At the other pole, she did indeed have symptoms similar to those of **hypomania** (talkative, slept less, was more active than at other times), but they weren't even severe enough for hypomania. Honey's "up" moods weren't elevated (or irritable, or expansive) to an abnormal extent (hypomanic episode criterion A)—they *were* her normal functioning. Furthermore, she had experienced far more cycles than would be typical for bipolar II disorder. We can therefore rule out any other bipolar or major depressive diagnosis.

Honey testified that she was either up or down most of the time (we're back to cyclothymia—criterion B). Because she was never psychotic, she could not qualify for a diagnosis such as **schizoaffective disorder** (D). She didn't use drugs or alcohol, ruling out a **substance-induced mood disorder** (E). Again, **bipolar I, bipolar II,** and **major depressive disorders** are ruled out due to the lack of relevant episodes. (However, because they involve so many swings of mood, either bipolar I or II with rapid cycling can sometimes be confused with cyclothymic disorder.) Mood shifts, impulsivity, and interpersonal problems can of course be found aplenty in **borderline personality disorder**, but we'd never diagnose a personality disorder when a major mental diagnosis was available.

Symptoms that were present much of the time would qualify Honey for CD. She had many mood swings; only infrequently was her mood neither high nor low. The only specifier allowed with CD, *with anxious distress*, didn't to me seem relevant to Honey's symptoms. With a GAF score of 70 on admission and 90 at follow-up, her diagnosis would be simple:

F34.0 [301.13]   Cyclothymic disorder

N94.3 [625.4] Premenstrual Dysphoric Disorder

A long history of disagreement over the reality of premenstrual dysphoria caused it to languish in the appendices of earlier DSM editions. At last, enough research has been published to bring it forth from the shadows.

Premenstrual symptoms to one degree or another affect about 20% of women of reproductive age. The severe form, premenstrual dysphoric disorder (PDD), affects up to 7% of women, often beginning in the teenage years. Throughout their reproductive years, these symptoms appear for perhaps a week out of each menstrual cycle. These women complain of varying degrees of dysphoric mood, fatigue, and physical symptoms that include sensitivity of breasts, weight gain, and abdominal swelling. Differentiation from major depressive episode and dysthymia relies principally on timing and duration.

The consequences of PDD can be serious: Such a patient could experience mood symptoms during an accumulated 8 years of her reproductive life. Some patients may be unaware how markedly their anger and other negative moods affect those around them, and many suffer from severe depression; perhaps 15% attempt suicide. Yet the typical patient doesn't receive treatment until she is 30, sometimes even later. Symptoms may be worse for older women, though menopause offers a natural endpoint (duration is sometimes extended by hormone replacement therapy). Overall, this condition ranks high among the seriously underdiagnosed mental disorders.

Risk factors for PDD include excessive weight, stress, and trauma (including a history of abuse); there appears to be a robust genetic component. Comorbid are anxiety disorders and other mood disorders, including bipolar conditions.

Dating as far back as 1944—the term *premenstrual tension* dates at least to 1928—the premenstrual syndrome (PMS) has had a long and tempestuous life. It's dismissed by many as pejorative, ridiculed by would-be comics, and disparaged even by some of those who practice gender politics. It should come as no surprise that it has been so ill received; as disorders go, PMS is remarkably vague and variously defined.

All told, PMS encompasses over a hundred possible symptoms, with no minimum number and no specific symptoms required; it's all anecdotal. Here are just a few: fluid retention (the symptom most often reported), especially in breasts and abdomen; craving for sweet or salty foods; muscle aches/pains, fatigue, irritability, tension, acne, anxiety, constipation or diarrhea, and insomnia; a change in sex drive; and feeling sad or moody or out of control. Most women will occasionally have one or two of these symptoms around the time of their periods—these symptoms are so common that, individually, they may be considered physiological rather than pathological. This fact causes some people to blame all such symptoms on PMS (it hardly ever goes by its full, nonabbreviated name); all women are in effect tarred with the same brush, when it is of crucial importance to note the exact symptoms, their timing, and their intensity.

Again, the critical difference is the presence of mood symptoms in PDD.

Essential Features of **Premenstrual Dysphoric Disorder**

For a few days before menstruating, a patient experiences pronounced mood shifts, depression, anxiety, anger, or other expressions of dysphoria. She will also admit to typical symptoms of depression, including trouble concentrating, loss of interest, fatigue, feeling out of control, and changes in appetite or sleep. She may have physical symptoms such as sensitivity of breasts, muscle pain, weight gain, and a sensation of abdominal distention. Shortly after menstruation begins, she snaps back to normal.

The Fine Print

The D's: • Duration (for several days around menstrual periods, for most cycles during the past year) • Distress or disability (social, occupational, or personal impairment) • Differential diagnosis (substance use—including hormone replacement therapy; physical disorders; major depressive disorder or dysthymia; ordinary grief/sadness)

Coding Note

DSM-5 says that the diagnosis can only be stated as *(provisional)* until you've obtained prospective ratings of two menstrual cycles. What you as a clinician decide to do with this is, of course, your business.

Amy Jernigan

"Look, I don't need you to tell me what's wrong. I *know* what's wrong. I just need you to fix it." One ankle crossed over the other, Amy Jernigan slouched in the consultation chair and gazed steadily at her clinician. "I brought a list of my symptoms, just so there won't be any confusion." She unfolded a half-sheet of embossed stationery.

"It always starts out 4 or 5 days before my period," she recited. "I begin by feeling uptight, like I'm waiting to take an exam I haven't studied for. Then, after a day or two, depression sets in and I just want to cry." She looked up and smiled. "You won't catch me doing that now—I'm always just fine after my period starts."

Still in her early 20s, Amy had graduated from a college near her home in the Deep South. Now, while waiting for her novel to sell, she did research for a political blogger. With another glance at the paper, she continued. "But before, I'm depressed, cranky, lazy as a hound dog in August, and I don't really give a shit about anything."

Amy's mother, an antifeminist who'd campaigned against the Equal Rights Amendment, had refused to validate Amy's premenstrual symptoms, though she might have had them herself. Amy's problems had begun in her early teens, almost from the time of her first period. "I'd be so pissed off, I'd drive away all my friends. Fortunately, I'm pretty outgoing, so they didn't—don't—stay lost for long. But reliably every month, my breasts get so sensitive they could read Braille. Then I know I'd better put a lock on my tongue, or the next week I'll be buying beers for everyone I know."

Amy tucked her list into her back pocket and sat up straight. "I hate being the feminist with PMS—I feel like a walking cliché."

Discussion of Amy Jernigan

As Amy said, she didn't need much discussion about what was wrong, though she didn't have her terms quite right. Her list of symptoms—depression, irritability, and tension (criterion B) and breast tenderness, lethargy, and loss of interest (C)—exceeds the requirement for a total of five or more. Amy herself indicated just how debilitating she considered the symptoms to be (D). The recurrence, the timing, and the absence of symptoms at times other than before her menses (A) complete a pretty airtight case. The duration of her low moods was too brief for either a **major depressive episode** or **dysthymia** (E). Of course, the usual investigation must be made to rule out any lingering thoughts that her symptoms could be due to **substance use** or **another medical condition** (E). I should note that, in the absence of a couple of months of prospective symptom recording, Amy's clinician needs to be extra careful to rule out major depressive disorder. It is awfully easy to ignore depressive symptoms that occur at other times of the month.

Amy's clinician would have to assess her mood through two subsequent periods to comply with criterion F. When she was ill, her GAF score would be 60, and her diagnosis should be as follows:

N94.3 [625.4]   Premenstrual dysphoric disorder (provisional)

The demand for prospective data before a definitive diagnosis can be made is unique in DSM-5, and has never been required in a prior edition of the DSM. The rationale is to ensure that the diagnosis is made with the best data possible; the fact that such a step is not required for more diagnoses may be a nod to the realities of clinical practice. Even so, we may have just experienced the first breeze of a gathering storm.

F34.8 [296.99] Disruptive Mood Dysregulation Disorder

New in DSM-5, disruptive mood dysregulation disorder (DMDD) showcases extremes of childhood. Most kids fight among themselves, but DMDD broadens the scope and intensity of battle. Minor provocations (insufficient cheese in a sandwich, a favorite shirt in the wash) can provoke these children to fly completely off the handle. In a burst of temper, they may threaten or bully siblings (and parents). Some may refuse to comply with chores, homework, or even basic hygiene. These outbursts occur every couple of days on average, and between them, the child's mood is persistently negative—depressed, angry, or irritable.

Their behavior places these children at enormous social, educational, and emotional disadvantage. Low assessments of functioning reflect the trouble they have interacting with peers, teachers, and relatives. They require constant attention from parents, and if they go to school at all, sometimes they need minders to ensure their own safety and that of others. Some suffer such intense rage that those about them actually fear for their lives. Even relatively mild symptoms may cause children to forgo many normal childhood experiences, such as play dates and party invitations. In one sample, a third had been hospitalized.

Perhaps as many as 80% of children with DMDD will also meet criteria for oppositional defiant disorder, in which case you would only diagnose DMDD. The diagnosis is more common in boys than in girls, placing it at odds with most other mood disorders, though right in line with most other childhood disorders. Although the official DSM-5 criteria remind us not to make the diagnosis prior to age 6, limited studies find that it is most common in preschool children. And it needs to be discriminated from teenage rebellion—the teens are a transitional period where mood symptoms are common.

The question has been asked: Why was DMDD not included in the same chapter with the disruptive, impulse-control, and conduct disorders? Of course, the original impetus was to give clinicians a mood-related alternative to bipolar I disorder. However, the prominent feature of persistently depressed (or irritable) behavior throughout the course of illness seems reason enough for placement with other mood disorders.

Partly because this diagnosis is intended for children, but mainly because I'm really worried about the validity of a newly concocted, poorly studied formulation (see the sidebar below), I'll not provide a vignette or further discussion at this time. At the same time, I'm really, *really* worried about all those kids who are being lumbered with a diagnosis of bipolar disorder, with attendant drug treatment.

How many disorders can you name that originated in an uncomfortable bulge in the number of patients being diagnosed with something else? I can think of exactly one, and here is how it came about.

Beginning in the mid-1990s, a few prominent American psychiatrists sufficiently relaxed the criteria for bipolar disorder to allow that diagnosis in children whose irritability was chronic, not episodic. Subsequently, the number of childhood bipolar diagnoses ballooned. Many other experts howled at what they perceived to be a subversion of the bipolar criteria; thus were drawn the battle lines for diagnostic war.

In aggregate, a number of features seem to set these youngsters well apart from traditional patients with bipolar disorder: (1) Limited follow-up studies find some increase in depression, not mania, in these children as they mature. (2) Family history studies find no excess of bipolar disorder in relatives of these patients. (3) The sex ratio is about 2:1 in favor of boys, which is disparate with the 1:1 ratio for bipolar disorder in older patients. (4) Studies of pathophysiology suggest that brain mechanisms may differentiate the two conditions. (5) The diagnosis of childhood bipolar disorder has been made far more often in the United States than elsewhere in the world. (6) Follow-up studies find far more manic or hypomanic episodes in children with bipolar disorder diagnosed according to traditional criteria than in those whose principal issue was with severe mood dysregulation.

The epic internecine battle among American mental health professionals has been chronicled in a 2008 *Frontline* program ("The Bipolar Child") on PBS and in a *New York Times Magazine* article by Jennifer Egan ("The Bipolar Puzzle," September 12, 2008). The dispute continues; meanwhile, the DMDD category was crafted to capture more accurately the pathology of severely irritable children. The DSM-5 committee struggled to differentiate the two conditions, and I suspect that the struggles have only just begun.

Essential Features of **Disruptive Mood Dysregulation Disorder**

For at least a year, several times a week, on slight provocation a child has severe tantrums—screaming or actually attacking someone (or something)—that are inappropriate for the patient's age and stage of development. Between outbursts, the child seems mostly angry, grumpy, or sad. The attacks and intervening moods occur across multiple settings (home, school, with friends). These patients have no manic episodes.

The Fine Print

Delve into the D's: • Duration and demographics (1+ years, and never absent longer than 3 months, starting before age 10; the diagnosis can only be made from age 6 through 17) • Distress or disability (symptoms are severe in at least one setting—home, school, with other kids—and present in other settings) • Differential diagnosis (substance use and physical disorders, major depressive disorder, bipolar disorders, oppositional defiant disorder, attention-deficit/hyperactivity disorder, behavioral outbursts consistent with developmental age)

Induced Mood Disorders

Substance/Medication-Induced Mood Disorders

Substance use is an especially common cause of mood disorder. Intoxication with cocaine or amphetamines can precipitate manic symptoms, and depression can result from withdrawal from cocaine, amphetamines, alcohol, or barbiturates. Note that for the diagnosis to be tenable, it must develop in close proximity to an episode of intoxication or withdrawal from the substance, which must in turn be capable of causing the symptoms.

Obviously, depression can occur with the misuse of alcohol and street drugs. (As DSM-5 notes, 40% or so of individuals with alcohol use disorder have depressive episodes, of which perhaps half are alcohol-induced, non-independent events.) However, even health care professionals can fail to recognize mood disorders caused by medications (see p. 643). That's why the case of Erin Finn below is a cautionary tale, probably encountered every working day in clinicians' offices around the world.

Essential Features of **Substance/Medication-Induced Depressive Disorder**

The use of some substance appears to have caused a patient to experience marked, persistent depressed mood or loss of interest in usual activities.

The Fine Print

For tips on identifying substance-related causation, see sidebar, page 95.

The D's: • Distress or disability (work/educational, social, or personal impairment) • Differential diagnosis (physical disorders, other depressive disorders, "ordinary" substance intoxication or withdrawal, delirium)

Coding Notes

Specify if:

> **With onset during {intoxication}{withdrawal}.** This gets tacked on at the end of your string of words.
> **With onset after medication use.** You can use this in addition to other specifiers. See sidebar, page 94.

Code depending on whether there is evidence that supports a mild or moderate/severe substance use disorder (see Tables 15.2 and 15.3 in Chapter 15).

Essential Features of **Substance/Medication-Induced Bipolar and Related Disorder**

The use of some substance appears to have caused a mood that is euphoric or irritable.

The Fine Print

For tips on identifying substance-related causation, see sidebar, page 95.

The D's: • Distress or disability (work/educational, social, or personal impairment) • Differential diagnosis (physical disorders, other bipolar disorders, schizoaffective disorder, "ordinary" substance intoxication or withdrawal, delirium)

Coding Notes

> **With onset during {intoxication}{withdrawal}.** This gets tacked on at the end of your string of words.
> **With onset after medication use.** You can use this in addition to other specifiers. See sidebar, page 94.

Code depending on whether there is evidence that supports a mild or moderate/severe substance use disorder (see Tables 15.2 and 15.3 in Chapter 15).

Erin Finn

Erin Finn came to the clinic straight from her job as media specialist at a political campaign. She'd taken part in her state's screening program for hepatitis C, which targeted people in her age group—reared before routine testing of the blood supply had reduced the incidence of the disease. Her test had come back positive. When the RNA polymerase test revealed a viral load, she'd agreed to a trial of interferon. "I sometimes feel tired, but I've had no other symptoms," she'd told her doctor.

Though solidly middle-class and conservatively dressed, Erin had actually had a number of possible exposures to hepatitis C. The most likely was a years-ago blood transfusion, but she'd also "had a wild-ish youth, experimented with injectable drugs a few times, even got a tattoo. It's more or less discreet—the tattoo, I mean."

Within a few days of starting the medication, she'd begun to complain of feeling depressed, first mildly, then increasing day by day. "It felt worse than that day last year when we thought we'd lost in the primary election," she told the interviewer. "It's been a horrible combination of sleeping poorly at night and never completely waking up during the day. And feeling draggy, and tired, and . . . " She groped for words while fiddling with the two campaign buttons pinned to her coat.

Originally hired to do data entry, Erin had been promoted to write campaign materials for brochures and television. But because she was depressed most of the day, her inability to concentrate had resulted in mistakes. "I'm a crap worker," she said, "always making simple mistakes in grammar and spelling. It'll be my fault if we lose in November."

After a moment, she added, "But I'm not suicidal, I'm not that dumb. Or desperate. But some days, I just wish I was dead." She thought for a moment. "Were dead!" she corrected herself. "And my boyfriend tells me I'm useless in bed. Along with everything else, I just don't seem to care about that any more, either."

Erin subsequently stopped the interferon, and her mood and other symptoms gradually returned to normal. "So the doctor thought I ought to try the interferon again, as a sort of challenge. At first, I said that was a total nonstarter! But then I got to worrying some more about cirrhosis, and thought I'd give it another shot. So to speak."

She shrugged as she rolled up her sleeve. "I guess hepatitis treatment has a lot in common with politics—neither of them's bean-bag."

Evaluation of Erin Finn

Erin's symptoms would rate her a diagnosis of (relatively mild) major depressive episode, even leaving out the fatigue (which we won't count because it antedated her use of interferon). Even without all those depressive symptoms, the mere fact of having such a pronounced low mood would fulfill the requirement for medication-induced depressive disorder criterion A. The timing was right (B1), and interferon is well known to produce depressive symptoms in a sizeable number of patients (though more often in those who have had previous mood episodes—B2). And, although it was hardly a controlled experiment, her depressive symptoms did clear up right away, once she stopped the interferon. DSM-5 doesn't specify a challenge test (sometimes such a test is inadvisable), but a return of Erin's depressive symptoms after she resumed the medication would forge the final cause-and-effect link.

OK, so we should consider other possible causes of her depression (criteria C and D). I'll leave that as an exercise for the reader. As for criterion E (distress and disability), res ipsa loquitur. When we turn to Table 15.2 in Chapter 15 for ICD-10 coding, her substance was "Other" (F19), and she had obviously used it only as prescribed, so there was no use disorder. Cross-indexing with the mood disorder column yields F19.94. The ICD-9 code comes from Table 15.3. I would give her GAF score as 55 on admission, 90 at discharge.

| F19.94 [292.84] | Interferon-induced depressive disorder, with onset after medication use |
| B18.2 [070.54] | Chronic hepatitis C |

Mood Disorders Due to Another Medical Condition

Many medical conditions can cause depressive or bipolar symptoms, and it is vital always to consider physical etiologies when evaluating a mood disorder. This is not only because they are treatable; with today's therapeutic options, most mood disorders *are* highly treatable. It is because some of the general medical conditions, if left inadequately treated too long, themselves have serious consequences—including death. And there are not a few that can cause manic symptoms. I've mentioned some of these in the "Physical Disorders That Affect Mental Diagnosis" table in the Appendix, though that table is by no means comprehensive.

Note this really important requirement: The medical condition has to have been the direct, *physiological* cause of the bipolar or depressive symptoms. *Psychological* causation (for instance, the patient feels understandably terrible upon being told "it's cancer") doesn't count, except as the possible precipitant for an adjustment disorder.

The vignette of Lisa Voorhees below illustrates the importance of keeping in mind that medical conditions can cause mood disorders.

Essential Features of **Depressive Disorder Due to Another Medical Condition**

A physical medical condition appears to have caused a patient to experience a markedly depressed mood or loss of interest or pleasure in most activities.

The Fine Print

For pointers on deciding when a physical condition may have caused a mental disorder, see sidebar, page 97.

The D's: • Duration (none stated, though it would not be fleeting) • Distress or disability (work/educational, social, or personal impairment) • Differential diagnosis (substance use disorders, other depressive disorders, delirium)

Coding Notes

Specify:

F06.31 [293.83] With depressive features. You cannot identify full symptomatic criteria for a major depressive episode.
F06.32 [293.83] With major depressive-like episode. You can.
F06.34 [293.83] With mixed features. Manic or hypomanic symptoms are evident but not predominant over the depressive symptoms.

It is only with DSM-5 that criteria have been written specifically differentiating medically induced bipolar from medically induced depressive disorders. What if you can't tell? Some mood disorders, in their early stages, may be too indistinct to call. You might then be reduced to diagnosing mood disorder due to a medical condition (F06.30) or substance-induced mood disorder (F19.94).

Essential Features of **Bipolar and Related Disorder Due to Another Medical Condition**

A physical medical condition appears to have caused a patient to experience both an elevated (or irritable) mood *and* an atypical increase in energy or activity, though full manic episode symptoms may not be present.

The Fine Print

For pointers on deciding when a physical condition may have caused a mental disorder, see sidebar, page 97.

The D's: • Duration (none stated, though it would not be fleeting) • Distress or disability (work/educational, social, or personal impairment) • Differential diagnosis (substance use disorders, other bipolar disorders, other mental disorders, delirium)

Coding Notes

Specify:

> **F06.33 [293.83] With manic- or hypomanic-like episode.** You can identify full symptomatic criteria for mania or hypomania.
> **F06.33 [293.83] With manic features.** Full mania or hypomania criteria are not met.
> **F06.34 [293.83] With mixed features.** Depressive symptoms are evident but not predominant over the manic symptoms.

Lisa Voorhees

By the time she arrived at the mental health clinic, Lisa Voorhees had already seen three doctors. Each of them had thought that her problems were entirely mental. Although she had "been 39 for several years," she was slender and smart, and she knew that she was attractive to men.

She intended to stay that way. Her job as personal secretary to the chairman of the department of English and literature at a large Midwestern university introduced her to a lot of eligible males. And that was where Lisa first noticed the problem that made her think she was losing her mind.

"It was this gorgeous assistant professor of Romance languages," she told the interviewer. "He was always in and out of the office, and I'd done everything short of sexual harassment to get him to notice me. Then one day last spring, he asked me out to dinner and a show. And I turned him down! I just wasn't interested. It was as if my sex drive had gone on sabbatical!"

For several weeks she continued to feel uninterested in men, and then one morning she "woke up next to some odious creep from the provost's office" she'd been avoiding for months. She felt disgusted with herself, but they had sex again anyway, before she kicked him out.

For the next several months, Lisa's sexual appetite would suddenly change every 2 or 3 weeks. Privately, she had begun to call it "The Turn of the Screw." During her active phase, she felt airy and light, and could pound away on her computer 12 hours a day. But the rest of the time, nothing pleased her. She was depressed and grouchy at the office, slept badly (and alone), and joked that her keyboard and mouse were conspiring to make her feel clumsy.

Even Lisa's wrists felt weak. She had bought a wrist rest to use when she was typing, and that helped for a while. But she could find neither splint nor tonic for the fluctuations of her sex drive. One doctor told her it was "the change" and prescribed estrogen; another diagnosed "manic–depression" and offered lithium. A third suggested pastoral counseling, but instead she had come to the clinic.

In frustration, Lisa arose from her chair and paced to the window and back.

"Wait a minute—do that again," the interviewer ordered.

"Do what? All I did was walk across the room."

"I know. How long have you had that limp?"

"I don't know. Not long, I guess. What with the other problems, I hardly noticed. Does it matter?"

It proved to be the key. Three visits to a neurologist, some X-rays, and an MRI later, Lisa's diagnosis was multiple sclerosis. The neurologist explained that multiple sclerosis sometimes caused mood swings; treatment for it was instituted, and Lisa was referred back to the mental health clinic for psychotherapy.

Evaluation of Lisa Voorhees

On paper, the various criteria sets make reasonably clear-cut the differences between mood disorders with "emotional" causes and those caused by general medical conditions or substance use. In practice, it isn't always obvious.

Lisa's mood symptoms alternated between periods of highs and lows. Although they lasted 2 weeks or longer, none of these extremes was severe enough to qualify as a **manic, hypomanic,** or **major depressive episode.** The depressed period was too brief for **dysthymia**; the whole episode had not lasted long enough for **cyclothymic disorder**; and there was no evidence of a **substance-induced mood disorder.**

Depressive (or bipolar) disorder due to another medical condition must fulfill two important criteria. The first is that symptoms must be directly produced by physiological mechanisms of the illness itself, not simply by an emotional reaction to having the illness. For example, patients with cancer of the head of the pancreas are known to have a special risk of depression, which doesn't occur just as a reaction to the news or continuing stress of having a serious medical problem.

Several lines of evidence could bear on a causal relationship between a medical condition and mood symptoms. A connection may exist if the mood disorder is more severe than the general medical symptoms seem to warrant or than the psychological impact would be on most people. However, such a connection would *not* be presumed if the mood symptoms begin before the patient learns of the general medical condition. Similar mood symptoms developing upon the disclosure of a *different* medical problem would argue against a diagnosis of either bipolar or depressive disorder due to another medical condition. By contrast, arguing for a connection would be clinical features different from those usual for a primary mood disorder (such as atypical age of onset). None of these conditions obtained in the case of Lisa Voorhees.

A known pathological mechanism that can explain the development of the mood symptoms in physiological terms obviously argues strongly in favor of a causal relationship. Multiple sclerosis, affecting many areas of the brain, would appear to satisfy this criterion. A high percentage of patients with multiple sclerosis have reported mood swings. Periods of euphoria have also been reported in these patients; anxiety may be more common still.

Many other medical conditions can cause depression. **Endocrine disorders** are important causes: Hypothyroidism and hypoadrenocorticalism are associated with depressive symptoms, whereas hyperthyroidism and hyperadrenocorticalism are linked with manic or hypomanic symptoms. **Infectious diseases** can cause depressive symptoms (many otherwise normal people have noted lassitude and low mood when suffering from a bout of the flu; Lyme disease has been getting a lot of attention recently). **Space-occupying lesions of the brain** (tumors and abscesses) have also been associated with depressive symptoms, as have **vitamin deficiencies.** Finally, about one-third of patients with **Alzheimer's disease, Huntington's disease,** and **stroke** may develop serious depressive symptoms.

The second major criterion for a mood disorder due to another medical condition is that the mood symptoms must not occur only during the course of a **delirium.** Delirious patients can have difficulties with memory, concentration, lack of interest, episodes of tearfulness, and frank depression that closely resemble major depressive disorder. Lisa presented no evidence that suggested delirium.

As to the specifier, we could choose between *with manic features* and *with mixed features* (see Essential Features, above). At different times, Lisa had both extremes of mood; neither predominated, so I'd go with . . . well, see below, along with a GAF score of 70. The code and name of the general medical condition would be included, as follows, with the name of the medical condition:

F06.34 [293.83]   Bipolar disorder due to multiple sclerosis, with mixed features

G35 [340]   Multiple sclerosis

Modifiers of Mood Diagnoses

Table 3.3 (on p. 168) shows at a glance when and how to apply each of the modifiers of mood disorders covered below.

Severity and Remission

Severity Codes

Neither major depressive episode, manic episode, nor hypomanic episode is codable (stop me if you've heard this before). Instead, we use each as the basis for other diagnoses. However, they do have severity codes attached to them, and the same severity codes are used for major depressive and manic episodes. Use these codes for the current or most recent major depressive episode in major depressive, bipolar I, or bipolar II disorders, or the current or most recent manic episode in the two bipolar disorders. (Hypomanic episode is by definition relatively mild, so it gets no severity specifier.)

The basic severity codes for manic and major depressive episodes are these:

Mild. Symptoms barely fulfill the criteria and result in little distress or interference with the patient's ability to work, study, or socialize.

Moderate. Intermediate between mild and severe.

Severe. There are several symptoms more than the minimum for diagnosis, and they markedly interfere with patient's work, social, or personal functioning.

Remission Codes

The majority of patients with bipolar disorders recover completely between episodes (and most of them will have subsequent episodes). Still, up to a third of patients with bipolar I do not recover completely. The figures for patients with major depressive disorder are not quite so grim. Following are two specifiers for current status of both these disorders, as well as bipolar II disorder and persistent depressive disorder (aka dysthymia).

In partial remission. A patient who formerly met full criteria and now either (1) has fewer than the required number of symptoms or (2) has had no symptoms at all, but for under 2 months.

In full remission. For at least 2 months, the patient has had no important symptoms of the mood episode.

Specifiers That Describe the Most Recent Mood Episode

The episode specifiers describe features of the patient's current or most recent episode of illness. No additional code number is assigned for these features; you just write out the verbiage. Again, Table 3.3 shows at a glance when you can use each of the following special qualifiers.

With Anxious Distress

Patients with bipolar I, bipolar II, cyclothymic, major depressive, or persistent depressive disorder may experience symptoms of high anxiety. These patients may have a greater than average potential for suicide and for chronicity of illness.

Essential Features of **With Anxious Distress**

During a major depressive/manic/hypomanic episode or dysthymia, the patient feels notably edgy or tense, and may be extra restless. Typically, it is hard to focus attention because of worries—"Something terrible could happen," or "I could lose control and [fill in the awful consequence] . . . "

Coding Notes

Specify severity: **mild** (2 symptoms of anxious distress), **moderate** (3 symptoms), **moderate–severe** (4–5 symptoms), **severe** (4–5 symptoms plus physical agitation)

See Table 3.3 for application.

There's something kind of funny here. We've been given a mood specifier that has its own severity scale, derived (as are manic and major depressive episodes) by counting symptoms. If there's any other place in DSM-5 where it's possible to have two separate severity ratings in the same diagnosis, I don't recall it. (Other specifiers have several symptoms to count; for example, why don't we also rate severity of *with melancholic features*?) Furthermore, it is at least theoretically possible for a patient to have mild depression with severe anxious distress. Of course, you can rate each part independently, but it could be confusing and it sounds a little silly. My approach would be to focus on the severity of the mood episode. The specifier will probably get along just fine on its own.

With Atypical Features

Not all seriously depressed patients have the classic vegetative symptoms typical of melancholia (see below). Patients who have atypical features seem almost the reverse: Instead of sleeping and eating too little, they sleep and eat too much. This pattern is especially common among younger (teenage and college-age) patients. Indeed, it is common enough that it might better be called *nonclassic depression*.

Two reasons make it important to specify *with atypical features*. First, because such patients' symptoms often include anxiety and sensitivity to rejection, they risk being mislabeled as having an anxiety disorder or a personality disorder. Second, they may respond differently to treatment than do patients with melancholic features. Atypical patients may respond to specific antidepressants (monoamine oxidase inhibitors), and may also show a favorable response to bright light therapy for seasonal (winter) depression.

Iris McMaster's bipolar II disorder included atypical features (p. 136).

Essential Features of **With Atypical Features**

A patient experiencing a major depressive episode feels better when something good happens ("mood reactivity," which obtains whether the patient is depressed or well). The patient *also* has other atypical symptoms: an increase in appetite or weight (the classic depressed patient reports a decrease), excessive sleeping (as opposed to insomnia), a feeling of being sluggish or paralyzed, and long-existing (not just when depressed) sensitivity to rejection.

The Fine Print

The *with atypical features* specifier cannot be used if your patient also has melancholia or catatonic features. See Table 3.3 for application.

With Catatonia

The catatonia specifier, first mentioned in Chapter 2 in association with the psychotic disorders (p. 100), can be applied to manic and major depressive (but not hypomanic) episodes of mood disorders as well. The definitions of the various terms are given in the sidebar on page 101. When you use it, you have to add a line of extra code after listing and coding the other mental disorder:

F06.1 [293.89]   Catatonia associated with [state the mental disorder]

I've given an example in the case of Edward Clapham (p. 102).

With Melancholic Features

The *with melancholic features* specifier refers to the classical "vegetative" symptoms of severe depression and a negative view of the world. Melancholic patients awaken too early in the morning, feeling worse than they do later in the day. They also have reduced appetite and lose weight. They take little pleasure in their usual activities (including sex) and are not cheered by the presence of people whose company they normally enjoy. This loss of pleasure is not merely relative, but total or nearly so. Brian Murphy (p. 124) is an example of such a patient; Noah Sanders (p. 141) is another.

Melancholic features are especially common among patients who first develop severe depression in midlife. This condition used to be called *involutional melancholia*, from the observation that it seemed to occur in patients who were in middle to old age (life's so-called "involutional" period). However, it is now recognized that melancholic features can affect patients of any age; they are especially likely to occur in psychotic depressions. Depression with melancholia usually responds well to somatic treatments such as antidepressant medication and ECT. Contrast this picture with that given for *with atypical features* (see above).

Again, see Table 3.3 for details of when to apply this specifier.

Essential Features of **With Melancholic Features**

In the depths of a major depressive episode, the patient cannot find pleasure in accustomed activities or feels no better if something good happens (OK, could be both). Such a patient also experiences some of these: a mood more deeply depressed than what you'd expect during bereavement; diurnal variation of mood (more depressed in the morning); terminal insomnia (awakening at least 2 hours early); change in psychomotor activity (sometimes agitated, more often slowed down); marked loss of appetite or weight; and guilt feelings that are unwarranted or excessive. This form of depression is extremely severe and can border on psychosis.

Coding Notes

You can apply this specifier to a major depressive episode, wherever it occurs: major depressive disorder (single episode or recurrent), bipolar I or II disorder, or persistent depressive disorder. See Table 3.3.

With Mixed Features

In 1921, Emil Kraepelin first described mixed forms of mania and depression. DSM-IV and its predecessors included a mixed episode among the mood disorders. Now that it's been retired, DSM-5 offers a *with mixed features* specifier to use with patients who within the same time frame have symptoms of depression *and* mania (or hypomania).

The features of the two opposite poles occur more or less at the same time, though some patients experience the gradual introduction (then fading away) of, say, depression into a manic episode.

However, researchers are only just ascertaining the degree to which such a patient differs from someone with "pure" episodic mania or depression. Patients who have mixed features appear to have more total episodes and more depressive episodes, and remain ill longer. They may tend to have more comorbid mental illness and greater suicide risk. Their work is more likely to be impaired. Patients with major depressive disorder who have mixed features are especially likely to develop a bipolar disorder in the future.

Despite this attention, we'll probably continue to use the *with mixed features* specifier less often than could be justified. Several studies suggest that a third or more of bipolar patients have at least one episode with mixed symptoms; some reports suggest that mixed mood states are more frequent in women than in men.

You can apply this specifier to episodes of major depression, mania, and hypomania (see Table 3.3). Because of the greater impairment and overall severity of mania symptoms, if you have a patient who meets full criteria for both mania and major depression, you should probably go with the diagnosis of bipolar I disorder with mixed features, rather than major depressive disorder with mixed features. Winona Fisk (p. 133) had bipolar I disorder with mixed features.

The criteria for *with mixed features* omit some of the mood symptoms found in manic and major depressive episodes. That's because they might conceivably *belong* on both lists, and hence do not indicate a mixed presentation. These symptoms include certain problems with sleep, appetite/weight, irritability, agitation, and concentration. Note, by the way, that the patient must meet *full* criteria for major depressive, manic, or hypomanic episode.

The criteria are silent as to how long each day (or, actually, the majority of days) the mixed features must be present, and I don't know of any data that would help us understand this question better. Right now, even a few minutes a day, repeated day after day, would seem enough to earn this specifier. Only additional research is going to help us understand whether that's a sensible time frame—or too short, or too long. Right now, that picture is decidedly mixed.

Essential Features of **With Mixed Features**

Here, there are two ways to go.

A patient with a manic or hypomanic episode also has some noticeable symptoms of depression most days: depressed mood, low interest or pleasure in activities, an activity level that is speeded up or slowed down, feeling tired, feeling worthless or guilty, and repeated thoughts about death or suicide. (See Coding Note.)

A patient with major depressive episode also has some noticeable symptoms of mania most days: heightened mood, grandiosity, increased talkativeness, flight of ideas, increased energy level, poor judgment (such as excessive spending, sexual adventures, imprudent financial speculations), and reduced need for sleep.

The Fine Print

The D: • Differential diagnosis (physical disorders, substance use disorders)

Coding Note

The impairment and severity of full-blown mania suggest that patients who simultaneously meet full episode criteria for *both* manic and depressive episodes should be recorded as having manic episode, with mixed features.

With Peripartum Onset

Over half of all women have "baby blues" after giving birth: They may feel sad and anxious, cry, complain of poor attention, and have trouble sleeping. This lasts a week or two and is usually of little consequence. But about 10% of women have enough symptoms to be diagnosed as having a depressive disorder; these people often have a personal history of mental disorder. An episode of hypomania may be especially likely after childbirth. Only about 2 out of 1,000 new mothers actually become psychotic.

The *with peripartum onset* specifier has the briefest Essential Features in this book. Though Elisabeth Jacks had a manic episode after giving birth (see p. 131), a major depressive episode would be much the more common response. *With peripartum onset* can apply to bipolar I and bipolar II disorders, to either type of major depressive disorder, or to brief psychotic disorder (see Table 3.3 for all applications except to brief psychotic disorder).

Essential Features of **With Peripartum Onset**

A female patient's mood disorder starts during pregnancy or within a month of giving birth.

Coding Notes

See Table 3.3 for application.

In the mood disorders, it's called *with peripartum onset*. However, when it occurs with brief psychotic disorder, it's called *with postpartum onset*, even though it's described there as occurring "during pregnancy or within 4 weeks postpartum." This is just one more little glitch that will probably get sorted out, by and by. Use it either way in any context, and you're still likely to be understood.

With Psychotic Features

Irrespective of the severity rating, some patients with manic or major depressive episodes will have delusions or hallucinations. (Of course, most of these patients you will have rated as being severely ill, but it is at least theoretically possible that someone could have just a few symptoms—including psychosis—that for whatever reason haven't hugely inconvenienced them.) Around half of patients with bipolar I disorder will have psychotic symptoms; far fewer patients with major depressive disorder will be psychotic.

Psychotic symptoms may be mood-congruent or mood-incongruent. Specify, if possible:

With mood-congruent psychotic features. The content of the patient's delusions or hallucinations is completely in accord with the usual themes of the relevant mood episode. For major depression, these include death, disease, guilt, delusions of nihilism (nothingness), personal inadequacy, or punishment that is deserved; for mania, they include exaggerated ideas of identity, knowledge, power, self-worth, or relationship to God or someone else famous.

With mood-incongruent psychotic features. The content of the patient's delusions or hallucinations is not in accord with the usual themes of the mood episode. For both mania and major depression, these include delusions of persecution, control, thought broadcasting, and thought insertion.

Essential Features of **With Psychotic Features**

The patient has hallucinations or delusions.

Coding Notes

Specify, if possible:

With mood-congruent psychotic features. The psychotic symptoms match what you'd expect from the basic manic or depressive mood (see above).
With mood-incongruent psychotic features. They don't match.

Specifiers That Describe Episode Patterns

Two specifiers describe the frequency or timing of mood episodes. Their appropriate uses are summarized below in Table 3.3, as are those for the other types of specifiers.

With Rapid Cycling

Typically, the bipolar disorders follow a more or less indolent course: a number of months (perhaps 3–9) of depression, followed by somewhat fewer months of mania or hypomania. Other than their number, the individual episodes meet full criteria for major depressive, manic, or hypomanic episodes. As patients age, the entire cycle tends to speed up, but most patients have no more than one up-and-down cycle per year, even after five or more complete cycles. Some patients, however, especially women, cycle much more rapidly than this: They may go from mania to depression to mania again within a few weeks. (Their symptoms meet full mood episode requirements—that's how they differ from cyclothymic disorder.)

Recent research suggests that patients who cycle rapidly are more likely to originate from higher socioeconomic classes; in addition, a past history of rapid cycling predicts that this pattern will continue in the future. Rapid cyclers may be more difficult to manage with standard maintenance regimens than other patients, and they may have a poorer overall prognosis. *With rapid cycling* can apply to bipolar I and bipolar II disorders.

Essential Features of **With Rapid Cycling**

A patient has four or more episodes per year of major depression, mania, or hypomania.

Coding Notes

To count as a separate episode, an episode must be marked by remission (part or full) for 2+ months or by a change in polarity (such as from manic to major depressive episode).

With Seasonal Pattern

Here is yet another specifier for mood disorders that has only been recognized in the last few decades. In the usual pattern, depressive symptoms (these are often also atypical) appear during fall or winter months and remit in the spring and summer. Patients with winter depression may report other difficulties, such as pain disorder symptoms or a craving for carbohydrates, during their depressed phase. Winter depressions occur more commonly in polar climates, especially in the far North, and younger people may be more susceptible. *With seasonal pattern* can apply to bipolar I and bipolar II disorders and to major depressive disorder, recurrent type. There may also be seasonality to manic symptoms, although this is far less well established. (Bipolar I patients may experience the seasonal pattern with one type of episode, not with the other.)

Sal Camozzi's bipolar II disorder included a seasonal pattern. His history is presented in Chapter 11 (p. 304).

Essential Features of **With Seasonal Pattern**

The patient's mood episodes repeatedly begin (and end) at about the same times of year. The seasonal episodes have been the only episodes for at least the past 2 years. Lifelong, seasonal episodes materially outnumber nonseasonal ones

The Fine Print

Disregard examples where there is a clear seasonal cause, such as being laid off every summer.

Putting It All Together: Coding and Labeling the Mood Disorders

Coding and labeling the mood disorders, especially major depressive disorder and bipolar I disorder, have always been complex undertakings—and DSM-5 and ICD-10 have further complicated them. Table 3.2 lays out the possible codes for bipolar I and major depressive disorders. A footnote to this table give two examples of how to label particular presentations of these disorders.

In addition to the three bipolar types listed in Table 3.2, there is also the possibility of bipolar I, unspecified type. That's mainly intended for the folks in the record room when we neglect to indicate the polarity of the most recent episode. We clinicians should ordinarily have little occasion to use this code. Because the episode type is unknown, no episode specifiers can apply.

Table 3.3 (p. 168) summarizes all the descriptors and specifiers that can apply to mood disorders, and indicates with which disorders each modifier can be used.

DSM-5 doesn't say that the depression of bipolar II disorder can have atypical, melancholic, or psychotic features. But neither does it say that it can't. *I* say that if you encounter a patient with bipolar II disorder who has any of those features, step right up and declare it. It'll do you a world of good.

TABLE 3.2. Coding for Bipolar I and Major Depressive Disorders

Severity	Bipolar I, current or most recent episode[a]			Major depressive, current or most recent episode	
	Manic	Hypomanic	Depressed	Single	Recurrent
Mild[b]	F31.11 [296.41]	F31.0 [296.40] (no severity, no psychosis for hypomanic episodes)	F31.31 [296.51]	F32.0 [296.21]	F33.0 [296.31]
Moderate[c]	F31.12 [296.42]		F31.32 [296.52]	F32.1 [296.22]	F33.1 [296.32]
Severe[d]	F31.13 [296.43]		F31.4 [296.53]	F32.2 [296.23]	F33.2 [296.33]
With psychotic features[e]	F31.2 [296.44]	—	F31.5 [296.54]	F32.3 [296.24]	F33.3 [296.34]
In partial remission[f]	F31.73 [296.45]	F31.71 [296.45]	F31.75 [296.55]	F32.4 [296.25]	F33.41 [296.35]
In full remission[g]	F31.74 [296.46]	F31.72 [296.46]	F31.76 [296.56]	F32.5 [296.26]	F33.42 [296.36]
Unspecified	F31.9 [296.40]		F31.9 [296.50]	F32.9 [296.20]	F33.9 [296.30]

Note. Here are two examples of how you put it together: Bipolar I disorder, manic, severe with mood-congruent psychotic features, with peripartum onset, with mixed features. Major depressive disorder, recurrent, in partial remission, with seasonal pattern. Note the order: name → episode type → severity/psychotic/remission → other specifiers.

[a]If the bipolar I type isn't specified, code as F31.9 [296.7].

[b]Mild. Meets the minimum of symptoms, which are distressing but interfere minimally with functionality.

[c]Moderate. Intermediate between mild and severe.

[d]Severe. Many serious symptoms that profoundly impede patient's functioning.

[e]If psychotic features are present, use these code numbers regardless of severity (it will almost always be severe, anyway). Record these features as mood-congruent or mood-incongruent (p. 164).

[f]Partial remission. Symptoms are no longer sufficient to meet criteria.

[g]Full remission. For 2 months or more, the patient has been essentially free of symptoms.

Other Specified and Unspecified Mood Disorders

F31.89 [296.89] Other Specified Bipolar and Related Disorder

Use other specified bipolar and related disorder when you want to write down the specific reason your patient cannot receive a more definite bipolar diagnosis. To prevent overuse and "medicalization" of the normal ebb and flow of mood, the patient must have symptoms that don't qualify for a more specific bipolar disorder diagnosis *and* that cause distress or interfere with the patient's normal functioning. DSM-5 gives a number of examples:

Short-duration hypomanic episodes (2–3 days) and major depressive episodes. Such a patient will have had at least one fully qualified major depressive episode, plus at least one episode of hypomania too brief (2–3 days) to justify a diagnosis of bipolar II disorder. Because the depression and hypomania don't occur together, a *with mixed features* designation wouldn't be appropriate.

TABLE 3.3. Descriptors and Specifiers That Can Apply to Mood Disorders

Disorder	Severity/ remission (p. 158)	With mixed features (p. 161)	With anxious distress (p. 159)	With catatonia[a] (p. 160)	With atypical features (p. 160)	With melancholic features (p. 161)	With peripartum onset (p. 163)	With psychotic features (p. 164)	With rapid cycling (p. 165)	With seasonal pattern (p. 165)
Major depression										
Single episode	×	×	×	×	×	×	×	×		
Recurrent	×	×	×	×	×	×	×	×		×
Bipolar I										
Most recent mania	×	×	×	×			×	×	×	×
Most recent depression	×	×	×	×	×	×	×	×	×	×
Most recent hypomania	×	×	×				×		×	×
Most recent unspecified										
Bipolar II										
Most recent hypomanic	×	×	×				×		×	
Most recent depressed	×	×	×	×	×	×	×	×	×	×
Cyclothymia			×							
Persistent (dysthymia)	×	×	×		×	×	×	×		

Note. This table can help you to choose the sometimes lengthy string of names, codes, and modifiers for the mood disorders. Start reading from left to right in the table, putting in any modifiers that apply in the order you come to them. Dysthymia can also have early or late onset, plus a variety of additional specifiers (p. 140).

[a]The catatonia specifier requires its own line of code and description. (See p. 100.)

Hypomanic episodes with insufficient symptoms and major depressive episodes. Such a patient will have had least one major depressive episode but no actual manic or hypomanic episodes, though there will have been at least one episode of *subthreshold hypomania*. That is, the high phase is long enough (4 days or more) but is a symptom or two shy of the number required for a hypomanic episode (elevated mood plus one or two of the other symptoms of a hypomanic episode, *or* irritable mood plus two or three of the other symptoms of hypomania). The hypomanic and major depressive symptoms don't overlap, so you can't call it major depressive episode with mixed features.

Hypomanic episode without prior major depressive episode. Here you'd classify (no surprise) someone who has had an episode of hypomania but who hasn't ever fully met criteria for a major depressive episode or a manic episode.

Short-duration cyclothymia. In a period less than 2 years (less than 12 months for a child or adolescent), such a patient will have had multiple episodes of both hypomanic symptoms and depressive symptoms, all of which will have been either too brief or have too few symptoms to qualify for a major depressive or hypomanic episode. Of course, there will be no manias and no symptoms of psychosis. Patients with short-duration cyclothymia will have symptoms for a majority of days and will have no symptom-free periods longer than 2 months.

Note that DSM-5 cautions us *not* to use just other specified bipolar disorder or other specified depressive disorder as the actual diagnosis. Rather, we are also supposed to state, in full, one of the many (often cumbersome) titles given in the bipolar list just above and the depressive list below. One thing is certain: Regardless of which of the several discrete terms we choose, there is just one code number for each of these two categories of uncertainty.

F31.9 [296.80] Unspecified Bipolar and Related Disorder

And here you'd include patients for whom you don't care to indicate the reason you aren't diagnosing a well-defined bipolar condition.

F32.8 [311] Other Specified Depressive Disorder

Use other specified depressive disorder in the same way as described above for other specified bipolar and related disorder. DSM-5 provides the following examples of other specified depressive disorder:

Recurrent brief depression. Every month for 12+ months, lasting from 2 to 13 days at a time, these patients have low mood plus at least four other symptoms of depression that aren't associated with menstruation. The patients have never fulfilled criteria for another mood disorder, and they've not been psychotic.

Short-duration depressive episode. These patients would meet criteria for major depressive episode except for duration—their episodes last 4–13 days. Here's the full run-down: depressed mood; at least four other major depressive symptoms; clinically significant distress or impairment; have never met criteria for other mood disorders; not currently psychotic; and don't meet criteria for other conditions.

Depressive episode with insufficient symptoms. These patients would meet criteria (duration, distress) for major depression, except that they have too few symptoms. They don't have another psychotic or mood disorder.

F32.9 [311] Unspecified Depressive Disorder

As for unspecified bipolar and related disorder, when you don't care to indicate the reason for a more secure diagnosis, you can use the unspecified depressive disorder category. The advantage: mood disorders "of uncertain etiology" have been used so often in the past as to undermine their value.

Whenever we clinicians encounter a patient with schizophrenia and postpsychotic depressive disorder, or one with a major depressive episode superimposed on a psychosis, we should think extra carefully about the diagnosis. Likewise, the occurrence of a manic episode in a patient who was formerly diagnosed as psychotic should cause us to wonder whether the original diagnosis was correct. In both cases, some of these patients may actually have bipolar I disorder, and not schizophrenia or another psychotic disorder at all. This would appear to be an ongoing problem, regardless of which edition of the DSM we are using.

CHAPTER 4

Anxiety Disorders

Quick Guide to the Anxiety Disorders

One or more of the following conditions may be diagnosed in patients who present with prominent anxiety symptoms; a single patient may have more than one anxiety disorder. As usual, the page number following each item indicates where a more detailed discussion begins.

Primary Anxiety Disorders

Panic disorder. These patients experience repeated panic attacks—brief episodes of intense dread accompanied by a variety of physical and other symptoms, together with worry about having additional attacks and other related mental and behavioral changes (p. 176).

Agoraphobia. Patients with this condition fear situations or places such as entering a store, where they might have trouble obtaining help if they became anxious (p. 179).

Specific phobia. In this condition, patients fear specific objects or situations. Examples include animals; storms; heights; blood; airplanes; being closed in; or any situation that may lead to vomiting, choking, or developing an illness (p. 182).

Social anxiety disorder. These patients imagine themselves embarrassed when they speak, write, or eat in public or use a public urinal (p. 185).

Selective mutism. A child elects not to talk, except when alone or with select intimates (p. 187).

Generalized anxiety disorder. Although they experience no episodes of acute panic, these patients feel tense or anxious much of the time and worry about many different issues (p. 191).

Separation anxiety disorder. The patient becomes anxious when separated from a parent or other attachment figure (p. 188).

Anxiety disorder due to another medical condition. Panic attacks and generalized anxiety symptoms can be caused by numerous medical conditions (p. 195).

Substance/medication-induced anxiety disorder. Use of a substance or medication has caused panic attacks or other anxiety symptoms (p. 193).

Other specified, or unspecified, anxiety disorder. Use these categories for disorders with prominent anxiety symptoms that don't fit neatly into any of the groups above (p. 198).

Other Causes of Anxiety and Related Symptoms

Obsessive–compulsive disorder. These patients are bothered by repeated thoughts or behaviors that can appear senseless, even to them (p. 200).

Posttraumatic stress disorder. A severely traumatic event, such as combat or a natural disaster, is relived over and over (p. 219).

Acute stress disorder. This condition is much like posttraumatic stress disorder, except that it begins during or immediately after the stressful event and lasts a month or less (p. 224).

Avoidant personality disorder. These timid people are so easily wounded by criticism that they hesitate to become involved with others (p. 553).

With anxious distress specifier for major depressive disorder. Some patients with major depressive disorder have much accompanying tension and anxiety (p. 159).

Somatic symptom disorder and **illness anxiety disorder**. Panic and other anxiety symptoms are often part of somatic symptom disorder and illness anxiety disorder (pp. 251 and 260).

Introduction

The conditions discussed in this chapter are characterized by anxiety and the behaviors by which people try to ward it off. Panic disorder, the various phobias, and generalized anxiety disorder are collectively among the most frequently encountered of all mental disorders listed in DSM-5. Yet, in discussing them, we must also keep in mind three other facts about anxiety.

The first of these is that a certain amount of anxiety isn't just normal, but adaptive and perhaps vital for our well-being and normal functioning. For example, when we are about to take an examination or speak in public (or write a book), the fear of failure spurs us on to adequate preparation. Similarly, normal fear lies behind our healthy regard for excessive debt, violent criminals, and poison ivy.

Anxiety is also a symptom—one that's encountered in many, perhaps most, mental disorders. Because it is so dramatic, we sometimes focus our attention on the anxiety to the exclusion of historical data and other symptoms (depression, substance use, and problems with memory, to name just a few) that are crucial to diagnosis. I've interviewed countless patients whose anxiety symptoms have masked mood, somatic symptom, or other disorders—conditions that are often not only highly treatable when they are recognized, but deadly when they are not.

The third issue I want to emphasize is that anxiety symptoms can sometimes indicate the presence of a substance use problem, another medical condition, or even a different mental disorder altogether (such as a mood, somatic symptom, cognitive, or substance-related disorder). These conditions should be considered for any patient who presents with anxiety or avoidance behavior.

Once again, I've eschewed DSM-5's organization, which seems to rely on the typical age of onset (most anxiety disorders begin when the patient is relatively young). Rather, I've started with panic attacks, because they are pervasive throughout the anxiety (and many other) disorders.

Panic Attack

Someone in the throes of a panic attack feels foreboding—a sense of disaster that is usually accompanied by cardiac symptoms (such as irregular or rapid heartbeat) and trouble breathing (shortness of breath, chest pain). The attack usually begins abruptly and builds rapidly to a peak; the whole, miserable experience usually lasts less than half an hour.

Here are several important facts about panic attacks:

- They are common (perhaps 30% of all adults have experienced at least one). In a 12-month period, over 10% of Americans will have one (though they are apparently about a third as common among Europeans).

- Women are more often affected than men.

- They can occur as isolated experiences in normal adults; in such cases, there is no diagnosis at all.

- Panic attacks may occur within a broad spectrum of frequency, from just a few episodes in the lifetime of some individuals to many times per week in others. Some people even awaken at night with *nocturnal* attacks.

- Untreated, they can be severely debilitating. Many patients change their behavior in reaction to the fear that the attacks mean they are psychotic or physically ill.

- Treatment is sometimes easy, perhaps just by providing a little reassurance or a paper bag to breathe into.

- But sometimes panic attacks mask other illnesses that range from mood disorders to heart attacks.

- Some panic attacks are triggered by specific situations, such as crossing a bridge or roaming a crowded supermarket. Such attacks are said to be *cued* or *situationally bound*. Others have no relationship to a specific stimulus but arise spontaneously, as in panic disorder. These are termed unexpected or *uncued*. A third type, *situationally predisposed* attacks, consists of attacks in which the patient often (but not invariably) becomes panic-stricken when confronted by the stimulus.

- The patient can be calm or anxious when the upswing in panic symptoms begins.

- By themselves, panic attacks are not codable. The criteria are given so that they can be identified and applied as a specifier to whatever disorder may be appropriate. Of course, they always occur in panic disorder, but there you don't have to specify them: they go with the territory.

Pathological panic attacks usually begin in a person's 20s. Panic attacks may occur without other symptoms (when they may qualify for a diagnosis of panic disorder) or in connection with a variety of other disorders, which may include agoraphobia, social anxiety disorder, specific phobia, posttraumatic stress disorder (PTSD), mood disorders, and psychotic disorders. They can also feature in anxiety disorder due to another medical condition and in substance-induced anxiety disorder.

Essential Features of **Panic Attack**

A panic attack is fear, sometimes stark terror, that begins suddenly and is accompanied by a variety of classic "fight-or-flight" symptoms, plus a few others—chest pain, chills, feeling too hot, choking, shortness of breath, rapid or irregular heartbeat, tingling or numbness, excessive perspiration, nausea, dizziness, and tremor. As a result, these people may feel unreal or be afraid that they are losing their minds or dying. At least four of the somatic sensations are required.

Coding Notes

Panic attack is not a codable disorder. It provides the basis for panic disorder, and it can be attached as a specifier to other diagnoses. These include posttraumatic stress disorder, other anxiety disorders, and other mental disorders (including eating, mood, psychotic, personality, and substance use disorders). They are even found in medical conditions affecting the heart, lungs, and gastrointestinal tract.

Shorty Rheinbold

Seated in the clinician's waiting room, Shorty Rheinbold should have been relaxed. The lighting was soft, the music soothing; the sofa on which he was sitting was comfortably upholstered. Angel fish swam lazily in their sparkling glass tank. But Shorty felt anything but calm. Perhaps it was the receptionist—he wondered whether she was competent to handle an emergency with his sort of problem. She looked something like a badger, holed up behind her computer. For several minutes he had been feeling worse with every heartbeat.

His heart was the key. When Shorty first sat down, he hadn't even noticed it, quietly ticking away, just doing its job inside his chest. But then, without any warning, it had begun to demand his attention. At first it had only skipped a beat or two, but after a minute, it had begun a ferocious assault on the inside of his chest wall. Every beat had become a painful, bruising thump that caused him to clutch at his chest. He tried to keep his hands under his jacket so as not to attract too much attention.

The pounding heart and chest pain could mean only one thing—after 2 months of attacks every few days, Shorty was beginning to get the message. Then, right on schedule, the shortness of breath began. It seemed to arise from his left chest area, where his heart was doing all the damage. It clawed its way up through his lungs and into his throat, gripping him around the neck so he could breathe only in the briefest of gulps.

He was dying! Of course, the cardiologist Shorty consulted the week before had assured him that his heart was as sound as a brass bell, but this time he knew it was about to fail. He couldn't fathom why he hadn't died before; he had feared it with every attack. Now it seemed impossible that he would survive this one. Did he even want to? That thought made him suddenly want to retch.

Shorty leaned forward so he could grip both his chest and his abdomen as unobtrusively as possible. He could hardly hold anything at all: The familiar tingling and numbness had started up in his fingers, and he could sense the shaking of his hands as they tried to contain the various miseries that had taken over his body.

He glanced across the room to see whether Miss Badger had noticed. No help was coming from that quarter; she was still pounding away at her keyboard. Perhaps all the patients behaved this way. Perhaps—suddenly, there *was* an observer. Shorty was watching himself! Some part of him had floated free and seemed to hang suspended, halfway up the wall. From this vantage point, he could look down and view with pity and scorn the quivering flesh that was, or had been, Shorty Rheinbold.

Now the Spirit Shorty saw that Shorty's face had become fiery red. Hot air had filled his head, which seemed to expand with every gasp. He floated farther up the wall and the ceiling melted away; he soared out into the brilliant sunshine. He squeezed his eyes shut but could not keep out the blinding light.

Depression is so often found in patients who complain of recurrent panic attacks that the association cannot be overemphasized. Some studies suggest that over half the patients with panic disorder also have major depressive disorder. Clearly, we must carefully evaluate for symptoms of a mood disorder everyone who presents with panic symptoms.

Evaluation of Shorty Rheinbold

Shorty's panic attack was typical: It began suddenly, developed rapidly, and included a generous helping of the required symptoms. His shortness of breath (criterion A4) and heart palpitations (A1) are classical panic attack symptoms; he also had chest pain (A6), lightheadedness (A8), and numbness in his fingers (A10). Shorty's fear that he would die (A13) is typical of the fears that patients have during an attack. The sensation of watching himself (depersonalization—A11) is a less common symptom of panic. He needed only four of these symptoms to substantiate the fact of panic attack.

Shorty's panic attack was uncued, which means that it seemed to happen spontaneously, without provocation. He was unaware of any event, object, or thought that triggered it. Uncued attacks are typical of **panic disorder**, which can also include cued (or situationally bound) attacks. The panic attacks that develop in **social anxiety disorder** and **specific phobia** are cued to the stimuli that repeatedly and predictably pull the trigger.

Panic attacks can occur in several **medical conditions**. One of these is acute myocardial infarction, the very condition many panic patients fear the most. Of course, when indicated patients with symptoms like Shorty's should be evaluated for myocardial infarction and other medical disorders. These include low blood sugar, irregular heartbeat, mitral valve prolapse, temporal lobe epilepsy, and a rare adrenal gland tumor called a pheochromocytoma. Panic attacks also occur during intoxication with several **psychoactive substances,** including **amphetamines**, **marijuana**, and **caffeine**. (Note that in addition, some patients misuse alcohol or sedative drugs in an effort to reduce the severity of their panic attacks.)

There is no code number associated with panic attack. I'll give Shorty's complete diagnosis below.

F41.0 [300.01] Panic Disorder

Panic disorder is a common anxiety disorder in which the patient experiences *unexpected* panic attacks (usually many, but always more than one) and worries about having another. Though the panic attacks are usually uncued, situationally predisposed attacks and cued/situationally bound attacks also occur (see definitions, above). A strong minority will have nocturnal panic attacks as well as those that occur while awake. Perhaps half of patients with panic disorder also have symptoms of agoraphobia (see p. 179), though many do not.

Panic disorder typically begins during the patient's early 20s. It is one of the most common anxiety disorders, found in 1–4% of the general adult population (10% is the approximate figure for panic attacks in general). It is especially common among women.

Essential Features of **Panic Disorder**

As a result of surprise panic attacks (see the preceding description), the patient fears that they will happen again or tries to avert further attacks by taking (ineffective) action, such as abandoning an once-favored activities or avoiding places where attacks have occurred.

The Fine Print

Don't forget the D's: • Duration (1+ months) • Distress or disability (as above) • Differential diagnosis (substance use and physical disorders, other anxiety disorders, mood and psychotic disorders, obsessive–compulsive disorder [OCD], PTSD, actual danger)

Shorty Rheinbold Again

Shorty opened his eyes to discover that he was lying on his back on the waiting room floor. Two people were bending over him. One was the receptionist. He didn't recognize the other, but he guessed it must be the mental health clinician who was supposed to interview him.

"I feel like you saved my life," he said.

"Not really," the clinician replied. "You're just fine. Does this happen often?"

"Every 2 or 3 days now." Shorty cautiously sat up. After a moment or two, he allowed them to help him to his feet and into the inner office.

Just when his problem had begun wasn't quite clear at first. Shorty was 24 and had spent 4 years in the Coast Guard. Since his discharge, he'd knocked around a bit, and then moved in with his folks while he worked in construction. Six months ago, he'd gotten a job as cashier in a filling station.

That was just fine, sitting in a glassed-in booth all day making change, running credit cards through the electronic scanner, and selling chewing gum. The wages weren't exciting, but he didn't have to pay rent. Even with eating out almost every evening, Shorty still had enough at the end of the week to take his girl out on Saturday nights. Neither one of them drank or used drugs, so even that didn't set him too far back.

The problem had begun the day after Shorty had been working for a couple of months, when the boss told him to go out on the wrecker with Bruce, one of the mechanics. They had stopped along the eastbound Interstate to pick up an old Buick Skylark with a blown head gasket. For some reason, they had trouble getting it into the sling. Shorty was on the traffic side of the truck, trying to manipulate the hoist in response to Bruce's shouted directions. Suddenly, a caravan of tractor-trailer trucks roared past. The noise and the blast of wind caught Shorty off guard. He spun around into the side of the wrecker, fell, and rolled to a stop, inches from huge tires rolling by.

Shorty's color and heart rate had returned to normal. The remainder of his story was easy enough to tell. He continued to go out on the wrecker, even though he felt scared, near panic every time he did so. He'd only go when Bruce was along, and he carefully avoided the traffic side of the vehicles.

But that wasn't the worst of the problem—he could always quit and get another job. Lately, Shorty had been having these attacks at other times, when he was least expecting them. Now nothing seemed to trigger the attacks; they just happened, though not when he was at home or in his glass cage at work. When he was shopping last week, he'd had to abandon the cart full of groceries he was buying for his mother. Now he didn't even want to go to the movies with his girl. For the last few weeks he had suggested that they spend Saturday night at her place watching TV instead. She hadn't complained yet, but he knew it was only a matter of time.

"I have just about enough strength to tough it out through the work day," Shorty said. "But I've got to get a handle on this thing. I'm too young to spend the rest of my life like a hermit in a cave."

Further Evaluation of Shorty Rheinbold

The fact that Shorty experienced panic attacks has already been established. They were originally associated with the specific situation of working around the wrecker. For months now, they occurred every few days, usually catching him unaware (panic disorder criterion A). Undoubtedly worried and concerned (B1), he had altered his activities with his girlfriend (B2). A number of **medical conditions** can cause panic attacks; however, a cardiologist had recently pronounced Shorty to be medically fit. **Substance-induced anxiety disorder** (C) is also eliminated by the history: Shorty didn't use drugs or alcohol. (However, watch out for patients who "medicate" their panic attacks with drugs or alcohol.) With no other mental disorder more likely (D), his symptoms fully support a diagnosis of panic disorder.

But wait, as they say, there's more, for which we'll have to consider the symptoms of agoraphobia. Recently, Shorty feared all sorts of other situations that involved being away from home—driving, shopping, even going to the movies (agoraphobia criterion A)—which nearly always provoked panic (C). As a result, he either avoided the situations or had to be accompanied by Bruce or by his girlfriend (D). Shorty's life space had already begun to contract as a result of his fears; without treatment, it would seem to be only a matter of time before he would have to quit his job and remain at home (G). These symptoms are typical; we won't quibble about the exact duration, because they are so severe (F). They'll fulfill the requirements for agoraphobia, provided that we can rule out other etiologies for his symptoms (H, I). Sure, we should ask to determine that driving him was the fear that help would be unavailable or that escape would be difficult (B), but knowing Shorty, I'm pretty sure of the answer.

The diagnosis of **specific phobia** or **social anxiety disorder** would seem unlikely, because the focus of Shorty's anxiety was not a single issue (such as enclosed places) or a social situation. Patients with **somatic symptom disorder** also complain of anxiety symptoms (though they aren't a diagnostic feature), but this is an unlikely diagnosis for a physically healthy man.

Although the vignette doesn't address this possibility, **major depressive disorder** is comorbid with panic disorder in half of the cases. The danger lies in the often dramatic anxiety symptoms overshadowing subtle depressive symptoms, so that the clinician overlooks them completely. When the criteria for both an anxiety and a mood disorder are met, they should both be listed. Other anxiety disorders can be comorbid in panic disorder patients; these include **generalized anxiety disorder** and **specific phobia**.

Shorty's mood was anxious, not depressed or irritable. I'd give him a GAF score of 61. His diagnosis would be as follows:

F41.0 [300.01]	Panic disorder
F40.00 [300.22]	Agoraphobia

It can be really hard to differentiate panic disorder and agoraphobia from other anxiety disorders that involve avoidance (especially specific phobia and social anxiety disorder). The final decision often comes down to clinical judgment, though the following sorts of information can help:

1. How many panic attacks does the patient have, and what type are they (cued, uncued, situationally predisposed)? Uncued attacks suggest panic disorder; cued attacks suggest specific phobia or social anxiety disorder. (But they can be intermixed.)
2. In how many situations do they occur? Limited situations suggest specific phobia or social anxiety disorder; attacks that occur in a variety of situations suggest panic disorder and agoraphobia.
3. Does the patient awaken at night with panic attacks? This is more typical of panic disorder.
4. What is the focus of the fear? If it is having a subsequent panic attack, panic disorder may be the correct diagnosis—unless the panic attacks occur only when the patient is, say, riding in an airplane, in which case you might correctly diagnose specific phobia, situational type.
5. Does the patient constantly worry about having panic attacks, even when in no danger of facing a feared situation (such as riding in an elevator)? This would suggest panic disorder and agoraphobia.

F40.00 [300.22] Agoraphobia

The *agora* was the marketplace to ancient Greeks. In contemporary usage, *agoraphobia* refers to the fear some people have of any situation or place where escape seems difficult or embarrassing, or where help might be unavailable if anxiety symptoms should occur. Open or public places such as theaters and crowded supermarkets qualify; so does travel from home. Persons with agoraphobia either avoid the feared place or situation entirely, or, if they must confront it, suffer intense anxiety or require the presence of a companion. In any event, agoraphobia is a concept the Greeks didn't have a word for; it was first used in 1873.

Agoraphobia usually involves such situations as being away from home; standing in a crowd; staying home alone; being on a bridge; or traveling by bus, car, or train. Agoraphobia can develop rapidly, within just a few weeks, in the wake of a series of panic attacks (see p. 173), when fear of recurrent attacks causes the patient to avoid leaving home or participating in other activities. Some patients develop agoraphobia without any preceding panic attacks.

In recent years, estimates of the prevalence of agoraphobia have risen to the neighborhood of 1–2%. As with panic disorder, women are more susceptible than men; the disorder usually begins in the teens or 20s, though some patients have their first symptoms after the age of 40. Often panic attacks precede the onset of the agoraphobia. It is strongly heritable.

Essential Features of **Agoraphobia**

These patients almost invariably experience inordinate anxiety or dread when they have to be alone or away from home. Potentially, there's an abundance of opportunity: riding a bus (or other mass transit), shopping, attending a theatrical entertainment. For some, it's as ordinary as walking through an open space (flea market, playground), being part of a crowd, or standing in a queue. When you explore their thinking, these people are afraid that escape would be impossible or that help (in the event of panic) unavailable. So they avoid such situations or confront them only with a trusted friend or, if all else fails, endure them with lots of suffering.

The Fine Print

Don't duck the D's: • Duration (6+ months) • Distress or disability (work/educational, social, or personal impairment) • Differential diagnosis (substance use and physical disorders, other anxiety disorders, mood and psychotic disorders, OCD, PTSD, social and separation anxiety disorders, situational phobias, panic disorder)

Lucy Gould

"I'd rather have her with me, if that's all right." Lucy Gould was responding to the clinician's suggestion that her mother wait outside the office. "By now, I don't have any secrets from her."

Since age 18, Lucy hadn't gone anywhere without her mother. In fact, in those 6 years she'd hardly been anywhere at all. "There's no way I could go out by myself—it's like entering a war zone. If someone's not with me, I can barely stand to go to doctor appointments and stuff like that. But I still feel awfully nervous."

The nervousness Lucy complained of hadn't included actual panic attacks; she never felt that she couldn't breathe or was about to die. Rather, she experienced an intense motor agitation that had caused her to flee from shopping malls, supermarkets, and movie theaters. Nor could she ride on public transportation; buses and trains both terrified her. She had the feeling, vague but always present, that something awful would happen there. Perhaps she would become so anxious that she would pass out or wet herself, and no one would be able to help her. She hadn't been alone in public since the week before her high school commencement. She had only been able to go up onto the platform to receive her diploma because she was with her best friend, who would know what to do if she needed help.

Lucy had always been a timid, rather sensitive girl. The first week of kindergarten, she had cried each time her mother left her by herself at school. But her father had insisted that she "toughen up," and within a few weeks she had nearly forgotten her terror. She'd subsequently maintained a nearly perfect attendance record at school. Then, shortly after her 17th birthday, her father died of leukemia. Her terror of being away from home had begun within a few weeks of his funeral.

To make ends meet, her mother had sold their house, and they had moved into a condominium across the street from the high school. "It's the only way I got through my last year," Lucy explained.

For several years, Lucy had kept house while her mother assembled circuit boards at an electronics firm outside town. Lucy was perfectly comfortable in that role, even though her mother was away for hours at a time. Her physical health had been good; she had never used drugs or alcohol; and she had never had depression, suicidal ideas, delusions, or hallucinations. But a year ago Lucy had developed insulin-dependent diabetes, which required frequent trips to the doctor. She had tried to take the bus by herself, but after several failures— once, in the middle of traffic, she had forced the rear door open and sprinted for home—she had given up. Now her mother was applying for disability assistance so that she could remain at home to provide the aid and attendance Lucy required.

Evaluation of Lucy Gould

Because of her fears, which were inordinate and out of proportion to the actual danger (criterion E), Lucy avoided a variety of situations and places, including supermarkets, malls, buses, and trains (A). If she did go, she required a companion (D). She couldn't state exactly what might happen—only that it would be awful and embarrassing (she might even lose bladder control) and that help might not be available (B). It is not unusual that her symptoms only came to light when another problem (diabetes) prevented her from staying at home; diabetes itself isn't associated with agoraphobic fears (H). OK, you'll have to read between the lines of the vignette to verify criteria C (the situations almost always provoke anxiety) and G (the patient experiences clinically important distress or impairment).

Lucy's symptoms were too varied for **specific phobia** or **social anxiety disorder**.

(Note also that in agoraphobia, the perceived danger emanates from the environment; in social anxiety disorder, it comes from the relationship with other people.) Her problem wasn't that she feared being left alone, as would be the case with **separation anxiety disorder** (although when she was five she clearly had had elements of that diagnosis). She hadn't had a major trauma, as would be the case in **PTSD** (the death of her father was traumatic, but her own symptoms didn't focus on reliving this experience). There is no indication that she had **OCD**. And so (finally!) we have disposed of criterion I.

Agoraphobia can accompany a variety of diagnoses, the most important of which are mood disorders that involve major depressive episodes. However, Lucy denied having symptoms of depression, psychosis, and substance use. Although she had diabetes, it developed many years after her agoraphobia symptoms became apparent. Besides, it's hard to imagine a physiological connection between agoraphobia and diabetes, and her anxiety symptoms were far more extensive than the realistic concerns you'd expect from the average diabetic individual.

Because Lucy had never experienced a discrete panic attack, she would not meet the criteria for panic disorder in addition to her agoraphobia. By the way, the fact that she was housebound would net her a low GAF score (31).

F40.00 [300.22]	Agoraphobia
E10.9 [250.01]	Insulin-dependent diabetes mellitus

Specific Phobia

Patients with specific phobias have unwarranted fears of specific objects or situations. The best recognized are phobias of animals, blood, heights, travel by airplane, being closed in, and thunderstorms. The anxiety produced by exposure to one of these stimuli may take the form of a panic attack or of a more generalized sensation of anxiety, but it is always directed at something specific. (However, these patients can also worry about what they might do—faint, panic, lose control—if they have to confront whatever it is they are afraid of.) Generally, the closer they are to the feared stimulus (and the more difficult it would be to escape), the worse they feel.

Patients usually have more than one specific phobia. A person who is about to face one of these feared activities or objects will immediately begin to feel nervous or panicky—a condition known as *anticipatory anxiety.* The degree of discomfort is often mild, however, so most people do not seek professional help. When it causes a patient to avoid feared situations, anticipatory anxiety can be a major inconvenience; it can even interfere with working. Patients with specific phobias involving blood, injury, or injection often experience what is called a *vasovagal response*; this means that reduced heart rate and blood pressure actually do cause the patients to faint.

In the general population, specific phobia is one of the most frequently reported anxiety disorders. Up to 10% of U.S. adults have suffered to some degree from one of these specific phobias. However, by no means would all of these people qualify for a DSM-5 diagnosis: The clinical significance of these reported fears is so hard to judge.

Onset is usually in childhood or adolescence; animal phobias especially tend to begin early. Some begin after a traumatic event, such as being bitten by an animal. A situational fear (such as being closed in or traveling by air) is more likely than other types of specific phobia to have a comorbid disorder such as depression and substance misuse, though comorbidity with a wide range of mental disorders is the rule. Females outnumber males, perhaps by a 2:1 ratio.

Essential Features of **Specific Phobia**

A specific situation or thing habitually causes such immediate, inordinate (and unreasonable) dread or anxiety that the patient avoids it or endures it with much anxiety.

The Fine Print

The D's: • Duration (6+ months) • Distress or disability (work/educational, social, or personal impairment) • Differential diagnosis (substance use and physical disorders, agoraphobia, social anxiety disorder, separation anxiety disorder, mood and psychotic disorders, anorexia nervosa, OCD, PTSD)

Coding Notes

Specify all types that apply with individual ICD-10 codes:

F40.218 [300.29] Animal type (snakes, spiders)
F40.228 [300.29] Natural environment type (thunderstorms, heights)
Blood–injection–injury type (syringes, operations):

F40.230 [300.29] Blood
F40.231 [300.29] Injections and transfusions
F40.232 [300.29] Other medical care
F40.233 [300.29] Injury

F40.248 [300.29] Situational type (traveling by air, being closed in)
F40.298 [300.29] Other type (situations where the person could vomit or choke; for children, loud noises or people wearing costumes)

Esther Dugoni

A slightly built woman of nearly 70, Esther Dugoni was healthy and fit, though in the last year or two she had developed a tremor characteristic of early Parkinson's disease. For the several years since she had retired from her job teaching horticulture in junior college, she had concentrated on her own garden. At the flower show the year before, her rhododendrons had won first prize.

But 10 days earlier, her mother had died in Detroit, over halfway across the country. She and her sister had been appointed co-executors. The estate was large, and she would have to make several trips to probate the will and dispose of the house. That meant flying, and this was why she had sought help from the mental health clinic.

"I can't fly!" she had told the clinician. "I haven't flown anywhere for 20 years."

Esther had been reared during the Depression; as a child, she had never had the opportunity to fly. With five children of her own to care for on her husband's school-teacher pay, she hadn't traveled much as an adult, either. She had made a few short hops years ago, when two of her children were getting married in different cities. On one of those trips, her plane had circled the field for nearly an hour, trying to land in Omaha between thunderstorms. The ride was wretchedly bumpy; the plane was full; and many of the passengers were airsick, including the men seated on either side of her. There was no one to help—the flight attendants had to remain strapped in their seats. She had kept her eyes closed and breathed through her handkerchief to try to filter out the odors that filled the cabin.

They finally landed safely, but it was the last time Esther had ever been up in an airplane. "I don't even like to go to the airport to meet someone," she reported. "Even that makes me feel short of breath and kind of sick to my stomach. Then I get sort of a dull pain in my chest and I start to shake—I feel that I'm about to die, or something else awful will happen. It all seems so silly."

Esther really had no alternatives to flying. She couldn't stay in Detroit until all of the business had been taken care of; it would take months. The train didn't connect, and the bus was impossible.

Evaluation of Esther Dugoni

Esther's anxiety symptoms were cued by the prospect of airplane travel (criterion A); even going to the airport inevitably produced anxiety (B), and she had avoided plane travel for years (C, E). She recognized that this fear was unreasonable ("silly"), and it embarrassed her (D); it was about to interfere with how she conducted her personal business (F).

Specific phobia is not usually associated with any **general medical condition** or **substance-induced disorder**. In response to delusions, patients with **schizophrenia** will sometimes avoid objects or situations (a telephone that is "bugged," food that is "poisoned"), but such patients do not have the required insight that their fears are unfounded. Of course, specific phobias must be differentiated from fears associated with other disorders (such as **agoraphobia**, **OCD**, **PTSD**, **social anxiety disorder**—G). Esther's clinician should ask about possible comorbid diagnoses. Pending that, and with a GAF score of 75, her diagnosis would be as given below. (Esther had only one phobia, a situational one; the average is three, each of which would be listed on a separate line with its own number.)

F40.248 [300.29]	Specific phobia, situational (fear of flying)
G20 [332.0]	Parkinson's disease, primary
Z63.4 [V62.82]	Uncomplicated bereavement

Fears involving animals of one sort or another are remarkably common. Children are especially susceptible to animal phobias, and many adults don't much care for spiders, snakes, or cockroaches. But a diagnosis of specific phobia, animal type, should not be made unless a patient is truly impaired by the symptoms. For example, you wouldn't diagnose a snake phobia in a prisoner serving a life sentence—under which circumstances confrontation with snakes and activity restriction as a result would be unlikely.

F40.10 [300.23] Social Anxiety Disorder

Social anxiety disorder (SAD) is a fear of appearing clumsy, silly, or shameful. Patients dread social gaffes such as choking when eating in public, trembling when writing, or being unable to perform when speaking or playing a musical instrument. Using a public urinal will cause anxiety for some men. Fear of blushing affects especially women, who may not be able to put into words what's so terrible about turning red. Fear of further choking is often acquired after an episode of choking on food; it can occur any time from childhood to old age. Some patients fear (and avoid) multiple such public situations.

Many people, men and women, have noticeable physical symptoms with SAD: blushing, hoarseness, tremor, and perspiration. Such patients may have actual panic attacks. Children may express their anxiety by clinging, crying, freezing, shrinking back, throwing tantrums, or refusing to speak.

Studies of general populations report a lifetime occurrence of SAD ranging from 4% to as high as 13%. However, if we consider only those patients who are truly inconvenienced by their symptoms, prevalence figures are probably lower. Whatever the actual figure, these findings contradict previous impressions that SAD is rare. Perhaps interviewers tend to overlook a common condition that patients silently endure. Though males outnumber females in treatment settings, women predominate in general population samples.

Onset is typically in the middle teens. The symptoms of SAD overlap with those of avoidant personality disorder; the latter is more severe, but both begin early, tend to last for years, and have some commonalities in family history. Indeed, SAD is reported to have a genetic basis.

Essential Features of **Social Anxiety Disorder**

Inordinate anxiety is attached to circumstances where others could closely observe the patient—public speaking or performing, eating or having a drink, writing, perhaps just speaking with another person. Because these activities almost always provoke disproportionate fear of embarrassment or social rejection, the patient avoids these situations or endures them with much anxiety.

The Fine Print

For children, these "others" must include peers, not just adults.

The D's: • Duration (6+ months) • Distress or disability (work/educational, social, or personal impairment) • Differential diagnosis (substance use and physical disorders, mood and psychotic disorders, anorexia nervosa, OCD, avoidant personality disorder, normal shyness, and other anxiety disorders—especially agoraphobia)

Coding Notes

Specify if:

> **Performance only.** The patient fears public speaking or performing, but not other situations.

Valerie Tubbs

"It starts right here, and then it spreads like wildfire. I mean, like real fire!" Valerie Tubbs pointed to the right side of her neck, which she kept carefully concealed with a blue silk scarf. "It" had been happening for almost 10 years, any time she was with people; it was worse if she was with a lot of people. Then she felt that everybody noticed.

Although she had never tried, Valerie didn't think that her reaction was something she could control. She just blushed whenever she thought people were watching her. It had started during a high school speech class, when she had to give a talk. She had become confused about the difference between a polyp and a medusa, and one of the boys had commented on the red spot that had appeared on her neck. She had quickly flushed all over and had to sit down, to the general amusement of the class.

"He said it looked like a bull's-eye," she said. Since then, Valerie had tried to avoid the potential embarrassment of saying anything to more than a handful of people. She had given up her dream of becoming a fashion buyer for a department store, because she couldn't tolerate the scrutiny the job would entail. Instead, for the last 5 years she had worked dressing mannequins for the same store.

Valerie said that it seemed "stupid" to be so afraid. It wasn't just that she turned red; she turned *beet*-red. "I can feel prickly little fingers of heat crawling out across my neck and up my cheek. My face feels like it's on fire, and my skin is being scraped with a rusty razor." Whenever she blushed, she didn't feel exactly panicky. It was a sense of anxiety and restlessness that made her wish her body belonged to someone else. Even the thought of meeting new people caused her to feel irritable and keyed up.

Evaluation of Valerie Tubbs

For years, Valerie had feared being embarrassed by the blushing that occurred whenever she spoke with other people (criteria A, B, C, and F in one sentence). Her fear was excessive (E), and she knew it—though insight isn't required for the diagnosis. With her reluctance to speak publicly (and her scarf), she avoided exposure to scrutiny (D). Her anxiety also prevented her from working at the job she would have preferred (G).

With no actual panic attacks, and in the absence of **anxiety disorder due to another medical condition** and **substance-induced anxiety disorder** (H), determining her disorder would come down to the differential diagnosis of phobias (I). In the absence of a typical history, we can quickly dismiss **specific phobia**. People who have **agoraphobia** may avoid dining out because they fear the embarrassment of having a panic attack in a public restaurant. Then you would only diagnose SAD if it had been present prior to the onset of the agoraphobia and was unrelated to it. (Sometimes even clinicians who specialize in diagnosing and treating the anxiety disorders can have trouble deciding between these two diagnoses.) Patients with **anorexia nervosa** avoid eating, but the focus is on their weight, not on the embarrassment that might result from gagging or leaving food on their lips.

It is important to differentiate SAD from the **ordinary shyness** that is so common among children and other young people; this shows the value of the criterion that symptoms must be present for at least half a year, required by DSM-5 for adults as well as for children. Also keep in mind that many people worry about or feel uncomfortable with social activities such as speaking in public (**stage fright** or **microphone fright**). They should not receive this diagnosis unless it in some important way affects their working, social, or personal functioning.

Social phobia (as SAD used to be called) is often associated with suicide attempts and **mood disorders**. Anyone with SAD may be at risk for self-treatment with **drugs** or **alcohol**; Valerie's clinician should ask carefully about these conditions. SAD has elements in common with **avoidant personality disorder**, which, often comorbid in these patients, may be a warranted diagnosis in a patient who is generally inhibited socially, is overly sensitive to criticism, and feels inadequate. Other mental disorders you might sometimes need to rule out—no problem for Valerie—would include **panic disorder**, **separation anxiety disorder**, **body dysmorphic disorder**, and **autism spectrum disorder**.

Valerie's fears involved far more than performances, so the specifier wouldn't apply. With a GAF score of 61, her diagnosis would be as follows:

F40.10 [300.23]　　　Social anxiety disorder

F94.0 [313.23] Selective Mutism

Selective mutism denotes children who remain silent except when alone or with a small group of intimates. The disorder typically begins during preschool years (ages 2–4), after normal speech has developed. Such a child, who speaks appropriately at home among family members but becomes relatively silent when among strangers, may not attract clinical attention until formal schooling begins. Although often shy, most such children have normal intelligence and hearing. When they do speak, they tend to use normal articulation, sentence structure, and vocabulary. The condition often improves spontaneously within weeks or months, though no one knows how to identify such a patient in advance of improvement.

Selective mutism is uncommon, with a prevalence of under 1 in 1,000; it appears to affect girls and boys about equally. Family history is often positive for social anxiety disorder and relatives with selective mutism. Comorbid conditions include other anxiety disorders (especially separation anxiety disorder and social anxiety disorder). They do *not* tend to have externalizing disorders, such as oppositional defiant or conduct disorder.

Essential Features of **Selective Mutism**

Despite speaking normally at other times, the patient regularly doesn't speak in certain situations where speech is expected, such as in class.

The Fine Print

The first month of a child's first year in school is often fraught with anxiety; exclude behaviors that occur during this time.

The D's: • Duration (1+ months) • Distress or disability (social or work/academic impairment) • Differential diagnosis (unfamiliarity with the language to be used, a communication disorder such as stuttering, psychotic disorders, autism spectrum disorder, social anxiety disorder)

F93.0 [309.21] Separation Anxiety Disorder

For years, separation anxiety disorder (SepAD) was diagnosed in childhood—and stayed there. More recently, however, evidence has accumulated that the condition also affects adults. This can happen in two ways. Perhaps one-third of children with SepAD continue to have symptoms of the disorder well into their adult years. However, some patients develop symptoms de novo in their late teens or even later—sometimes even beginning in old age. SepAD has a lifetime prevalence of about 4% for children and 6% for adults; for adults, the 12-month prevalence is nearly 2%. It is more common in females than in males, though boys are more likely to be referred for treatment.

In children, SepAD may begin with a precipitant such as moving to a new home or school, a medical procedure or serious physical diagnosis, or the loss of an important friend or pet (or a parent). Symptoms often show up as school refusal, but younger children may even show reluctance at being left with a sitter or at day care. Children may enlist physical complaints, imagined or otherwise, as justification for remaining home with parents.

Adults, too, may fear that something horrible will happen to an important attachment figure—perhaps a spouse, or even a child. As a result, they are reluctant to leave home (or any place of safety); they may fear even sleeping alone, and they experience nightmares about separation. When apart from the principal attachment figure, they may need to telephone or otherwise touch base several times a day. Some may try to ensure safety by setting up a routine of following the other person.

When the onset is early in childhood, this condition is likely to remit; with later onset, symptoms are more likely to continue into adulthood and to confer more severe disability (though the intensity may wax and wane). Children with SepAD tend to drift into subclinical forms or nonclinical status. Most adults and children also have other disorders (especially mood, anxiety, and substance use disorders), though SepAD is often the condition present the longest.

Children with SepAD often have parents with an adult form of the same disorder, and, as with most anxiety disorders, there is a strong genetic component.

Essential Features of **Separation Anxiety Disorder**

Because they fear what might happen to a parent or someone else important in their lives, these patients resist being alone. They imagine that the parent will die or become lost (or that *they* will), so that even the thought of separation can cause anxiety, nightmares, or perhaps vomiting spells or other physical complaints. They are therefore reluctant to attend school, go out to work, or to sleep away from home—perhaps even in their own beds.

The Fine Print

The D's: • Duration (6+ months in adults, though extreme symptoms—such as total school refusal—could justify diagnosis after a shorter duration; 4+ weeks in children) • Distress or disability (work/educational, social, or personal impairment) • Differential diagnosis (mood disorders, other anxiety disorders, PTSD)

Nadine Mortimer

At age 24, Nadine Mortimer still lived at home. The only reason for her evaluation, she told the clinician, was that her mother and stepfather had just signed on to join the Peace Corps; she, Nadine, would be left behind. "I just *know* I won't be able to stand it." She sobbed into her Kleenex.

Being alone had frightened Nadine from the time she was very small. She thought she could trace it back to her father's death: He was a mechanic who drove a racing car for fun until the weekend he encountered a wall at the far turn of their hometown track. Her mother's response was strangely stoic. "I think I took on the job of grieving for both of us," Nadine commented. Within the year, her mother had remarried.

Her first day of first grade, Nadine had been so fearful that her mother had stayed in the classroom. "I was afraid something terrible would happen to her too, and I wanted to be there, for safety." After several weeks, Natalie had been able to tolerate being left, but the following year, she threw up when Labor Day rolled around. After a few miserable weeks in second grade, she was withdrawn and home-schooled.

In 10th grade, she was reading and doing math at 12th-grade level. "But my socialization skills were near nil. I'd never even been to a sleepover at another girl's house," she said. So her parents bribed her with a cell phone and a promise that she could call any time. By the time Nadine was in junior college—hardly farther away than her high school—she'd negotiated for a smart phone with a GPS device; now she could track her mother's whereabouts to within a few feet. With that, she said, she could "roam comfortably, stores and whatnot, as long as I could check Mom's location whenever I wished." Once, when her battery died, she had suffered a panic attack.

Nonetheless, she still didn't graduate from junior college, and after a semester she returned home to be with her mother. "I know it seems weird," she told the interviewer, "but I always imagine that someday she won't come home to me. Just like Daddy."

Evaluation of Nadine Mortimer

From the time she started school (criterion B), Nadine had had clear symptoms of SepAD. She worried that harm might befall her mother and was severely distressed when they were separated; she'd vomited at the mere prospect of a new school year (A). As a result, she had almost no friends and had never slept away from home (C). There was no sign of other disorders to exclude (D).

Modified by her adult status, many of these same symptoms persisted—panic symptoms when she couldn't keep close tabs on her mother, from whom she refused to live apart. She even retained the same fear of harm befalling her mother if they ever were separated. The prospect of her parents' leaving for a new career deeply affected her. Even if Nadine hadn't had symptoms as a child, her adult disorder was troubling enough to qualify for the diagnosis of SepAD.

A significant problem remains in the differential diagnosis of SepAD: How does one distinguish it from **agoraphobia**? There is some overlap, but patients with SepAD are afraid of being away from a parent or other significant person, whereas the fear for a person with agoraphobia is of being in a place from which escape will be difficult. The mute testimony of her smart phone suggests that Nadine's anxiety was of the former type, not the latter. I would put her current GAF score at 45.

F93.0 [309.21]   Separation anxiety disorder

The DSM-IV criteria for SepAD employed a number of behaviors only appropriate to children; perhaps this explains why it wasn't recognized in adults earlier. Even now, panic symptoms may sometimes draw clinicians off the scent of adult SepAD.

F41.1 [300.02] Generalized Anxiety Disorder

Generalized anxiety disorder (GAD) can be hard to diagnose. The symptoms are relatively unfocused; the nervousness is low-key and chronic; there are no panic attacks. Furthermore, it is, after all, just worry, and that's something that touches all of us. But there are differences. Ordinary worry is somehow less serious; we are able (well, most of the time) to put it aside and concentrate on other, more immediate issues. The worry of GAD often starts of its own accord, seemingly without cause. And GAD worry is at times hard to control. It carries with it a collection of physical symptoms that pile onto the sense of agitated restlessness in a cascade of misery.

Although some patients with GAD may be able to state what it is that makes them nervous, others cannot. GAD worry is typically about far more issues ("everything") than objective facts can justify. The disorder typically begins at about 30 years of age; many patients with GAD have been symptomatic for years without coming to the attention of a clinician. Perhaps this is because the degree of impairment in GAD is often not all that severe. Genetic factors play an important role in the development of GAD. It is found in up to 9% of the general adult population (lifetime risk), and, as with nearly every other anxiety disorder, females predominate.

Essential Features of **Generalized Anxiety Disorder**

Hard-to-control, excessive worrying about a variety of issues—health, family problems, money, school, work—results in physical and mental complaints: muscle tension, restlessness, becoming easily tired and irritable, experiencing poor concentration, and trouble with insomnia.

The Fine Print

The D's: • Duration (on most days for 6+ months) • Distress or disability (work/educational, social, or personal impairment) • Differential diagnosis (substance use and physical disorders, mood disorders, other anxiety disorders, OCD, PTSD, realistic worry)

Bert Parmalee

For most of his adult life, Bert had been "a worry-wart." At age 35, he still had dreams that he was flunking all of his college electrical engineering courses. But recently he had felt that he was walking a tightrope. For the past year he had been the administrative assistant to the chief executive officer of a Fortune 500 company, where he had previously worked in product engineering.

"I took the job because it seemed a great way to move up the corporate ladder," he said, "but almost every day I have the feeling my foot's about to slip off the rung."

Each of the company's six ambitious vice-presidents saw Bert as a personal pipeline to the CEO. His boss was a hard-driving workaholic who constantly sparked ideas and wanted them implemented yesterday. Several times he had told Bert that he was pleased with his performance. In fact, Bert was doing the best job of any administrative assistant he had ever had, but that didn't seem to reassure Bert.

"I've felt uptight just about every day since I started this job. My chief expects action and results. He has zero patience for thinking about how it should all fit together. Our vice-presidents all want to have their own way. Several of them hint pretty broadly that if I don't help them, they'll put in a bad word with the boss. I'm always looking over my shoulder."

Bert had trouble concentrating at work; at night he was exhausted but had trouble getting to sleep. Once he did, he slept fitfully. He had become chronically irritable at home, yelling at his children for no reason. He had never had a panic attack, and he didn't think he was depressed. In fact, he still took a great deal of pleasure in the two activities he enjoyed most: Sunday afternoon football on TV and Saturday night lovemaking with his wife. But recently, she had offered to take the kids to her mother's for a few weeks, to relieve some of the pressure. This only resurrected some of his old concerns that he wasn't good enough for her—that she might find someone else and leave him.

Bert was slightly overweight and balding, and he looked apprehensive. He was carefully dressed and fidgeted a bit; his speech was clear, coherent, relevant, and spontaneous. He denied having obsessions, compulsions, phobias, delusions, or hallucinations. On the MMSE, he scored a perfect 30. He said that his main problem—his only problem—was his nagging uneasiness.

Valium made him drowsy. He had tried meditating, but it only allowed him to concentrate more effectively on his problems. For a few weeks he had tried having a cocktail before dinner; that had both relaxed him and prompted worries about alcoholism. Once or twice he even went with his brother-in-law to an Alcoholics Anonymous meeting. "Now I've decided to try dreading one day at a time."

Evaluation of Bert Parmalee

Bert worried about multiple aspects of his life (his job, being an alcoholic, losing his wife); each of these worries was excessive for the facts (criterion A). The excessiveness of his worries would differentiate them from the usual sort of anxiety that is not pathological. Despite repeated efforts (meditation, medication, reassurance), he had been unable to control these fears (B). In addition, he had at least four physical or mental symptoms (only three are required): trouble concentrating (C3), fatigue (C2), irritability (C4), and sleep disturbance (C6). He had been having difficulty nearly every day for longer than the required 6 months (A). And his symptoms caused him considerable distress, perhaps even more than is usual for patients with GAD (D).

One of the difficulties in diagnosing GAD is that so many other conditions must be excluded (E). A number of **physical conditions** can cause anxiety symptoms; a complete workup of Bert's anxiety would have to consider these possibilities. From the information contained in the vignette, a **substance-induced anxiety disorder** would appear unlikely.

Anxiety symptoms can be found in nearly every category of mental disorder, including **psychotic, mood** (depressed or manic), **eating, somatic symptom**, and **cognitive disorders**. From Bert's history, none of these would seem remotely likely (F). For example, an **adjustment disorder with anxiety** would be eliminated because Bert's symptoms met the criteria for another mental disorder.

It is important that the patient's worry and anxiety not focus solely on feature of another mental disorder, especially another anxiety disorder. For example, it shouldn't be "merely" worry about weight gain in **anorexia nervosa**, about contamination (**OCD**), separation from attachment figures (**separation anxiety disorder**), public embarrassment (**social anxiety disorder**), or having physical symptoms (**somatic symptom disorder**). Nevertheless, note that a patient can have GAD in the presence of another mental disorder—most often, mood and other anxiety disorders—provided that the symptoms of GAD are independent of the other condition.

GAD is one of those conditions that offers no specifiers, or even indicators of severity, so Bert's diagnosis, other than a GAF score of 70, would be a plain vanilla:

F41.1 [300.02] Generalized anxiety disorder

It is reasonable to ask this question: Does diagnosing GAD in a depressed patient help with your evaluation? After all, the anxiety symptoms may disappear once the depression has been sufficiently treated. The value, I suppose, is that flagging the anxiety symptoms gives a more complete picture of the patient's pathology. Also, you may have to treat the anxiety symptoms independently later on.

Substance/Medication-Induced Anxiety Disorder

When the symptoms of anxiety or panic can be attributed to the use of a chemical substance, make the diagnosis of substance/medication-induced anxiety disorder. It can occur during acute intoxication (or heavy use, as with caffeine) or during withdrawal (as with alcohol or sedatives), but the symptoms must be more severe that you'd expect for ordinary intoxication or withdrawal, and they must be serious enough to warrant clinical attention.

Many substances can produce anxiety symptoms, but those most commonly associated are marijuana, amphetamines, and caffeine. See Table 15.1 in Chapter 15 for a summary of the substances for which intoxication or withdrawal can be expected to create anxiety. If more than one substance is involved, you'd code each separately. Quite frankly, these disorders are probably rare.

Essential Features of **Substance/Medication-Induced Anxiety Disorder**

The use of some substance appears to have caused the patient to experience anxiety symptoms or panic attacks.

The Fine Print

For tips on identifying substance-related causation, see sidebar, page 95.

The D's: • Distress or disability (work/educational, social, or personal impairment) • Differential diagnosis (ordinary substance intoxication or withdrawal, delirium, physical disorders, mood disorders, and other anxiety disorders)

Coding Notes

Specify:

> **With onset during {intoxication}{withdrawal}.** This gets tacked on at the end of your string of words.
> **With onset after medication use.** You can use this in addition to other specifiers.

For specific coding procedures, see Tables 15.2 and 15.3 in Chapter 15.

Bonita Ramirez

Bonita Ramirez, a 19-year-old college freshman, was brought to the emergency room by two friends. Alert, intelligent, and well informed, she cooperated fully in providing the following information.

Bonita's parents both held graduate degrees and were well established in their professions. They lived in a well-to-do suburb of San Diego. Bonita was their oldest child and only daughter. Strictly reared in the Catholic faith, she hadn't been allowed to date until a year before. Until sorority rush week, the only alcohol she had tasted had been Communion wine. By her account and that of her companions, she had been happy, healthy, and vivacious when she arrived on campus a fortnight earlier.

Two weeks had made a remarkable difference. Bonita now sat huddled on the examination table, feet drawn up beneath her. With her arms wrapped around her knees, she trembled noticeably. Although it was only September, she wore a sweater and complained of feeling cold. She kept reaching for the emesis basin beside her, as though she might need it again.

Her voice quavered as she said that nothing like this had ever happened to her before. "I had some beer last week. It didn't bother me at all, except I had a headache the next morning."

This evening there had been a "big sister, little sister" party at the sorority Bonita had just pledged. She had drunk some beer, and that had prompted her to take a few hits from the marijuana cigarette they were passing around. The beer must have numbed her throat, because she had been able to draw the smoke deep into her lungs and hold it, the way her friends had showed her.

For about 10 minutes Bonita hadn't noticed anything at all. Then her head began to feel tight, as though her hair was a wig that didn't fit right. Suddenly, when she tried to inhale, her chest "screamed in pain," and she became instantly aware that she was about to die. She tried to run, but her rubbery legs refused to support her.

The other girls hadn't had much experience with drug reactions, but they called one of the men from the fraternity house next door, who came over and tried to talk Bonita down. After an hour, she still felt the panicked certainty that she would die or go mad. That was when they decided to bring her to the emergency room.

At length she said, "They said it would relax me and expand my consciousness. I just want to contract it again."

Evaluation of Bonita Ramirez

Bonita's history—she was healthy until the ingestion of a substance that is known to produce anxiety symptoms, especially in a naïve user—is a dead giveaway for the diagnosis (criteria A, B). Other drugs that commonly produce anxiety symptoms include **amphetamines**, which can also produce panic attack symptoms, and **caffeine** when used heavily. However, because anxiety symptoms can be encountered at some point during the use of most substances, you can code an anxiety disorder secondary to the use of nearly any of them, provided that the anxiety symptoms are worse than you would expect for ordinary **substance withdrawal** or **intoxication**. Because she required emergency evaluation and treatment, we would judge this to be the case for Bonita (E).

Despite the proximity of the development of her symptoms to substance use (C), her clinician would want to be sure that she did not have **another medical condition** (or **treatment with medication** for a medical condition) that could also explain her anxiety symptoms.

Although she was severely panicked when she arrived at the emergency room, I would score Bonita's GAF as a relatively high 80, because her symptoms had caused her no actual disability (plenty of distress) and should be transient; other diagnosticians might disagree. She had not used pot before, so she had no use disorder, and her code comes from the "none" row for cannabis in Table 15.3.

F12.980 [292.89]   Cannabis-induced anxiety disorder, with onset during intoxication

F06.4 [293.84] Anxiety Disorder Due to Another Medical Condition

Many medical disorders can produce anxiety symptoms, which will usually resemble those of panic disorder or generalized anxiety disorder. Occasionally, they may take the form of obsessions or compulsions. Most anxiety symptoms won't be caused by a medical disorder, but it is supremely important to identify those that are. The symptoms of an untreated medical disorder can evolve from anxiety to permanent disability (consider the dangers of a growing brain tumor).

Essential Features of **Anxiety Disorder Due to Another Medical Condition**

A physical medical condition appears to have caused panic attacks or marked anxiety.

The Fine Print

For pointers on deciding when a physical condition may have caused a disorder, see sidebar, page 97.

The D's: • Distress or disability (work/educational, social, or personal impairment) • Differential diagnosis (substance use disorders, delirium, mood disorders, other anxiety disorders, adjustment disorder)

Coding Notes

In recording the diagnosis, use the name of the responsible medical condition, and list *first* the medical condition, with its code number.

Millicent Worthy

"I wonder if we could just leave the door open." Millicent Worthy got up from the chair and opened the examining room door. She had fidgeted throughout the first part of the interview. Part of that time, she had hardly seemed to be paying attention at all. "I feel better not being so closed in." Once she finally settled down, she told this story.

Millicent was 24 and divorced. She had never touched drugs or alcohol. In fact, until about 4 months ago, she'd been well all her life. She had visited a mental health clinic only once before, when she was 12: Her parents were having marital problems, and the entire family had gone for family counseling.

She had first felt nervous while tending the checkout counter at the video rental outlet where she worked. She felt cramped, hemmed in, as if she needed to walk around. One afternoon, when she was the only employee in the store and she had to stay behind the counter, her heart began to pound and she perspired and became short of breath. She thought she was about to die.

Over the next several weeks, Millicent gradually became aware of other symptoms. Her hand had begun to shake; she noticed it one day at the end of her shift when she was adding up the receipts from her cash register. Her appetite was voracious, yet in the past 6 weeks her weight had dropped nearly 10 pounds. She still loved watching movies, but lately she felt so tired at night that she could barely keep awake in front of the TV. Her mood had been somewhat irritable.

"As I thought about it, I realized that all this started about the time my boyfriend and I decided to get married. We've been living together for a year, and I really love him. But I'd been burned before, in my first marriage. I thought that might be what was bothering me, so I gave back his ring and moved out. If anything, I feel worse now than before."

Several times during the interview Millicent shifted restlessly in her chair. Her speech was rapid, though she could be interrupted. Her eyes seemed to protrude slightly, and although she had lost weight, a fullness in her neck suggested a goiter. She admitted that she was having trouble tolerating heat. "There's no air conditioner in our store. Last summer it was no problem—we kept the door open. But now it's terrible! And if I wore any less clothing to work, they'd have to give me a desk in the adult video section."

Millicent's thyroid function studies proved to be markedly abnormal. Within 2 months an endocrinologist had brought her hyperactive thyroid under control, and her anxiety symptoms had disappeared completely. Six months later, she and her fiancé were married.

Evaluation of Millicent Worthy

Millicent had at least one panic attack (criterion A); her distress was palpable (E). The only remaining requirements would involve ruling out other causes of her problem.

If she had had repeated panic attacks and if the symptoms of her goiter had been overlooked, she could have been misdiagnosed as having **panic disorder**. Her restlessness could have been misinterpreted as **generalized anxiety disorder**; her feelings of being closed in sound like a **specific phobia**. (Even Millicent interpreted her own symptoms as psychological, C.) Such scenarios reinforce the wisdom of placing physical conditions at the top of the list of differential diagnoses.

Irritability, restless hyperactivity, and weight loss also suggest a **manic episode**, but these are usually accompanied by a subjective feeling of high energy, not fatigue. Millicent's rapid speech could be interrupted; in bipolar mania, often it cannot. Her lack of previous depressions or manias would also militate against any mood disorders. Her history rules out a **substance/medication-induced anxiety disorder**. And her attention span and orientation were good, so that we can disregard delirium (D). Finally, we know that the physiological effects of hyperthyroidism can cause anxiety symptoms of the sort Millicent experienced (B).

The broken engagement was noted not because it seemed a cause of her anxiety symptoms, but because her relationship with her fiancé was a problem that should be addressed as part of the overall treatment plan. I'd put her GAF score at an almost-healthy, but still-needs-to-be-addressed 85.

E05.00 [242.00]	Hyperthyroidism with goiter without thyroid storm
F06.4 [293.84]	Anxiety disorder due to hyperthyroidism
Z63.0 [V61.10]	Estrangement from fiancé

F41.8 [300.09] Other Specified Anxiety Disorder

Patients who have prominent symptoms of anxiety, fear, or phobic avoidance that don't meet criteria for any specific anxiety disorder can be coded as having other specified anxiety disorder—and the reason for not including them in a better-defined category should be stated. DSM-5 suggests several different possibilities:

Insufficient symptoms. This would include panic attacks or GAD with too few symptoms.

The presentation is atypical.

Cultural syndromes. DSM-5 mentions several in an appendix on page 833.

F41.9 [300.00] Unspecified Anxiety Disorder

CHAPTER 5

Obsessive–Compulsive and Related Disorders

Quick Guide to the Obsessive–Compulsive and Related Disorders

Patients who are preoccupied with obsessional ideas or certain repetitive behaviors may qualify for the disorders listed here. As in earlier chapters, the page number following each item indicates where a more detailed discussion begins.

Obsessive–compulsive disorder. These patients are bothered by repeated thoughts or behaviors that appear senseless, even to them (p. 200).

Body dysmorphic disorder. In this disorder, physically normal patients believe that parts of their bodies are misshapen or ugly (p. 204).

Hoarding disorder. An individual accumulates so many objects (perhaps of no value) that they interfere with life and living (p. 207).

Trichotillomania (hair-pulling disorder). Pulling hair from various parts of the body is often accompanied by feelings of "tension and release" (p. 210).

Excoriation (skin-picking) disorder. Patients so persistently pick at their skin that they traumatize it (p. 212).

Obsessive–compulsive and related disorder due to another medical condition. Obsessions and compulsions can be caused by various medical conditions (p. 215).

Substance/medication-induced obsessive–compulsive and related disorder. Various substances can lead to obsessive–compulsive symptoms that don't fulfill criteria for any of the above-mentioned disorders (p. 214).

Other specified, or unspecified, obsessive–compulsive and related disorder. Use one of these categories to code disorders with prominent anxiety symptoms that do not fit neatly into any of the groups above (p. 216).

Introduction

This chapter—new to the DSMs—pulls together disorders that have in common intrusive thoughts and time-consuming, repetitive behaviors: skin picking, hoarding, checking for body defects, and of course the classic component symptoms of obsessive–compulsive disorder (OCD). These behaviors aren't all unwanted—at least not at first, as with the pursuit of physical perfection (body dysmorphic disorder) or an accumulation of goods (hoarding). However they begin, the behaviors eventually become symptoms—burdensome to those whose once voluntary acts have morphed into duties that are performed at the cost of anxiety and distress.

A number of other features bind together this seemingly disparate collection of conditions: onset when young, similar comorbidity, a family history of OCD, similar treatment response, and hints of dysfunction in the frontostriatal brain circuitry (caudate hyperactivity).

F42 [300.3] Obsessive–Compulsive Disorder

Obsessions are recurring thoughts, beliefs, or ideas that dominate a person's mental content. They persist despite the fact that the person may believe they are unrealistic and tries to resist them. *Compulsions* are acts (either physical or mental) performed repeatedly in a way that the person may realize is neither appropriate nor useful. So why do them? For the most part, the aim is to neutralize the obsessional thinking. Note, then, that repeated thoughts can themselves sometimes be compulsions, if their purpose is to reduce the obsessional anxiety.

Compulsions can be comparatively simple, such as uttering or thinking a word or phrase of protection against an obsessive thought. But some are almost unbelievably complex. For instance, some elaborate dressing, bedtime, or washing rituals, if not performed exactly as specified by intricate rules, must be repeated until the patient gets it right. Of course, that sort of behavior can soak up hours every day.

Most patients have both obsessions and compulsions, which usually result in anxiety and dread. And most patients recognize them as being irrational and want to resist. OCD comprises four major symptom patterns, whose features sometimes overlap.

- The most common is a fear of contamination that leads to excessive handwashing.

- Doubts ("Did I turn off the cooktop?") lead to excessive checking: The patient returns repeatedly to be sure that the cooktop is well and truly cold.

- Obsessions without compulsions constitute a less common pattern.

- Obsessions and compulsions slow some patients down to the point that it can take them hours just to finish breakfast or other daily routines.

Obsessions about symmetry (putting things into a specific order, counting things) and forbidden thoughts (sacrilegious ideas, sexual taboos) also commonly occur.

One feature that helps classify patients with OCD is their degree of insight. Most patients are pretty well aware that their behavior is odd or peculiar; in fact, they are often embarrassed by it and try to hide it. But others—perhaps 10–25% of all patients with OCD—either have never recognized the irrationality of their behavior or have now to some degree lost that insight. Poor insight often indicates a worse prognosis. A few patients have so little that they are actually delusional; however, their OCD can be distinguished from delusional disorder by the presence of their obsessions (you don't need to give them an additional psychotic diagnosis). Note that children often don't have the experience to judge the reasonableness of their own behavior; therefore, insight specifiers often don't apply to them.

OCD is clinically important because it is usually chronic and often debilitating. Though symptoms may wax and wane, it puts patients at risk for celibacy or marital discord and interferes with performance at school and work. Comorbidity is the rule, with two-thirds of patients experiencing major depression. Perhaps 15% attempt suicide.

Men and women are about equally likely to be affected by OCD. Its prevalence, which may be as high as 2% in the general population, is reported to be greater in higher socioeconomic classes and in individuals of high intelligence. OCD is strongly familial (risk for first-degree relatives is 12%, about six times normal) and probably at least in part inherited. However, it is still unclear how genetics and environmental influences interact.

OCD typically begins in adolescence (males) or young adult life (females), but it often takes a decade or more before patients come to clinical attention. When it begins before puberty, compulsions may start first, often accompanied by tics and comorbid disorders.

Tic Specifier

DSM-5 has added a new specifier concerning a patient's experience with chronic (but not transient) tic disorder. These patients, usually male, tend to have a very early onset of OCD—often before the age of 11. They are especially likely to obsess over issues of exactness and symmetry; their compulsions concern ordering and arranging things. Some studies seem to suggest that a chronic tic disorder may reduce patients' response to antidepressant medications (though not to cognitive-behavioral therapy), and that antipsychotic drugs may help. However, it isn't clear that the history of tics denotes a patient who is more seriously ill. The tic specifier will apply to about a fourth of patients with OCD.

The December 2008 issue of *The Atlantic* reported asking for a term that would describe the irresistible impulse to rearrange that which someone else has already loaded into a dishwasher. Numerous readers suggested "obsessive compulsive dishorder."

Essential Features of **Obsessive–Compulsive Disorder**

The patient has distressing obsessions or compulsions (or both!) that occupy so much time they interfere with accustomed routines.

The Fine Print

Obsessions are recurring, unwanted ideas that intrude into awareness; the patient usually tries to suppress, disregard, or neutralize them.

Compulsions are repeated physical (sometimes mental) behaviors that follow rules (or respond to obsessions) in an attempt to alleviate distress; the patient may try to resist them. The behaviors are unreasonable, meaning that they don't have any realistic chance of helping the obsessional distress.

The D's: • Distress or disability (typically, the obsessions and/or compulsions occupy an hour a day or more or cause work/educational, social, or personal impairment) • Differential diagnosis (substance use and physical disorders, "normal" superstitions and rituals that don't actually cause distress or disability, depressive and psychotic disorders, anxiety and impulse-control disorders, Tourette's disorder, obsessive–compulsive personality disorder)

Coding Notes

Specify degree of insight:

> **With good or fair insight.** The patient realizes that the OCD thoughts and behaviors are definitely (or probably) not true.
> **With poor insight.** The patient thinks that the OCD concerns are probably true.
> **With absent insight/delusional beliefs.** The patient strongly believes that the OCD concerns are true.

Specify if:

> **Tic-related.** The patient has a lifetime history of a chronic tic disorder.

Leighton Prescott

Pausing for a moment, Leighton Prescott leaned forward to straighten a stack of journals on the interviewer's desk. The chapped skin on the backs of his hands was the color of dusty bricks. Apparently satisfied, he resumed his narrative.

"I would get this feeling that there could be semen on my hands and that it might be transferred to a woman and get her pregnant, even if I only shook hands with her. So I started washing extra carefully each time I masturbated."

Leighton was a 23-year-old graduate student in plant physiology. Though he was enormously bright and dedicated to science, his grades had slipped badly over the past few months. He attributed this to the handwashing rituals. Whenever he had the thought that he might have contaminated his hands with semen, he felt compelled to scrub them vigorously.

A year earlier, this had only meant 3 or 4 minutes with a bar of soap and water as hot as he could stand it. Soon he required a nail brush; still later he was brushing his hands and wrists as well. Now an elaborate ritual had evolved. First he scraped under his nails with a blade; then he used the brush on them. He then lathered surgical soap up to his elbows and scrubbed with a different brush for 15 minutes per arm. Then he would have to start over with his nails, because semen he had scrubbed off his arms might have lodged under them. If he had the thought that he had not performed one of the steps exactly right, he would have to start all over again. In recent weeks this had become the norm.

"I know it seems crazy," he said with a glance at his hands. "I'm a biologist. That part of me knows that spermatozoa can't live longer than a few minutes on the skin. But if I don't wash, the pressure just builds up and up, until I have to wash—washing is the only thing that relieves the anxiety."

Leighton didn't think he was depressed, though he was appropriately concerned about his symptoms. His sleep and appetite had been normal; he had never felt guilty or suicidal.

"Just stupid, especially when my girl stopped seeing me. I used the bathroom in a restaurant where I took her to eat. After 45 minutes, she had to send the manager in for me." He laughed without much humor. "She said she might see me again, if I'd clean up my act."

Evaluation of Leighton Prescott

Leighton's obsessions and compulsions (criterion A) both easily fulfilled the requirements for OCD. He tried to suppress the recurrent thoughts about contamination, which he recognized were the unreasonable products of his own mind (good insight). He felt compelled to ward off these ideas by repetitive handwashing, which he acknowledged was grossly excessive. By the time he came for help, his symptoms occupied several hours each day, interfered with his schooling and social life, *and* caused him severe distress (B). He had no other identifiable mental disorder that might account for his symptoms (D).

An important step in evaluating anyone for OCD is to determine whether the patient's focus of concern is pathological. For example, someone who lives in a ghetto or a war zone might be prudent to triple-lock the doors and frequently check security. Had Leighton been excessively concerned about numerous real-life problems (such as passing his exams or succeeding with his girlfriend), he might instead warrant a diagnosis of **generalized anxiety disorder**.

Though repetitive behavior is also characteristic of **Tourette's disorder** and **temporal lobe epilepsy**, patients with **other medical conditions** rarely present with obsessions or compulsions (C). However, occasionally a person will develop obsessions or compulsions as a result of **substance use**.

Inquire carefully about past or present tics, reported in about one-quarter of all patients with OCD. Not only is there a relationship between OCD and Tourette's disorder, but an outsized percentage of patients with OCD (though not Leighton) report a history of chronic tics.

Obsessional thinking or compulsive behavior can be found in a variety of other mental disorders. People may obsessively pursue any number of activities, such as **gambling**, **drinking**, and **sex**. The differential diagnosis also includes **body dysmorphic disorder** (the patient obsesses about body shape) and **illness anxiety disorder** (the focus is health). Patients with **psychotic disorders** sometimes maintain their obsessional ideas to a delusional degree. And of course there is something a bit obsessive in the eating behaviors of patients with **anorexia nervosa** and **bulimia nervosa**.

Perhaps 20% of patients with OCD have premorbid obsessional traits. Because of its name, **obsessive–compulsive personality disorder** (see p. 558) can be confused with OCD. Patients with only the personality disorder may not have obsessions or compulsions at all. They are perfectionistic and become preoccupied with rules, lists, and details. These people may accomplish tasks slowly because they keep checking to be sure it is being performed exactly right, but they do not have the desire to resist these behaviors. OCD and obsessive–compulsive personality disorder can coexist, in which case the OCD is often extra severe. Some clinicians believe that the border zone between OCD and **schizotypal personality disorder** is also a common problem in differential diagnosis.

Leighton's clinician needs to ensure that he doesn't have one of the (numerous) other conditions that often accompany OCD. Besides the two personality disorders just mentioned, I'd especially check for mood disorders (either depressive or bipolar) and anxiety disorders (generalized anxiety disorder, social anxiety disorder, and panic disorder).

Although most patients with OCD recognize that their obsessions and compulsions are unreasonable or excessive, some lose insight as the illness wears on. Leighton recognized that he was being unreasonable; we'll code him accordingly. With a GAF score of 60, his diagnosis would be the following:

F42 [300.3]   Obsessive–compulsive disorder, with good insight

---

As many as half of patients with OCD have an accompanying mood disorder. Some only show their obsessional symptoms when they are in the midst of a severe depression. Patients with OCD are also highly likely to have an accompanying anxiety disorder. (Indeed, OCD was itself classified as an anxiety disorder in earlier DSMs.)

F45.22 [300.7] Body Dysmorphic Disorder

Patients with body dysmorphic disorder (BDD) worry that there is something wrong with the shape or appearance of a body part—most often breasts, genitalia, hair, or the nose or some other portion of the face. The ideas these patients have about their bodies are not delusional; as in illness anxiety disorder, they are overvalued ideas. At one time the disorder was called *dysmorphophobia*; although some clinicians may still call it that, it isn't a phobia at all (irrational *fear* doesn't really enter into it).

This disorder can be devastating. Although they frequently request medical procedures (such as dermabrasion) or plastic surgery to correct their imagined defects, patients are often dissatisfied with the results. For that reason, surgery is usually contraindicated in these patients. They may also seek reassurance (which helps only briefly), try to hide their perceived deformities with clothing or body hair, or avoid social situations; some even become housebound. The preoccupation causes clinically important distress of other sorts—depressed mood, for example, even suicide ideas and attempts. Insight varies, though it's mostly poor.

In the general population, the rate of BDD is probably about 2%. It may account for as many as 10% of patients who consult a dermatologist and a third of patients seeking rhinoplasty. Though patients with BDD are relatively young (it tends to begin during the teen years), incidence may peak again after menopause. Although the question is not settled, men and women are probably about equally affected. However, males are more often concerned about genitals and hair.

Essential Features of **Body Dysmorphic Disorder**

In response to a miniscule, sometimes invisible physical flaw, the patient repeatedly checks in a mirror, asks for reassurance, or picks at patches of skin—or makes mental comparisons with other people.

The Fine Print

The D's: • Distress or disability (work/educational, social, or personal impairment) • Differential diagnosis (substance use and physical disorders, mood and psychotic disorders, anorexia nervosa or other eating disorders, OCD, illness anxiety disorder, ordinary dissatisfaction with personal appearance)

Coding Notes

Specify if:

> **With muscle dysmorphia.** These people believe that their bodies are too small or lack adequate musculature.

Specify degree of insight:

> **With good or fair insight.** The patient realizes that the BDD thoughts and behaviors are definitely (or probably) not true.

> **With poor insight.** The patient thinks that the BDD concerns are probably true.
> **With absent insight/delusional beliefs.** The patient strongly believes that the BDD concerns are true.

Muscle Dysmorphia Specifier

The muscle dysmorphia specifier for BDD is found almost exclusively in men. Such a man believes that he is too small or slightly built. As a result, he will often take dieting or weight lifting to extremes, and may misuse anabolic steroids or other drugs. (These patients may also be concerned about other body features—skin, hair, or whatever.)

Cecil Crane

Cecil Crane was only 24 when he was referred. "He came in here last week asking for a rhinoplasty," said the plastic surgeon on the telephone, "but his nose looks perfect to me. I told him that, but he insisted there was something wrong with it. I've seen this kind of patient before—if I operate, they're never satisfied. It's a lawsuit waiting to happen."

When Cecil appeared a few days later, he had the most beautiful nose the clinician had ever seen, apart from one or two Greek statues. "What seems to be wrong with it?"

"I was afraid you'd ask that," said Cecil. "Everybody says that."

"But you don't believe it?"

"Well, they look at me funny. Even at work—I sell suits at Macy's—I sometimes feel that the customers notice. I think it's this bump here."

Viewed from a certain angle, the area Cecil pointed out bore the barest suggestion of a convexity. He complained that it had cost him his girlfriend, who always said it looked fine to her. Weary of Cecil's trying to look at his profile in every mirror he passed and banging on about plastic surgery all the time, she'd finally sought greener pastures.

Cecil felt unhappy, though not depressed. He admitted that he was making a mess of his life, but he had nevertheless maintained his interests in reading and going to the movies. He thought his sex interest was good, though he'd had no chance to test it since the departure of his girlfriend. His appetite was good, and his weight was about average for his height. His flow of thought was unremarkable; its content, aside from his concern for his nose, seemed quite ordinary. He even admitted that it was possible that his nose was less ugly than he feared, though he thought that unlikely.

Cecil couldn't say exactly when his worry about his nose began. It may have been about the time he started shaving. He recalled frequently gazing at a silhouette of his profile that had been cut from black paper during a seashore vacation with his family. Although numerous relatives and friends had remarked that it was a good likeness, something about the nose had bothered him. One day he had taken it down from the wall and, with a pair of scissors, he'd tried to put it to rights. Within moments the nose lay in snippets on the kitchen table, and Cecil was grounded for a month.

"I sure hope the plastic surgeon is a better artist than I am," he commented.

Evaluation of Cecil Crane

The criteria for BDD are straightforward. Cecil was preoccupied with his flawless nose (criterion A), which caused him enough distress to seek surgery—and lose his girlfriend (C). More than one person had tried to assure him that his nose was rather ordinary, so his distress evidently exceeded normal concerns regarding appearance. And he appeared to need the constant checking in the mirror (B). Despite the full range of symptoms, there are several disorders in the differential diagnosis to consider.

In **illness anxiety disorder**, it isn't appearance that preoccupies the patient; rather, it is fear of having a disease. In **anorexia nervosa**, patients have distorted self-image, but only in the context of concern about overweight. In the **somatic type** of **delusional disorder,** patients lack insight that their complaints might be unreasonable, whereas Cecil was willing to entertain the notion that others might see his nose differently. (However, some patients with BDD completely lack insight; then the differentiation turns on the content of the delusion, which in delusional disorder will involve the function of or sensations in body parts, not their appearance.) Complaints from patients with **schizophrenia** about appearance are often bizarre (one woman reported that when she looked into the mirror, she noticed that her head had been replaced by a mushroom). In **gender dysphoria**, patients' complaints are limited to the conviction that they should have been born the opposite sex.

None of these was the focus of Cecil's concern (D, E). However, his clinician would do well to look carefully for **social phobia**, **obsessive–compulsive disorder**, and **major depressive disorder**, all of which can be comorbid with body dysmorphic disorder. Pending investigation for these disorders, Cecil's full diagnosis would be as given below, with a GAF score of 70:

F45.22 [300.7]   Body dysmorphic disorder, with fair insight

F42 [300.3] Hoarding Disorder

Over a thousand years ago, the Beowulf legend referred to a *hoard* as a mass of something valuable (especially money or other treasure) laid by for future use. Nowadays, we stand this definition on its head to mean worthless stuff that's kept beyond all practical use.

The motivations behind hoarding can be varied. Some people believe their things are valuable when they're not. Others may be imitating behavior they've encountered in family members (a genetic component is also suspected). Still others apparently feel comforted by the presence of things they've grown used to having, or that they think they may need later. Whatever the instigation, a hoarder's living space becomes cluttered, perhaps eventually filling up completely. (If living areas remain habitable, it's probably because someone else tidies up the mess.) One social consequence of hoarding is that children dread having visitors to the home; they sure don't learn the basics of housekeeping there! There are now online support groups for hoarders' children, who are otherwise left with their own hopeless attempts at coping with the unsanitary, the unsightly, and the unsafe.

A condition that's said to affect 2–5% of the general population, hoarding disorder is new in DSM-5. It was once considered a possible variant of OCD, but in fact not even 20% of hoarders meet OCD criteria—partly because they don't consider their symptoms to be intrusive, unpleasant, or distressing. Indeed, distress often develops only when they are forced to get rid of the stuff they've so laboriously brought home.

Hoarding disorder comprises several special types: people who hoard books, or animals (think a houseful of cats), or food that is—ugh!—way past its pull date. Animal hoarders also save other things, which may at least have the advantage of better sanitation. The disorder begins young and worsens with time, so that it is more often found among older adults; males may outnumber females. It appears to be strongly hereditary.

Essential Features of **Hoarding Disorder**

These patients are in the grip of something powerful: the overwhelming urge to accumulate stuff. They experience trouble—indeed, distress—when trying to discard their possessions, even those that appear to have little value (sentimental or otherwise). As a result, things pile up, cluttering up living areas to render them unusable.

The Fine Print

The D's: • Duration (not stated, other than "persistent") • Distress or disability (work/educational, social, or personal impairment) • Differential diagnosis (substance use and physical disorders, mood and psychotic disorders, dementia, OCD, normal collecting

Coding Notes

Specify if:

> **With excessive acquisition.** If symptoms are accompanied by excessive collecting, buying, or stealing of items that are not needed or for which there is no space available.

Specify degree of insight:

> **With good or fair insight.** The patient realizes that these thoughts and behaviors cause problems.
> **With poor insight.** The patient mostly believes that hoarding isn't a problem.
> **With absent insight/delusional beliefs.** The patient strongly believes that hoarding isn't a problem.

Langley Collyer

More than half a century later, the Collyer case remains celebrated in the annals of hoarding.

Though well educated (Columbia University) and a talented pianist, Langley Collyer probably never held gainful employment. He and his older brother, Homer, lived in the Harlem house left them by their parents, an obstetrician and his wife who were first cousins. Trained as a lawyer, Homer worked for a time, but his vision deteriorated and he suffered from arthritis. So, as they grew older, the brothers lived on their inherited money. They didn't require much: They had no gas, electricity, or telephone service. Even the water was eventually turned off. For decades, they essentially camped out indoors.

Langley would walk miles to the store for supplies that he'd bring home in a wagon, pulled along by a string. On these journeys, he also collected much of the debris that ultimately invaded their living space. Though he wore clothes long out of fashion, Langley was not completely asocial. As reported from accounts of those who knew him, he was pleasant, at times grateful for company. He even admitted that he was too reclusive.

In 1947, at age 61, Langley died, crushed under the weight of the booby trap he'd designed and installed over a period of years to prevent criminals from stealing the brothers' possessions. Finding the doorways stuffed with 10-foot-high walls of bailed newspaper and other debris, police had to chop their way in. It took them over 2 weeks to find Langley's body, which lay just 10 feet from where Homer had subsequently also died—of starvation.

After the bodies had been removed, the house was cleared of its holdings. Workers found dressmaker's dummies, sheets of Braille, a doll carriage, bicycles, a photograph of Mickey Rooney, old advertisements, firearms and ammunition, parts for old radios, chunks of concrete, and shoelaces. The brothers had stored some of their body waste in jars. There was a two-headed baby preserved in formaldehyde (probably an artifact from their father's medical practice), a canoe, a dismantled Model T automobile, two pipe organs, thousands of empty tin cans, and 14 pianos. There were also tons of newspapers, saved so that Homer could catch up on the news, once he regained his sight. In all, the house eventually yielded 180 tons of junk, with everything covered in decades of dust.

Evaluation of Langley Collyer

The analysis of Langley's condition requires a little forgiveness. That's because, candidly, we must infer one criterion important for hoarding disorder: that no **other medical disorder** could better explain the symptoms (criterion E). Langley and Homer famously refused to seek medical attention; hence Homer's crippling arthritis and, perhaps, his blindness. But Langley eschewed alcohol and drugs, and he appeared well enough for decades until the very end of his life—when it all came, quite literally, crashing down.

Hoarding can occur as a symptom of **OCD**, but as with most patients who hoard, we have no evidence of actual obsessions or (other) compulsions (F). Although there is no evidence for another mental disorder, neither have we positive evidence that Langley did not suffer from, say, **major depressive disorder** (it and OCD are often comorbid with hoarding disorder).

As for the other requirements of the syndrome, Langley was undeniably a collector whose accumulated tonnage didn't just impinge upon but engulfed the living space of the two hermit brothers (A, B, C). It imperiled their own health and that of any public service personnel who might be required to enter to give assistance; failing to maintain a safe environment satisfies the stress or impairment requirement (D).

In the absence of direct testimony from Langley, we cannot know how deeply he understood his condition, so we must ignore the insight specifiers. However, we can probably agree that his collecting habits qualify for the specifier *with excessive acquisition*—as is the case in the vast majority of hoarders. Although we are no longer able to code something on the order of "personality disorder, diagnosis deferred," if Langley were a living patient I'd make some sort of note in my summary to that effect—to alert me, or some other clinician down the road, that there was more diagnostic work to be done. I'd give him a GAF score of 60.

F42 [300.3]   Hoarding disorder, with excessive acquisition

F63.3 [312.39] Trichotillomania (Hair-Pulling Disorder)

Trichotillomania comes from the Greek meaning "passion for pulling hair." As with pyromania and kleptomania, many such patients (but not all) feel a mounting tension until they succumb to the urge. Then, when they pull out the hair, they experience release. Usually beginning in childhood, hair-pullers repeatedly extract their own hair, beards, eyebrows, or eyelashes. Less often, they will pull hair from armpits, the pubic area, or other body locations. They usually don't report pain associated with the hair pulling, although they may note a tingling sensation.

Some people put the hair into their mouths, and about 30% swallow it. If the hair is long, it can accumulate in the stomach or intestines as a bezoar (hairball) that may require surgical removal. Patients may be referred to mental health professionals by dermatologists, who note patchy hair loss.

Onset of trichotillomania is usually in childhood or adolescence. (When it begins in an adult, it may be associated with psychosis.) The condition tends to wax and wane, but is usually chronic.

Trichotillomania is embarrassing to patients, who tend to be secretive, so it's unclear just how common it is. Some hair pulling can be found in up to 3% of the adult population, especially women, though far fewer (probably under 1%) meet full criteria for the disorder. It is far more common in females than in males, and it is especially common in people with intellectual disability. Hair pullers also tend to crack their knuckles, bite their nails, or excoriate themselves.

The feeling of tension before hair pulling, and release or relief of stress afterwards, still characterizes many sufferers (though it is no longer a requirement for diagnosis). But patients who have the "tension and release" aspect of hair pulling may be in for a more severe course of the illness than those who don't report this feature.

Essential Features of **Trichotillomania**

Repeated pulling out of the patient's own hair results in bald patches and attempts to control the behavior.

The Fine Print

The D's: • Duration ("recurrent") • Distress or disability (work/educational, social, or personal impairment) • Differential diagnosis (substance use and physical disorders, mood and psychotic disorders, body dysmorphic disorder, OCD, ordinary grooming)

Rosalind Brewer

"I don't know why I do it, I just do it." Rosalind Brewer had been referred to the mental health clinic by her dermatologist. "I get to feeling sort of uptight, and if I just pop one little strand loose, somehow it relieves the tension." She selected a single strand of her long blonde hair, twined it neatly twice around her forefinger, and tweaked it out. She gazed at it a moment before dropping it onto the freshly vacuumed carpet.

Rosalind had been pulling out her hair for nearly half her 30 years. She thought it had started during her sophomore or junior year in high school, when she was studying for final exams. Perhaps the tingling sensation on her scalp had helped her stay awake; she didn't know. "Now it's a habit. I've always only pulled the hairs from the very top of my head."

The top of Rosalind's head bore a round, almost bald spot about the size of a silver dollar. Only a few broken hairs and a sparse growth of new hair sprouted there. It looked like a tiny tonsure.

"It used to make my mom really angry. She said I'd end up looking like Dad. She'd order me to stop, but you know kids. I used to think I had her by the short hairs." She laughed a little. "Now that I want to stop, I can't."

Rosalind had sucked her thumb until the age of 8, but otherwise her childhood hadn't been remarkable. Her physical health was good; she had no other compulsive behaviors or obsessive thinking. She denied using drugs or alcohol. Although she had no significant symptoms of depression, she admitted that her hair pulling was a serious problem for her. She could wear a hairpiece to hide her bald spot, but the knowledge that it was there had kept her from forming any close relationships with men.

"It's bad enough looking like a monk," Rosalind said. "But this thing has got me living like one, too."

Evaluation of Rosalind Brewer

Rosalind's symptoms of repeated hair pulling (criterion A) included the classic "tension and release" that used to be required for a diagnosis of trichotillomania, but now is only a frequent feature. She had no evidence of a **dermatological disorder** or other **general medical condition** (D) that might explain the condition (she was referred by a dermatologist). The mental conditions that might be confused with trichotillomania would include **OCD,** in which compulsions are performed not as an end to themselves, but as a means of preventing anxiety. Hair pulling is sometimes found in **body dysmorphic disorder**, but all would agree that Rosalind had a cosmetic flaw. **Factitious disorder**, another possibility, would be ruled out because Rosalind gave no indication that she wanted to be a patient. She had no **psychosis** or other evident mental disorder (especially **mood disorder**, E), except for her distress (C) at her inability to stop (B).

With a GAF score of 70, her complete diagnosis would be straightforward:

F63.3 [312.39]   Trichotillomania

L98.1 [698.4] Excoriation (Skin-Picking) Disorder

Excoriation (skin-picking) disorder usually begins by adolescence, though sometimes later. These patients spend much time—perhaps hours each day—digging at their skin. Most will focus on head or face; fingernails tend to be the instruments of choice, though some people employ tweezers. Tension prior to the act, as with other disorders of impulse such as pyromania, is a frequent finding in these patients. Then the act of picking may yield gratification; subsequent embarrassment or shame can delay treatment. Infections are common, sometimes producing ulceration. Patients may use cosmetics to conceal the scarring and excoriations; some will avoid social events as a result.

Other consequences can be dire. One patient picked so persistently at his neck and scalp that he picked right through his skull and developed an epidural abscess. The resultant quadriplegia resolved only partially; confined to a wheelchair, he ultimately resumed picking. Of course, this is the extreme; however, scarring and less harmful infections are common. Many patients will expend an hour or more each day engaged in picking behavior or its consequences.

A third of patients with excoriation disorder currently have some other mental disorder, most notably trichotillomania, a mood disorder, or OCD; some bite their nails. Nearly half of patients with body dysmorphic disorder also pick at themselves. Excoriation is found in people with developmental disabilities, especially in those with Prader–Willi syndrome (see sidebar, p. 215).

For a "new" disorder (though it was described as early as 1889, its DSM-5 listing is its first appearance as an official mental disorder), excoriation disorder is surprisingly common; its prevalence is probably 2% or more. It tends to begin in adolescence and runs a chronic course. By a large majority, these patients tend to be female; many have relatives similarly afflicted.

Essential Features of **Excoriation (Skin-Picking) Disorder**

The patient frequently tries to stop the repeated digging, scratching, or picking at skin, which has caused lesions.

The Fine Print

The D's: • Duration (recurring) • Distress or disability (work/educational, social, or personal impairment) • Differential diagnosis (substance use and physical disorders, psychotic disorders, OCD, body dysmorphic disorder, stereotypic movement disorder)

Brittany Fitch

The evidence was stark: Brittany Fitch's face was replete with pits and scars. A few of her lesions were still inflamed, and one on her forehead had scabbed over. She'd covered her fingernails with tape.

When she was 11, Brittany had developed acne, which her mother would "relieve" by squeezing the pustules and blackheads. Brittany endured long minutes standing with her head wedged into a corner, her mother's muscular fingers digging away "as if for gold," Brittany would recall years later. Released at last, she'd run to the bathroom and dab cool water on her smarting, spotted face. She'd hated her mother.

Now in college, Brittany had taken over the squeezing and picking job, though she knew it only led to more damaged skin. Several times a week she'd attack herself, usually just a few minutes at a time, but longer if she was alone in the bathroom. She felt drawn to mirrors to inspect, to criticize her face; those inspections, inevitably, ushered in further bouts of destruction. Because she felt ashamed of the damage she'd wreaked, she avoided dating. It had been 6 months since she'd attended a play or a concert, even by herself.

"I hope you can help me," she said with a wry smile. "More than anything, I want to stop being my mother."

Evaluation of Brittany Fitch

Brittany's condition isn't hard to diagnose. The spots and scars (criterion A) and the taped fingernails (B) told much of the story, and her clinic visit testified to the distress her symptoms were causing (C). The most important question at this point would be this: Could **another mental (or medical) disorder** explain her symptoms? For that, her clinician would have to dig a little deeper, so to speak, into her history to make sure she didn't have **OCD** (E). Of course she didn't have **body dysmorphic disorder**: Her skin condition was perfectly evident to anyone who looked.

As long as her clinician could find no evidence of a **medical condition** (such as scabies or some other dermatological disease) or a **substance use disorder** (such as use of cocaine or methamphetamines, in which the sensation of bugs crawling on or under the skin can precipitate picking, D), Brittany's diagnosis seems secure. I would base her GAF score (60) on the degree of social disability she experienced.

L98.1 [698.4]   Excoriation disorder

Substance/Medication-Induced Obsessive–Compulsive and Related Disorder

Reports link obsessive–compulsive symptoms to use of codeine, cocaine, ecstasy, and methamphetamine. If these criteria look an awful lot like those for substance-induced anxiety disorders, it's because the two sections were one and the same in DSM-IV. That's one reason I've elected not to include an additional vignette here. The other is that these conditions are probably vanishingly rare.

A principal example is the foraging behavior noted in users of crack cocaine. For a few hours at most, heavy users will inspect the carpet or bare floor looking for bits of the drug they might have dropped. It always occurs as a withdrawal phenomenon, and though they realize it is in vain, they feel helpless to resist.

Essential Features of **Substance/Medication-Induced Obsessive–Compulsive and Related Disorder**

The use of some substance appears to have caused obsessions, compulsions, hoarding, hair pulling, excoriation, or other recurring symptoms concerning the patient's own body.

The Fine Print

For tips on identifying substance-related causation, see sidebar, page 95.

The D's: • Distress or disability (work/educational, social, or personal impairment) • Differential diagnosis (ordinary substance intoxication or withdrawal, delirium, physical disorders, OCD, anxiety disorders)

Coding Notes

Specify:

> **With onset during {intoxication}{withdrawal}.** This gets tacked on at the end of your string of words.
> **With onset after medication use.** You can use this in addition to other specifiers.

For specific coding procedures, see Tables 15.2 and 15.3 in Chapter 15.

F06.8 [294.8] Obsessive–Compulsive and Related Disorder Due to Another Medical Condition

Occasionally you'll encounter obsessive–compulsive symptoms that are associated with another medical condition. Of course, association doesn't prove causation, but an etiological relationship has been claimed for Japanese B encephalitis and arachnoid cyst, among others.

Obsessive–compulsive symptoms are also found with Sydenham's chorea, which results from streptococcus infection in children. Much has been written about the pediatric autoimmune neuropsychiatric disorders associated with streptococcal infection (PANDAS), in which young children develop obsessions and compulsions as well as tics and other symptoms, but without the motor disorder of chorea. After years of study, a lot still isn't known—including whether PANDAS is an actual entity, and whether the alleged association is even genuine. (In 2013, a young man was arrested for planning to bomb his own high school near Portland, Oregon. In his defense, he cited OCD due to PANDAS.)

Prader–Willi syndrome is a rare (about 1 in 50,000) disorder associated with a portion of DNA mission from chromosome 15. The condition may be identified at birth with genetic testing of markedly hypotonic babies. Though some individuals with this syndrome have borderline normal intelligence, mild to moderate intellectual disability is common. Patients typically have short stature and hypogonadism; insatiable appetite often results in severe obesity. Some have mood symptoms and problems with impulse control. Patients with Prader–Willi have also been reported to have hoarding behavior, foraging for food, skin picking, and obsessions with cleanliness—almost a clean sweep of the disorders this chapter comprises.

Essential Features of **Obsessive–Compulsive and Related Disorder Due to Another Medical Condition**

A physical condition appears to have caused a patient to have obsessions, compulsions, hoarding, hair pulling, excoriation, or other recurrent symptoms concerning the patient's own body.

The Fine Print

For pointers on deciding when a physical condition may have caused a mental disorder, see sidebar, page 97.

The D's: • Distress or disability (work/educational, social, or personal impairment) • Differential diagnosis (substance use disorders, delirium, mood and anxiety disorders, OCD)

Coding Notes

Depending on presentation, specify:

> **With appearance preoccupations.** For symptoms similar to body dysmorphic disorder.
> **With obsessive–compulsive disorder-like symptoms.**
> **With hoarding symptoms.**
> **With hair-pulling symptoms.**
> **With skin-picking symptoms.**

F42 [300.3] Other Specified Obsessive–Compulsive and Related Disorder

This category (which you use, remember, when a patient has obsessive–compulsive features but doesn't fully qualify for a diagnosis, and you want to say *why*) might be appropriate in several situations, including these:

> **Symptoms similar to body dysmorphic disorder, but with actual flaws.** The flaws are there, all right, but the concern seems excessive.

> **Obsessional jealousy.** Without qualifying for any other mental disorder, the patient is distressed (or impaired) by a partner's infidelity; as a result, repetitive behavior or thoughts occur.

> **Symptoms similar to body dysmorphic disorder, but without repetitive behaviors.**

F42 [300.3] Unspecified Obsessive–Compulsive and Related Disorder

The patient has obsessions or compulsions or other behaviors that belong in this chapter, and you *don't* care to explain yourself.

CHAPTER 6

Trauma-
and Stressor-Related Disorders

Quick Guide to Trauma- and Stressor-Related Disorders

Various types of stress and trauma are responsible for the disorders we'll consider in this chapter. By now, you know the drill: The page number following each item indicates where a more detailed discussion begins.

Primary Trauma- and Stressor-Related Disorders

Reactive attachment disorder. There is evidence of pathogenic care in a child who habitually doesn't seek comfort from parents or surrogates (p. 231).

Disinhibited social engagement disorder. There is evidence of pathogenic care in a child who fails to show normal reticence in the company of strangers (p. 231).

Posttraumatic stress disorder. These adolescents or adults repeatedly relive a severely traumatic event, such as combat or a natural disaster (p. 219).

Posttraumatic stress disorder in preschool children. Children repeatedly relive a severely traumatic event, such as car accidents, natural disasters, or war (p. 223).

Acute stress disorder. This condition is much like posttraumatic stress disorder, except that it begins during or immediately after the stressful event and lasts a month or less (p. 224).

Adjustment disorder. Following a stressor, an individual develops symptoms that disappear once the cause of stress has subsided (p. 228).

Other specified, or unspecified, trauma- and stressor-related disorder. Patients whose stress or trauma appears related to other presentations may be classified in one of these categories (pp. 233, 234).

Other Problems Related to Trauma or Stress

Problems related to abuse or neglect. An astonishing number of Z-codes (V-codes in ICD-9) cover the categories of difficulties that arise from neglect or from physical or sexual abuse of children or adults (p. 594).

Separation anxiety disorder. The patient becomes anxious when separated from parent, other attachment figure, or home (p. 188).

Introduction

Another new chapter for the DSMs incorporates certain diagnoses formerly listed as anxiety, developmental, or adjustment disorders. The unifying factor here is that something traumatic or stressful in the patient's history appears to be at least partly responsible for the symptoms that develop. It is part of a trend toward grouping together patients of any age who have the right mix of symptoms, rather than separating patients by developmental stage.

Many diagnoses include statements about what is *not* causative, but here is the only full DSM-5 section that presumes any etiology at all, let alone one rooted in the psychology of a pathological developmental process.

In the instances of reactive attachment and disinhibited social engagement disorders, there must be evidence of pathogenic care; for posttraumatic stress disorder (PTSD) and its cousins, a horrific event; for adjustment disorder a stressful—well, stressor. The respective criteria sets permit us to check off the fulfilled criteria and go on our way, perhaps thinking that we've solved the puzzle.

While we rejoice that we've successfully determined a cause–effect relationship, nagging at the back of our minds must be a sense that there is more to the story. Otherwise, why do some people become symptomatic while others, exposed to the (as nearly as we can tell) exact same stimulus, go untrammeled on their way? Furthermore, studies have demonstrated that, sooner or later, significant stressors will visit the majority of us. Shouldn't we conclude that the stimulus in question is necessary, but not sufficient, for the outcome observed?

At least this DSM-5 chapter has herded most of these etiology-specific diagnoses into one corral, where we can keep a watchful eye on them.

F43.10 [309.81] Posttraumatic Stress Disorder

Many people who survive severely traumatic events will develop PTSD. Survivors of combat are the most frequent victims, but it is also encountered in those who have experienced other disasters, both natural and contrived. These include rape, floods, abductions, and airplane crashes, as well as the threats that may be posed by a kidnapping or hostage situation. Children can have PTSD as a result of inappropriate sexual experience, whether or not actual injury has occurred. PTSD can be diagnosed even in those who have only learned about severe trauma (or its threat) suffered by someone to whom they are close—children, spouses, other close relatives. One or two in every 1,000 patients who have undergone general anesthesia have afterwards reported awareness of pain, anxiety, helplessness, and the fear of impending death during the procedure; up to half of them may subsequently develop PTSD symptoms. Implicitly excluded from the definition are stressful experiences of ordinary life, such as bereavement, divorce, and serious illness. Awakening from anesthesia while your surgery is still in progress, however, would qualify as a traumatic event, as would learning about a spouse's sudden, accidental death or a child's life-threatening illness. Watching TV images of a calamity would not be a sufficient stressor (except if the viewing was related to the person's job).

After some delay (symptoms usually don't develop immediately after the trauma), the person in some way relives the traumatic event and tries to avoid thinking about it. There are also symptoms of physiological hyperarousal, such as an exaggerated startle response. Patients with PTSD also express negative feelings such as guilt or personal responsibility ("I should have prevented it").

Aside from the traumatic event itself, other factors may play a role in the development of PTSD. Individual factors include the person's innate character structure and genetic inheritance. Relatively low intelligence and low educational attainment are positively associated with PTSD. Environmental influences include relatively low socioeconomic status and membership in a minority racial or ethnic group.

In general, the more horrific or more enduring the trauma, the greater will be the likelihood of developing PTSD. The risk runs to one-quarter of the survivors of heavy combat and two-thirds of former prisoners of war. Those who have experienced natural disasters such as fires or floods are generally less likely to develop symptoms. (Overall *lifetime* prevalence of PTSD is estimated at about 9%, though European researchers usually report lower overall rates.) Older adults are less likely to develop symptoms than are younger ones, and women tend to have somewhat higher rates than do men. About half the patients recover within a few months; others can experience years of incapacity.

In children, the general outline is pretty much the same as the five general points given in the list of typical symptoms, though the emphasis on symptom numbers differs, as discussed below (p. 223).

Mood, anxiety, and substance use disorders are frequently comorbid. A new specifier reflects findings that in perhaps 12–14% of patients, dissociation is important in the development and maintenance of PTSD symptoms.

Essential Features of **Posttraumatic Stress Disorder**

Something truly awful has happened. One patient has been gravely injured or perhaps sexually abused; another has been closely involved in the death or injury of someone else; a third has only learned that someone close experienced an accident or other violence, whereas emergency workers (police, firefighters) may be traumatized through repeated exposure.

As a result, for many weeks or months these patients:

- Repeatedly relive their event, perhaps in nightmares or upsetting dreams, perhaps in intrusive mental images or dissociative flashbacks. Some people respond to reminders of the event with physiological sensations (racing heart, shortness of breath) or emotional distress.
- Take steps to avoid the horror: refusing to watch films or television or to read accounts of the event, or pushing thoughts or memories out of consciousness.
- Turn downbeat in their thinking: with persistently negative moods, they express gloomy thoughts ("I'm useless," "The world's a mess," "I can't believe anyone.") They lose interest in important activities and feel detached from other people. Some experience amnesia for aspects of the trauma; others become numb, feeling unable to love or experience joy.
- Experience symptoms of hyperarousal: irritability, excessive vigilance, trouble concentrating, insomnia, or an intensified startle response.

The Fine Print

The D's: • Duration (1+ months) • Distress or disability (work/educational, social, or personal impairment) • Differential diagnosis (substance use and physical disorders [especially traumatic brain injury], mood and anxiety disorders, normal reactions to stressful events)

Coding Notes

Specify if:

With delayed expression. Symptoms sufficient for diagnosis didn't accumulate until at least six months after the event.
With dissociative symptoms:
Depersonalization. This indicates feelings of detachment, as though dreaming, from the patient's own mind or body.
Derealization. To the patient, the surroundings seem distant, distorted, dreamlike, or unreal.

Barney Gorse

"They're gooks! The place is staffed with gooks!"

Someone sitting behind Barney Gorse had dropped a book onto the tile floor, and that had set him off. Now he had backed into a corner in the waiting room of the mental health clinic. His pupils were widely dilated, and perspiration stood out on his forehead. He was panting heavily. He pointed a shaky finger at the Asian student who stood petrified on the other side of the room. "Get this goddamn gook out of here!" He made a fist and lumbered off in the direction of the student.

"Hang on, Barney. It's OK." Barney's new therapist took him firmly by the elbow and led him to a private office. They sat there in silence for a few minutes, while Barney's breathing gradually returned to normal and the clinician reviewed his chart.

Barney Gorse was 39 now, but he had been barely 20 when his draft number came up and he joined the Ninth Infantry Division in Vietnam. At that time President Nixon was "winding down the war," which made it seem all the more painful when Barney's squad was hit by mortar fire from North Vietnamese regulars.

He had never talked about it, even during "anger displacement" group therapy with other veterans. Whenever he was asked to tell his story, he would fly into a rage. But something truly devastating must have happened to Barney that day. The reports mentioned a wound in the upper thigh; he had been the only member of his squad to survive the attack. He had been awarded a Purple Heart and a full pension.

Barney hadn't been able to remember several hours of the attack at all. And he had always been careful to avoid films and television programs about war. He said he'd had enough of it to last everybody's lifetime; in fact, he had gone to some lengths to avoid thinking about it. He celebrated his discharge from the Army by getting drunk, which was how he remained for 6 years. When he finally sobered up, he turned to drugs. Even they hadn't been enough to obliterate the nightmares that still haunted him; he awakened screaming several times a week. Sudden noises would startle him into a panic attack.

Now, thanks to disulfiram and a chaplain in the county jail where he had been held as a persistent public nuisance, Barney had been clean and sober for 6 months. On the condition that he would seek treatment for his substance use, he had been released. The specialists in substance misuse treatment had quickly recognized that he had other problems, and that had led him here.

Last week when they met, the therapist had reminded him again that he needed to dig into his feelings about the past. Barney had responded that he didn't have any feelings; they'd dried up on him. For that matter, the future didn't look so good, either: "Got no job, no wife, no kids. I just wasn't meant to have a life." He got up and put his hand on the doorknob to leave. "It's no use. I just can't talk about it."

Evaluation of Barney Gorse

Let's summarize and restate the criteria that must be fulfilled to diagnose PTSD.

1. There must be *severe trauma* (criterion A). Barney's occurred in the context of combat, but a variety of civilian stressors can also culminate in death, serious injury, or sexual abuse. Two features must be present for the stressor to be considered sufficiently traumatic: (a) It must involve the fact or threat of death, severe wounds or injuries, or sexual violation; and (b) it must be personally experienced by the patient in some way—through direct observation (not viewed on TV), through personal involvement, or through information obtained after the fact that it involved a relative or close friend. A first responder (police officer, ambulance attendant) could also qualify through repeated exposure to consequences of the horrific event (think workers at Ground Zero shortly after 9/11). Divorce and death of a spouse from cancer, though undeniably stressful, are relatively commonplace and expected; they don't qualify.

2. Through some intrusive mechanism, the patient *relives the stress*. Barney had flashbacks (B3), during which he imagined himself actually back in Vietnam. He also experienced rather intense responses to an external cue (seeing a staff member who, to him, resembled a Viet Cong soldier). Less dramatic forms of recollection include recurrent ordinary memories, dreams, and any other reminder of the event that results in distress or physiological symptoms.

3. The patient attempts (wittingly or not) to achieve *emotional distance* from the stressful event by avoiding reminders of the trauma. The reminders can be either internal (feelings, thoughts) or external (people, places, activities). Barney refused to watch movies and TV programs or to talk about Vietnam (C).

4. The patient experiences expressions (two or more) of *negative mood and thoughts* related to the trauma. Barney's included amnesia for much of his time in combat (D1), a persistently negative frame of mind ("I wasn't meant to have a life"—D4), and the lack of positive mood states (his feelings had "dried up" on him, D7).

5. Finally, for PTSD, patients must have at least two symptoms of *heightened arousal and reactivity* associated with the traumatic event. Barney suffered from insomnia (E6) and a severe startle response (E4); others may experience general irritability, poor concentration, or excessive vigilance. As with all symptoms, the clinician would have to determine that these symptoms of arousal had not been apparent before Barney's Vietnam trauma.

Barney's symptoms had persisted far longer than the required minimum of 1 month (F); were obviously stressful and impaired his functioning in a number of areas (G); and could not be attributed to the direct effects of substance use—now that he'd been clean and sober for half a year (H).

The experience of severe trauma in combat and the typical symptoms would render any other explanation for Barney's symptoms unlikely. A patient with **intermittent explosive disorder** might become aggressive and lose control, but wouldn't have the history of trauma. Still, clinicians must always be alert to the possibility of another **medical condition** (H) that might produce anxiety symptoms and could be diagnosed instead of or in addition to PTSD. For example, head injuries would be relatively common among veterans of combat or other violent trauma; we'd have to mention and code any accompanying brain injury. Situational **adjustment disorder** shouldn't be confused with PTSD: The severity of the trauma would be far less, and the effects would be transient and less dramatic.

In PTSD, comorbidity is the rule rather than the exception. Barney had used drugs and alcohol; his clinician would have gathered additional information about use of other substances and mentioned them in his diagnostic summary. Of combat veterans who have PTSD, half or more also have a problem with a **substance use disorder**, and use of multiple substances is common. Anxiety disorders (**phobic disorders**, **generalized anxiety disorder**) and mood disorders (**major depressive disorder** and **dysthymia**) are likewise common in this population. **Dissociative amnesia** may also occur. Any coexisting **personality disorder** would be explored, but it is hard to make a definitive diagnosis when a patient is acutely ill from PTSD. **Malingering** is also a diagnosis to consider whenever there appears to be a possibility of material gain (insurance, disability, legal problems) resulting from an accident or physical attack.

Although the vignette is imprecise on this point, Barney's symptoms probably began by the time he was discharged from the military, so he would not rate the specifier *with delayed onset*. The vignette doesn't provide encouragement to add *with prominent dissociation*. I'd give him a GAF score of 35. Pending further information on substance use, Barney's diagnosis would read as follows:

F43.10 [309.81]	Posttraumatic stress disorder
F10.20 [303.90]	Alcohol use disorder, moderate, in early remission
Z60.2 [V60.3]	Lives alone
Z56.9 [V62.29]	Unemployed

There is still considerable controversy over the specifier *with delayed expression*. Many experts deny that symptoms of PTSD can begin many months or years after the trauma. Nonetheless, it is there to use, should you ever find it appropriate.

Posttraumatic Stress Disorder in Preschool Children

There can be no doubt that preschool children are sometimes exposed to traumatic events. Mostly, these are car accidents, natural disasters, and war—in short, all the benefits contemporary life has to offer. The question is, do very young children respond with typical PTSD symptoms? The best evidence would seem to indicate that they do, but with a likelihood much lower (0–12%) than for older children.

Table 6.1 compares the DSM-5 criteria for PTSD in young children, PTSD in adults, and acute stress disorder (to be discussed next). The revamped criteria for PTSD in young children are, as we would hope, more sensitive to symptoms in this age group. Based on interviews with parents, they yield rates in children who have survived severe burns of 25% and 10% at 1 month and 6 months, respectively.

F43 [308.3] Acute Stress Disorder

Based on the observation that some people develop symptoms immediately after a traumatic stress, acute stress disorder (ASD) was devised several decades ago. Even then, this wasn't exactly new information; something similar was noted as far back as 1865, just after the U.S. Civil War. For many years it was termed "shell shock." Like PTSD, ASD can also be found among civilians. Overall rates of ASD, depending on the nature of the trauma and personal characteristics of the individual, center on 20%.

Though the number and distribution of symptoms is different, the criteria embody the same elements required for PTSD:

- Exposure to an event that threatens body integrity

- Reexperiencing the event

- Avoidance of stimuli associated with the event

- Negative changes in mood and thought

- Increased arousal and reactivity

- Distress or impairment

The symptoms usually begin as soon as the patient is exposed to the event (or learns about it), but they must be experienced farther out than 3 days after the stressful event to fulfill the criterion for duration. This gets us to a period of time beyond the stressful event itself and its immediate aftermath. Should symptoms last longer than 1 month, they are no longer acute and no longer constitute ASD. Then many patients will be rolled over into a diagnosis of PTSD. This is the fate of as many as 80% of patients with ASD. However, patients with PTSD don't usually enter through the ASD doorway; most are identified farther along the road than one month.

TABLE 6.1. Comparison of PTSD in Preschool Children, PTSD in Adults, and Acute Stress Disorder

Child PTSD	Adult PTSD	Acute Stress Disorder
Trauma		
Direct experience	Direct experience	Direct experience
Witness (not just TV)	Witness	Witness
Learn of	Learn of	Learn of
	Repeat exposure (not just TV)	Repeat exposure (not just TV)
Intrusion symptoms (1/5)[a]	*Intrusion symptoms (1/5)*	*All symptoms (9/14)*
• Memories	• Memories	• Memories
• Dreams	• Dreams	• Dreams
• Dissociative reactions	• Dissociative reactions	• Dissociative reactions
• Psychological distress	• Psychological distress	• Psychological distress *or* physiological reactions
• Physiological reactions	• Physiological reactions	
Avoid/Neg. emotions (1/6)	*Avoidance (1/2)*	
• Avoids memories	• Avoids memories	• Avoids memories
• Avoids external reminders	• Avoids external reminders	• Avoids external reminders
	Negative emotions (2/7)	
		• Altered sense of reality of self or surroundings
	• Amnesia	• Amnesia
	• Negative beliefs	
	• Distortion → self-blame	
• Negative emotional state	• Negative emotional state	
• Decreased interest	• Decreased interest	
• Social withdrawal	• Detached from others	
• Decreased positive emotions	• No positive emotions	• No positive emotions
Physiological (2/5)	*Physiological (2/6)*	
• Irritable, angry	• Irritable, angry	• Irritable, angry
	• Reckless, self-destructive	
• Hypervigilance	• Hypervigilance	• Hypervigilance
• Startle	• Startle	• Startle
• Poor concentration	• Poor concentration	• Poor concentration
• Sleep disturbance	• Sleep disturbance	• Sleep disturbance
Duration		
>1 month	>1 month	3 days–1 month

[a]Fractions indicate the number of symptoms required of the number possible in the following list.

Essential Features of **Acute Stress Disorder**

Something truly awful has happened—grave injury or sexual abuse, or perhaps the traumatic death or injury of someone else. (It could have come about through learning another has experienced violence or injury, or through repeated exposure for an emergency worker.) As a result, for up to a month the patient experiences many symptoms such as intrusive memories or bad dreams; dissociative experiences such as flashbacks or feeling unreal; the inability to experience joy or other love; amnesia for parts of the event; attempts to avoid reminders of the event (refusing to watch films or television or to read accounts of the event); pushing thoughts or memories out of consciousness. The patient may also experience symptoms of hyperarousal: irritability, hypervigilance, trouble concentrating, insomnia, or an intense startle response.

The Fine Print

The D's: • Duration (3 days to 1 month) • Distress or disability (work/educational, social, or personal impairment) • Differential diagnosis (substance use and physical disorders (especially traumatic brain injury), panic disorder, mood disorders, dissociative disorders, PTSD)

Marie Trudeau

Marie Trudeau and her husband, André, sat in the intake interviewer's office. Marie was the patient, but she spent most of the time rubbing the knuckles of one hand and gazing vacantly into the room. André did most of the talking.

"I just can't believe the change in her," he said. "A week ago, she was completely normal. Never had anything like this in her life. Heck, she's never had anything wrong with her. Then, all of a sudden, boom! She's a mess."

At André's exclamation, Marie jerked around to face him and rose half out of her chair. For a few seconds she stood there, frozen except for her gaze, which darted from one side of the room to the other.

"Aw, geez, I'm sorry, honey. I forgot." He put his arm around her. Grasping her shoulders firmly but gently, he eased her back into the chair. He held her there until she began to relax her grip on his arm.

A week earlier, Marie had just finished her gardening and was sitting in the back yard with a lemonade, reading a book. When she heard airplane engines, she looked up and saw two small planes flying high overhead, directly above her. "My God," she thought, "they're going to collide!" As she watched in horror, they did collide.

She could see perfectly. The sun was low, highlighting the two planes brilliantly against the deep blue of the late afternoon sky. Something seemed to have been torn off one of them—the news media later reported that the right wing of one plane had ripped right through the cockpit of the other. Thinking to call 911, Marie picked up her portable phone, but she didn't dial. She could only watch as two tiny objects suddenly appeared beside the stricken airplanes and tumbled toward her in a leisurely arc.

"They weren't objects, they were people." It was the first time she had spoken during the interview. Marie's chin trembled, and a lock of hair fell across her eye. She didn't try to brush it back.

As she continued to watch, one of the bodies hurtled into her yard 15 feet from where she was sitting. It buried itself 6 inches deep in the soft earth behind her rose bushes.

What happened next, Marie seemed to have blanked out completely. The other body landed in the street a block away. Half an hour later, when the police knocked on her door, they found her in the kitchen peeling carrots for supper and crying into the sink. When André arrived home an hour after that, she seemed dazed. All she would say was "I'm not here."

In the 6 days since, Marie hadn't improved much. Although she might start a conversation, something would appear to distract her, and she would usually trail off in midsentence. She couldn't focus much better on her work at home. Amy, their 9-year-old daughter, seemed to be taking care of *her*. Sleep had slipped to a restless struggle, and three nights running Marie had awakened from a dream, trying to cry out but managing only a terrified squeak. She kept the blinds in the kitchen closed, so she wouldn't even have to look into the back yard.

"It's like someone I saw in a World War II movie," André concluded. "You'd think she'd been shell-shocked."

Evaluation of Marie Trudeau

Anxiety and depressive symptoms are nearly universal following a severe stress. Usually these are relatively short-lived, however, and do not include the full spectrum of symptoms required for ASD. This diagnosis should only be considered when major symptoms last 3 days or more after personal exposure to a horrific event. Such an event was the plane crash Marie witnessed (criterion A2). She was dazed (B6) and emotionally unresponsive (B5), and could not recall what had happened during part of the accident (B7). When she could sleep at all (B10), she had nightmares (B2); she also avoided looking into the back yard (B9), startled easily (B14), and even in the interviewer's office appeared hypervigilant (B12). From her inability to finish conversations, we infer poor concentration (B13), as she was distracted by intrusive recollections of the event (B1). As far as we are aware, she had had none of these symptoms (DSM-5 requires 9 of the 14 symptoms listed in criterion B) prior to witnessing the accident. Since then, just a week earlier (C), she had been unable to carry on with her work at home (D).

Would any other diagnosis be possible? According to André, Marie's previous health had been good, reducing the likelihood of **another medical condition** (E). We aren't told whether she used alcohol or drugs, though the fact that she was drinking lemonade at the time of the crash could suggest that she did not. (OK, I'm definitely out on a limb here; her clinician needs to rule out a **substance use disorder**.) **Brief**

psychotic disorder would be ruled out by the lack of delusions, hallucinations, or disorganized behavior or speech.

Patients with ASD are likely to have severe depressive symptoms ("survivor's guilt"), to the point that a concomitant diagnosis of **major depressive disorder** may sometimes be justified; Marie deserves further investigation along those lines. Until then, with a GAF score of 61, her diagnosis would be straightforward:

F43.0 [308.3]   Acute stress disorder

Adjustment Disorder

Patients with adjustment disorder (AD) may be responding to one stress or to many; the stressor may happen once or repeatedly. If the stressor goes on and on, it can even become chronic, as when a child lives with parents who fight continually. In clinical situations, the stressor has usually affected only one person, but it can affect many (think flood, fire, and famine). However, almost any relatively commonplace event could be a stressor for someone. Those most often cited for adults are getting married or divorced, moving, and financial problems; for adolescents, they are problems at school. Whatever the nature of the stressor, patients feels overwhelmed by the demands of something in the environment.

As a result, they develop emotional symptoms such as low mood, crying spells, complaints of feeling nervous or panicky, and other depressive or anxiety symptoms—which must not, however, meet criteria for any defined mood or anxiety disorder. Some patients have mainly behavioral symptoms—especially ones we might think of as conduct symptoms, such as driving dangerously, fighting, or defaulting on responsibilities.

The course is usually relatively brief; DSM-5 criteria specify that the symptoms must not persist longer than 6 months after the end of the stressor or its consequences. (Some studies report that a large minority of patients continue to have symptoms longer than the 6-month limit.) Of course, if the stressor is one that will be ongoing, such as a chronic illness, it may take a very long time for the patient to adjust.

Although AD has been reported in 10% or more of adult primary care patients, and in huge percentages of mental health patients, one recent study found a prevalence of only 3%; many of these patients were being inappropriately treated with psychotropic medications, and in only two cases had the AD diagnosis been made. The discrepancies probably rest on the rather poorly developed criteria and on the (mistaken) view of AD as a residual diagnosis.

AD is found in all cultures and age groups, including children. It may be more firmly anchored in adults than in adolescents, whose early symptoms often evolve into other, more definitive mental disorders. The reliability and validity of AD tend to be quite low. In a recent study, in under two-thirds of patients receiving the clinical diagnosis of AD could it be subsequently confirmed with ICD-10 criteria.

Personality disorders or cognitive disorders may make a person more vulnerable to stress, and hence to AD. Patients in whom AD is diagnosed often misuse substances as well.

Essential Features of **Adjustment Disorder**

A stressor causes someone to develop depression, anxiety, or behavioral symptoms—but the response exceeds what you'd expect for most people in similar circumstances. After the stressor has ended, the symptoms might drag on, but not longer than 6 more months.

The Fine Print

The D's: • Duration (starts within 3 months of stressor's onset, stops within 6 months of stressor's end) • Distress or disability (work/educational, social, or personal impairment) • Differential diagnosis (just about everything you can name: substance use and physical disorders, mood and anxiety disorders, trauma-related disorders, somatic symptom disorder, psychotic disorders, conduct and other behavior disorders, milder reactions to life's stresses, normal bereavement)

Coding Notes

Specify:

> **F43.21 [309.0] With depressed mood.** The patient is mainly tearful, sad.
> **F43.22 [309.24] With anxiety.** The patient is mainly nervous, tense, or fearful of separation.
> **F43.23 [309.28] With mixed anxiety and depressed mood.** Symptoms combine the preceding.
> **F43.24 [309.3] With disturbance of conduct.** The patient behaves inappropriately or unadvisedly, perhaps violating societal rules, norms, or the rights of others.
> **F43.25 [309.4] With mixed disturbance of emotions and conduct.** The clinical picture combines emotional and conduct symptoms.
> **F43.20 [309.9] Unspecified.** Use for other maladaptive stress-related reactions, such as physical complaints, social withdrawal, work or academic inhibition.

Specify if:

> Acute. The condition has lasted less than 6 months.
> Persistent (or chronic). 6+ months duration of symptoms, though still not lasting more than 6 months after the stressor has ended.

Clarissa Wetherby

"I know it's temporary, and I know I'm overreacting. I sure don't want to, but I just feel upset!"

Clarissa Wetherby was speaking of her husband's new work schedule. Arthur Wetherby was foreman on a road-paving crew whose current job was to widen and resurface a portion of the interstate highway just a few miles from the couple's house. Because the section the crew was working on involved an interchange with another major highway, the work had to be done at night.

For the past 2 months, Arthur had slept days and gone to work at 8:00 P.M. Clarissa worked the day shift as cashier in a restaurant. Except on weekends, when he tried to revert to a normal sleep schedule so he could be with her, they hardly ever saw one another. "I feel like I've been abandoned," she said.

The Wetherbys had been married only 3 years, and they had no children. Each partner had been married once before; each was 35. Neither drank or used drugs. Clarissa's only previous encounter with the mental health system had occurred 7 years earlier, when her first husband had left her for another man. "I respected his right not to continue living a lie," she said, "but I felt terribly alone and humiliated."

Clarissa's symptoms now were much as they had been then. Most of the time when she was at work, she felt "about normal" and maintained good interest in what she was doing. But when alone at home in the evenings, she would be overwhelmed by waves of sadness. These left her virtually immobilized, unable even to turn on the television for company. She often cried to herself and felt guilty for giving in to her emotions. "It's not as if someone had died, after all." Although she had some difficulty getting to sleep at night, she slept soundly in the morning. Her weight was constant, her appetite was good, and she had no suicidal ideas or death wishes. She did not report any problems with her concentration. She denied ever having mania symptoms.

The previous time she'd sought help, she had remained depressed and upset until a few weeks after the divorce was final. Then she seemed suddenly able to put it behind her and begin dating once again.

"I know I'll feel better, once Arthur gets off that schedule," she said. "I guess it just makes me feel worthless, playing second fiddle to an overpass."

Evaluation of Clarissa Wetherby

As she herself recognized, Clarissa's reaction to the stress of her husband's work schedule might be considered extreme by some observers. That is one of the important points of this diagnosis: The patient's misery seems disproportionate to the apparent degree of the stress that has caused it (criterion B1). Her history provides a clue as to the source of her reaction: She was reminded of that awful time when her previous husband abandoned her—for good, and under circumstances that she considered humiliating. It is important, however, always to consider carefully whether a patient's reaction occurs as a **nonpathological response** to a genuine danger, which was not the case with Clarissa.

The time course of Clarissa's symptoms was right for AD: They developed shortly after she learned about Arthur's new work schedule (A). Although we have no way of knowing how long this episode might last, her previous episode ended after a few months, when the aftermath of her divorce had subsided (E). Of course, bereavement didn't enter into her differential diagnosis (D).

Note that AD is not intended as a residual diagnosis, though it is often used that way. Nonetheless, it does come at the end of a long differential diagnosis that comprises every other condition listed in DSM-5 (C). For Clarissa, the symptoms of mood disorder were the most prominent. She had never been manic, so could not qualify for a **bipolar disorder.** She had low mood, but only when alone in the evenings (not most of the day). She maintained interest in her work (rather than experiencing loss of interest in nearly all activities). Without at least one of these symptoms, there could not be a diagnosis of **major depressive disorder**, regardless of her guilt feelings, low energy, and trouble getting to sleep at night. Of course, her symptoms had lasted far less than 2 years, ruling out **dysthymia.** Although she remained fully functional at work, she was seriously distressed, fulfilling the severity requirement.

The question of **PTSD** (and **acute stress disorder**) often arises in the differential diagnosis of AD. Each of those diagnoses requires that the stressor threaten serious harm and that the patient react with a variety of responses; Clarissa did not fulfill these conditions. She similarly did not have symptoms that would suggest **generalized anxiety disorder**, another diagnosis prominent in the differential for AD. A **personality disorder** may worsen (and hence become more apparent) with stress, but there is no hint that Clarissa had any lifelong character pathology. I'd assign her a GAF score of 61.

F43.21 [309.0]   Adjustment disorder, with depressed mood, acute

Although some data support the utility of AD, which has been used clinically for decades, I recommend reserving it as a diagnosis of "almost last resort." There are several reasons for this warning.

For one thing, we probably too often use it when we simply have no better idea of what is going on. For another, the DSM-5 criteria do not tell us how we are to differentiate ordinary events from those that are stressful enough to cause depression, anxiety, or aberrant behavior. I suspect that an event is singled out solely on the basis that it causes emotional or behavioral problem, and that seems to me a tad circular.

F94.1 [313.89] Reactive Attachment Disorder

F94.2 [313.89] Disinhibited Social Engagement Disorder

In two apparently rare but extremely serious disorders, children who have been mistreated (by accident or design) respond by becoming either extremely withdrawn or pathologically outgoing. For neither disorder do we have a lot of information, placing these two among the least well understood of mental disorders that affect children (or adults, for that matter).

Each disorder is conceived as a reaction to an environment in which the child experiences caregiving that is inconstant (frequent change of parent or surrogate) or pathological (abuse, neglect). One of two patterns then develops.

In reactive attachment disorder (RAD), even young infants withdraw from social contacts, appearing shy or distant. Inhibited children will resist separation by tantrums or desperate clinging. In severe cases, infants may exhibit failure-to-thrive syndrome, with head circumference, length, and weight hovering around the 3rd percentile on standard growth charts.

By contrast, a child's response in disinhibited social engagement disorder (DSED) borders on the promiscuous. Small children eschew normal wariness and boldly approach strangers; instead of clinging, they may instead appear indifferent to the departure of a parent. In both subtypes, the abnormal responses are more obvious when the main caregiver is absent.

Factors that indicate increased risk for either RAD or DSED include being reared in an orphanage or other institution; protracted hospitalizations; multiple and frequent changes in caregivers; severe poverty; abuse (the gamut of physical, emotional, and sexual); and a family riven by death, divorce, or discord. Complications associated with these disorders include stunted physical growth, low self-esteem, delinquency, anger management issues, eating disorders, malnutrition, depression or anxiety, and later substance misuse.

In either disorder, a constant, nourishing relationship with a sensitive caregiver is required to reestablish adequate physical and emotional growth. Without such a remedy, the conditions tend to persist into adolescence. There has been almost no follow-up into adult life; despite a dearth of reliable information, you will (of course) find websites.

DSM-IV listed these two conditions as subcategories of one disorder. Because of differences in symptoms, course, treatment response, and other correlates, DSM-5 now treats them as separate diagnoses—despite their supposed common etiology. However, some children will appear withdrawn when very young, then become disinhibited later, whereas others have symptoms of both conditions simultaneously. The upshot is that some observers find the dichotomy a bit forced.

Essential Features of **Reactive Attachment Disorder**

Adverse child care (abuse, neglect, caregiving insufficient or changed too frequently) has apparently caused a child to withdraw emotionally; the child neither seeks nor responds to soothing from an adult. Such children will habitually show little emotional or social response; far from having positive affect, they may experience periods of unprovoked irritability or sadness.

The Fine Print

The presumption of causality stems from the temporal relationship of the traumatic child care to the disturbed behavior.

The D's: • Demographics (begins before age 5; child has developmental age of at least 9 months) • Differential diagnosis (autism spectrum disorder, intellectual disability, depressive disorders)

Coding Notes

Specify if:

> **Persistent.** Symptoms are present longer than 1 year.
> **Severe.** All symptoms are present at a high level of intensity.

Essential Features of **Disinhibited Social Engagement Disorder**

Adverse child care (abuse, neglect, caregiving insufficient or changed too frequently) has apparently caused a child to become unreserved in interactions with strange adults. Such children, rather than showing typical first-acquaintance shyness, will little hesitate to leave with a strange adult; they don't "check in" with familiar caregivers, and readily become excessively familiar. In so doing, they may cross normal cultural and social boundaries.

The Fine Print

The presumption of causality stems from the temporal relationship of the traumatic child care to the disturbed behavior.

The D's: • Demographics (child has developmental age of at least 9 months) • Differential diagnosis (autism spectrum disorder, intellectual disability, ADHD)

Coding Notes

Specify if:

> **Persistent.** Symptoms are present longer than 1 year.
> **Severe.** All symptoms are present at a high level of intensity.

F43.8 [309.89] Other Specified Trauma- or Stressor-Related Disorder

This diagnosis will serve to categorize those patients for whom there is an evident stressor or trauma, but who for a specific, stated reason don't fulfill criteria for any of the standard diagnoses already mentioned above. DSM-5 gives several examples, including two forms of adjustment-like disorders (one form with delayed onset and another with prolonged duration relative to adjustment disorder). Others are as follows:

Persistent complex bereavement disorder. For at least a year, a patient experiences intense grief for someone close who has died. There may be yearning and preoccupation of thoughts for the person, or continuing ruminations over the circumstance of death. A number of other symptoms express the patient's loss of identity and reactive distress. Proposed criteria and discussion are given in Section III of DSM-5 on page 789.

Various cultural syndromes. You'll find a number of these in an appendix in DSM-5, page 833.

F43.9 [309.9] Unspecified Trauma- or Stressor-Related Disorder

This diagnosis will serve to categorize those patients for whom there is an evident stressor or trauma, but who don't fulfill criteria for any of the standard diagnoses already mentioned above, and for whom you do not care to specify the reasons why the criteria are not fulfilled.

CHAPTER 7

Dissociative Disorders

Quick Guide to the Dissociative Disorders

Dissociative symptoms are principally covered in this chapter, but there are some conditions (especially involving loss or lapse of memory) that are classified elsewhere. Yep, the page number following each item indicates where a more detailed discussion begins.

Primary Dissociative Disorders

Dissociative amnesia. The patient cannot remember important information that is usually of a personal nature. This amnesia is usually stress-related (p. 239).

Dissociative identity disorder. One or more additional identities intermittently seize control of the patient's behavior (p. 245).

Depersonalization/derealization disorder. There are episodes of detachment, as if the patient is observing the patient's own behavior from outside. In this condition, there is no actual memory loss (p. 237).

Other specified, or unspecified, dissociative disorder. Patients who have symptoms suggestive of any of the disorders above, but who do not meet criteria for any one of them, may be placed in one of these two categories (p. 248).

Other Causes of Marked Memory Loss

When dissociative symptoms are encountered in the course of other mental diagnoses, a separate diagnosis of a dissociative disorder is not ordinarily given.

Panic attack. Some patients panic may experience depersonalization or derealization as part of an acute panic attack (p. 173).

Posttraumatic stress disorder. A month or more following a severe trauma, the patient may not remember important aspects of personal history (p. 219).

Acute stress disorder. Immediately following a severe trauma, patients may not remember important aspects of personal history (p. 224).

Somatic symptom disorder. Patients who have a history of somatic symptoms that cannot be explained on the basis of known disease mechanisms can also forget important aspects of personal history (p. 251).

Non-rapid eye movement sleep arousal disorder, sleepwalking type. Sleepwalking resembles the dissociative disorders, in that there is amnesia for purposeful behavior. But it is classified elsewhere in order to keep all the sleep disorders together (p. 331).

Borderline personality disorder. When severely stressed, these people will sometimes experience episodes of dissociation, such as depersonalization (p. 545).

Malingering. Some patients consciously feign symptoms of memory loss. Their object is material gain, such as avoiding punishment or obtaining money or drugs (p. 599).

Introduction

Dissociation occurs when one group of normal mental processes becomes separated from the rest. In essence, some of an individual's thoughts, feelings, or behaviors are removed from conscious awareness and control. For example, an otherwise healthy college student cannot recall any of the events of the previous 2 weeks.

As with so many other mental symptoms, you can have dissociation without disorder; if it's mild, it can be entirely normal. (Perhaps, for example, while enduring a boring lecture, you once daydreamed about your weekend plans, unaware that you've been called on for a response?) There's also a close connection between the phenomena of dissociation and hypnosis. Indeed, over half the people interviewed in some surveys have had some experience of a dissociative nature.

Episodes of dissociation severe enough to constitute a disorder have several features in common:

- They usually begin and end suddenly.

- They are perceived as a disruption of information that is needed by the individual. They can be *positive*, in the sense of something added (for example, flashbacks) or *negative* (a period of time for which the person has no memory).

- Although clinicians often disagree as to their etiology, many episodes are apparently precipitated by psychological conflict.

- Although they are generally regarded as rare, their numbers may be increasing.

- In most (except depersonalization/derealization disorder), there is a profound disturbance of memory.

- Impaired functioning or a subjective feeling of distress is required only for dissociative amnesia and depersonalization/derealization disorder.

Conversion symptoms (typical of the somatic symptom disorders) and dissociation tend to involve the same psychic mechanisms. Whenever you encounter a patient who dissociates, consider whether such a diagnosis is also warranted.

F48.1 [300.6] Depersonalization/Derealization Disorder

Depersonalization can be defined as a sense of being cut off or detached from oneself. This feeling may be experienced as viewing one's own mental processes or behavior; some patients feel as though they are in a dream. When a patient is repeatedly distressed by episodes of depersonalization, and there is no other disorder that better accounts for the symptoms, you can diagnose depersonalization/derealization disorder (DDD).

DSM-5 offers another route to that diagnosis: through the experience of *derealization*, a feeling that the exterior world is unreal or odd. Patients may notice that the size or shape of objects has changed, or that other people seem robotic or even dead. Always, however, the person retains insight that it is only a change in perception—that the world itself has remained the same.

Because about half of all adults have had at least one such episode, we need to place some limits on who receives this diagnosis. It should not be made unless the symptoms are persistent or recurrent, and unless they impair functioning or cause pretty significant distress (this means something well beyond the bemused reflection, "Well, *that* was weird!"). In fact, depersonalization and derealization are much more commonly encountered as symptoms than as a diagnosis. For example, derealization or depersonalization is one of the qualifying symptoms for panic attack (p. 173).

Episodes of DDD are often precipitated by stress; they may begin and end suddenly. The disorder usually has its onset in the teens or early 20s; usually it is chronic. Although still not well studied, prevalence rates in the general population appear to be around 1–2%, with males and females nearly equal.

Essential Features of **Depersonalization/Derealization Disorder**

A patient experiences depersonalization or derealization, but reality testing remains intact throughout. (For definitions, see p. 237).

The Fine Print

The D's: • Distress or disability (work/educational, social, or personal impairment) • Differential diagnosis (substance use and physical disorders, mood or anxiety disorders, psychotic disorders, trauma- and stressor-related disorders, other dissociative disorders)

Francine Parfit

"It feels like I'm losing my mind." Francine Parfit was only 20 years old, but she had already worked as a bank teller for nearly 2 years. Having received several raises during that time, she felt that she was good at her job—conscientious, personable, and reliable. And healthy, though she'd been increasingly troubled by her "out-of-body experiences," as she called them.

"I'll be standing behind my counter and, all of a sudden, I'm also standing a couple of feet away. I seem to be looking over my own shoulder as I'm talking with my customer. And in my head I'm commenting to myself on my own actions, as if I were a different person I was watching. Stuff like 'Now she'll have to call the assistant manager to get approval for this transfer of funds.' I came to the clinic because I saw something like this on television a few nights ago, and the person got shock treatments. That's when I began to worry something really awful was wrong."

Francine denied that she had ever had blackout spells, convulsions, blows to the head, severe headaches, or dizziness. She had smoked pot a time or two in high school, but otherwise she was drug- and alcohol-free. Her physical health had been excellent; her only visits to physicians had been for immunizations, Pap smears, and a preemployment physical exam 2 years ago.

Each episode began suddenly, without warning. First Francine would feel quite anxious; then she'd notice that her head seemed to bob up and down slightly, out of her control. Occasionally she felt a warm sensation on the top of her head, as if someone had cracked a half-cooked egg that was dribbling yolk down through her hairline. The episodes seldom lasted longer than a few minutes, but they were becoming more frequent—several times a week now. If they occurred while she was at work, she could often take a break until they passed. But several times it had happened when she was driving. She worried that she might lose control of her car.

Francine had never heard voices or had hallucinations of other senses; she denied ever feeling talked about or plotted against in any way. She had never had suicidal ideas and didn't really feel depressed.

"Just scared," she concluded. "It's so spooky to feel that you've sort of died."

Evaluation of Francine Parfit

The sensation of being an outside observer of yourself can be quite unsettling; it is one that many people who are not patients have had a time or two. What makes Francine's experience stand out is the fact that it returned often enough (criterion A1) and forcibly enough to cause her considerable distress—enough to seek an evaluation, at any rate (C). (She was a little unusual in that her episodes didn't seem to be precipitated by stress; in many people, they are.) Notice that she described her experience "as if I were a different person," not "I am a different person." This tells us that she retained contact with reality (B).

Francine's experiences and feelings were much like those of Shorty Rheinbold (p. 174), except that his occurred as symptoms of **panic disorder.** A variety of other conditions include depersonalization as a symptom: **posttraumatic stress disorder, anxiety, cognitive, mood, personality,** and **substance-related disorders; schizophrenia;** and **epilepsy** (D, E). However, Francine did not complain of panic attacks or have symptoms of other disorders that could account for the symptoms.

Note a new feature in DSM-5: Francine could also have received this diagnosis if she had experienced only symptoms of derealization. With a GAF score of 70, her diagnosis would be:

F48.1 [300.6]   Depersonalization/derealization disorder

Though it goes unmentioned in DSM-5, a collection of symptoms called the *phobic anxiety depersonalization syndrome* sometimes occurs, especially in young women. In addition to depression, such patients, not surprisingly, have phobias, anxiety, and depersonalization. This condition may be a variant of major depressive disorder, with atypical features.

F44.0 [300.12] Dissociative Amnesia

There are two main requirements for dissociative amnesia (DA): (1) The patient has forgotten something important, and (2) other disorders have been ruled out. Of course, the central feature is the inability to remember significant events. Over 100 years ago, clinicians like Pierre Janet recognized several patterns in which this forgetting can occur:

Localized (or circumscribed). The patient has recall for none of the events that occurred within a particular time frame, often during a calamity such as a wartime battle or a natural disaster.

Selective. Certain portions of a time period, such as the birth of a child, have been forgotten. This type is less common.

The next three types are much less common, and may eventually lead to a diagnosis of dissociative identity disorder (see below):

Generalized. All of the experiences during the patient's entire lifetime have been forgotten.

Continuous. The patient forgets all events from a given time forward to the present. This is now extremely rare.

Systematized. The patient has forgotten certain classes of information, such as that relating to family or to work.

DA begins suddenly, usually following severe stress such as physical injury, guilt about an extramarital affair, abandonment by a spouse, or internal conflict over sexual issues. Sometimes the patient wanders aimlessly near home. Duration ranges widely, from minutes to perhaps years, after which the amnesia usually ends abruptly with complete recovery of memory. In some individuals, it may occur again, perhaps more than once.

DA has still received insufficient study, so too little is known about demographic patterns, family occurrence, and the like. Beginning during early adulthood, it is most commonly reported in young women; it may occur in 1% or less of the general population, though recent surveys have pegged it somewhat higher. Many patients with DA have reported childhood sexual trauma, with a high percentage who cannot remember the actual abuse.

Dissociative Fugue

In the subtype of DA known as dissociative fugue, the amnesic person suddenly journeys from home. This often follows a severe stress, such as marital strife or a natural or human-made disaster. The individual may experience disorientation and a sense of perplexity. Some will assume a new identity and name, and for months may even work at a new occupation. However, in most instances the episode is a brief episode of travel, lasting a few hours or days. Occasionally, there may be outbursts of violence. Recovery is usually sudden, with subsequent amnesia for the episode.

Dissociative fugue is another of those extraordinarily interesting, rare disorders—fodder for novels and motion pictures—about which there has been little in the way of recent research. For example, little is known about sex ratio or family history. This is a part of the reason (after its general rarity) that accounts for the demotion of dissociative fugue from an independent diagnosis in DSM-IV to a mere subtype of dissociative amnesia in DSM-5. DSM-5 notes, by the way, that the greatest prevalence of fugue states is among patients with dissociative identity disorder.

Essential Features of **Dissociative Amnesia**

Far beyond common forgetfulness, there is a loss of recall for important personal (usually distressing or traumatic) information.

The Fine Print

The D's: • Distress or disability (work/educational, social, or personal impairment) • Differential diagnosis (substance use and physical disorders, cognitive disorders, trauma- and stressor-related disorders, dissociative identity disorder, somatic symptom disorder, ordinary forgetfulness)

Coding Note

If relevant, specify:

> **F44.1 [300.13] With dissociative fugue**

Holly Kahn

A mental health clinician presented the following dilemma to a medical center ethicist.

A single 38-year-old woman had been seen several times in the outpatient clinic. She had complained of depression and anxiety, both of which were relatively mild. These symptoms seemed focused on the fact that she was 38 and unmarried, and "her biological clock was ticking." She had had no problems with sleep, appetite, or weight gain or loss, and had not thought about suicide.

For many months Holly Kahn had so longed for a child that she intentionally became pregnant by her boyfriend. When he discovered what she had done, he broke off contact with her. The following week she miscarried. Stuck in her boring, unrewarding job as a sales clerk in a store that specialized in teaching supplies, she said she'd come to the clinic for help in "finding meaning for her life."

The oldest girl in a Midwestern family, Holly had spent much of her adolescence caring for younger siblings. Although she had attended college for 2 years during her mid-20s, she had come away with neither degree nor career to show for it. In the last decade, she had lived with three different men; her latest relationship had lasted the longest and had seemed the most stable. She had no history of drug abuse or alcoholism and was in good physical health.

The clinician's verbal description was of a plain, no longer young (and perhaps never youthful), heavy-set woman with a square jaw and stringy hair. "In fact, she looks quite a lot like this." The clinician produced a drawing of a woman's head and shoulders. It was somewhat indistinct and smudged, but the features did fit the verbal description. The ethicist recognized it as a flyer that had recently received wide distribution. The copy below the picture read: "Wanted by FBI on suspicion of kidnapping."

A day-old infant had been abducted from a local hospital's maternity ward. The first-time mother, barely out of her teens, had handed the baby girl to a woman wearing an operating room smock. The woman had introduced herself as a nursing supervisor and said she needed to take the baby for a final weighing and examination before the mother could take her home. That was the last time anyone could remember seeing either the woman or the baby. The picture had been drawn by a police artist from a description given by the distraught mother. A reward was being offered by the baby's grandparents.

"The next-to-last time I saw my patient, we were trying to work on ways she could take control over her own life. She seemed quite a bit more confident, less depressed. The following week she came in late, looking dazed. She claimed to have no memory of anything she had done for the past several days. I asked her whether she'd been ill, hit on the head, that sort of thing. She denied all of it. I started probing backward to see if I could jog her memory, but she became more and more agitated and finally rushed out. She said she'd return the next week, but I haven't seen her since. It wasn't until yesterday that I noticed her resemblance to the woman in this picture."

The therapist sat gazing at the flyer for a few seconds, then said: "Here's my dilemma. I think I know who committed this really awful crime, but I have a privileged relationship with the person I suspect. Just what is my ethical duty?"

Evaluation of Holly Kahn

Whether Holly took the baby is not the point here. At issue is the cause of her amnesia, which was her most pressing recent problem (criterion A). She had been under stress because of her desire to have a baby, and this could have provided the stimulus for her amnesia. The episode was itself evidently stressful enough that she broke off contact with her clinician (B).

There is no information provided in the vignette that might support other (mostly biological) causes of amnesia (D). Specifically, there was no **head trauma** that might have induced a **major neurocognitive disorder due to traumatic brain injury. Substance-induced neurocognitive disorder, persistent** would be ruled out by Holly's history of no substance use (C). Her general health had been good and there was no history of abnormal physical movements, reducing the likelihood of **epilepsy.** Although she had had a miscarriage, too much time had passed for a **postabortion psychosis** to be a possibility. Some patients with amnesia are also mute; they may be misdiagnosed as having **another medical condition** with **catatonic symptoms.** And, just to be complete, we should note that her loss of memory is far more striking and significant than **ordinary forgetfulness,** which is what we humans experience all the time.

There was no history of a recent, massive trauma that might indicate **acute stress disorder.** If she was **malingering,** she did it without an obvious motive (had she been trying to avoid punishment for a crime, simply staying away from the medical center would have served her better). It certainly wouldn't appear to be a case of normal **daydreaming.** Holly was clear about her personal identity, and she did not travel from home, so she would not qualify for the **dissociative fugue** subtype diagnosis. Although we must be careful not to make a diagnosis in a patient we have not personally interviewed and for whom we lack adequate collateral information, if what material we do have is borne out by subsequent investigation, her diagnosis would be as below. I'd give her GAF score as 31.

F44.0 [300.12]   Dissociative amnesia

John Doe

When the man first walked into the homeless shelter, he hadn't a thing to his name, including a name. He'd been referred from a hospital emergency room, but he told the clinician on duty that he'd only gone there for a place to stay. As far as he was aware, his physical health was good. His problem was that he didn't remember a thing about his life prior to waking up on a park bench at dawn that morning. Later, when filling out the paperwork, the clinician had penciled in "John Doe" as the patient's name.

Aside from the fact that he could give a history spanning only about 8 hours, John Doe's mental status exam was remarkably normal. He appeared to be in his early 40s. He was dressed casually in slacks, a pink dress shirt, and a nicely fitting corduroy sports jacket with leather patches on the elbows. His speech was clear and coherent; his affect was generally pleasant, though he was obviously troubled at his loss of memory. He denied having hallucinations or delusions ("as far as I know"), though he pointed out logically enough that he "couldn't vouch for what kind of crazy ideas I might have had yesterday."

John Doe appeared intelligent, and his fund of information was good. He could name five recent presidents in order, and he could discuss recent national and international events. He could repeat eight digits forward and six backwards. He scored 29 out of 30 on the MMSE, failing only to identify the county in which the shelter was located. Although he surmised (he wore a wedding ring) that he must be married, after half an hour's conversation he could remember nothing pertaining to his family, occupation, place of residence, or personal identity.

"Let me look inside your sports jacket," the clinician said.

John Doe looked perplexed, but unbuttoned his jacket and held it open. The label gave the name of a men's clothing store in Cincinnati, some 500 miles away.

"Let's try there," suggested the clinician. Several telephone calls later, the Cincinnati Police Department identified John Doe as an attorney whose wife had reported him missing 2 days earlier.

The following morning John Doe was on a bus for home, but it was days before the clinician heard the rest of the story. A 43-year-old specialist in wills and probate, John Doe had been accused of mingling the bank accounts of clients with his own. He had protested his innocence and hired his own attorney, but the Ohio State Bar Association stood ready to proceed against him. The pressure to straighten out his books, maintain his law practice, and defend himself in court and against his own state bar had been enormous. Two days before he disappeared, he had told his wife, "I don't know if I can take much more of this without losing my mind."

Evaluation of John Doe

John Doe was classically unable to recall important autobiographical information—in fact, all of it (criterion A). It is understandable—and required (B)—that this troubled him.

Neither at the time of evaluation nor at follow-up was there evidence of alternative disorders (D). John had not switched repeatedly between identities, which would rule out **dissociative identity disorder** (you wouldn't diagnose the two disorders together). Other than obvious amnesia, there was no evidence of a **cognitive disorder.** At age 43, a new case of **temporal lobe epilepsy** would be unlikely, but a complete evaluation should include a neurological workup. Of course, any patient who has episodes of amnesia must be evaluated for **substance-related disorders** (especially as concerns alcohol, C).

Conscious imitation of amnesia in **malingering** can be very difficult to discriminate from the amnesia involved in DA with dissociative fugue. However, although John Doe did have legal difficulties, these would not have been relieved by his feigning amnesia. (When malingering appears to be a possibility, collateral history from relatives or friends of previous such behavior or of **antisocial personality disorder** can help.) A history of lifelong multiple medical symptoms might suggest **somatic symptom disorder.** John had no cross-sectional features that would suggest either a **manic episode** or **schizophrenia**, in either of which wandering and other bizarre behaviors can occur.

Epilepsy is always mentioned in the differential diagnosis of the dissociative disorders. However, epilepsy and dissociation should not be hard to tell apart in practice, even without the benefit of an EEG. Epileptic episodes usually last no longer than a few minutes and involve speech and motor behavior that are repetitive and apparently purposeless. Dissociative behavior, on the other hand, may last for days or longer and involves complex speech and motor behaviors that appear purposeful.

Although John Doe's case is not quite classical (he did not assume a new identity and adopt a new life), he did travel far from home and purposefully set about seeking shelter. That sets up the specifier for his diagnosis. And by the way, his GAF score would be 55.

F44.1 [300.13]	Dissociative amnesia, with dissociative fugue
Z65.3 [V62.5]	Investigation by state bar association

Note that the fugue subtype has a different code number than plain old dissociative amnesia. This reflects the fact that, in ICD-10 *and* in ICD-9, a fugue state is a diagnosis separate and apart from dissociative amnesia. So the number change isn't a mistake.

F44.81 [300.14] Dissociative Identity Disorder

In dissociative identity disorder (DID), which previously achieved fame as multiple personality disorder, the person possesses at least two distinct identities. Ranging up to 200 in number, these identities may have their own names; they don't even have to be of the patient's own gender. Some may be symbolic, such as "The Worker." They can vary widely in age and style: If the patient is normally shy and quiet, one identity may be outgoing or even boisterous. The identities may be aware of one another to some degree, though only one interacts with the environment at a time. The transition from one to another is usually sudden, often precipitated by stress. Most of them are aware of the loss of time that occurs when another identity is in control. However, some patients aren't aware of their peculiar state until a close friend points out the alterations in character with time.

Of particular diagnostic note are states of pathological *possession*, which can have characteristics similar to DID. They may be characterized by the patient as a spirit or other external being that has taken over the person's functioning. If this behavior is part of a recognized, accepted religious practice, it will not usually qualify for diagnosis as DID. However, a person who has recurrent possession states that cause distress and otherwise conform to DSM-5 criteria may well qualify for diagnosis. Of course, we would not diagnose DID in a child on the basis of having an imaginary playmate.

Affecting up to 1% of the general population, DID is diagnosed much more commonly by clinicians in North America than in Europe. This fact has engendered a long-running dispute. European clinicians (naturally) claim that the disorder is rare, and that by paying so much attention to patients who dissociate, New World clinicians actually encourage the development of cases. At this writing, the dispute continues unresolved.

The onset of this perhaps too-fascinating disorder is usually in childhood, though it is not commonly recognized then. Most of the patients are female, and many may have been sexually abused. DID tends toward chronicity. It may run in families, but the question of genetic transmission is also unresolved.

Essential Features of **Dissociative Identity Disorder**

A patient appears to have at least two clearly individual personalities, each with unique attributes of mood, perception, recall, and control of thought and behavior. The result: a person with memory gaps for personal information that common forgetfulness cannot begin to explain.

The Fine Print

The D's: • Distress or disability (work/educational, social, or personal impairment) • Differential diagnosis (substance use and physical disorders, mood or anxiety disorders, psychotic disorders, trauma- and stressor-related disorders, other dissociative disorders, religious possession states accepted in non-Western cultures, childhood imaginary playmates/fantasy play)

Effie Jens

On her first visit to the mental health clinic, Effie cried and talked about her failing memory. At age 26—too young for Alzheimer's—she felt senile on some days. For several months she had noticed "holes in her memory," which sometimes lasted 2 or 3 days. Her recall wasn't just spotty; for all she knew about her activities on those days, she might as well have been under anesthesia. However, from telltale signs—such as food that had disappeared from her refrigerator and recently arrived letters that had been opened—she knew she must have been awake and functioning during these times.

On the proceeds of the property settlement from her recent divorce, Effie lived alone in a small apartment; her family lived in a distant state. She enjoyed quiet pastimes, such as reading and watching television. She was shy and had trouble meeting people; there was no one she saw often enough to help her account for the missing time.

For that matter, Effie wasn't all that clear about the details of her earlier life. She was the second of three daughters of an itinerant preacher; her early childhood memories were a jumble of labor camps, cheap hotel rooms, and Bible-thumping sermons. By the time she reached age 13, she had attended 15 different schools.

Late in the interview, she revealed that she had virtually no memory of the entire year she was 13. Her father's preaching had been moderately successful, and they had settled for a while in a small town in southern Oregon—the only time she had started and finished a year in the same school. But what had happened to her during the intervening months? Of that time, she recalled nothing whatsoever.

The following week Effie came back, but she was different. "Call me Liz," she said as she dropped her shoulder bag onto the floor and leaned back in her chair. Without further prompting, she launched into a long, detailed, and dramatic recounting of her activities of the last 3 days. She had gone out for dinner and dancing with a man she had met in the grocery store, and afterwards they had hit a couple of bars together.

"But I only had ginger ale," she said, smiling and crossing her legs. "I never drink. It's terrible for the figure."

"Are there any parts of last week you can't remember?"

"Oh, no. She's the one who has amnesia."

"She" was Effie Jens, whom Liz clearly regarded as a person quite different from her own self. Liz was happy, carefree, and sociable; Effie was introspective and preferred solitude. "I'm not saying that she isn't a decent human being," Liz conceded, "but you've met her—don't you think she's just a tad mousy?"

Although for many years she had "shared living space" with Effie, it wasn't until after the divorce that Liz had begun to "come out," as she put it. At first this had happened for only an hour or two, especially when Effie was tired or depressed and "needed a break." Recently Liz had taken control for longer and longer periods of time; once she had done so for 3 days.

"I've tried to be careful, it frightens her so," Liz said with a worried frown. "I've begun to think seriously about taking control for all time. I think I can do a better job. I certainly have a better social life."

Besides being able to recount her activities during the blank times that had driven Effie to seek care, Liz could give an eyewitness account of all of Effie's conscious activities as well. She even knew what had gone on during Effie's "lost" year, when she was 13.

"It was Daddy," she said with a curl of her lip. "He said it was part of his religious mission to 'practice for a reenactment of the Annunciation.' But it was really just another randy male groping his own daughter, and worse. Effie told Mom. At first, Mom wouldn't believe her. And when she finally did, she made Effie promise never to tell. She said it would break up the family. All these years, I'm the only other one who's known about it. No wonder she's losing her grip—it even makes me sick."

Evaluation of Effie Jens

Effie's two personalities (criterion A) are fairly typical of DID: One was quiet and unassuming, almost mousy, whereas the other was much more assertive. (Effie's history was atypical in that more personalities than two are the rule.) What happened when Liz was in control was unknown to Effie, who experienced these episodes as amnesia. This difficulty with recall was vastly more extensive than you'd expect of common forgetfulness (B). It was distressing enough to send Effie to the clinic (C).

Several other causes of amnesia should be considered in the differential diagnosis of this condition. Of course, any possible **medical condition** must first be ruled out, but Effie/Liz had no history suggestive of either a **seizure disorder** or **substance use** (we're thinking of alcoholic blackouts and partial seizures here). Even though Effie (or Liz) had a significant problem with amnesia, it was not her *main* problem, as would be the case with **dissociative amnesia**, which is less often recurrent and does not involve multiple, distinct identities. Note, too, the absence of any information that Effie belonged to a cultural or religious group whose practices included trances or other rituals that could explain her amnesia (D).

Schizophrenia has often been confused with DID, primarily by laypeople who equate "split personality" (which is how many have come to characterize schizophrenia) with multiple personality disorder, the old name for DID. However, although bizarre behavior may be encountered in DID, none of the identities is typically psychotic. As with other dissociative disorders, discrimination from **malingering** can be difficult; information from others about possible material gain provides the most valuable data. Effie's history was not typical for either of these diagnoses.

Some patients with DID will also have **borderline personality disorder.** The danger is that only the latter will be diagnosed by a clinician who mistakes alternating personae for the unstable mood and behavior typical of borderline personality disorder. **Substance-related disorders** sometimes occur with DID; neither Effie nor Liz drank alcohol (E). Her GAF score would be 55.

F44.81 [300.14]	Dissociative identity disorder
Z63.5 [V61.03]	Divorce

F44.89 [V300.15] Other Specified Dissociative Disorder

This category is for patients whose symptoms represent a change in the normally integrative function of identity, memory, or consciousness, but who do not meet criteria for one of the specific dissociative disorders listed above. Here are some examples; a particular condition should be stated after the other specified diagnosis is given.

Identity disturbance due to prolonged and intense coercive persuasion. People who have been brainwashed or otherwise indoctrinated may develop mixed dissociative states.

Acute dissociative reactions to stressful events. DSM-5 mentions that these often last just a few hours, though less than a month, and are characterized by mixed dissociative symptoms (depersonalization, derealization, amnesia, disruptions of consciousness, stupor).

Dissociative trance. Here the person loses focus on the here and now, and may behave automatically. (A person's engaging in an accepted religious or cultural ritual would not qualify as an example of dissociative trance.)

F44.9 [V300.15] Unspecified Dissociative Disorder

This diagnosis will serve to categorize those patients for whom there are evident dissociative symptoms, but who don't fulfill criteria for any of the standard diagnoses already mentioned above, and for whom you do not care to specify the reasons why the criteria are not fulfilled.

CHAPTER 8

Somatic Symptom and Related Disorders

Quick Guide to the Somatic Symptom and Related Disorders

When somatic (body) symptoms are a prominent reason for evaluation by a clinician, the diagnosis will often be one of the disorders (or categories) listed below. As usual, the page number following each item indicates where a more detailed discussion begins.

Primary Somatic Symptom Disorders

Somatic symptom disorder. Formerly called somatization disorder, this chronic condition is characterized by unexplained physical symptoms. It is found almost exclusively in women (p. 251).

Somatic symptom disorder, with predominant pain. The pain in question has no apparent physical or physiological basis, or it far exceeds the usual expectations, given the patient's actual physical condition (p. 257).

Conversion disorder (functional neurological symptom disorder). These patients complain of isolated symptoms that seem to have no physical cause (p. 262).

Illness anxiety disorder. Formerly called hypochondriasis, this is a disorder in which physically healthy people have an unfounded fear of a serious, often life-threatening illness such as cancer or heart disease—but little in the way of somatic symptoms (p. 260).

Psychological factors affecting other medical conditions. A patient's mental or emotional issues influence the course or care of a medical disorder (p. 266).

Factitious disorder imposed on self. Patients who want to occupy the sick role (perhaps they enjoy the attention of being in a hospital) consciously fabricate symptoms to attract attention from health care professionals (p. 268).

Factitious disorder imposed on another. A person induces symptoms in someone else, often a child, possibly for the purpose of gaining attention (p. 269).

Other specified, or unspecified, somatic symptom and related disorder. These are catch-all categories for patients whose somatic symptoms fail to meet criteria for any better-defined disorder (p. 275).

Other Causes of Somatic Complaints

Actual physical illness. Psychological causes for physical symptoms should be considered only after physical disorders have been eliminated.

Mood disorders. Pain with no apparent physical cause is characteristic of some patients with major depressive disorder (p. 122) and bipolar I disorder, current or most recent episode depressed (p. 129). Because they are treatable and potentially life-threatening, these possibilities must be investigated early.

Substance use. Patients who use substances may complain of pain or other physical symptoms. These may result from the effects of substance intoxication (p. 411) or withdrawal (p. 402).

Adjustment disorder. Some patients who are experiencing a reaction to environmental circumstances will complain of pain or other somatic symptoms (p. 228).

Malingering. These patients know that their somatic (or psychological) symptoms are fabricated, and their motive is some form of material gain, such as avoiding punishment or work, or obtaining money or drugs (p. 599).

Introduction

For centuries, clinicians have recognized that physical symptoms and concerns about health can have emotional origins. DSM-III and its successors have gathered several alternatives to organic diagnoses under one umbrella. Collectively, these are now called the somatic symptom and related disorders, because their presentations resemble somatic (bodily) disease. Like so many other groups of disorders discussed in this book, these conditions are not bound together by common etiologies, family histories, treatments, or other factors. This chapter is simply another convenient collection—in this case, of conditions that are concerned primarily with physical symptoms.

Several sorts of problems can suggest somatic symptom disorder. These include the following:

- Pain that is excessive or chronic

- Conversion symptoms (see sidebar below)

- Chronic, multiple symptoms that seem to lack an adequate explanation

- Complaints that don't improve, despite treatment that helps most patients

- Excessive concern with health or body appearance

Patients with somatic symptom and related disorders have usually been evaluated (perhaps many times) for physical illness. These evaluations often lead to testing and treatments that are expensive, time-consuming, ineffective, and sometimes dangerous. The result of such treatment may be only to reinforce the patients' fearful belief in some nonexistent medical illness. At some point, health care personnel recognize that whatever is wrong has strong emotional underpinnings, and refer these patients for mental health evaluation.

It is important to acknowledge that, with the obvious exception of factitious disorder, these patients are not faking their symptoms. Rather, they often believe that they have something seriously wrong; this belief can cause them enormous anxiety and impairment. Without meaning to, they inflict great suffering on themselves and on those around them.

On the other hand, we must also remember that the mere presence of a somatic symptom disorder does not ensure against the subsequent development of another medical condition. These patients can also develop other forms of mental disturbance.

F45.1 [300.82] Somatic Symptom Disorder

The DSM-5 criteria for somatic symptom disorder (SSD) require only a single somatic symptom, but it must cause distress or markedly impair the patient's functioning. Nonetheless, the classical patient has a pattern of multiple physical and emotional symptoms that can affect various (often many) areas of the body, including pain symptoms, problems with breathing or heartbeat, abdominal complaints, and/or menstrual disorders. Of course, conversion symptoms (body dysfunctioning such as paralysis or blindness that has no anatomical or physiological cause) may also be encountered. Treatment that usually helps symptoms that are caused by actual physical disease is usually ineffective in the long run for these patients.

SSD* begins early in life, usually in the teens or early 20s, and can last for many

---

*Much of the information presented here and elsewhere in this chapter is based on studies of patients defined by DSM-IV criteria. When DSM-5 criteria were written, there simply weren't data available for disorders defined by the new criteria.

years—perhaps the patient's entire lifetime. Often overlooked by health care professionals, this condition affects about 1% of all women; it occurs less often in men, though the actual ratio is unknown, considering that the definition of SSD has only just been written. SSD may account for 7–8% of mental health clinic patients and perhaps nearly that percentage of hospitalized mental health patients. It has a strong tendency to run in families. Transmission is probably both genetic and environmental; SSD may be more frequent in patients with low socioeconomic status and less education.

Half or more of patients with SSD have anxiety and mood symptoms. There is an ever-present danger that clinicians will diagnose an anxiety or mood disorder and ignore the underlying SSD. Then the all-too-common result is that the patient receives treatment specific for the mood or anxiety disorder, rather than an approach that might actually address the underlying SSD.

Essential Features of **Somatic Symptom Disorder**

Concern about one or more somatic symptoms leads the patient to express a high level of health anxiety by investing excessive time in health care or being excessively worried as to the seriousness of symptoms.

The Fine Print

The D's: • Duration (6+ months) • Differential diagnosis (DSM-5 does not state one; I would cite substance use and physical disorders, mood or anxiety disorders, psychotic or stress disorders, dissociative disorders)

Coding Notes

Specify if:

> **With predominant pain.** For patients who complain mainly of pain. See the additional discussion on page 257.
> **Persistent.** If the course is marked by serious symptoms, lots of impairment, and a duration greater than 6 months.

Consider the following behaviors related to seriousness of patient's symptoms: excessive thoughts, persistent high anxiety, excessive energy/time expended. Now rate severity:

> **Mild.** One of these behaviors.
> **Moderate.** 2+.
> **Severe.** 2+, along with numerous somatic complaints (or one extremely severe complaint).

In my own professional lifetime, this mental disorder has borne four different names. *Hysteria* was created over 2,000 years ago by the Greeks, who famously believed that its symptoms arose from a uterus that wandered throughout the body, producing pain or stopping the breath or clogging the throat. That ancient term remained in use until the middle of the 20th century, when it received a new label and a more complicated definition.

Briquet syndrome was coined to honor the 19th-century French physician who first described the disorder's typical polysymptomatic presentation. For diagnosis, it required 25 symptoms (of a possible 60), each of which the clinician had to determine to be unsubstantiated by physical or laboratory examination. The list included pseudoneurological symptoms (such as temporary blindness and aphonia), but also emotional symptoms such as depression, anxiety attacks, and hallucinations—plus a lot more.

Twenty-five symptoms were just too many for some clinicians. In 1980, the authors of DSM-III devised the term *somatization disorder* to highlight new criteria that reduced the number of symptoms, along the way discarding all the mental and emotional symptoms from the Briquet symptoms list. DSM-III-R and DSM-IV further redefined and shortened the list ("dumbed it down," some would say). The Briquet symptoms yielded excellent results in terms of isolating a group of patients who later did *not* turn out to have actual physical disease and who responded well to psychological and behavioral treatment. Even with the simpler somatization disorder symptoms, however, few patients were ever diagnosed; perhaps clinicians didn't want to take the trouble, or perhaps the symptoms were simply too restrictive for practical purposes.

Now, with SSD, we are back where we started: A single symptom, attended by a certain degree of concern on the part of the patient, will suffice for a DSM-5 diagnosis. It is noteworthy that as the names have progressively lengthened, the criteria sets have been getting shorter—with the obvious exception of hysteria itself, which was a seat-of-the-pants diagnosis that entailed identifying but a single symptom, often of the pseudoneurological "conversion" type. It remains to be seen how well the DSM-5 criteria for SSD will discriminate these patients from those with other diagnoses in the somatic symptoms and related disorders group, and from patients with physical illness. But I fear that we really may have truly come full circle, to the point where we are once again in danger of misidentifying people whose symptoms are perplexing, even mysterious, but which may well presage ultimate physical disease.

There's one other issue that deserves our scrutiny: Nowhere do the DSM-5 criteria require that other causes of the patient's symptoms be ruled out. That places the SSD criteria in select company (intellectual disability, personality disorders, substance use disorders, anorexia nervosa, and the paraphilic disorders) as requiring no consideration of a differential diagnosis.

Here's the bottom line. I can indeed make this part of DSM-5 *truly* easy: Don't use it! Until the data are in that persuade me SSD is a useful concept that promotes the well-being of my patients, I will personally continue to use either the old DSM-IV somatization disorder guidelines (see the next sidebar, p. 256) or the even older Briquet syndrome criteria. And here's my guarantee: Any patient diagnosed by either of these standards will also qualify for a diagnosis of DSM-5 SSD.

Cynthia Fowler

When Cynthia Fowler told her story, she cried. At age 35, she was talking with the most recent in her series of health care professionals. Her history was a complicated one; it began in her mid-teens with arthritis that seemed to move from one joint to another. She had been told that these were "growing pains," but the symptoms had continued to come and go over the intervening 20 years. Although she was subsequently diagnosed as having various types of arthritis, laboratory tests never substantiated any of them. A long succession of treatments had proven fruitless.

In her mid-20s, Cynthia was evaluated for left flank pain, but again nothing was found. Later, abdominal pain and vomiting spells were worked up with gastroscopy and barium X-rays. Each of these studies was normal. A histamine antagonist was added to her growing list of medications, which by now included various anti-inflammatory agents, as well as prescription and over-the-counter analgesics.

Cynthia had thought at one time that many of her symptoms were aggravated by her premenstrual syndrome, which she had recognized in herself after reading about it in a women's magazine. She had invariably been irritable with cramps before her period, which used to be so heavy that she would sometimes stay in bed for several days. When she was 26, therefore, she'd had a total hysterectomy. Six months later, persistent vomiting led to endoscopy; other than adhesions, no abnormalities were found. Alternating diarrhea and constipation then caused her to experiment with a series of preparations to regulate her bowel movements.

When she was questioned about sex, Cynthia shifted uncomfortably in her chair. She didn't care much for it and had never experienced a climax. Her lack of interest was no problem to her, though each of her three husbands had complained a lot. When she was a young teenager, something sexual might have happened to her, she finally admitted, but that was a part of her life she really couldn't recall. "It's as if someone cut a whole year out of my diary," she explained.

When she was 2 and her brother was 6 months old, Cynthia's father had deserted the family. Her mother subsequently worked as a waitress and lived with a succession of men, some of whom she married. When Cynthia was 12, her mother escaped from one of Cynthia's stepfathers; she then placed the two children in foster care.

One way or another, each of Cynthia's former clinicians had disappointed her. "None of the others knew how to help me. But I just know you'll find out what's wrong. Everyone says you're the best in town." Through her tears, she managed a confident smile.

Evaluation of Cynthia Fowler

At a glance, we can affirm that Cynthia had distressing somatic symptoms (criterion A) that for years (C) had occupied a great deal of time and effort (B). That, in essence, earns her a DSM-5 diagnosis of SSD. However, I'd prefer to analyze her condition in light of the old DSM-IV somatization disorder guidelines (again, see the sidebar, p. 256).

Cynthia needed to have at least eight symptoms across the four symptom areas, and she did: pain (abdominal, flank, joint, and menstrual); gastrointestinal (diarrhea, vomiting); sexual (excessive menstrual bleeding, sexual indifference); and a lone pseudoneurological symptom (amnesia). The DSM-IV criteria require that these symptoms not be explainable on the basis of physical disease, and that they impair the patient's functioning in some way—I don't think I'll get much disagreement there, either. They started well before she turned 30, and there is nothing to suggest that she was intentionally feigning them. Q.E.D.

Even so, as with nearly every mental disorder, **another medical condition** is the first possibility that I would seek to rule out. Among the medical and neurological disorders to consider are multiple sclerosis, spinal cord tumors, and diseases of the heart and lungs. Cynthia had already been worked up for a variety of medical conditions and had been prescribed multiple medications, none of which had done her much good. Judging by the last paragraph of the vignette, her previous clinicians might have been at a loss to diagnose or treat her effectively.

Setting Cynthia's experience apart from patients with actual physical disease are (1) the number and variety of the symptoms (though neither is required by SSD criterion A); (2) the absence of an adequate explanation for the symptoms based on history, lab findings, or physical examination; and (3) inadequate relief from treatments that are ordinarily helpful for the symptoms in question. Note once again that although the SSD criteria allow a diagnosis based on far fewer symptoms than Cynthia had, her history is typical of a group of patients whom clinicians have been attempting to help for millennia.

Certain other somatic symptom and related disorders require discussion. In **SSD with predominant pain**, the patient focuses on severe, sometimes incapacitating somatic pain. Although Cynthia complained of pain in a variety of locations, it was only one aspect of a much broader picture of somatic illness. Patients with **illness anxiety disorder** (formerly hypochondriasis) can have multiple physical symptoms, but their concern focuses on the fear of having a specific physical disease, not, as with Cynthia, particular symptoms. Cynthia did not have any classical physical conversion symptoms (e.g., stocking or glove anesthesia, hemiparalysis), but many patients with SSD do. Then **conversion disorder (functional neurological symptom disorder)** enters the differential diagnosis. However, as with SSD with predominant pain, conversion disorder should not be diagnosed in any patient who fulfills criteria for the more encompassing SSD. In addition, Cynthia's amnesia might qualify for the diagnosis of **dissociative amnesia** if it were the predominant problem.

You should always inquire carefully about **substance-related disorders**, which are found in one-quarter or more of patients with SSD. And when patients come to the attention of mental health providers, it is often because of a concomitant mood disorder or anxiety disorder.

Many patients with SSD also have one or more **personality disorders.** Especially prevalent is **histrionic** personality disorder, though **borderline** and **antisocial** personality disorders may also be diagnosed. Cynthia's words to the clinician in the last paragraph suggest a personality disorder, but with insufficient information, I'd defer that diagnosis for now. There's no way to code it out, so I would mention "possible personality disorder," or some such verbiage, in my summary.

With a GAF score of 61, Cynthia's current diagnosis would read as follows:

F45.1 [300.82]   Somatic symptom disorder

Here's an outline of the DSM-IV somatization disorder (SD):

- From an early age, these patients have numerous physical complaints that wax and wane, with new ones often beginning as old ones resolve. With treatment typically ineffective, patients tend to switch health care providers in search of cure.
- The wide variety of possible symptoms fall into several groups.
  - Pain (several different sites are required): in the head, back, chest, abdomen, joints, arms or legs, or genitals; or related to body functions, such as urination, menstruation, or sexual intercourse
  - Gastrointestinal (other than pain): bloating, constipation, diarrhea, nausea, vomiting spells (except during pregnancy), or intolerance of several foods (nominally, three or more)
  - Sexual or reproductive systems (other than pain): difficulty with erection or ejaculation, irregular menses, excessive menstrual flow, or vomiting that persists throughout pregnancy
  - Pseudoneurological (not pain): blindness, deafness, double vision, lump in throat or trouble swallowing, inability to speak, poor balance or coordination, weak or paralyzed muscles, retention of urine, hallucinations, numbness to touch or pain, seizures, amnesia (or any other dissociative symptom), or loss of consciousness (other than fainting)
- The typical patient will have eight or more symptoms, with four (or more) from the pain group, two from the gastrointestinal group, and at least one each from the other two groups. Most patients will have far more symptoms than eight. Symptoms require treatment or impair social, personal, or occupational functioning.
- DSM-IV required an onset by age 30, but most patients have been ill from their teens or early 20s on. SD symptoms must be unexplained by any medical condition (including substance misuse). Patients who also have actual physical illnesses often react to them with greater anxiety than you might expect.
- Of course, actual physical illness should be first on the list of differential diagnoses. And, because SD can be difficult to treat, there are many other mental and emotional disorders that need to be ruled out. These include mood or anxiety disorders, psychotic disorders, and dissociative or stress disorders. Substance use disorders can be comorbid with SD. I would include factitious disorder and malingering on the differential list, but these belong very near the bottom.

With Predominant Pain Specifier for Somatic Symptom Disorder

Some patients with SSD experience mainly pain, in which case the specifier *with pre-dominant pain* is indicated. DSM-IV called it pain disorder, an independent condition with its own criteria. (From here on, I refer to it as SSD–Pain.) Whatever we call it, we need to keep in mind these facts:

- Pain is subjective—individuals experience it differently.
- There is no gross anatomical pathology.
- Measuring pain is hard.

So it's hard to know that a patient who complains of chronic or excruciating pain, and apparently lacks adequate objective pathology, has a mental disorder at all. (In DSM-5, patients who have actual pain but show excessive concern can be diagnosed with SSD–Pain.)

The pain in question is usually chronic and often severe. It can take many forms, but especially common is pain in the lower back, head, pelvis, or temporomandibular joint. Typically, SSD–Pain doesn't wax and wane with time and doesn't diminish with distraction; it may respond only poorly to analgesics, if at all.

Chronic pain interferes with cognition, causing people to have trouble with memory, concentration, and completing tasks. It is often associated with depression, anxiety, and low self-esteem; sleep may be disturbed. Such patients may experience slower response to stimuli; fear of worsening pain may reduce their physical activity. Of course, work suffers. In over half the cases, chronic pain is managed inadequately by clinicians.

SSD–Pain usually begins in the 30s or 40s, often following an accident or some other physical illness. It is more often diagnosed in women than in men. As its duration extends, it often leads to increasing incapacity for work and social life, and sometimes to complete invalidism. Although some form of pain affects many adults in the general population—perhaps as high as 30% in the United States—no one knows for sure the prevalence of SSD–Pain.

Ruby Bissell

Ruby Bissell placed a hand on each chair arm and shifted uncomfortably. She had been talking for nearly half an hour, and the dull, constant ache had worsened. Pushing up with both hands, she hoisted herself to her feet. She winced as she pressed a fist into the small of her back; the furrows on her face added a decade to her 45 years.

Although Ruby had had this problem for nearly 6 years, she wasn't sure exactly when it began. It could have started when she helped to move a patient from the operating table to a gurney. But the first orthopedist she ever consulted explained that her pulled ligament was mild, so she continued to work as an operating room nurse for nearly a year. Her back hurt whether she was sitting or standing, so she'd had to resign from her job; she couldn't maintain any physical position longer than a few minutes at a time.

"They let me do supervisory work for a while," she said, "but I had to quit that, too. My only choices were sitting or standing, and I have to spend part of each hour flat on my back."

From her solidly blue-collar parents, Ruby had inherited a work ethic. She'd supported herself from the age of 17, so her forced retirement had been a blow. But she couldn't say she felt depressed about it. In fact, she had never been very introspective about her feelings and couldn't really explain how she felt about many things. She did deny ever having hallucinations or delusions; aside from her back pain, her physical health had been good. Although she occasionally awakened at night with back pain, she had no real insomnia; appetite and weight had been normal. When the interviewer asked whether she had ever had death wishes or suicidal ideas, she was a little offended and strongly denied them.

A variety of treatments had made little difference in Ruby's condition. Pain medication provided almost no relief at all, and she had quit them all before she could get hooked. Physical therapy made her hurt all the more, and an electrical stimulation unit seemed to burn her skin.

A neurosurgeon had found no anatomical pathology and explained to Ruby that a laminectomy and spinal fusion were unlikely to improve matters. Her own husband's experience had caused her to distrust any surgical intervention. He had been injured in a trucking accident a year before her own difficulty began; his subsequent laminectomy had left him not only disabled for work, but impotent. With no children to support, the two lived in reasonable comfort on their combined disability incomes.

"Mostly we just stay at home," Ruby remarked. "We care a lot for each other. Our relationship is the one part of my life that's really good."

The interviewer asked whether they were still able to have any sort of a sex life. Ruby admitted that they did not. "We used to be very active, and I enjoyed it a lot. After his accident, and he couldn't perform, Gregory felt terribly guilty that he couldn't satisfy me. Now my back pain would keep me from having sex, regardless. It's almost a relief that he doesn't have to bear all the responsibility."

Evaluation of Ruby Bissell

For several years (far longer than the 6 months required by SSD criterion C), Ruby had complained of severe pain (A) that had markedly affected her life, especially her ability to work. She had clearly spent a great deal of time and effort (B) trying to manage her pain. There, in a nutshell, we've covered the three requirements for SSD–Pain.

Although the criteria don't require us to rule out other causes, we're responsible clinicians, so of course we will do so anyway. Principally, we need to know that her pain wasn't caused by **another medical condition.** The vignette makes clear that she had been thoroughly evaluated by her orthopedist, who determined that she did not have pathology adequate to account for the severity of her symptoms. (Even if she did have some defined pathology, SSD–Pain might also be suspected if the distribution, timing, or description of the pain was atypical of a physical illness.)

Could Ruby have been **malingering**? This question is especially relevant to anyone who receives compensation for a work-related injury. However, Ruby's suffering seemed genuine, and the vignette gives no indication that she was physically more able-bodied at leisure that at work. Her referral had not been made within a legal context, and she cooperated fully with the examination. Furthermore, malingering would not seem consistent with her long-held work ethic.

Pain is often a symptom of **depression**; indeed, many practitioners will automatically recommend a course of antidepressant medication for nearly anyone who complains of severe or chronic pain. Although Ruby denied feeling especially depressed, her pain symptoms could still be a stand-in for a mood disorder. But she had no suicidal ideas, disturbance of sleep, or disturbance of appetite that would support such a diagnosis. Although patients with substance-related disorders will sometimes fabricate (or imagine) pain in order to obtain medications, Ruby had been careful to avoid becoming dependent on analgesics.

Several other somatic symptom disorders should be briefly considered. People with **illness anxiety disorder** tend to have symptoms other than pain, and they fluctuate with time. Pain is not a symptom typical of **conversion disorder.** People with **adjustment disorder** will sometimes have physical symptoms, but such conditions are associated with identifiable precipitants and disappear with the stressor.

DSM-5 doesn't require us to identify psychological factors that could underlie pain. Indeed, the presumption that there be a psychological mechanism is no longer a criterion for SSD. It is useful, however, to think about possible psychological factors that could contribute to the production or maintenance of a given patient's pain experience. Ruby's history includes several such possibilities. These included her perception of her husband's feeling about his impotence, her anxiety at being left as the sole breadwinner, and possibly her own resentment at having worked since she was a teenager. (Many patients have multiple psychological considerations.)

Psychological factors that might be causing or worsening Ruby's pain thus include stress resulting from relationships, work, and finances. With her GAF score of 61, her diagnosis would be as follows:

F45.1 [300.82]	Somatic symptom disorder, with predominant pain
Z65.8 [V62.89]	Health problems and disability in husband

An occasional patient like Ruby will be completely unable to describe the emotional component of pain. The inability to verbalize the emotions one feels has been termed *alexithymia*, Greek for "without expression of mood."

F45.21 [300.7] Illness Anxiety Disorder

People with illness anxiety disorder (IAD) are terribly worried that they might have a serious illness. Their anxiety persists despite medical evidence to the contrary and reassurance from health care professionals. Common examples include fear of heart disease (which might start with an occasional heart palpitation) and of cancer (ever wonder about that mole—it seems to have darkened a bit?). These patients are not psychotic: They may agree temporarily that their symptoms could be emotional in origin, though they quickly revert to their fearful obsessing. Then they reject any suggestion that they do not have physical disease, and may even become outraged and refuse mental health consultation.

Many such patients have physical symptoms that would qualify them for somatic symptom disorder, as just discussed. However, about a quarter of such patients have all the concern about being sick, but not much in the way of somatic symptoms. Occasionally patients will have demonstrable organic disease, but their hypochondriacal symptoms are out of proportion to the seriousness of the actual medical condition. To delineate these patients more clearly, the condition has been renamed (*hypochondria* is considered pejorative), and new criteria have been written.

Though known for centuries, IAD still hasn't been carefully studied; for example, it isn't even known whether it runs in families. By all accounts, however, it is fairly common (perhaps 5% of the general population), especially in the offices of non-mental health practitioners. It tends to begin in the 20s or 30s, with peak prevalence at about 30 or 40. It is probably about equally frequent in men and women. Although they do not have high rates of current medical illnesses, such patients report a high prevalence of childhood illness.

Historically, hypochondriasis has been a source of fun for cartoonists and playwrights (read Molière's *The Imaginary Invalid*), but in reality the disorder causes genuine misery. Although it can resolve completely, it more often runs a chronic course, for years interfering with work and social life. Many patients go from doctor to doctor in the effort to find someone who will relieve them of the serious disorders they feel sure they have; for a few, like Molière's poor creature, Argan, it leads to complete invalidism.

Essential Features of **Illness Anxiety Disorder**

Despite the absence of serious physical symptoms, the patient is inordinately concerned about being ill. High anxiety coupled with a low threshold for alarm yields recurring behaviors concerning health (seeking reassurance, checking over and over for physical signs). Some patients cope instead by avoiding hospitals and medical appointments.

The Fine Print

The D's: • Duration (6+ months, though the concerns may vary) • Differential diagnosis (substance use and physical disorders, mood or anxiety disorders, psychotic or stress disorders, body dysmorphic disorder, somatic symptom disorder)

Coding Notes

Specify subtype:

> **Care-seeking type.** The patient uses medical services more than normal.
> **Care-avoidant type.** Due to heightened anxiety levels, the patient avoids seeking medical care.

Julian Fenster

"Wow! That chart must be 2 inches thick." Julian Fenster was being checked in for his third emergency room visit in the past month. "That's just Volume 3," the nurse told him.

At age 24, Julian lived with his mother and a teenage sister. Years ago, he'd started attending a college several hundred miles away. After only a semester, he'd moved back home. "I didn't want to be that far from my doctors," he remarked. "When you're trying to prevent heart disease, you can't be too careful." With a practiced hand, he adjusted the blood pressure cuff around his upper arm.

When Julian was a young teenager, his dad had died. "His death was self-inflicted," Julian pointed out. "He'd had rheumatic fever as a child, which gave him an enlarged heart. And the only thing he ever exercised was his right to eat anything fried, including Twinkies. And he smoked—he was a proud two-pack-a-day man. Look where that got him."

None of these health risks applied to Julian, who was nothing if not careful about what he put into his body. He had spent hours searching the Internet for information on diet, and he'd attended a lecture by Dean Ornish. "I've followed a plant-based diet ever since," Julian said. "I'm especially keen on tofu. And broccoli."

Julian had never complained much of symptoms—just the odd palpitation, maybe "hot flushes" on an especially humid day. "I don't feel bad," he explained. "I just feel scared."

This time, he'd heard a report on NPR about young people with heart disease. It had startled him so much he'd dropped the dish he had been putting into the cupboard. Without even cleaning up the mess, he caught the next bus to the ER.

Julian agreed that he needed a different approach to his health care needs, and thought he might be willing to give cognitive-behavioral therapy a try. "But first," he asked, "could you check my blood pressure just once more?"

Evaluation of Julian Fenster

The requirements for IAD are not onerous; Julian met them handily. He had a dispro-portionate concern for a condition he had been assured he did not have (criterion A). He had both high anxiety and a low threshold for alarm (it took only a report on the radio to frighten him into the ER once again, C). His actual symptoms weren't just mild—they were pretty much nonexistent (B)—so we can rule out **somatic symptom disorder.** He invested huge amounts of time in trolling the Internet for health information (D). Finally, he had had these symptoms far longer than the 6-month minimum required (E) for the diagnosis of IAD.

As with any other condition discussed in this chapter (other than the disparaged [by me] somatic symptom disorder), the first issue on our list to rule out is **another medical condition**: Marked, if not inordinate, health anxiety is pretty common in med-ical outpatients. Physical illnesses can be easy to miss, especially if the patient has had a long history of complaints that seem without physical basis. However, Julian's symptoms had been evaluated over and again, to the point that there was little danger anything had been missed. Still, even people with hypochondriacal behavior are not immortal, so physical disorders would remain a significant rule-out that his clinicians must always keep in mind.

Anxious concern about health can occur in other mental disorders, but we can find some differences to help discriminate. Among these are **body dysmorphic disorder** and anxiety and related disorders (for example, **generalized anxiety disorder**, **panic disor-der**, and **obsessive–compulsive disorder**). Julian had no symptoms suggesting any of these. When somatic concerns emerge in **schizophrenia**, they tend to be delusional and bizarre ("My brain is turning to bread"). In **major depressive disorder**, they are ego-syntonic but may be influenced by melancholia ("My bowels have turned to cement"). As keen as I am on looking for depression in almost every mental health patient, I don't see depressive symptoms here. I'd give him a GAF score of 65.

The girth of Julian's chart would support the care-seeking subtype specifier.

F45.21 [300.7]   Illness anxiety disorder, care-seeking type

Conversion Disorder (Functional Neurological Symptom Disorder)

Let's define a conversion symptom as (1) a change in how the body functions when (2) no causative physical or physiological malfunctioning can be found. These symptoms are often termed *pseudoneurological*, and they include both sensory and motor symp-toms—with or without impaired consciousness.

Conversion symptoms usually don't conform to the anatomical pattern we'd expect for a condition with a well-defined physical cause. An example would be a *stocking anesthesia*, in which the patient complains of numbness of the foot that ends abruptly in a line encircling the lower leg. The actual pattern of nerve supply to the foot is quite dif-ferent; it would not occasion numbness defined by such a neat line. Other examples of sensory conversion symptoms include blindness, deafness, double vision, and hallucinations. Examples of motor deficits that are conversion symptoms include impaired balance or staggering gait (at one time called *astasia-abasia*), weak or paralyzed muscles, lump in throat or trouble swallowing, loss of voice, and retention of urine.

For decades, criteria for conversion disorder required the clinician to judge that causation by an emotional conflict or specific psychological stress cause the conversion symptom (for example, a man develops blindness after finding his wife in bed with a neighbor). DSM-5 has abandoned this requirement, in view of the potential for disagreement as to causation: One clinician may see a "causal link" between nearly any two events, while another strenuously argues against any such connection.

Conversion symptoms occur widely, throughout various medical populations; up to one-third of adults have had at least one such symptom lifetime. However, conversion disorder is rarely diagnosed in mental health patients—perhaps in only 1 of 10,000. It is usually a disorder of young people and is probably far more common among women than men. It is somewhat more likely to be found in patients who are undereducated and medically unsophisticated, and who live where medical practice and diagnosis are still emerging. It may be diagnosed more often among patients seen in consultation in a general hospital.

Note that the criteria don't require patients to undergo laboratory or imaging tests. The requirement is only that, after a careful physical and neurological evaluation, the patient's symptom cannot be explained by a known medical or neurological disease process. The stocking anesthesia I have mentioned above would fill that requirement; so would total blindness in a patient whose pupils constrict in response to a bright light. There is a rich and entertaining literature of clinical tests for pseudoneurological symptoms.

Having a conversion symptom may not allow meaningful predictions about a patient's future course. Follow-up studies find that many people who have had a conversion symptom do not have a mental disorder. Years later, many are well, with no physical or mental disorders. Some have somatization (or somatic symptom) disorder or another mental disorder. A few turn out to have an actual physical (sometimes neurological) illness, including brain or spinal cord tumors, multiple sclerosis, or a variety of other medical and neurological disorders. Although clinicians have undoubtedly improved in their ability to discriminate conversion symptoms from "real disease," it remains distressingly easy to make mistakes.

Essential Features of **Conversion Disorder**

The patient's symptom or symptoms—changes in sensory or voluntary motor functioning—seem clinically inconsistent with any known medical illness.

The Fine Print

A "normal" exam or a bizarre test result isn't enough to affirm the diagnosis; there must be positive supportive evidence. Such evidence would include a change in findings from positive to negative when a different test is used (or the patient is distracted), or impossible findings such as tunnel vision.

The D's: • Distress or disability (work/educational, social, or personal impairment) • Differential diagnosis (substance use and physical disorders, mood or anxiety disorders, body dysmorphic and dissociative disorders)

Coding Notes

Specify if:

> **Acute episode.** Symptoms have lasted under 6 months.
> **Persistent.** Symptoms have lasted 6+ months.

Specify: {With}{Without} psychological stressor

Specify type of symptom:

> **F44.4 [300.11] With weakness or paralysis; with abnormal movement** (tremor, dystonia, abnormal gait); **with swallowing symptoms;** or **with speech symptom**
> **F44.5 [300.11] With attacks or seizures**
> **F44.6 [300.11] With anesthesia or sensory loss;** or **with special sensory symptom** (hallucinations or other disturbance of vision, hearing, smell)
> **F44.7 [300.11] With mixed symptoms**

There's something missing from the DSM-5 criteria for conversion disorder. In DSM-IV, we clinicians had to rule out intentional production of symptoms—specifically, malingering and factitious disorder. Although we are still asked to assure ourselves that no other diagnosis better explains the symptom, those two diagnoses aren't explicitly mentioned. In my opinion, this is a good thing, because it's hard (sometimes impossible) to determine for sure that a patient is faking. But with conversion symptoms, we should always keep the possibility in mind and do all we can to rule it out, along with every other confounding diagnosis.

Rosalind Noonan

Rosalind Noonan came to her university's student health service because of a stutter. This was remarkable because she was 18 and she had only been stuttering for 2 days.

It had begun on Tuesday afternoon during her women's issues seminar. The class had been discussing sexual harassment, which gradually led to a consideration of sexual molestation. To foster discussion, the graduate student leading the seminar asked each participant to comment. When Rosalind's turn came, she stuttered so badly that she gave up trying to talk at all.

"I still ca-ca-ca-can't understand it," she told the interviewer. "It's the first time I've ever had this pr-pr-pro-pro—difficulty."

Rosalind was a first-year student who had decided to major in psychology, she said, "to help me learn more about myself." What she already knew included the following.

Rosalind had no information about her biological parents. She had been adopted when she was only a week old by a high school physics teacher and his wife, who had no other children. Her father was a rigid and perfectionistic man who dominated both Rosalind and her mother.

As a young child, Rosalind was overly active; during her early school years she'd had difficulty focusing her attention. She would probably have qualified for a diagnosis of attention-deficit/hyperactivity disorder, but the only evaluation she had ever had was from their family physician, who thought it was "just a phase" that she would soon outgrow. Despite that lack of diagnostic rigor, when she was 12 she did begin to grow out of it. By the time she entered high school, she was doing nearly straight-A work.

Although she had had many friends in high school and had dated extensively, she'd never had a serious boyfriend. Her physical health had been excellent, and her only visits to doctors had been for immunizations. Her mood was almost always bright and cheerful; she had no history of delusions or hallucinations, and she had never used drugs or alcohol. "I g-g-grew up healthy and happy," she protested. "That's why I d-d-d-don't understand this!"

"Hardly anyone reaches adulthood without having some problems." The interviewer paused for a response, but received none, and so continued: "For example, when you were a child, did anyone ever approach you for sex?"

Rosalind's gaze seemed to lose focus as tears trickled from her eyes. Haltingly at first, then in a rush, the following story emerged. When she was 9 or 10, her parents had become friendly with a married couple, both English teachers at her father's school. When she was 14, the woman had suddenly died; subsequently, the man was invited for dinner on a number of occasions. One evening he consumed too much wine and was put to bed on their living room sofa. Rosalind awakened to find him lying on top of her in her bed, his hand covering her mouth. She was never certain whether he actually entered her, but her struggles apparently caused him to ejaculate. After that, he left her room. He never again returned to their home.

The following day she confided her story to her mother, who at first assured Rosalind that she must have been dreaming. When confronted with the evidence of the stained sheets, her mother urged her to say nothing about the matter to her father. It was the last time the subject had ever been discussed in their house.

"I'm not sure what we thought Daddy would do if he found out," Rosalind commented, with notable fluency, "but we were both afraid of him. I felt I'd done something to be punished for, and I suppose Mom must have worried he'd attack the other teacher."

Evaluation of Rosalind Noonan

Rosalind's stuttering is a classic conversion symptom: It suggested or mimicked a medical condition, and its sudden, de novo appearance at college age wasn't what we'd expect for the stuttering of **speech fluency disorder** (criteria A, B). Many clinicians would agree that it was precipitated by the stress of discussing long-buried sexual abuse. This aspect of the disorder—the putative psychological factors related to the symptoms—is one criterion for diagnosis that has been eliminated from the DSM-5 revision. However, it is still something to note when you encounter it.

The most serious mistake a clinician can make in this context is to diagnose conversion disorder when the symptom is caused by **another medical condition** (C). Some very peculiar symptoms eventually turn out to have a medical basis. However, the abrupt onset of stuttering in an adult is almost certain to have no identifiable organic cause. The fact that Rosalind's difficulty disappeared during the discussion would be additional evidence that this was a conversion symptom.

Rosalind stated that her health had always been good, but her clinician would nonetheless be well advised to ask about other symptoms that could indicate **somatic symptom disorder**, in which conversion symptoms are so commonly encountered. The fact that she focused on the symptom, rather than on the fear of having some serious disease, would eliminate **illness anxiety disorder** (hypochondriasis) from consideration. Although pain is not excluded in the criteria, by convention conversion symptoms don't usually include pain; when pain occurs as a symptom that is caused or increased by psychological factors, the diagnosis is likely to be **somatic symptom disorder, with predominant pain.** Another condition in which conversion symptoms are sometimes encountered is **schizophrenia**, but there was no evidence that Rosalind had ever been psychotic. Neither was there evidence that she had consciously feigned her symptom, which would rule out **factitious disorder** and **malingering.**

Rosalind was concerned about her stuttering (D), which is quite the opposite from the unconcerned indifference (sometimes called *la belle indifférence*) often associated with conversion symptoms. Although many of these patients will also have a diagnosis of **histrionic**, **dependent**, **borderline**, or **antisocial personality disorder**, there was no indication of any of these in Rosalind's case. As in somatic symptom disorder, **mood**, **anxiety**, and **dissociative disorders** are often associated with conversion disorder.

Although Rosalind was terribly stressed by the sexual molestation, her overall functioning was overall pretty good; hence her GAF score would be 75. The type of symptom and presumed psychological stressor are detailed in the final diagnosis:

F44.4 [300.11]   Conversion disorder, with speech symptom (stuttering), acute episode, with psychological stressor (concerns about molestation)

F54 [316] Psychological Factors Affecting Other Medical Conditions

Mental health professionals deal with all sorts of problems that can influence the course or care of a medical condition. The diagnosis of psychological factors affecting other medical conditions can be used to identify such patients. Although it is coded as a mental disorder and with mental disorders, it does not actually constitute one, so I've not provided a full vignette—just a few snippets to illustrate how the diagnosis might be applied. In truth, this condition should have been given a Z-code and stuck in the back with other such conditions, but that wasn't a possibility: ICD-10 makes the rules. Still, it doesn't belong up in the front seat, either.

Essential Features of **Psychological Factors Affecting Other Medical Conditions**

A physical symptom or illness is affected by a psychological or behavioral factor that precipitates, worsens, interferes with, or extends the patient's need for treatment.

The Fine Print

The D's: • Differential diagnosis (other mental disorders, such as panic disorder, mood disorders, other somatic symptom and related disorders, posttraumatic stress disorder)

Coding Notes

Specify current severity:

> **Mild.** The factor increases medical risk.
> **Moderate.** The factor worsens the medical condition.
> **Severe.** It causes an ER visit or hospitalization.
> **Extreme.** It results in severe, life-endangering risk.

Code the name of the relevant medical condition first.

Some Examples

DSM-IV included six specific categories of factors that could change the course of a medical condition. Partly because they were hardly ever used, DSM-5 has ditched these categories. However, I've used them as examples that might alert clinicians to the sorts of issue that can affect treatment decisions. If more than one psychological factor is present, choose the one most prominent.

> **Mental disorder.** For 15 years Philip's compliance with treatment for schizophrenia has been spotty. Now his voices warn him to refuse dialysis.

> **Psychological symptoms (insufficient for a DSM-5 diagnosis).** With few other mental symptoms, Alice's mood has been so low that she hasn't bothered filling prescriptions for her type II diabetes.

Personality traits or coping style. Gordon's lifelong hatred of authority figures has led him to reject his doctor's recommendation for a stent.

Maladaptive health behaviors. Weighing nearly 400 pounds, Tim knows that he should avoid sweetened drinks, but nearly every day his love of Big Gulps wins out.

Stress-related physiological response. April's job as the Governor's spokesperson is so demanding that she's had to double up on her antihypertensive drugs.

Other or unspecified psychological factors. Harold's religion prohibits him from accepting a blood transfusion. In Nanja's culture, a woman mustn't allow any man not her husband to see her unclothed; her internist is Derek.

Of course, you might find a psychological factor or two at play in nearly any medical condition. To use this diagnosis effectively, reserve it for situations in which it is clear that the psychological factor is adversely influencing the course of the illness.

F68.10 [300.19] Factitious Disorder

Factitious means something artificial. In the context of mental health patients, it means that a disorder looks like bona fide disease, but isn't. Such patients accomplish this by simulating symptoms (for example, complaining of pain) or physical signs (for instance, warming a thermometer in coffee or submitting a urine specimen that's been supplemented with sand). Sometimes they will complain of psychological symptoms, including depression, hallucinations, delusions, anxiety, suicidal ideas, and disorganized behavior. Because they are subjective, manufactured mental symptoms can be very hard to detect.

DSM-5 includes two subtypes of factitious disorder: one in which behaviors affect the person of the perpetrator, and one in which the behaviors affect another individual.

Factitious Disorder Imposed on Self

People affected by factitious disorder imposed on self (FDIS) can have remarkably dramatic symptoms, accompanied by outright lying about the severity of the distress. The overall pattern of signs and symptoms may be atypical for the alleged illness, and some patients change their stories upon retelling; either sort of evidence of inconsistency aids identification. Other patients with FDIS, however, know a lot about the symptoms and terminology of disease, which can make their behavior harder to detect. Some willingly undergo many procedures (some of them painful or dangerous) to continue in the patient role. With treatment that is ordinarily adequate to address their "disease," their symptoms either do not remit or evolve into new complications.

Once hospitalized, patients with FDIS often tend to complain bitterly and to argue with staff members. They characteristically remain hospitalized for a few days, have few if any visitors, and leave against medical advice once their tests prove negative. Many travel from city to city in the quest for medical care. The most persistent travelers and confabulators among these are sometimes said to have Münchausen's syndrome, named for the fabled baron who told outrageous lies about his adventures.

Contrary to its immediate predecessor, DSM-5 doesn't require speculation as to possible motives for FDIS (or its sibling, FDIA, discussed below)—a blessing for those clinicians who reject the implication that they can read minds. It is enough to detect a pattern of such behavior in a patient whose behavior involves no other person.

Patients with FDIS differ profoundly from malingerers, who may show some of the same behaviors—silting a urine specimen, embellishing the subjective reports of their suffering. However, malingerers do these things to qualify for financial compensation (such as insurance payments), to obtain drugs, or to avoid work, punishment, or, in days gone by, military service. The motivation in FDIS is apparently more complex: These patients may need the feeling of being cared for, of duping medical personnel, or simply of receiving a whole lot of attention from important people. For whatever reason, they manufacture physical or psychological symptoms in a way that they may claim they cannot control.

The diagnosis of FDIS is made by excluding physical disease and other disorders. (Although it is conceivable that a patient might manufacture a personality disorder, I know of no such cases.) However, many patients with FDIS also have genuine personality disorders.

This disorder begins early in life. No one knows how rare it is, though it is probably more common in males than in females. Often it starts with a hospitalization for genuine physical problems. It results in severe impairment: These people are often unemployed and do not maintain close ties with family or friends. Their lives are complicated (and sometimes put at risk) by tests, medications, and unnecessary surgical procedures.

Factitious Disorder Imposed on Another

A condition that has been around for only a few years, factitious disorder imposed on another (FDIA) has just now emerged from an appendix to enter the body of the DSM (there's a somewhat unsettling image). It used to be called factitious disorder (or Münchausen's) *by proxy*, because the symptoms are not endured by the patient. Rather, it is the caregiver who both causes factitious symptoms in another person and bears the diagnosis. That "other" is almost always a child, though my Medline search revealed the occasional elderly person and at least one dog.

Three-quarters, sometimes more, of the perpetrators are female—usually the mothers of children exhibiting the symptoms. Because many of these people have a background in health care, it can be hard to catch them out. When apprehended, they often turn out to have a mood or personality disorder, or both; actual psychosis is rare. Some perpetrators have a history of FDIS.

Some parents with FDIA appear to believe that the children are ill; they tend to behave as "doctor addicts" who need the attention that comes with having a desperately ill child. These people usually limit themselves to the false reporting of signs and symptoms of disease, such as seizures or apnea. Others, however, will actually induce symptoms—most commonly by suffocation or poisoning, but also by falsifying urine or stool samples or other lab specimens. Perhaps half the victims have a real physical illness, in addition.

Overall, FDIA is rare, with an annual incidence of just 0.4–2 per 100,000 population. This translates to perhaps 600 new cases in the United States each year. Most are not single parents; often they are described as exemplary parents, though they may react inappropriately (for example, excitement) upon receiving bad news. Three-quarters of instances of FDIA occur in hospitals.

Victims are about equally male and female. Though most are under age 5, some are older. As you might expect, when a teen is involved, there is often a degree of collusion with the perpetrator. The death rate overall is an appalling 10%, most often when poisoning or suffocation is involved.

Medical personnel may be persuaded to prescribe for the child treatment that is unneeded and perhaps harmful. Indeed, the doctor may be the one most taken in; an occasional physician even becomes angry at staff members who accumulate evidence of the caregiver's perfidy. Indeed, some experts recommend against informing the doctor when covert surveillance is planned, to lessen the risk that the perpetrator will be tipped off.

The suspicions of medical personnel may be alerted by a parent who seems insufficiently concerned about a sick child, by symptoms that seem to make no sense, or by a child whose symptoms continue despite treatment that should be adequate. In some cases, however, the parent perpetrator appears so distraught that the physician remains steadfastly unaware of the potential for foul play. Then the injuries will continue until the perpetrator is apprehended, the child dies, or with the march of time, the perpetrator moves on to involve a younger child. In one survey, over 70% of victims sustained disfigurement or permanent disability.

Patients with factitious disorder sometimes take on symptoms of new (and often poorly investigated) illnesses—the "disorder *du jour*" phenomenon. The criteria for the diagnoses are not very specific, and the patients are difficult to manage and often disagreeable. It is far too easy to dismiss them with a diagnosis of factitious disorder without first taking steps to ensure that we have first ruled out every other possible causative mental (and physical) condition.

I'd also point out that here in the differential diagnosis, I've used the term *malingering*—a rare occurrence in this book. Why is that? Surely people malinger other symptoms and disorders. Of course they can, and sometimes do. But I feel strongly that it is incumbent on clinicians to be extremely chary of malingering as a diagnostic formulation.

Essential Features of **Factitious Disorder**

To present a picture of someone who is ill, injured, or impaired, {the patient}{another person, acting for the patient} feigns physical or mental symptoms or signs of illness, or induces a disease or injury. This behavior occurs even without evident benefits (such as financial gain, revenge, or avoiding legal responsibility).

The Fine Print

The D's: • Differential diagnosis (substance use and physical disorders, mood or anxiety disorders, psychotic disorders, trauma- and stressor-related disorders, dissociative and cognitive disorders, malingering)

Coding Notes

Diagnose:

Factitious disorder imposed on self. The perpetrator is also the patient.
Factitious disorder imposed on another. The perpetrator and victim are separate individuals. (The perpetrator receives the factitious disorder code; the victim receives a Z-code reflecting the abuse.)

For either type, specify:

Single episode.
Recurrent episodes.

Jason Bird

Jason Bird carried no health care card—he claimed he had lost his billfold to a mugger a few hours before he came to the emergency room of a Midwestern hospital late one Saturday night, complaining of crushing substernal chest pain. Although his electrocardiogram (EKG) was markedly abnormal, it did not show the changes typical of an acute myocardial infarction. The cardiologist on call, noting his ashen pallor and obvious distress, ordered him admitted to the cardiac ICU, then waited for the cardiac enzyme results.

The following day, Jason's EKG was unchanged, and the serum enzymes showed no evidence of heart muscle damage. His chest pain continued. He complained loudly that he was being ignored. The cardiologist urgently requested a mental health consultation.

At age 47, Jason was a slightly built man with a bright, shifting gaze and a 4-day growth of beard. He spoke with a nasal Boston accent. His right shoulder bore the tattoo of a boot and the legend "Born To Kick Ass." Throughout the interview he frequently complained of chest pain, but he breathed and talked normally, and he showed no evident anxiety about his medical condition.

He said he had grown up in Quincy, Massachusetts, the son of a physician. After high school he had attended college for several years, but found he was "too creative" to stick with a profession or a conventional job. Instead, he had turned to inventing medical devices, and numbered among his successes a positive-pressure respirator that bore his name. Although he had made several fortunes, he had lost nearly everything to his penchant for playing the stock market. He had been visiting in the area, relaxing, when the chest pain struck.

"And you've never had it before?" asked the interviewer, looking through the chart.

Jason denied that he'd had any previous heart trouble. "Not even a twinge. I've always been blessed with good health."

"Ever been hospitalized?"

"Nope. Well, not since a tonsillectomy when I was a kid."

Further questioning was similarly unproductive. As the interviewer left, Jason was demanding extra meal service.

Playing a hunch, the interviewer began telephoning emergency room physicians in the Boston area to ask about a patient with Jason's name or peculiar tattoo. The third try struck pay dirt.

"Jason Bird? I wondered when we'd hear from him again. He's been in and out of half the facilities in the state. His funny-looking EKG—probably an old MI—looks pretty bad, so he always gets admitted, but there's never any evidence that anything acute is going on. I don't think he's addicted. A couple of years ago, he was admitted for a genuine pneumonia and got through a week without pain medication and with no withdrawal symptoms. He'll stay in the ICU a couple of days and rag on the staff. Then he'll split. He seems to enjoy needling medical people."

"He told me that he was the son of a physician and that he was a wealthy inventor."

The voice on the other end of the line chuckled. "The old respirator story. I checked into that one when he was admitted here for the third time. That was a different Bird altogether. I don't know that Jason's ever invented anything in his life—other than his medical history. As for his father, I think he was a chiropractor."

Returning to the ward to add a note to the chart, the interviewer discovered that Jason had discharged himself against advice and departed, leaving behind a letter of complaint to the hospital administrator.

Evaluation of Jason Bird

Jason illustrates the principal difficulty of diagnosing factitious disorder: The criteria depend heavily on the clinician's ability to determine that the signs and symptoms presented are intentionally falsified (criterion A). Sometimes that's easy, as when you find the patient scratching open a wound or parking the thermometer on a radiator. But often the intent to deceive must be inferred, as in Jason's case, from a string of visits to diverse health care facilities for the same complaint. Jason's EKG did not change and his cardiac enzymes were not elevated, so his interviewer inferred that Jason was feigning or markedly exaggerating his chest pain. That assumption may have been correct, but it was supported not by proof, only by reports from the emergency room.

Jason presented himself as ill (B), even in the absence of external motivation such as monetary gain or escape from punishment (C). That was important, for such behavior is the principal ingredient that differentiates factitious disorder from **malingering**— which of course we must consider, if only to refute it. Malingering carries with it no criteria, but we commonly agree that it occurs when a person consciously pretends to have a disorder in order to gain something of value: money (from insurance, a lawsuit, compensation); drugs (from a sympathetic physician); avoidance of a conviction for a crime; or release from, for example, military service. For Jason, no such gain was apparent.

The list of other differential diagnoses is predictable. Most important, of course, FDIS must be differentiated from **physical illnesses.** This was soon accomplished in Jason's case. Then other mental disorders must be ruled out. Patients with **somatic symptom disorder** may also complain of symptoms that have no apparent organic basis. Those with **antisocial personality disorder** may lie about symptoms, but they usually have some material gain in mind (to avoid punishment, to obtain money). Some patients with **schizophrenia** have a bizarre lifestyle that could be confused with the wanderings of classic Münchausen's syndrome, but their content of thought will usually include clear delusions and hallucinations. Patients who feign psychological symptoms may look as though they have **dementia** or **brief psychotic disorder.** None of these disorders could be supported by Jason's history or cross-sectional presentation.

Several other disorders may accompany FDIS. These include **substance-related disorders** (involving sedatives and analgesics) and **dependent, histrionic,** and **borderline personality disorders.** Many patients with FDIS have a serious personality disorder, but of course we have far too little information for such a diagnosis in Jason's case. We'd need to mention the possibility in the summary we dictate. With a GAF score of 41, here is how I'd diagnose Jason Bird:

F68.10 [300.19]   Factitious disorder imposed on self

Claudia Frankel

Police reports are usually pretty dry; they don't often moisten the eye. The Frankel case proved the exception to that rule.

When Rose Frankel was only 2 years old, she began to experience intestinal and other symptoms that would fill the next 6 years of her life. It started with spells of vomiting that seemed intractable to treatment. In all, she was carried back and forth to the pediatrician's office, and frequently to the hospital, some 200 times. Each visit led to new tests, new attempts at treatment that led nowhere. She had undergone nearly two dozen operative procedures, and swallowed numerous medications for diarrhea, infections, seizures, and spells of vomiting, when finally nurses on the pediatric intensive care unit noticed that Rose would appear to be on the mend until her mother, Claudia, arrived and would take her to a private room. They'd hear Rose crying, and her health would take another turn for the worse—sometimes, just when she was thought ready for discharge.

In all, Rose suffered nearly a dozen serious infections; one of them, a life-threatening sepsis, involved multiple organisms. Through it all, Claudia worked closely with their family doctor. They would speak in person or on the phone several times a day, and Dr. Bhend often spoke of Claudia as his "good right arm" in trying to get to the bottom of the calamity that was engulfing their patient.

During the 4 years of her medical ordeal, the only time that Rose remained healthy longer than a month was when Claudia left town to nurse her own mother, during what proved to be that old lady's final illness. For the last few weeks of her kindergarten year, Rose bloomed. But she sickened again, shortly after Grandma died and Claudia returned home.

Several on the hospital nursing staff were beyond suspicious. Once, they'd found a bottle of Ipecac discarded in the room Rose had occupied. On another occasion, a monitoring device that three staff members had checked within the hour had been found turned off. As they told the investigating officers, most staff members had concluded that Claudia was directly responsible for her daughter's illness, so they hid a camera in the private room Claudia always used during Rose's many admissions. When he found out, Dr. Bhend, concerned about the loss of trust, warned Claudia of the "impending sting." That afternoon, she checked Rose out of the hospital, and they were lost to follow-up. The staff revealed the full details to the police, who opened a file but were never able to pull together solid information.

FDIA is just one of the new DSM-5 disorders that was included in an appendix of DSM-IV as a possible diagnosis that needed further study. Also making the big time after years of study are premenstrual dysphoric disorder, mild neurocognitive disorder, binge-eating disorder, and (my personal favorite) caffeine withdrawal. Welcome aboard, all!

Evaluation of Claudia Frankel

Two of the criteria required for a diagnosis of factitious disorder were easily satisfied. There was nothing to suggest an external reward for Claudia's behavior such as financial gain (criterion C), and she certainly did present Rose as being impaired (D). Two others we have to take on faith: although the circumstantial evidence was strong that Rose's symptoms were fabricated, the staff just missed nailing down the proof (A). And, we cannot be sure that Claudia had no other mental disorder such as a delusional disorder that could better explain her behavior (D). Therefore, our current diagnosis should be treated as provisional. I would make a note in her chart to the effect that further investigation would be needed in regard to a personality disorder; in ICD-10, we can no longer code "diagnosis deferred" in that category.

Assigning Claudia's GAF score prompts some discussion. Should we base our judgment on the fact that she was able to function well in most areas of her life, or on the effect of her behavior on Jennifer and on their relationship? In my opinion, the disastrous consequences of her impaired judgment would be the deciding factor here; hence the very low GAF score of 30. However, others might see her situation quite differently and choose to argue.

Note that Rose herself would be given the code Z69.010 [V61.21] to reflect the fact that she had suffered from physical abuse by a parent.

F68.10 [300.19]   Factitious disorder imposed on another (provisional)

F45.8 [300.89] Other Specified Somatic Symptom and Related Disorder

This category is for patients whose somatic symptoms do not fulfill criteria for any of the somatic symptom and related disorders discussed above, but about which we have some information. Any diagnosis suggested here has not as yet been studied enough for formal inclusion in DSM-5, and should be considered provisional. Keep in mind that with more information, such a patient may qualify for a diagnosis in a different chapter or for another diagnosis in this one.

Pseudocyesis. The word *pseudocyesis* means "false pregnancy," and it refers to patients' incorrect belief that they are pregnant. They develop signs of pregnancy such as protruding abdomen, nausea, amenorrhea, and breast engorgement—and even symptoms such as the sensation of fetal movement and labor pains.

Brief illness anxiety disorder. Duration less than 6 months.

Brief somatic symptom disorder. I'll leave the definition as homework.

F45.9 [300.82] Unspecified Somatic Symptom Disorder

Use this category for cases in which full criteria for any of the disorders discussed in this chapter are not met, and you do not wish to specify a reason or a possible presentation.

CHAPTER 9

Feeding and Eating Disorders

DSM-5's chapter on feeding and eating disorders has mushroomed. It now contains diagnoses appropriate to children (and infants) as well as adults. And the sheer number of conditions has doubled—and then some.

Quick Guide to the Feeding and Eating Disorders

As usual, the page number following each item indicates where a more detailed discussion begins.

Primary Feeding and Eating Disorders

Each of the primary feeding and eating disorders involves abnormal behaviors concerning the act of consumption. Anorexia nervosa is less common than is bulimia nervosa, and both are less common than the newbie, binge-eating disorder. The overall prevalence of these three disorders may be increasing. The three remaining specific disorders were transplanted from the old childhood/adolescence section of DSM-IV.

Anorexia nervosa. Despite the fact that they are severely underweight, these patients see themselves as fat (p. 277).

Bulimia nervosa. These patients eat in binges, then prevent weight gain by self-induced vomiting, purging, and exercise. Although appearance is important to their self-evaluations, they do not have the body image distortion characteristic of anorexia nervosa (p. 281).

Binge-eating disorder. These patients eat in binges, but do not try to compensate by vomiting, exercising, or using laxatives (p. 284).

Pica. The patient eats material that is not food (p. 288).

Rumination disorder. The person persistently regurgitates and re-chews food already eaten (p. 289).

Avoidant/restrictive food intake disorder. An individual's failure to eat enough leads to weight loss or a failure to gain weight (p. 291).

Other specified, or unspecified, feeding or eating disorder. Use one of these categories for a disorder of feeding or eating that does not meet the criteria for any of those mentioned above (p. 292).

Other Causes of Abnormal Appetite and Weight

Mood disorders. Patients with a major depressive episode (or dysthymia) can experience either anorexia with weight loss or increased appetite with weight gain (pp. 122 and 138).

Schizophrenia and other psychotic disorders. Bizarre eating habits are occasionally encountered in psychotic patients (p. 64).

Somatic symptom disorder. Complaints of marked weight fluctuation and appetite disturbance may be encountered in these patients (p. 251).

Simple obesity. This is not a DSM-5 diagnosis (there's no evidence that it is associated with any defined mental or emotional pathology). But emotional problems that contribute to the development or maintenance of obesity can be coded as psychological factors affecting other medical conditions (p. 266). There is now also a separate medical code for overweight or obesity.

Introduction

Eating too little and eating too much have probably caused trouble as long as there have been eaters. Nearly everyone has pursued one of these behaviors at one time or another. But like so many behaviors, when carried to extremes, they can be dangerous; sometimes they turn deadly. Although the criteria crisply distinguish one from another, patients can move back and forth between the disorders and subclinical presentations.

Anorexia Nervosa

Recognized for nearly 200 years, anorexia nervosa (AN) has three main components. The patient (1) restricts food intake to the point of markedly reduced body weight, yet (2) remains inordinately concerned about obesity or weight gain, and (3) has the distorted self-perception of being overweight. Other symptoms are elaborations of maladaptive eating behaviors—food restriction, excessive exercise, and vomiting or other methods of purging. Although many female patients stop menstruating, the absence of menses doesn't provide a meaningful distinction, so it's been dropped as a criterion. Patients with AN may have abnormal vital signs (slow heart rate, low blood pressure); abnormal lab values and other tests can also occur (anemia, loss of bone density, EKG changes).

AN carries with it serious health consequences. Although two-thirds of community sample patients have remitted at 5 years, mortality (due to substance use, suicide, and malnutrition) is about six times that of the general population. Clinical populations may (no surprise) fare worse. Those who binge and then purge to maintain low weight tend to be older, to be sicker, and to have worse outcomes than those who only restrict their intake, yielding the two clinical subtypes. Crossover between subtypes often occurs, however (more often *from* the restrictor type than *to* it), limiting predictive validity. Depression and anxiety are frequently concomitants.

AN affects a bit under 1% of the female population; the rate for males is perhaps a third of that. It is more common among adolescent and young adults, especially those who are figure skaters or gymnasts (women) or jockeys or long-distance runners (men). The restricting type is the more usual. The concordance rate is higher in identical than in fraternal twins, indicating a degree of genetic underpinning.

More patients with AN are seen by family practitioners than by mental health specialists.

Essential Features of **Anorexia Nervosa**

These patients are usually young women who (1) eat so little that many look skeletal, yet (2) remain fearful of obesity or weight gain and (3) have the distorted self-perception that they are fat.

The Fine Print

Some patients may not admit to fear of overweight, but take steps anyway to avert weight gain.

The D's: • Duration (note that the diagnostic criteria don't actually specify duration; however, we are required to specify the subtype that applies to the previous 3 months, which suggests a minimum duration) • Differential diagnosis (substance use and physical disorders, mood or anxiety disorders, obsessive–compulsive disorder, somatic symptom disorder, bulimia nervosa)

Coding Notes

Specify type that applies to the previous 3 months:

> **F50.02 [307.1] Binge-eating/purging type.** The patient has repeatedly purged (vomited; misused enemas, laxatives, or diuretics) or eaten in binges.
> **F50.01 [307.1] Restricting type.** The patient has not recently binged or purged.

Based on body mass index (BMI; kg/meter^2), specify severity (level may be increased, depending on functional impairment). For adults, levels are as follows:

Mild. BMI of 17 or more.
Moderate. BMI of 16–17.
Severe. BMI of 15–16.
Extreme. BMI under 15.

Specify if:

In partial remission. For what DSM-5 calls "a sustained period" (p. 339), the patient is no longer significantly underweight, but still is overly concerned about weight or still has misconceptions about body weight/shape.
In full remission. For "a sustained period," the patient has met no criteria for AN.

Marlene Richmond

A statuesque blonde (5 feet 7 inches tall), Marlene Richmond weighed just over 80 pounds on the day she was admitted to the hospital. Dressed in a jogging suit and leg warmers, she spent part of the initial interview doing deep knee bends. Information for her history was also provided by her older sister, who accompanied her to the hospital.

Marlene grew up in a small town in southern Illinois. Her father, who drilled wells for a living, had a drinking problem. Her mother, severely overweight, started numerous fad diets but never had much success with any of them. One of Marlene's earliest memories was her own resolve that she would not grow up to be like either of her parents.

The concerns of her 10th-grade social circle revolved around appearance, clothing, and diet. That year alone, Marlene dropped 15 pounds from her highest weight ever, which was 125 pounds; even then she complained to her friends that she was too fat. Throughout her high school career, she remained fascinated by food. She took both introductory and advanced home economics. She spent much of her time in computer science class devising a database that would count the calories in any recipe.

Whenever she was allowed to do so, Marlene ate in her room while watching television. If forced to eat with the family, she spent much of the meal rearranging the food on her plate or mashing it with a fork and taking the smallest bites that wouldn't fall through the tines.

"It's not as if I'm not hungry," she said during her admission interview. "I think about food most of the time. But I look so bloated and disgusting—I can't stand to see myself in the mirror. If I eat even a little bit too much, I feel so stuffed and guilty that I have to bring it back up."

Two years earlier, Marlene had started vomiting whenever she thought she had overeaten. At first she would stick her finger or the end of a pencil down her throat;

once she tried some Ipecac she found in the medicine cabinet at a friend's house. She soon learned simply to vomit at will, without any chemical or mechanical aids. She also reduced her weight with diuretics and laxatives. The diuretics helped her shave off a pound or two, but they left her so thirsty that she would soon gain it back. Once or twice a week, she would binge on high-carbohydrate food (she preferred corn chips and cola), then vomit up what she had eaten.

Other than her remarkable thinness and pallor, which was subsequently attributed to anemia, Marlene's appearance at admission was normal. She stopped exercising when the clinician requested it, but she asked whether the hospital had a stair-step exerciser she could use later. Her mood was cheerful and her flow of thought logical. She had no delusions or hallucinations, though she admitted that she was terrified of gaining weight. However, she denied having any other phobias, obsessions, or compulsions; she had never had a panic attack. Most of her spontaneous comments concerned menu planning and cooking; she volunteered that she might like to become a dietitian. She appeared bright and attentive, and made a perfect score on the MMSE.

Marlene's only health concern was that she hadn't had a menstrual period for 5 or 6 months. She knew she wasn't pregnant because she hadn't even had a date for a year. "I think I'd be more attractive if I could just lose another couple of pounds," she said.

Evaluation of Marlene Richmond

Despite the fact that she was markedly underweight for her height (criterion A), Marlene continued to express inappropriate concerns about gaining weight (B). Her disgust at her own image in the mirror suggests the distorted view patients with AN have of themselves (C). Her loss of weight was profound enough that she had not had a menstrual period for several months. Although not all patients take active steps to avoid weight gain (some only restrict intake), Marlene's vomiting and use of diuretics and laxatives are classic for AN.

Loss of appetite and weight are commonly found in a variety of **medical illnesses** (liver disease, severe infections, and cancer, to name but a few); these must be ruled out by appropriate medical history and tests. Because the symptoms of AN are so distinctive, it is rarely confused with other mental disorders.

Loss of weight and anorexia can be encountered in **somatic symptom disorder,** but for *that* diagnosis, a patient must show excessive concern about the symptoms— and Marlene's attitude seemed the antithesis of concern. Patients with **schizophrenia** will sometimes have peculiar eating habits, but unless they become dangerously underweight and have the typical distortion of self-image, both diagnoses should not be made. **Hunger strikes** are usually brief and occur in the context of trying to influence the behavior of others for personal or political benefit. Patients with **bulimia nervosa** usually maintain body weight at an acceptable level. Despite the fact that Marlene binged and purged, neither bulimia nervosa nor **binge-eating disorder** should be diagnosed when bingeing and purging occur only during AN. However, some patients who initially have AN later become bulimic. Bulimia nervosa may also be diagnosed if there is a history of binge–purge cycles that occur during times the patient does not meet criteria for AN.

Several mental disorders are often associated with AN. **Major depressive disorder** could be diagnosed if Marlene had had symptoms of mood disorder. **Panic disorder, agoraphobia, obsessive–compulsive disorder,** and **substance use** may also complicate diagnosis and treatment. Patients with AN may also fear eating in public, though you wouldn't give an additional diagnosis of **social anxiety disorder** if the anxiety symptoms are strictly limited to eating behaviors. Specific **personality disorders** have not been identified, but patients with AN are reported to be somewhat rigid and perfectionistic.

Marlene's history of binge–purge cycles would fit the specifier of binge-eating/purging type, which we'll add in coding. Her GAF score would be 45; her full diagnosis would be as follows:

E44.0 [263.0]	Malnutrition, moderate
F50.02 [307.1]	Anorexia nervosa, binge-eating/purging type

F50.2 [307.51] Bulimia Nervosa

Let's start by sketching an idealized mealtime. Wouldn't it involve the pleasant anticipation of sharing good food with friends, savoring every bite while lingering at the table for fellowship and conversation? That's just not the way for people with bulimia nervosa (BN), whose dining experiences tend toward the polar opposite. Typically, in response to feelings of depression or stress, they gobble their food, consuming quantities far in excess of a normal meal. Because they're ashamed of their way-out-of-control behavior, they eat alone. And then they head to the bathroom and throw it all up. Their own self-evaluation involves body shape and how they look; in that, they resemble patients with anorexia nervosa. What they don't have is the distorted view of being fat when they are not.

Starting in their late teens or early 20s, patients with BN will wolf down prodigious quantities of food once a week or more, often past the point of uncomfortable satiety. (These binges can be discontinuous; for example, occasionally one is interrupted by travel between dining venues.) The fact that these patients are generally about normal in weight (some are overweight, but not obese) would be surprising, were it not for their compensatory behavior. Besides vomiting, which some do so often that the enamel wears off their lower teeth, they may use laxatives or other drugs; others exercise excessively, just as in anorexia nervosa. Still others fast between binges. But nearly all vomit.

BN is more common than anorexia nervosa, affecting 1–2% of adult women (men much less so). (The crossover rate with anorexia nervosa is in the 10% neighborhood.) It is more frequently found in people whose professions and activities emphasize slim body lines—gymnastics, figure skating, dance, modeling. For unknown reasons, the incidence has probably decreased somewhat over the past 20 years. Like patients with other eating disorders, patients with BN often have comorbid conditions (especially mood and anxiety disorders, but also problems with impulse control and substance use).

With time, nearly half of patients with BN recover fully, and another quarter improve. But that final quarter settle into chronic bulimic behavior. Although mortality rates are higher than average for any comparison age group, the condition is less lethal than AN. The suicide rate, however, is higher than in the general population. Table 9.1 compares BN with anorexia nervosa and with binge-eating disorder, discussed next.

Essential Features of **Bulimia Nervosa**

A patient has lost control over eating, consuming in binges much more food than is normal for a similar time frame. Fasting, vomiting, extreme physical workouts, and the abuse of laxatives or other drugs may be used to control weight.

The Fine Print

The D's: • Duration (weekly for 3+ months) • Differential diagnosis (substance use and physical disorders, mood or anxiety disorders, obsessive–compulsive disorder, somatic symptom disorder, anorexia nervosa, traditional Thanksgiving meal)

Coding Notes

Specify if:

> **In partial remission.** For what DSM-5 calls "a sustained period," the patient meets some but not all BN criteria.
> **In full remission.** For "a sustained period," no BN criteria have been met.

Based on the number per week of episodes of inappropriate compensatory behavior, specify severity (level may be increased, depending on functional impairment):

> **Mild.** 1–3 episodes/week.
> **Moderate.** 4–7.
> **Severe.** 8–13.
> **Extreme.** 14+.

Bernadine Hawley

"I eat when I'm depressed, and I'm depressed when I eat. I'm totally out of control." As she told her story, Bernadine Hawley frequently dabbed at her eyes with a wad of tissues. She was single and 32, and she taught second grade. She had never before sought mental health care.

During her first 2 years in college, Bernadine had been moderately anorectic. Convinced that she was too fat, she starved and purged herself down to a scant 98 pounds, strung out along her 5-foot-5-inch frame. In those years she was always hungry and would often go on food binges, during which she would "clean out the refrigerator—

TABLE 9.1. Comparison of Three Eating Disorders

	Anorexia nervosa	Bulimia nervosa	Binge-eating disorder
Eats in binges	No	Yes	Yes
Self-perception	Abnormal (perceives self as fat)	Influenced by body weight, shape	Not remarkable
Compensates with exercise, purging	Yes	Yes	No
Body weight is low	Yes	No	No
Feels lack of control	No	Yes	Yes

mine or anyone else's." She later admitted, "I must have looked pretty sparse." By the time she finished college, her weight had returned to a steady 120 pounds, controlled by self-induced vomiting.

During the intervening 10 years, Bernadine had followed a binge-and-purge pattern. On the average, twice a week she would come home from work, assemble a meal for three, and consume it. She preferred sweets and starches—at a sitting she might consume two lasagna TV dinners, a quart of frozen yogurt, and a dozen sugar donuts, none of which required much effort to prepare. Between courses she vomited up nearly all she took in. If she didn't feel like "cooking," she went out for fast food, wolfing down as many as four Big Macs in half an hour. What she relished seemed to be not the taste but the act of consumption; one evening she ate a stick of butter dipped in confectioner's sugar. In a fit of remorse, she once calculated that during a single evening's binge, she had consumed and regurgitated over 10,000 calories.

She also frequently purged herself with laxatives. The laxatives were effective, but expensive enough that Bernadine felt constrained to steal them. To minimize the chances of detection, she was careful to shoplift only one package at a time. She managed always to keep at least a 3-month supply on the shelf at the back of her closet.

Bernadine was the only child of a Midwestern couple she described as "solidly dysfunctional." Because her parents never celebrated the date of their anniversary, she assumed that her own conception had precipitated the marriage. Her mother worked in a bank and was cold and controlling; her father, a barber, drank. In the resulting marital strife, Bernadine was alternately censured and ignored. She'd had friends as a child and as an adult, though some of her girlfriends complained that she was overly concerned with her weight and figure. From the few times she'd tried it in college, she'd discovered that she had a healthy appetite for sex. But feelings of shame and embarrassment about her bulimia had kept her from forming any long-lasting relationships. She was often lonely and sad, though these feelings never lasted longer than a few days.

Although Bernadine admitted that her weight was currently normal, she was very concerned about it. She clipped low-fat recipes and belonged to a health club. She had often told herself she would give everything she owned to get rid of her bingeing.

Recently she had offered a dentist $2,000 to wire her jaws shut. The dentist had pointed out the obvious difficulty that she might then starve, and referred her to the mental health clinic.

Evaluation of Bernadine Hawley

As is true for many patients with BN, Bernadine's disorder began with behavior typical of moderate **anorexia nervosa.** She currently would not qualify for that diagnosis, however (her weight was normal, and she did not have a distorted self-image—criterion E). During her later binge–purge episodes, she lost control and ate far more than normal (A1 and A2). She also maintained weight by vomiting and using laxatives (B). Friends had pointed out that she focused excessively on her figure and weight (D). Her episodes occurred more often than weekly and had lasted far longer than the 3-month minimum (C).

Shoplifting isn't a criterion for BN, but the two often occur together. Though any history of stealing should raise the possibility of **antisocial** or **borderline personality disorder,** no evidence for either is given in the vignette. When criteria for **kleptomania** are met, it should also be diagnosed.

Rarely, **neurological disorders** (some epilepsies, Kleine–Levin syndrome) can present with overeating. Excessive appetite can also occur in **major depressive disorder with atypical features.** Bernadine showed no evidence of either of these conditions. She did not misuse **alcohol or drugs,** though many patients with BN do.

Bernadine engaged in overeating and purging a couple of times per week; this would rate her a severity level of mild. However, the vignette gives no indication of her overall functionality, so we have to base her GAF score of 61 strictly on her eating behaviors. Her clinician should dig deeply to inquire whether her eating behavior had had an impact on personal relationships and her work experience. If so, and if it was severe, we'd want to increase the severity level of both her BN (it's permitted under DSM-5 guidelines) and her GAF score (encouraged under my guidelines). Right now, her diagnosis would read:

F50.2 [307.51]   Bulimia nervosa, mild

F50.8 [307.51] Binge-Eating Disorder

When it comes to food, who among us has never overindulged? (In good conscience, perhaps no one should cast the first scone.) An extra wedge of pie at Thanksgiving, a triple-dip cone after lunch, and we are left, replete and groaning, vowing to sin no more. Heap on extra portions by the plateful, garnish with shame, warm and serve ad lib, and you have the recipe for binge-eating disorder (BED).

Overeating behavior usually starts during the teens or early 20s, sometimes on the heels of a diet. The two central features are the rate of consumption (total amounts can be prodigious) and the sense of loss of control over eating behavior. Patients don't have specific cravings, and their selections can be both varied and varying with time. Unlike patients with anorexia or bulimia nervosa, patients with BED don't usually go back and forth from other eating disorders.

Though BED is a newcomer among officially recognized diagnoses (DSM-IV said it required more study), it is the most common of the eating disorders, affecting about 2% of adults and perhaps half that many adolescents. It occurs nearly twice as often in women as in men, and for some reason is especially prevalent in people with type 2 diabetes. Although it is often associated with obesity, only about one-quarter of overweight patients have BED. However, obese people are far more likely than the general population to experience episodes of binge eating; those who do have BED may find it especially hard to lose weight.

This partly heritable condition often begins as a diet winds down. The eating binges typically occur when the person is feeling glum or anxious, and they often involve delicious foods high in fat, sugar, salt, and guilt. Rapid eating forestalls satiety until too much has been consumed, leading to an uncomfortable, overfull feeling. Bingeing may occur secretly as a consequence of shame and embarrassment, which contribute even more to distress and problems with quality of life than does the simple fact of obesity.

Essential Features of **Binge-Eating Disorder**

A patient has lost control, consuming in binges much more food than is normal in a similar time frame. During a binge the patient will eat too fast, too much (until painfully full), yet in the absence of actual hunger. The bingeing causes guilt (sometimes, depression) and solitary dining (to avoid embarrassment), but it does *not* result in behaviors (such as vomiting and excessive exercise) designed to make up for overeating.

The Fine Print

The D's: • Duration (weekly for 3+ months) • Distress over eating behavior • Differential diagnosis (mood disorders, bulimia or anorexia nervosa, ordinary overweight)

Coding Notes

Specify if:

> **In partial remission.** For what DSM-5 calls "a sustained period," the patient has eaten in binges less often than once a week.
>
> **In full remission.** For "a sustained period," the patient has met no criteria for BED.

Specify severity (level may be increased, depending on functional impairment):

Mild. 1–3 binges/week.
Moderate. 4–7.
Severe. 8–13.
Extreme. 14+.

Monica Hudgens

"I know I'm obese by anyone's standards," Monica Hudgens told her internist, "and I'm doing it to myself."

Even as a child, Monica was overweight. Now, at 5 feet 3 inches, she weighed 210 pounds. "I'm 37 now; for years, my BMI has been tracking with my age."

Monica's bingeing started years ago, on the heels of a busted relationship. Now, at least twice a week, she would cook supper—she especially loved pasta with hazelnuts. She'd devour one helping, then gobble down another, then another. Even if she wasn't still hungry, she'd then have ice cream ("At *least* two servings—I just scarf it down, no thinking involved") and cookies. Though she felt stuffed ("with nosh and remorse"), she never vomited up what she had eaten; she'd never used laxatives or other drugs to purge. Washing the dishes afterwards, she was often surprised to realize that only 30 minutes had elapsed.

"I've always been large. But until the last couple of years, I've dieted pretty hard. Now I just seem to have given up," Monica said as she touched the bran muffin hidden in her purse. She denied any history of substance misuse; other than the obesity, the internist pronounced her healthy.

Born and reared on the West Coast, Monica had been married and divorced; she now lived with her 15-year-old son, Roland, whose weight was normal. She tended to binge on weekends, when she wasn't working. It had worsened since Roland developed his own set of friends and was "off doing his own thing."

Monica's self-image was mixed: "I have a terrific sense of humor and a really pretty face, but I know I'm huge. My ex-husband loved hiking in the mountains, but in the end, he decided he didn't want to be married to one."

Monica worked as a radio announcer for her local public broadcasting affiliate. Her "final straw" moment occurred when she was almost offered a better job. "A producer for cable TV heard me on the radio and liked my voice. But when we met for coffee, he lost interest." She looked sad, but then, with just a hint of a smile, she added, "Can't you just see me on TV? It'd have to be wide-screen."

Evaluation of Monica Hudgens

In a meal, Monica ate far more than most people would in similar circumstances, and she clearly voiced her loss of control ("I've given up . . . no thinking involved" (criteria A1, A2). These binge episodes occurred at least once a week and had lasted many months (D). During an episode, she ate rapidly ("gobbled down" her food), felt uncomfortably full, and ate when she wasn't physically hungry (B1, B2, B3). She also expressed contempt for her own eating behavior and ate alone (B4, B5); this might be due to embarrassment, though the vignette doesn't make that point clear. Only three of the criterion B symptoms are required for diagnosis. Her distress (C) was apparent from her first statement to the clinician. Monica would not qualify for an alternative eating disorder diagnosis: the absence of purging and other behavior to compensate for her overeating (E) would rule out **bulimia nervosa**, and her weight would obviously put paid to **anorexia nervosa**. However, she fully earned the diagnosis of BED.

Some **medical illnesses** that involve heavy eating have already been mentioned in connection with bulimia nervosa. In addition to those, Monica showed no evidence of **Prader–Willi syndrome** (caused by deletion of several genes from chromosome 15), in which the patient is often markedly overweight and eats voraciously. However, that condition is usually apparent from childhood and is associated with low intelligence. Monica also denied ever using marijuana; **cannabis intoxication** is sometimes attended by increased appetite.

Most patients with BED also have a history of other DSM-5 diagnoses, especially mood and anxiety disorders and problems with substance use; for many, a substance use disorder is concurrent. Any second diagnosis predicts that the patient will have more severe BED symptoms. Monica should be fully evaluated for **major depressive disorder with atypical features**, which can involve overeating and weight gain.

Monica only binged a couple of times a week, which the severity criteria say should rate her at mild. However, I thought I detected a note of desperation in what she told the clinician. Despite a relatively healthy GAF score of 61, I'm going to assign her a severity level of moderate. Does anyone want to argue?

F50.8 [307.51]	Binge-eating disorder, moderate
E66.9 [278.00]	Obesity

Whereas a bright line separates most physical disorders from normal, an astonishing number of mental disorders are basically just everyday behavior writ large. Disordered eating, substance use, depression, anxiety, somatic symptoms, and even personality disorders are made up of bits of behavior that perfectly normal people experience at one time or another. DSM-5 uses several features to discriminate diagnosable pathology from the everyday.

Number of symptoms. If you occasionally feel a bit anxious, welcome to life in the 21st century! If you have episodes that include marked anxiety, shortness of breath, heart palpitations, sweating, and weakness, you may have panic disorder.

Level of distress. Many (perhaps most) DSM-5 diagnoses include a statement that the disorder causes the patient (or associates) to feel markedly distressed . . .

Impairment . . . and if they're not distressed, they're impaired in work, social, or personal contexts.

Time. Other factors being held constant, a minimum *duration* or *frequency* of symptoms may be needed for a diagnosis. For example, consider dysthymia (duration) and cyclothymic disorder (duration plus frequency).

Severe sequels. These include suicide or suicide attempts, profound loss of weight, and violent acting out.

Exclusions. Most disorders require that we rule out medical illnesses and substance use; for BED, we exclude patients who have anorexia nervosa or bulimia nervosa. For most, there are other mental disorders to consider in our differential.

Some criteria sets get by with one of these mechanisms; others use a belt and suspenders approach. A few utilize most or all of these categories, in effect adding thumbs through the belt loops for added security.

The remaining conditions in this chapter are noted primarily in children. Two (pica and rumination disorder) occur during normal early childhood development. We really don't know how often they occur in adults, but they seem to have relatively little presence in most mental health populations. Ergo, no vignettes.

Pica

Pica, or the consumption of non-nutritional substances, has been commonly reported in young children and pregnant women. The list of consumables is lengthy, and the variety at times astonishing—dirt, chalk, plaster, soap, paper, and even (rarely) feces. One patient from India had consumed quantities of iron nails and glass beads. Pica has been related to iron deficiency, though other minerals (zinc, for one) may be implicated. Of course, various complications can ensue, among them lead toxicity and the ingestion of various parasites that live in soil and other inedible matter. The behavior is sometimes recognized only when the patient comes to surgery for a bowel obstruction.

Patients with autism spectrum disorder and intellectual disability are especially prone to pica—a risk that increases with the severity of each disorder. Affected children may come from a background of low socioeconomic status and neglect. The behavior usually begins by 2 years of age and remits during adolescence, or when the presumed iron (or other mineral) deficiency is corrected. Note that if pica does occur in the context of another mental or medical disorder, it must be sufficiently severe to warrant additional clinical care.

However, the literature is also replete with examples of people whose abnormal dietary intake began when they were already grown. Pica often runs through the family histories of affected adults, whose own history may have begun when they were children. It has traditionally been associated with pregnancy (though a prevalence of only 0.02% was found in a survey of pregnant Danish women), but is also found in patients with schizophrenia.

Medical specialists tend to think of pica as rare, but you'll find a lot of it if you investigate the right population. For example, it was diagnosed in a majority of patients who presented with gastrointestinal blood loss that led to iron-deficiency anemia. Pagophagia (ice craving—no, not ice *carving*) is especially common among patients with iron deficiency. In such instances, as well as in cases of schizophrenia, intellectual disability, and autism spectrum disorder, before you made the diagnosis, you'd have to persuade yourself that the patient needed additional clinical attention as the result of the pica.

Derived from the magpie, a black-and-white bird whose scientific genus is *Pica*, this term for a type of abnormal eating behavior dates back at least 400 years. Perhaps someone watching actual magpies collect mud for nests assumed that they were eating it.

As far as four millennia ago and across countless cultures, humans have chewed and swallowed clay. Researchers don't know why it happens; hypotheses include a putative detoxifying role of clay and micronutrients absorbed from the clay.

Essential Features of **Pica**

The patient persists in eating dirt or something else that isn't food.

The Fine Print

The D's: • Duration and demographics (1+ months in someone who is at least 2 years old) • Differential diagnosis (nutritional deficits, developmentally normal behavior, psychotic disorders, practice endorsed by the person's culture)

Coding Notes

Specify if: **In remission.**

Code by patient's age:

F98.3 [307.52] Pica in children
F50.8 [307.52] Pica in adults

F98.21 [307.53] Rumination Disorder

During *rumination*, an individual regurgitates a bolus of food from the stomach and chews it again. This occurs by the mechanism of retrograde peristalsis, and it is a normal part of the digestive process for cattle, deer, and giraffes—they are, after all, ruminants. But in humans it is abnormal and potentially problematic, and it is called rumination disorder (RD). It is also uncommon, most often developing in infants after they begin eating solid foods. Boys are more often affected than are girls.

Most people who ruminate will later reswallow the food. Some, however—especially infants and those with intellectual disability—instead spit it out, risking malnutrition, failure to thrive (in infants), and vulnerability to disease. Mortality rates as high as 25% have been reported. RD can go undiagnosed for years, perhaps because we don't think to ask.

The cause isn't known, though the usual suspects have been suggested. Possible etiologies include the organic (it may be a symptom of gastroesophageal reflux), the psychological (it may reflect a disordered mother–baby relationship), and the behavioral (it may be reinforced by the attention it attracts).

Of individuals with intellectual disability who live in institutions, 6–10% are sometimes affected; an occasional adult without such disability has been reported. RD has also been associated with bulimia nervosa, though patients with both disorders are less likely to reswallow the food. In most cases the behavior subsides spontaneously, though it can persist throughout life. Reportedly, one such adult ruminator was Samuel Johnson, the 18th-century lexicographer whose acquaintances commented on his "cud-chewing" behavior.

Note that, like pica (and a host of other conditions throughout the chapters of DSM-5), RD that occurs in the context of another mental or medical disorder must be sufficiently severe to warrant additional clinical care.

RD and pica are two of a relatively few DSM-5 conditions that require no criteria for clinical significance. That is, unless they occur in the context of another mental disorder, there is no requirement for some statement of harm, distress, additional investigation, or impaired functioning to the patient or to other people. Therefore, there isn't any bright line separating the behavior from what's normal.

Essential Features of **Rumination Disorder**

For at least a month, the patient has been regurgitating food.

The Fine Print

The D's: • Duration (1+ months) • Differential diagnosis (physical disorders, intellectual disability, other eating disorders)

Pica and RD are now listed with anorexia and bulimia nervosa, which is where they started out in DSM-III. DSM-IV placed them with other disorders that typically begin in childhood. Welcome home, pica and RD!

F50.8 [307.59] Avoidant/Restrictive Food Intake Disorder

Many young children (nearly half) experience some degree of difficulty with feeding, but most outgrow it. Those who don't may have a form of avoidant/restrictive food intake disorder (ARFID), the latest iteration of what used to be called feeding disorder of infancy or early childhood. The new name reflects the fact that we don't really know why some patients eat too little to remain healthy, only that it happens—and not always early in childhood.

The behavior may commence in the context of parent–child conflict centered around eating. Neglect, abuse, and parental psychopathology (depression, anxiety states, or personality disorders, for example) have also been adduced as causes. However, the vast majority are probably due to some sort of medical disorder. Among these are physical barriers to the act of chewing and swallowing and hypersensitivity to certain aspects of food such as texture, taste, and appearance. Indeed, DSM-5 encourages us to notice that children with ARFID fall into three principal categories: those who basically don't care about eating; those who restrict their diet due to sensory issues (certain foods are just unappetizing); and those who don't eat because of an unpleasant experience (perhaps they've choked when trying to swallow). In any case, the consequences of the behavior extend this definition well beyond the everyday picky eater.

Most children with ARFID are under the age of 6, but could even an adult ever be so diagnosed? There's nothing in the DSM-5 criteria to prevent it, but you won't find examples thick on the ground.

Essential Features of **Avoidant/Restrictive Food Intake Disorder**

With no abnormality of self-image, the patient eats too little to maintain adequate nutrition or weight (for children, to grow or gain weight). As a result, the patient may need tube feeding or added nourishment. Social and personal life may also be disrupted.

The Fine Print

The D's: • Differential diagnosis (medical conditions, accepted cultural practices, unavailability of food, mood or anxiety disorders, anorexia nervosa, psychotic or factitious disorders)

Coding Notes

Specify if: **In remission.** The patient hasn't met criteria for what DSM-5 calls "a sustained period of time."

F50.8 [307.59] Other Specified Feeding or Eating Disorder

Numerous patients fall outside the definitions of the major feeding and eating disorders; many of them are seriously ill. (It is also critically important to make sure that such a patient doesn't have another definitive condition, such as a mood disorder, schizophrenia, somatic symptom disorder, or any disorder caused by another medical condition.) Below are several that can be specified by name, following the "other specified" numbers and label.

Atypical anorexia nervosa. Some patients lose considerable weight, fear becoming fat, and believe they look fat, yet their weight remains normal.

Bulimia nervosa (of low frequency or limited duration). A patient who fulfills most criteria for bulimia nervosa doesn't binge often or long enough to meet the time criteria.

Night eating syndrome. Episodes of binge eating occur at night while the patient is in some stage of sleep; the next day, the patient may forget doing so.

Purging disorder. Without binge eating, the patient repeatedly engages in purging behavior (intentionally vomits or uses drugs) to affect weight or appearance.

F50.9 [307.50] Unspecified Feeding or Eating Disorder

As with unspecified diagnoses in other sections of DSM-5, use unspecified feeding or eating disorder when the patient does not meet full criteria for one of the diagnoses described above, and you do not wish to be more specific.

CHAPTER 10

Elimination Disorders

Quick Guide to the Elimination Disorders

Encopresis. At the age of 4 years or later, the patient repeatedly passes feces into inappropriate places (p. 294).

Enuresis. At the age of 5 years or later, there is repeated voiding of urine (it can be voluntary or involuntary) into bedding or clothing (p. 293).

Introduction

Encopresis and enuresis most often occur separately, but sometimes they travel together, especially in a child who has been seriously neglected or emotionally deprived. You can encounter either diagnosis as *primary* (symptoms have been present throughout the child's development) or as *secondary* (toilet training was initially successful). Abnormalities of the genitourinary and/or gastrointestinal tracts are often suspected but only rarely found, so that a careful medical history is usually enough to help you make the correct diagnosis.

F98.0 [307.6] Enuresis

By a ratio of 4:1, primary enuresis (the child has never been dry) is more common than secondary enuresis. It is limited to bedwetting; daytime bladder control is unaffected. Parents of children referred to a mental health professional have usually tried the common remedies—fluid restriction before bedtime, midnight toilet use—without success. Because the children typically wet several times a week, they are too embarrassed to sleep over with friends.

   In some children, enuresis is associated with non-rapid eye movement sleep, which occurs especially during the first 3 hours of sleep. In others, trauma such as hospitalization or separation from parents may precipitate secondary enuresis, which can occur more than once per night or randomly throughout the period of sleep. Although some enuretic children have urinary tract infections or physical anomalies (which would mean that we *wouldn't* make the diagnosis of enuresis), for most the etiology remains unknown. Although the formal criteria state that the wetting can be done on purpose, it is accidental and embarrassing for the vast majority of children.

There are strong genetic ties: About three-fourths of affected children have a first-degree relative with a history of enuresis. Having two enuretic parents strongly predicts that a child will be affected.

Before age 6, boys and girls are about equally represented (overall, around 5–10% of young children are affected). In older children, enuresis is more frequent in boys. The prevalence falls off with maturation, so that it affects only about 1% of adolescents. Adults who wet the bed are likely to continue doing so lifelong.

Essential Features of **Enuresis**

Without known cause, a patient repeatedly urinates into clothing or bedding.

The Fine Print

The D's: • Duration and demographics (2+ times/week for 3+ months in someone 5 years of age or older) • Distress (or frequency as above) • Differential diagnosis (medication side effects and physical disorders)

Coding Notes

Specify the type:

> **Nocturnal only**
> **Diurnal only**
> **Nocturnal and diurnal**

F98.1 [307.7] Encopresis

Patients with encopresis move their bowels in inappropriate places, such as into their clothing or onto the floor. There are two types. One is associated with chronic constipation, which causes fissures around the anus. Defecation therefore causes pain, which the child seeks to forestall by withholding stool. Then the stool hardens (worsening the fissures), and liquid feces leak from the impacted rectum into clothing and bedclothes.

The less common type, without constipation, is often a matter of secrecy and denial. Children hide their otherwise normal stools in unusual locations—behind the toilet, in bureau drawers—and then claim not to know how they got there. Encopresis without constipation is often associated with stress and other family psychopathology. Some of these children may have been abused physically or sexually.

Encopresis affects about 1% of elementary school-age children; boys predominate by a 6:1 ratio.

Essential Features of **Encopresis**

The patient recurrently defecates in improper locations or in clothes.

The Fine Print

The D's: • Duration and demographics (1+ times/month for 3+ months in someone 4 years or older) • Differential diagnosis (laxative use and physical disorders)

Coding Notes

Specify type:

With constipation and overflow incontinence
Without constipation and overflow incontinence

Other Specified Elimination Disorder

Use the other specified elimination disorder category for symptoms of encopresis or enuresis that do not meet the full diagnostic criteria, in cases where you wish to state the reason. Use the following diagnostic codes:

N39.498 [788.39] With urinary symptoms

R15.9 [787.60] With fecal symptoms

Unspecified Elimination Disorder

Use the unspecified elimination disorder category for symptoms of encopresis or enuresis that do not meet the full diagnostic criteria, in cases where you do not wish to state the reason. Use the following diagnostic codes:

R32 [788.30] With urinary symptoms

R15.9 [787.60] With fecal symptoms

CHAPTER 11

Sleep–Wake Disorders

Quick Guide to the Sleep–Wake Disorders

Once again, the DSM has an updated classification—this time, a more complicated structure that reflects advances in the field. In this Quick Guide, I have arranged the disorders rather differently from DSM-5's ordering, in order to emphasize the most prevalent underlying diagnoses. (I know it's boring, but the page number following each item indicates where a more detailed discussion begins.)

Sleeping Too Little (Insomnia)

Insomnia is often a symptom; sometimes it is a presenting complaint. Only occasionally is it a diagnosis independent of a major mental disorder or another medical condition (see sidebar, p. 301).

I can't overstate how important it is to evaluate first whether another mental disorder or medical condition could be the cause of insomnia.

Insomnia disorder. It can be comorbid with a medical condition (p. 301), primary (when there's no discernible cause; p. 307), or comorbid with another sleep disorder or mental disorder (p. 303). The last is most often encountered in patients suffering from major depressive episodes (p. 122), manic episodes (p. 129), or even panic attacks (p. 173).

Substance/medication-induced sleep–wake disorder, insomnia type. Most of the commonly misused psychoactive substances, as well as a variety of prescription medicines, can interfere with sleep (p. 346).

Sleep apnea. Although most patients with breathing problems such as sleep apnea complain of hypersomnia, some instead have insomnia. Three principal types are listed: obstructive sleep apnea hypopnea, central sleep apnea, and sleep-related hypoventilation (pp. 318, 321).

Sleeping Too Much (Hypersomnolence)

You might think that the term *hypersomnia* means *only* that a patient sleeps too much. However, it can also indicate drowsiness at a time when the patient should be alert. A new word, *hypersomnolence*, has been introduced to make sure that we're thinking of both meanings.

Hypersomnolence disorder. Excessive drowsiness or sleepiness can accompany mental or medical disorders, or other sleep disorders; sometimes it's primary (p. 309).

Narcolepsy. These people experience a crushing need to sleep, regardless of time of day, causing them to fall asleep almost instantly—sometimes, even when standing. They may also have sleep paralysis, sudden loss of strength (cataplexy), and hallucinations as they fall asleep or awaken (p. 313).

Substance/medication-induced sleep–wake disorder, daytime sleepiness type. The use of a substance is less likely to produce hypersomnolence than insomnia, but it can happen (p. 346).

Sleep apnea. What DSM-5 calls breathing-related sleep disorders commonly result in day-time drowsiness. Three principal types are listed, as noted above for insomnia (pp. 318, 321).

Circadian Rhythm Sleep–Wake Disorders

There's a mismatch between someone's biological clock and the environment. Five principal subtypes are listed:

Delayed sleep phase type. Falling asleep and waking later than desired (p. 324).

Advanced sleep phase type. Falling asleep and waking earlier than desired (p. 324).

Irregular sleep–wake type. Falling asleep and waking at irregular times (p. 325).

Non-24-hour sleep–wake type. Falling asleep and waking (usually) progressively later than desired (p. 324).

Shift work type. Sleepiness associated with changes in work schedule (p. 325).

Jet lag. Feeling sleepy or "hung over" after crossing time zones is no longer considered a sleep disorder; it's a physiological fact of modern life. Nonetheless, I've covered it briefly in a sidebar (p. 323).

Parasomnias and Other Disorders of Sleep

In these disorders, something abnormal happens in association with sleep (or the stages of sleep), or during the times when the patient is falling asleep or waking up.

Non-rapid eye movement (non-REM) sleep arousal disorder, sleep terror type. These patients cry out in apparent fear during the first part of the night. Often they don't really wake up at all. This behavior is considered pathological only in adults, not children (p. 333).

Non-REM sleep arousal disorder, sleepwalking type. Persistent sleepwalking usually occurs early in the night (p. 331).

Non-REM sleep arousal disorder, confusional arousals. Patients partially awaken, but they don't walk about and don't appear fearful. This isn't an official DSM-5 disorder, but people experience it anyway (p. 335).

Rapid eye movement (REM) sleep behavior disorder. These patients awaken from REM sleep to speak or thrash about, sometimes injuring themselves or bed partners (p. 343).

Nightmare disorder. Bad dreams trouble some people more than others (p. 340).

Restless legs syndrome. The irresistible need to move one's legs during periods of inactivity (especially evenings/nights) leads to fatigue and other behavioral/emotional sequels (p. 336).

Substance/medication-induced sleep–wake disorder, parasomnia type. Alcohol and other substances (during intoxication or withdrawal) can cause various problems with sleep (p. 346).

Other specified, or unspecified, sleep disorder. These categories are for problems of insomnia, hypersomnolence, or general sleep issues that cannot be fitted into any of the categories above (p. 349).

Introduction

Sleep is basic behavior for humans, as for all other animals. Keep in mind these points about the normal sleep of humans:

1. Normality takes in a wide range. This refers to the amount of sleep, how long it takes to fall asleep and to awaken, and what happens in between.

2. When sleep is abnormal, it can have profound consequences for health.

3. An individual's sleep changes throughout the life cycle. Everyone knows that babies sleep most of the time. As people age, they take more time to fall asleep, they require less sleep, and they awaken more often throughout the night. I've heard it said that 9-year-olds sleep the best of anyone. Too bad: Everyone reading this is over the hill, sleep-wise.

4. Sleep isn't uniform; it varies in depth and quality throughout the night. The

two principal phases of sleep are rapid eye movement (REM) sleep, during which most dreaming takes place, and non-REM sleep. Various disorders can be related to these phases of sleep.

5. Many people who sleep less soundly or more briefly than they think they should don't have an actual disorder of sleep.

6. Even today, sleep disorder criteria are based principally upon clinical findings. EEG and other sleep laboratory studies may be confirmatory, but they are required for diagnosis in just a few of the conditions described here.

Sleep specialists divide sleep disorders into *dyssomnias* and *parasomnias*. A patient with a *dyssomnia* sleeps too little, too much, or at the wrong time, but the sleep itself—what there is of it—is pretty normal. In a *parasomnia*, the quality, quantity, and timing of sleep are essentially normal. But something abnormal happens during sleep itself, or during the times when the patient is falling asleep or waking up; motor, cognitive, or autonomic nervous system processes become active during sleep or during the transitions between sleep and wakefulness, and all hell breaks loose.

Consider, for example, sleep apnea (dyssomnia) versus nightmares (parasomnia). Both occur during sleep, but nightmares are usually problematic because they are scary, not because they interfere with sleeping or impair wakefulness the next day, as is often the case with sleep apnea.

Sleeping Too Much or Too Little

F51.01 [307.42] Insomnia Disorder

What most of us understand by *insomnia* is this: sleep that is too brief or is unrestful. Some people with insomnia may not realize just how tense they are. Some cases may start as insomnia secondary to another medical condition, such as pain from a broken hip. The hip heals, but the patient has become accustomed to the idea of being unable to sleep at night. In other words, insomnia can be learned behavior. Indeed, many medical illnesses can lead to the symptoms of insomnia disorder.

Some patients with insomnia may use their beds for activities other than sleeping or having sex—eating and watching TV, for example. These associations condition them to be wakeful when they are in bed; it's part of what clinicians call *poor sleep hygiene*. These patients may discover the source of the problem when their sleep improves during weekends, during holidays, or on a vacation, when they've escaped their usual habits and habitats. Whatever the cause, insomnia can persist forever if it isn't effectively addressed. Insomnia disorder (ID) is found especially in older patients and in women.

Many people complain of unrefreshing (or nonrestorative) sleep, or of being awake, when their bed partners swear they have slept all night. For this reason, the statement that insomnia is "sleeping too little" still isn't quite right; rather, insomnia is the *complaint* of sleeping too little. But these people do have problems that should not be belittled. Giving them time to state what is on their minds is important in seeking the etiology of their difficulties.

Note that the definition of ID requires that the patient experience clinically important distress or disability as a result. Although the distress may be experienced during the nighttime, any resulting disability is most likely to be experienced during the daytime—reduced effectiveness at work, interpersonal conflict at home, daytime fatigue and sleepiness, and the like. Anyone who complains of difficulty sleeping, but who does *not* report distress or disability, should not receive the diagnosis of ID. Even with those restrictions, that still leaves up to 10% of the adult population affected by ID. It is a bit more common among women than men.

DSM-5 specifies that we should use the diagnosis of ID for any patient who fulfills the diagnostic criteria, whether or not there is a coexisting mental, medical, or other sleep–wake disorder—as long as the patient's ID is sufficiently serious that it requires independent clinical attention. I'll illustrate with three vignettes.

Essential Features of **Insomnia Disorder**

It's mainly quality or amount of sleep that causes complaint: trouble getting to sleep, staying asleep, or awaking too early without again falling asleep. Occasionally, sleep is just plain not refreshing. The following day, the patient feels fatigued, grumpy, or has poor concentration or otherwise impaired functioning.

The Fine Print

The D's: • Duration (3+ nights a week for 3+ months) • Distress or disability (work/ educational, social, or personal impairment) • Differential diagnosis (substance use and physical disorders, mood or anxiety disorders, psychotic disorders, posttraumatic stress disorder, other sleep–wake disorders, poor sleep hygiene, or too little available sleep time)

Coding Notes

Specify if:

>   **Episodic.** Duration 1–3 months (any shorter-duration insomnia disorder would actually have to be coded as other specified insomnia disorder, p. 349).
>   **Persistent.** Duration 3+ months.
>   **Recurrent.** 2+ episodes in 1 year.

Specify if:

With non-sleep disorder mental comorbidity.
With other medical comorbidity.
With other sleep disorder.

In each case, specify the coexisting disorder.

Nobody knows how common complaints of insomnia are in a patient who isn't otherwise sick (that is, who has neither another medical nor another mental condition). Such patients are probably a tiny minority of those a mental health professional encounters. Perhaps these people are more likely to seek help from a primary medical care provider. Although texts say that persistent insomnia is fairly common, they must seek treatment from family practitioners or internists: of over 15,000 mental health patients I have examined, exactly 1 had what I considered primary ID (without another medical or mental disorder).

Insomnia Disorder, with Other Medical Comorbidity

Many medical illnesses are associated with sleep problems (mostly insomnia). Such problems are usually ones of restlessness, increased sleep onset latency, and frequent awakenings during the night. The medical issues cited—which can produce discomfort day or night—include the following:

- Fever resulting from a variety of infections.

- Pain caused by headache (especially some migraines), rheumatoid arthritis, cancer, persistent nocturnal penile erections, or angina.

- Itching caused by a variety of systemic and skin disorders.

- Breathing problems resulting from asthma or chronic obstructive pulmonary disease (COPD), restricted lung capacity (due to obesity, pregnancy, or spinal deformities), or cystic fibrosis.

- Endocrine and metabolic diseases, including hyperthyroidism, liver failure, and kidney disease.

- Sleeping in one position enforced, for example, by wearing a cast.

- Neuromuscular disorders, such as muscular dystrophy and poliomyelitis.

- Movement and other neurological disorders, such as Huntington's disease, torsion dystonia, Parkinson's disease, and some seizure disorders.

Hoyle Garner

Hoyle Garner was 58 when he sought treatment for his insomnia. His wife, Edith, accompanied him to the appointment. Together, they ran a "mom and pop" grocery store.

Several years earlier, Hoyle had learned that he had emphysema. A series of pulmonary function tests had prompted his doctor to ask him to quit smoking. After 3 weeks, he had gained 10 pounds and couldn't concentrate well enough to add up the receipts from the store each night. "I was depressed and uptight, and I couldn't sleep 2 hours without waking up and wanting a cigarette," said Hoyle.

"I begged him to start smoking again," said Edith. "When he did, it was a relief for both of us."

Hoyle quit seeing the doctor, and his sleep returned to normal. Within the past few months, however, he'd begun awakening several times during the course of the night. Some nights this happened as often as every hour. He felt restless and uncomfortable, with some of the same anxiety he'd experienced the time he tried to quit smoking. A few times he tried sitting on the edge of the bed to have a cigarette, but it didn't seem to help. And anyway, Edith complained about the smell of smoke in the night. They still ran their grocery, and Hoyle was having no trouble at all with his columns of figures. He never drank more than a single beer, usually in the afternoon.

"Waking up doesn't bother him much," Edith complained. "He usually goes right back to sleep again. He doesn't even feel sleepy the next day. But it leaves me wide awake, wondering how soon he'll wake up again."

Edith's hours awake had given her plenty of opportunity to observe her husband. After he slept quietly for half an hour or so, his breathing seemed to become rapid and shallow. It never stopped for longer than a few seconds, and he never snored. They had tried having him sleep with extra pillows (it had helped her Uncle Will with his heart failure), but it hadn't eased Hoyle's sleeping any, and it "kinda hurt his neck."

"I hope we can get to the bottom of this," Edith concluded. "It doesn't seem to bother him very much, but I've got to get some sleep."

Shameless advertisement: How do you decide that one event has caused another? Of course, in clinical diagnosis, it's hard ever to be certain. But several features can help you decide with a reasonable degree of confidence that *A* has caused *B*. I've discussed these issues (and much more) in my book *Diagnosis Made Easier*, now in its second edition (The Guilford Press, 2014).

Evaluation of Hoyle Garner

Hoyle's main problem was with sleep, which showed up as frequent awakenings, several times every night, for months (ID criteria A2, C, D) despite sufficient opportunities for sleep (E). Although for him the effects were less than earth-shaking (insomnia due to COPD typically doesn't produce daytime drowsiness), his wife complained quite a lot. And the effect of someone's insomnia on a bed partner or caregiver is one of the symptoms that tells us we have a problem deserving consideration (B).

The features of Hoyle's insomnia would not suggest a severe **mood disorder**, which could produce early morning awakening. Besides, a mild mood disorder, or **adjustment disorder with depressed mood,** is typically associated with trouble falling asleep. Based on Edith's observations of his sleep, Hoyle did not have (F) a variety of **narcolepsy** or **sleep apnea** (do check for sleep apnea in any patient with insomnia with other medical comorbidity; a small number will have two disorders). He was taking no medications at the time, but many patients with medical illnesses will be doing that; then, you'll have to rule out **substance-induced insomnia.**

Hoyle also had tobacco use disorder, which was probably responsible for the emphysema in the first place; it would be hard to attribute his insomnia to a physiological consequence of nicotine (G). When he was trying to quit smoking, he clearly experienced tobacco withdrawal, and he continued to smoke despite his COPD (see p. 461). I'd give him a GAF score of 61. His complete diagnosis would be as follows:

F51.01 [307.42]	Insomnia disorder, with pulmonary emphysema, persistent
J43.9 [492.8]	Pulmonary emphysema
F17.200 [305.1]	Tobacco use disorder, moderate

Note that DSM-5 no longer asks us to specify whether insomnia is "due to" a comorbid physical or mental disorder. It is enough to say that they coexist. That's because it can be extraordinarily difficult to determine whether one has actually caused the other. We are allowed (indeed, encouraged) to diagnose any disorder whose symptoms are severe enough to justify independent clinical attention.

Insomnia Disorder, with Non-Sleep Disorder Mental Comorbidity

When it is a symptom of some other mental disorder, insomnia is often directly proportional to the severity of the other diagnosis. And, logically enough, sleep usually improves with resolution of the underlying condition. Meanwhile, patients sometimes abuse hypnotic and other medications. Here's a brief overview:

Major depressive episodes. Insomnia is probably most often a symptom of a mood disorder. In fact, sleep disturbance may be one of the earliest symptoms of depression. Insomnia is especially likely to affect depressed elderly patients. In severe depression, terminal insomnia (awakening early in the morning and being unable to get back to sleep) is characteristic—and a truly miserable experience.

Trauma- and stressor-related disorders. Criteria for acute stress disorder and for posttraumatic stress disorder specifically mention sleep disturbance as a symptom.

Panic disorder. Panic attacks may occur during sleep.

Adjustment disorder. Patients who have developed anxiety or depression in response to a specific stressor may lie awake worrying about a particular stressor or the day's events.

Somatic symptom disorder. Many somatizing patients will complain of problems with sleep, especially initial and interval insomnia.

Cognitive disorders. Most demented patients have some degree of sleep disturbance. Typically, this involves interval awakening: They will wander at night and suffer from reduced alertness during the day.

Manic and hypomanic episodes. In a 24-hour period, manic and hypomanic patients typically sleep less than they do when they are euthymic. However, they do not *complain* of insomnia. They feel rested and ready for more activity; it's their families and friends who become concerned (and fatigued). If such patients do complain, it is usually of lengthened sleep onset latency—the time it takes to fall asleep.

Schizophrenia. When they are becoming ill, delusions, hallucinations, or anxiety may keep patients with schizophrenia preoccupied later and later into the night. Total sleep time may remain constant, but they arise progressively later, until most of their sleeping occurs during the day. DSM-5 doesn't provide a way to code a circadian rhythm sleep–wake disorder related to a mental disorder; ID related to schizophrenia (or, perhaps, other specified insomnia disorder) would be about the best we could do.

Obsessive–compulsive personality disorder. This personality disorder is commonly cited as associated with insomnia.

Anxiety or mania may mask an insomnia that occurs in the course of another mental disorder. Patients may not recognize a sleep deficit until they fall asleep at the wheel or suffer an industrial accident. On the other hand, there's a risk that clinicians could focus on the problem with sleep and underdiagnose the associated mental problem.

Sal Camozzi

"I'm just not getting enough sleep to play." Sal Camozzi was a third-year student who attended a small liberal arts college in southern California on a football scholarship.

Now it was early November, midway through the season, and he didn't think he could maintain the effort. He had always kept regular hours and "eaten healthy," but for over a month he had been awakening at 2:30 every morning.

"I might as well be setting an alarm," he said. "My eyes snap open and there I am, worrying about the next game, or passing chemistry, or whatever. I'm only getting 5 hours at night, and I've always needed 8. I'm getting desperate."

For a while Sal had tried over-the-counter sleep medications. They helped a little, but mainly they made him feel groggy the next day. He gave them up; he had always avoided alcohol and drugs, and hated the feeling of chemicals in his body.

Sal had had something of the same problem the previous fall, and the one before that. Then he'd had the same difficulty with sleep; his appetite had fallen off, too. Neither time had things been as severe as now, however. (This year he had already lost 10 pounds; as a linebacker, he needed to keep his weight up.) Sal also complained that he just didn't seem to enjoy life in general the way he usually did. Although his interest in football and his concentration on the field had diminished, it hadn't been as bad last year, and he had finished the season with respectable statistics.

One summer during high school, Sal had felt listless and slept too much. He'd been tested for infectious mononucleosis and found to be physically well. He was his normal self by the time school started that fall.

Last spring and the one before had been a different matter. When Sal went out for baseball, he seemed to explode with energy, batted .400, and played every game. He didn't sleep much then, either, when he came to think of it, though 5 hours a night had seemed plenty. "I had loads of energy and never felt happier in my life. I felt like another Babe Ruth."

The coach had noted that Sal had been "terrific during baseball season, all hustle, but he talked too much. Why doesn't he put the same effort into football?"

Primary (as in a primary insomnia) is one of those funny words that have taken on meanings different from that which most speakers of English understand. In the clinical world, *primary* means an illness or symptom for which no cause can be found. Of course, that doesn't mean that there *isn't* a cause; it's just that no one's sure what it is. In this context, *primary* doesn't mean that one condition is more important than another, or that one begins earlier than something else. (The World Health Organization also uses *primary* to mean a disorder that attacks the brain directly or preferentially, as opposed to those that attack the brain only as one of several body organs or systems.) The DSM-5 doesn't use *primary* in any official sense at all, but clinicians do, to differentiate disorders for which we can state a cause from those for which we can't.

Clinicians also use the term *functional* to describe disorders for which they can find no basis in brain anatomy, chemistry, or physiology. Most mood disorders and psychoses are called *functional*; that is, we still don't know why or how they have developed. If you think this is confusing, consider some of the other words deployed throughout the medical world to mean "I haven't the faintest idea what's behind it": *essential*, as in essential hypertension; *idiopathic*, as in idiopathic thrombocytopenic purpura; *cryptogenic* (literally, "hidden cause"). Sometimes we say *psychogenic*, which gives the illusion that we have found the cause, but that it's often only in our minds (or dreams).

No wonder clinicians in training don't sleep well.

Evaluation of Sal Camozzi

From Sal's history, his sleep disorder wasn't related to **substance use** or to any **physical illness.** There was similarly no evidence for **another sleep disorder.**

Sal's sleep difficulty was actually only the tip of his depressive iceberg. The first thing to look for would be other symptoms of a **major depressive episode.** Although he didn't complain of feeling depressed in so many words, he did report a general loss of zest for life. Besides that and the insomnia, Sal had also lost his appetite, interest, and concentration. Together, his symptoms would barely meet criteria for a major depressive episode. The history did not touch on death wishes or suicidal ideas; it should have.

Besides depression, the obvious episodes of high mood would need to be considered in the diagnosis. Sal had had several periods when he felt unusually happy, his energy level increased, he talked a great deal, and his need for sleep fell off. Especially in contrast to his present mood, his self-esteem was markedly increased (he noted that he "felt like Babe Ruth"). This change in his mood was pronounced enough that others noticed and commented on it, but it did not compromise his functioning or require hospitalization—if so, we'd instead have diagnosed a manic episode. His symptoms would fulfill criteria for a **hypomanic episode.**

All of this adds up to a diagnosis of **bipolar II disorder** (see p. 135); Sal's current episode would of course be depressed. He would nearly meet criteria for the specifier *with melancholic features*, but his history of repeated depressions beginning in the same season of the year (fall) and consistently either resolving or switching to hypomania during another season (spring) would be typical for the specifier *with seasonal pattern*. Although Sal may have had one episode of depression when he was in high school that did not fit this pattern, most of the episodes did, which is the requirement. And the last 2 years fit the mold exactly.

Sal's sleeplessness would have been clinically significant even without the bipolar II disorder (ID criteria A, B), since it caused fatigue and occurred several nights a week (C). But here's the rub: It had persisted for just over a month—perhaps 60 days shy of the 3 months required by DSM-5 for ID. Now Sal fit the DSM-IV criteria, and Sal hasn't changed; only the criteria have. What to do?

To me, it seems unreasonable that a person who has a disorder that, by definition, is relatively short-lived (patients with seasonal mood disturbance become ill and recover with the seasons) cannot qualify for the additional diagnosis of ID. So, with the understanding that the criteria are only guidelines, not handcuffs, I'm going to stick with my original evaluation of Sal. Whether you agree with or reject my judgment, his case can still help guide us through the maze of the diagnostic criteria. (If you do disagree, you could code his sleep disorder as G47.09 [780.52], other specified insomnia disorder, brief insomnia disorder.)

Sal's GAF score would be 55. We are instructed to list the associated mental (or medical) disorder right after the sleep disorder, so as to make the association clear. I wanted to list first the mood disorder, because it is the more critical to treat, but at least I did put them contiguously. (OK, it's hard to do otherwise when there are only two items to list.)

F31.81 [296.89]	Bipolar II disorder, depressed, with seasonal pattern
F51.01 [307.42]	Insomnia disorder, with bipolar II disorder

To a considerable extent, it's a matter of taste whether to diagnose a sleep disorder that occurs with another mental condition. DSM-5 notes that this is appropriate when the problem with sleep is serious enough to justify an evaluation in its own right. If the patient's presenting complaint is the sleep problem, I'd consider it evidence of clinical importance. However, these situations are often unclear and usually require judgment. In the example of a mood disorder, any problem with sleep is almost certainly a symptom that will resolve once the depression has been adequately treated. Therefore, no one could be faulted for diagnosing only the mood disorder.

[Primary] Insomnia Disorder

Another type of ID—in which the person has no apparent other condition to which the insomnia can be attributed—is actually the one most often diagnosed. Still, the "plain vanilla" type should be one of exclusion, used only after other possibilities (including insomnia caused by substance use; see p. 346) have been ruled out.

Just because we cannot discern the cause of insomnia, of course, doesn't mean there is no cause; it's just that we cannot pinpoint it. Sometimes insomnia may start because noise or some other stimulus inhibits sleep. (When sleeplessness is due to a noisy environment or one otherwise not conducive to sleep, it isn't technically insomnia. It's called, would you believe, environmental sleep disorder—but not by DSM-5.)

Another contributing factor is being active right up until bedtime. Vigorous exercise and arguments are just two of the sort of activities that can promote sleeplessness; people need quiet time to get into a relaxed frame of mind needed for sleep onset. Once insomnia is underway, muscle tension from lying awake and persistent negative thoughts ("I'm a terrible sleeper") perpetuate the problem. The result is hours of frustration at night, plus fatigue and dysphoria the following day.

How often does this type—it used to be called *primary insomnia*—occur? No one really knows. Though perhaps a quarter of adults are unhappy with their sleep, probably a percentage down in the single digits would qualify for an ID diagnosis. It is especially found in older people and in women. Over time, it can vary, but it usually follows a chronic course.

Curtis Usher

"It's almost spooky. It doesn't seem to make any difference what time I go to bed—9:30, 10:00, 10:30. Whatever, my eyes click open at 2:00 in the morning, and that's it for the rest of the night."

Curtis Usher had had this problem off and on for years. Recently, it was more often on. "Actually, I guess it's usually the worst during the week. Whenever I lie there, I'm worrying about work."

Curtis was a project manager at an advertising agency. It was a wonderful job when times were flush, which they hadn't been for several years. Curtis's boss was a bit of a tyrant, who enjoyed saying that he didn't have headaches; he caused them. Curtis didn't have headaches, but he didn't get much sleep, either.

At age 53, Curtis was a healthy man of regular habits. He had lived alone since his wife divorced him 3 years earlier, with the complaint that he was dull. Occasionally his current girlfriend stayed overnight in his studio apartment, but most evenings he spent lying on his bed watching public television until he couldn't stay awake any longer. He never drank or used drugs, and his mood was good; neither he nor anyone else in his family had ever had any mental health problems.

"I don't take naps during the day," Curtis summed up, "but I might as well. I'm sure not getting much done at work."

Evaluation of Curtis Usher

Curtis clearly had trouble sleeping—it would seem to include both initial and terminal components (ID criteria A1, A3)—that had lasted far longer than the required 3 months (D). From what Curtis related, it occurred several times a week (C) and was reducing his efficiency at work (B). Other than an occasional sleepover with his girlfriend, no other information suggests circumstances that would interfere with his opportunities for sleep (E).

The real challenge is to decide whether Curtis's insomnia was stand-alone or whether we would need to include in our coding some underlying problem that was destroying his sleep. Although the vignette doesn't cover every possibility, it does touch upon some of the major points.

Curtis probably did not have **another mental disorder** (H). His mood had been too good for a **major depressive episode.** Although he worried about work, we have no information to suggest that he had the wide-ranging anxiety typical of **generalized anxiety disorder.** He didn't drink or use drugs (G); there is no information to exclude a **personality disorder**, but these are probably infrequent as a sole cause of a sleep disorder.

We have only Curtis's own word on his good health to confirm that he did not have **another medical condition** (also criterion H); his clinician should refer him for a medical evaluation. What about other sleep disorders (F)? Curtis didn't nap, which would seem to rule out **narcolepsy. Sleep apnea** also seems unlikely: his former wife had cited dullness, not snoring, among her complaints. **Circadian rhythm sleep–wake disorder, delayed sleep phase type** would result in awakening late rather than early, and he didn't get sleepy early, as would be the case with the **advanced sleep phase type.** The vignette contains no information that would support a parasomnia diagnosis such as **nightmare disorder**, or a **non-REM sleep arousal disorder** such as **sleep terrors** or **sleepwalking.**

Two mechanisms could help account for Curtis's insomnia. His work-related anxiety would be one (his boss was demanding, and times were tough in his industry). Alternatively, he often reclined on his bed while watching TV. The association of this waking-related activity with bed (poor sleep hygiene) could be conditioning him to stay awake.

Pending the outcome of a medical evaluation, here's how I'd diagnose Curtis (with a GAF score of 65, with a Z-code to indicate an area that needs work):

F51.01 [307.42]	Insomnia disorder, persistent
Z72.9 [V69.9]	Lifestyle problem (poor sleep hygiene)

Generalized anxiety disorder is important in the differential diagnosis of ID. Like those with this anxiety disorder, patients with ID also lie awake worrying. (The difference is that their anxieties are focused on their inability to sleep as well as think they should.) Also watch for "masked depression": Inquire carefully about other vegetative symptoms (appetite, weight loss) of a major depressive episode when you are evaluating patients who appear to have only ID.

F51.11 [307.44] Hypersomnolence Disorder

Sleep experts have adopted the term *hypersomnolence* in place of the familiar *hypersomnia*, and here's why: The new term better describes the fact that these conditions can result either in excessive sleep or in a less-than-optimal quality of wakefulness. The latter includes trouble waking up or remaining fully awake, sometimes called *sleep inertia*—the sensation of just not being able to fully awaken (or stay that way) when we need to be fully alert. Hypersomnolence disorder (HD) includes conditions of hypersomnolence that occur with medical, mental, or other sleep disorders, and some that are apparently free-standing.

People with HD tend to fall asleep easily and rapidly (often in 5 minutes or less), and they may sleep late the next day. Although total sleep time is likely to be 9 or more hours in 24, they may feel so chronically tired and sleepy that even after a normal night's sleep they take daytime naps. These tend to be long and unrefreshing; they don't improve things much. Such people tend to have trouble awakening in the morning, and they may be groggy and have peculiar problems with disorientation, memory, and alertness. In their state of reduced alertness, they may behave more or less automatically, performing behaviors for which they have poor later recall.

Although we don't have a lot of information about HD, it probably occurs about equally in males and females and begins when they are relatively young, usually in their teens or 20s. It may affect up to 1% of the general population.

Though the cause of HD isn't always apparent, there are a number of known associations. Hypocretin deficiency occurs less often in cases of HD than in narcolepsy with cataplexy, though on average, its level is less than that for the general population. Also common is a gene allele (HLA DQB1*0602, for anyone keeping score at home), though no one is in a position to say that HD is strictly a genetic phenomenon. Some patients with HD may be experiencing difficulty coping with stress; others may be trying to compensate for a sense of something lacking in their lives. In any event, the outcome is total sleep time that far exceeds the norm, causing these people sometimes to take medications. Central nervous system stimulants can help reduce daytime sleepiness; however, tranquilizers are likely to make matters worse.

HD can occur with or without medical illnesses or other mental disorders, but we should not diagnose it if it occurs *only* with another sleep–wake disorder.

Essential Features of **Hypersomnolence Disorder**

The patient complains of severe daytime drowsiness even after 7+ hours of sleep, repeatedly naps or falls asleep each day, has difficulty remaining fully awake, or sleeps long (9+ hours a night) but doesn't sleep well (it isn't refreshing).

The Fine Print

The D's: • Duration (3+ times a week for 3+ months) • Distress or disability (work/educational, social, or personal impairment) • Differential diagnosis (substance use and physical disorders, other sleep–wake or mental disorders, normal sleep)

Coding Notes

Specify if:

   Acute. Duration under 1 month.
   Subacute. Duration 1–3 months.
   Persistent. Duration 3+ months.

Specify if:

   With mental disorder.

With medical condition.

With another sleep disorder. Don't make the diagnosis at all if hypersomnolence occurs *only* with another sleep disorder.

In each case, code the coexisting disorder.

Specify severity, depending on number of days with difficulty maintaining daytime alertness:

Mild. 1–2 days a week.
Moderate. 3–4 days a week.
Severe. 5+ days a week.

Colin Rodebaugh

From the time he was 15, Colin Rodebaugh had dreamed of becoming an architect. He had read biographies of Christopher Wren and Frank Lloyd Wright; in the summers, he worked around construction projects to learn how materials went together. Now he was 23 and in his second year of architectural school, and he couldn't stay awake during class.

"I might as well have weights tied to my eyelids," he said. "For the last 6 months, two or three times a day, I just have to take a nap. It could be in class, any time. It even happened once when I was making love to my girlfriend—not after, but during!"

Colin complained that he was tired all the time, but his health appeared to be excellent. His father, a family practitioner in Arizona, had insisted that he have a complete physical exam. Colin had been specifically questioned about any history of sudden weakness, loss of consciousness, or seizure disorder, none of which he had had. His mother practiced clinical psychology in Oregon, and she was ready to vouch for his mental health.

"I get plenty of sleep at night—at least 9 hours. That's not the problem. It's that I hardly ever feel rested, no matter how much sleep I've had. If I do take a nap, I wake up feeling almost as groggy as when I nodded off."

Even apart from Colin's sleep problem, school was a frustration. Although he was technically proficient, he'd discovered that he didn't have the eye for design of some of his classmates. During the past semester, he had realized that what talent he had lay in drafting, not design. His advisor hadn't argued with him when they had discussed a possible career change.

Evaluation of Colin Rodebaugh

As with insomnia, the first task in evaluating hypersomnolence is to rule out the many conditions that could be causing it. Although the vignette does not contain all the information Colin's clinician would need, it hits the high points.

Physical illnesses are probably the most important considerations for this differential diagnosis. Based on a recent workup and physical exam, Colin appeared to be healthy. Furthermore, there had been no history of sudden weakness or lapses of consciousness that might indicate **psychomotor epilepsy.** (According to DSM-5 criterion F, a patient can have a medical condition and still receive a diagnosis of HD, as long as the medical condition doesn't fully explain the problem with sleep.) We have no information about substance use (E); Colin's clinician would have to evaluate that. At least his mother, who was a mental health professional, felt that there was no indication of another mental disorder (also F).

Narcolepsy is another sleep disorder that causes daytime sleepiness (D). But such individuals are typically refreshed by their brief naps, whereas Colin felt groggy. His clinician could ask Colin's girlfriend whether he snored or had other symptoms suggestive of **sleep apnea. Insufficient nighttime sleep** seems so obvious a possibility that it is sometimes overlooked (suspect it in patients who sleep less than 7 hours a night). Colin felt that he got plenty of sleep, and at 9 hours a night or more, we wouldn't consider him sleep-deprived (A).

As far as we can tell from the vignette, Colin's sleep disorder had lasted about 6 months, and it occurred nearly every day—certainly every day he was in class (B, C). I'd definitely include in his evaluation some mention of the problem he was having with school; it could help point the way to a therapeutic intervention. His GAF score would be about 65.

F51.11 [307.44]	Hypersomnolence disorder, persistent, severe
Z55.9 [V62.3]	Inadequate school performance

A teenage or college-age boy who's grumpy and likes to sleep in? Stop the presses!

Well, if the behavior is due to Kleine–Levin syndrome (KLS)—one of myriad disorders subsumed under HD, with medical condition—it can be both unusual and distressing. Just how unusual? With fewer than 500 patients ever reported worldwide, KLS may be the rarest condition (by several orders of magnitude) mentioned in DSM-5. If ever you encounter such a patient, here's what you should expect to find.

Eighty percent of KLS cases begin during the teen years. By a 2:1 or 3:1 ratio, males predominate, though it may be more severe when it occurs in females. All patients experience profound hypersomnolence—sleeping 12–24 hours a day (mean and median are each 18 hours). In addition, nearly everyone experiences altered cognition: derealization, perplexity, perhaps loss of concentration or memory problems (some patients have complete amnesia for the episodes). Patients become churlish or argumentative and irritable, especially if prevented from sleeping. Four out of five have a change in eating behavior: specifically, voracious overeating (way past the point of feeling full), without, however, the purging behavior that is typical of patients with bulimia nervosa.

In two out of three cases, speech is also abnormal: Patients become mute or lack spontaneous speech; or they speak only in monosyllables; or speech is slow, slurred, or

incoherent. Nearly half also experience hypersexuality—some expose themselves or masturbate openly, or make inappropriate sexual advances to others. At the same time, nearly
half report depressed mood, which usually remits at the end of each episode. Indeed,
between episodes, nearly all patients appear completely normal.

The cause of KLS is unknown. Sometimes it begins with an infection, perhaps one as
mild as a cold; some cases are precipitated by a stroke, a tumor, or another neurological
disorder such as multiple sclerosis. Episodes last 1–3 weeks, and typically recur several
times a year. This pattern persists for perhaps 8 years, or an average of 12 episodes. Then,
for no apparent reason, just as it began, it often simply disappears. Those who continue to
have episodes often find them greatly moderated.

If you do see such a patient, write up the case history for publication—and send me
a copy.

Narcolepsy

Narcolepsy is a syndrome of excessive sleepiness that has been recognized since about
1880. The classic presentation includes four symptoms: sleep attacks, cataplexy, hallucinations, and sleep paralysis. Most people don't have all of these symptoms, though
the clinical picture can appear strange enough that patients are sometimes mistakenly
diagnosed as having a non-sleep-related mental disorder.

- REM periods begin within a few minutes of the onset of sleep, instead of the
  usual hour and a half. (In older patients, sleep latency tends to increase.) Often
  they will even intrude upon the normal waking state, resulting in the irresistible
  urge to sleep. These sleep attacks tend toward brevity, lasting from a few minutes to over an hour. In contrast to the grogginess that patients with hypersomnolence disorder often experience, the sleep is refreshing—except for children,
  who may awaken feeling tired. Then there follows a refractory period of an hour
  or more, during which the patient will remain completely awake. Sleep attacks
  can be triggered by stress or by emotional experiences (usually "positive" ones,
  such as jokes and laughter). The resulting daytime drowsiness is often the earliest complaint of patients with narcolepsy.

- The most dramatic symptom is *cataplexy*—a sudden, brief episode of paralysis that can affect nearly all voluntary muscles, though sometimes just specific
  muscle groups, such as the jaw or the knees. When all muscles are affected, the
  patient may collapse completely. If fewer muscle groups are involved or if the
  attack is brief, cataplexy may go almost unnoticed. Episodes of cataplexy may
  occur with sleep attacks, but they can be separate, without loss of consciousness.
  Often they are precipitated by intense emotion, such as laughter, weeping, or
  anger, or even by orgasm. Cataplexy usually develops within a few months of
  the onset of hypersomnia. (Brain lesions such as tumors, infections, or injury

can cause some people to experience cataplexy without having other symptoms of narcolepsy.)

Young children, especially those who have been only briefly ill, may not have classical cataplexy; rather, they experience episodes of jaw movement, grimacing, or sticking out of the tongue that can occur even without evidence of emotional triggers. These attacks gradually morph into more classical cataplexy.

- Hallucinations, which are mainly visual, may be the first symptoms of narcolepsy. They hint that REM sleep is suddenly intruding upon the waking state, because hallucinations occur when the patient is going to sleep or awakening.

- Sleep paralysis can be frightening: The patient has the sensation of being awake but unable to move, speak, or even breathe adequately. Sleep paralysis is associated with anxiety and fear of dying; it usually lasts less than 10 minutes and may be accompanied by visual or auditory hallucinations.

REM is a relatively shallow stage of sleep. The acronym stands for *rapid eye movement*—behind closed lids, our dreaming eyes track back and forth—which is when most of the dreams that we can recall also occur. During normal REM sleep, our skeletal muscles become paralyzed, which we ordinarily don't notice because we are safely asleep. REM sleep occurs throughout the night, usually beginning about 90 minutes after we first drop off, and it constitutes 20–25% of total sleep time. During REM sleep, heart rate and breathing are irregular; dreams are intense and tend to be remembered; erections of the penis or clitoris occur.

A typical history that includes at least three of the four classic symptoms (as described above) is good presumptive evidence for narcolepsy. But because it's a chronic disorder that can be difficult to manage and implies lifelong treatment, the diagnosis should be confirmed by appropriate lab studies. In that regard, the neuropeptide hypocretin (sometimes it's called orexin) has recently been implicated. Produced in the lateral hypothalamus, it promotes wakefulness. Patients with narcolepsy often have much less of it than normal, probably because some of the neurons that produce it have been destroyed by an autoimmune process. These findings are robust enough that they have crept into the criteria for this disorder.

Strongly hereditary, narcolepsy affects males and females about equally. Though uncommon, it is far from rare, affecting about 1 person in 2,000. It typically starts when the patient is a child or adolescent, but nearly always by the age of 30. Once begun, it usually develops slowly and steadily. It can lead to depression, impotence, trouble at work, and even accidents in the street or on the job. Complications include weight gain and the misuse of substances in an attempt to maintain daytime alertness. Mood disorders and generalized anxiety disorder are sometimes comorbid.

The italicized word pairs below are nearly homophones, but note carefully the differences. *Cataplexy* is from Greek, and it means "to strike down"; it is a brief—usually 2 minutes or less—symptom of narcolepsy. *Catalepsy* ("to hold down") is the prolonged form of immobility that occurs in catatonia.

Hypnagogic and *hypnopompic* are two terms widely used to describe events that take place when one is going to sleep or waking up, respectively (Greek: *hypn* = "sleep," *agogue* = "leader," *pomp* = "sending away"). And note the spellings: hypn*a* and hypn*o*—yet another gift from the Greeks.

Essential Features of **Narcolepsy**

The patient cannot resist attacks of daytime sleep, which are associated with cataplexy (see the preceding sidebar), low cerebrospinal fluid hypocretin, and decreased REM sleep latency on nighttime polysomnography. Cataplexy is usually associated with strong emotion, such as laughter.

The Fine Print

The D's: • Duration (several times a month for 3+ months) • Differential diagnosis (substance use and physical disorders, mood disorders, sleep apnea)

Coding Notes

Specify:

> G47.419 [347.00] Narcolepsy without cataplexy but with hypocretin deficiency
> G47.411 [347.01] Narcolepsy with cataplexy but without hypocretin deficiency (rare)
> G47.419 [347.00] Autosomal dominant cerebellar ataxia, deafness, and narcolepsy; or autosomal dominant narcolepsy, obesity, and type 2 diabetes
> G47.429 [347.10] Narcolepsy secondary to another medical condition
> G47.8 [780.59] Other specified sleep–wake disorder: Narcolepsy with cataplexy with hypocretin deficiency; or other specified sleep–wake disorder: Narcolepsy with cataplexy with unknown hypocretin status

(The last two narcolepsy conditions are probably among the most common we encounter, yet they are not specifically addressed in DSM-5. These "other specified" codes are what we'll have to use—at least for now.) For each type, code also the underlying medical condition.

Specify severity:

Mild. Cataplexy under once a week; only 1–2 naps per day.
Moderate. Cataplexy 1–7 times per week; multiple naps per day, troubled night-time sleep.
Severe. Cataplexy that is resistant to medications; multiple attacks per day, troubled nighttime sleep.

Emma Flowers

"It's been happening like this for several years. Only now it's worse," said Eric Flowers, Emma's husband. He had brought her to the clinic because she no longer felt she could drive safely.

Emma herself was slumped in the interview chair next to him. Her chin rested on her chest, and her left arm hung down at her side. She had been soundly asleep for several minutes. "If she hadn't been sitting down, she'd have fallen down," said Eric. "I've had to catch her half a dozen times."

As a teenager, Emma had had vivid, sometimes frightening dreams that occurred as she was going to sleep, even if it was only a brief afternoon nap. By the time she married Eric, she was having occasional "sleep attacks," when she would find the urge to lie down and take a brief nap irresistible. Over the next several years, these naps became more frequent. Now, at age 28, Emma was napping for 10 minutes or so every 3–4 hours during the day. Her nighttime sleep seemed entirely normal to her, but Eric reflected that she sometimes jerked or moved around a good deal in her sleep.

It was the falling attacks that had prompted this evaluation. At first Emma noticed only a sort of weakness in her neck muscles when she felt sleepy. Over the course of a year the weakness had increased, until now it affected every voluntary muscle in her body. It could happen at any time, but usually it was associated with the onset of sudden sleepiness. At these times she seemed to lose all of her strength, sometimes so suddenly that she didn't even have time to sit down. Then she would collapse, right where she had been standing, though she would often retain full consciousness. Today it had happened while she was sitting down. Once it had happened while she was trying to park her car. She had seen a neurologist the month before, but an EEG had revealed no evidence of a seizure disorder, and an MRI was normal.

Emma stirred, yawned, and opened her eyes. "I did it again, didn't I?"

"Feeling better?" asked her husband.

"I always do, don't I?"

Evaluation of Emma Flowers

This vignette illustrates most of the typical symptoms of narcolepsy: repeated attacks of irresistible sleep (criterion A) during the day; cataplexy (which does not invariably cause the patient to fall, and during which the patient may remain awake) (B1a). Some patients have vivid dreams that occur during the onset of sleep, and sleep paralysis, which also occurs unnoticed during normal REM sleep.

Sleep apnea also causes daytime sleepiness, but it usually occurs in male patients who are middle-aged or older. Differential diagnosis should also include all the other possible causes of excessive somnolence: **substance-induced sleep disorders; major depressive episode with atypical features**; various **cognitive disorders** (especially delirium); and a panoply of **medical illnesses**, such as hypothyroidism, epilepsy, hypoglycemia, myasthenia gravis, multiple sclerosis, and rarer **neurological conditions** such as Kleine–Levin and Prader–Willi syndromes. Emma's clinician should, of course, consider each of these. Don't disregard plain vanilla **insufficient sleep** and **circadian rhythm sleep–wake disorder, delayed sleep phase type**—both staples of adolescence.

Although Emma's clinical symptoms fulfill the DSM-5 requirements for narcolepsy, for us to determine the coding type, she would have to submit to a lumbar puncture for a measurement of cerebrospinal fluid hypocretin. I'm not sure that she (or many other patients) would willingly submit to the procedure for such limited benefit. Narcolepsy with cataplexy is almost always associated with reduced hypocretin, so, with a GAF score of 60, her diagnosis would almost certainly turn out to be this:

G47.8 [780.59]   Narcolepsy with cataplexy with unknown hypocretin status

---

DSM-5 notes that laboratory validators have become increasingly used in evaluating and diagnosing the sleep disorders, to the extent that they are now required for some conditions. One of these, the *multiple sleep latency test*, is an evaluation done by polysomnography in a sleep laboratory. First described by Dement and Carskadon in 1977, it is the standard by which we are now advised to judge hypersomnolence. Here's how it works:

During the patient's normal waking time, in a quiet, darkened room, an EEG is recorded during naps. After 20 minutes, the patient is awakened, then asked to nap again 2 hours later. This is repeated every 2 hours for a total of four or five sessions. Each episode of sleep is interrupted as soon as REM is detected, so as to preserve REM pressure for subsequent episodes. The times until the patient falls asleep (sleep latency) are averaged, yielding the score used for diagnosis. A score of 5 minutes is generally considered significant for the diagnosis of narcolepsy, though times tend to increase somewhat with age.

The multiple sleep latency test is not specific for narcolepsy: Positive scores are found in some people with sleep apnea or sleep deprivation, and even in a few (2–4%) people who have no symptoms at all.

Breathing-Related Sleep Disorders

G47.33 [327.23] Obstructive Sleep Apnea Hypopnea

Central Sleep Apnea

Apnea is easy: It means simply the absence of breathing. *Hypopnea*—shallow or infrequent breathing—has been variously defined. By convention, it now refers to a period of at least 10 seconds during which air flow is reduced by 30% or more and oxygen saturation of the blood is reduced by at least 4%.

As you have probably guessed, there is also a mixed form. It begins with a central apnea and ends in an obstructive apnea.

Here are two sleep–wake disorders that can kill. For periods lasting 10 seconds to a minute or longer during sleep (never while a patient is awake), airflow through the upper respiratory passages of these patients stops completely. Gas exchange falls off, affording sufferers a little taste of suffocation every time they go to bed.

In the more common obstructive type, the chest heaves as the sleeper tries to inhale, but tissues in the mouth and pharynx prevent the normal flow of air. The struggle can rage for up to 2 minutes, culminating in an extraordinarily loud snore. All of this may be inapparent to the patient, but a bed partner is usually well aware. Most patients experience far more than 30 of these episodes per night.

In the less common central type (which comprises a number of possible etiologies), the patient simply stops making any effort to breathe—the diaphragm just takes a rest, so to speak. Snoring can be present, but it is usually not prominent. Affected men may complain especially of hypersomnolence, women of insomnia. Note that patients don't need to have symptoms to qualify for this diagnosis; polysomnographic findings alone will be enough. However, patients typically note that they awaken at night, short of breath, and consequently feel sleepy the next day. This condition is found with the chronic use of opioids or with severe neurological or medical illnesses—disorders you are unlikely to encounter outside a critical care ward. (Cheyne–Stokes breathing is found in people who have had recent stroke and heart failure.)

Regardless of type, the blood of a patient with sleep apnea becomes depleted of oxygen until breathing starts again. Often patients are not aware of these events at all, though some may awaken partly or completely. Besides snoring and daytime drowsiness, there are often problems with hypertension and cardiac arrhythmias; patients may also complain of morning headaches and impotence. During the night, some people become markedly restless, kicking at bedclothes (or bed partners), standing up, or even walking. Other sequelae include irritability and cognitive impairment, as shown by distractibility, problems with perception or memory, or bewilderment. Patients may also experience heavy sweating, hallucinations when going to sleep, sleep talking, or sleep terrors. Nocturia (getting up at night to urinate) is often associated with sleep apnea, though no one knows why.

Obstructive sleep apnea hypopnea affects perhaps 5% of the general population, increasing with age to about 20% at 65. Besides old age, risk factors include obesity (shirt collar size over 16½ for adult men), African American ethnicity, and (the mutually exclusive) male gender and pregnancy. It is highly familial, with a genetic basis. Enlarged tonsil tissue can put even young children at risk.

Because sleep apnea is potentially lethal, always consider it in the differential diagnosis of either hypersomnolence or insomnia. Rapid detection and management can be life-saving. Although an observant bed partner can provide evidence of sleep apnea that is almost definitive, confirmatory polysomnography is now required for diagnosis.

The symptoms are similar for the two types, and discrimination depends on specific polysomnography findings, so I've provided only one vignette.

The criteria make central sleep apnea one of the few DSM diagnoses that you can't substantiate on purely clinical grounds. In fact, no clinical features at all are described. Though mental retardation, now intellectual disability, previously involved an IQ test, even that requirement (for severity levels) has been dumped by DSM-5. Still, with the sleep disorder requirements, I worry that we may be witnessing the beginnings of change to a world where mental health diagnosis is no longer a clinical discipline, but one that makes its home in the laboratory.

Essential Features of **Obstructive Sleep Apnea Hypopnea**

A patient complains of daytime sleepiness that results from nighttime breathing problems: (often long) pauses in breathing, followed by loud snores or snorts. Polysomnography reveals obstructive apneas and hypopneas.

The Fine Print

Diagnosis requires at least 5 apneas or hypopneas per hour, unless the history reveals no nocturnal breathing symptoms or daytime sleepiness; then, there must be 15 apnea/hypopnea episodes per hour.

The D's: There are none.

Coding Notes

Code severity, based on number of apneas/hypopneas per hour:

Mild. Fewer than 15.
Moderate. 15–30.
Severe. 30+.

Essential Features of **Central Sleep Apnea**

For each hour of sleep, the patient's polysomnography shows 5+ central sleep apneas.

The Fine Print

The D's: • Differential diagnosis (other sleep–wake disorders)

Coding Notes

Specify:

G47.31 [327.21] Idiopathic central sleep apnea
R06.3 [786.04] Cheyne–Stokes breathing (a pattern of rising and falling depth of breathing, with frequent arousals; see text)
G47.37 [780.57] Central sleep apnea comorbid with opioid use

Code severity based on number of apneas/hypopneas per hour and degree of oxygen saturation and sleep fragmentation. DSM-5 doesn't provide any further guidance.

Roy Dardis

"I guess it's been going on 30 years and more," said Lily Dardis. She meant her husband's snoring. "I used to sleep soundly myself, so it didn't bother me. Lately, I've had arthritis that's kept me awake. Roy rattles the windows."

Lying awake nights waiting for the painkiller to take effect, Lily had opportunities for minutely studying her husband's sleeping habits. As someone who slept on his back, Roy had always been a noisy breather at night. But every 5 minutes or so, his respirations dropped off to nothing. After 20 or 30 seconds, during which his chest would pitch and heave, he'd finally break through with an enormous snort. This would be rapidly followed by several additional louder-than-usual snores. "It's a wonder the neighbors don't complain," Lily said.

Roy Dardis was a tall man of enormous bulk—a testament to Lily's country cooking. He guessed he'd always snored some; his brother, with whom he had shared a room as a child, used to tease him about it. Of course, as he jokingly pointed out, the racket never bothered him because he slept right through it. Roy's complaint was that he just didn't feel rested. He tended to nod off, whether he was at work or watching TV, which left him grumpy.

In the mornings, Roy often awakened with a headache that seemed localized to the front of his head. Two cups of strong coffee usually took care of the headache.

Evaluation of Roy Dardis

Lily Dardis presented strong evidence that Roy had sleep apnea: She observed that Roy had many periods when he would stop breathing, then resume with an extra-loud snore. From her description of his struggles to breathe during the apneic periods, this would appear to be an obstructive type of sleep apnea. Roy's bulk, morning headaches, and complaints about dropping off to sleep during the day are also typical of sleep apnea. A clinician should ask any patient like Roy about hallucinations when going to sleep, changes in personality (irritability, aggression, anxiety, depression), loss of sex interest, impotence, night terrors, and sleepwalking; each of these is encountered with varying frequency in sleep apnea. Patients also often have heart disease, high blood pressure, stroke, and alcohol use, though some of these are undoubtedly complications rather than causes.

Other causes of hypersomnolence should be considered, though they would not seem likely in Roy's case. Daytime sleepiness and hypnagogic hallucinations occur in **narcolepsy**, but Roy had no cataplexy and his daytime naps were not refreshing. Of course, many otherwise normal people snore, and this should be considered in the differential diagnosis of any patient whose chief complaint is snoring.

Despite Roy's typical history, sleep lab studies must be pursued; in addition to the diagnostic requirement for polysomnography, his blood oxygen saturation during an attack of apnea should be evaluated. Other mental disorders (especially **mood** and **anxiety disorders**) and **substance-related disorders** should be evaluated. Some of these—notably **major depressive disorder**, **panic disorder**, and **major neurocognitive disorder**—may be found as associated diagnoses.

Roy had a GAF score of 60. We're supposed to score severity based on polysomnography. But on clinical grounds I would judge that Roy was at least moderately impaired by his disorder, and that's the level I'd put down—at least until he received some testing:

G47.33 [327.23]   Obstructive sleep apnea hypopnea, moderate
E66.9 [278.00]   Obesity

Sleep-Related Hypoventilation

Health and comfort demand steady regulation of our blood gases: oxygen (O_2) high, which means 95% or higher; carbon dioxide (CO_2) just right—not too high, not too low—in the range of 23–29 milliequivalents per liter. Our bodies accomplish this by means of a simple feedback loop: Low O_2 or high CO_2 signals the brain's respiratory center that our lungs need to work harder. In people with sleep-related hypoventilation, however, the chemoreceptors and the medullary (brainstem) neuronal network fail to send the right sort of signal, so breathing remains shallow. When awake, these folks can compensate by intentionally breathing faster or deeper, but during sleep, that strategy fails and breathing becomes shallower still. Symptoms are usually worse during sleep, and periods of apnea, when breathing stops completely, usually occur.

This condition is found especially in people who are severely overweight or who have disorders such as muscular dystrophy, poliomyelitis, amyotrophic lateral sclerosis, and tumors or other lesions of the spinal cord or central nervous system. Most adult patients (usually men ages 20–50) don't complain of breathing problems, but they do report the insidious development of daytime drowsiness, fatigue, morning headache, frequent nocturnal awakenings, and unrefreshing sleep. They may also have ankle edema and the blue skin tone that indicates oxygen deficit. Even small doses of sedatives or narcotics can make already inadequate breathing much worse. Tragically, it can affect small children, too (see the next sidebar).

Despite the many clues such as daytime sleepiness, fatigue, and morning headache, the DSM-5 criteria set rests entirely on results of polysomnography. The syndrome is uncommon, so I've provided no vignette.

Essential Features of **Sleep-Related Hypoventilation**

A patient's polysomnography shows periods of reduced breathing and high CO_2 levels.

The Fine Print

The D's: • Differential diagnosis (other sleep–wake disorders)

Coding Notes

Specify:

> **G47.34 [327.24] Idiopathic hypoventilation**
> **G47.35 [327.25] Congenital central aveolar hypoventilation**
> **G47.36 [327.26] Comorbid sleep-related hypoventilation** (due to a medical disorder such as lung disease, obesity, or muscular dystrophy)

Code severity based on CO_2 and O_2 saturation.

Even in research reports, sleep-related hypoventilation is sometimes called Ondine's curse. The name refers to the legend of Ondine (sometimes Undine), a water nymph who falls in love with a knight. Ondine knows that she will lose her immortality if she should marry a human and bear him a child. In thrall to love, she takes the plunge anyway, and sure enough, she begins to age. As her beauty slips away, so goes her husband's affection. When she finds him snoring in the arms of another woman, she reminds him that he had sworn "faithfulness with every waking breath." She then utters the curse that he will keep breathing only so long as he remains awake. When he inevitably falls asleep, he dies.

We aren't told how the curse of a now mortal Ondine could retain its force, and it remains unexplained why the term is usually attached specifically to the congenital form of hypoventilation. But in roughly 1 of 50,000 live births—traceable to a sporadic mutation in PHOX2B, an autosomal dominant gene on chromosome 4—the child simply doesn't breathe when sleeping. These children usually die young, though recently, with tracheostomy and nighttime mechanically assisted breathing, some have survived to relatively normal adulthood.

Circadian Rhythm Sleep–Wake Disorders

The word *circadian* comes from the Latin meaning "about 1 day." It refers to the body's cycles of sleep, temperature, and hormone production, which are generated in the suprachiasmatic nucleus of the brain's anterior hypothalamus. When there are no external time cues (natural daylight or artificial reminders like clocks), the free-running human cycle is actually about 24 hours, 9 minutes—a discrepancy too small to cause most of us any serious difficulty. But sometimes a misalignment between our natural body rhythms and the demands of our work or social lives results in unwanted sleeplessness or drowsiness, or both.

The normal circadian sleep–wake cycle changes throughout life. It lengthens during adolescence; that's one reason why teenagers are prone to late nights and sleeping in. It shortens again in old age, causing older people to fall asleep in the evening while reading or watching television, and making both shift work and jet lag harder on them.

Whatever happened to jet lag? In DSM-IV, it was one of the possible circadian rhythm subtypes. But because it is so common, brief, and (really, when you think about it) pretty darned normal to our jet-setting sensibilities, it has been removed from the pantheon of DSM disorders. Still, it might be useful to mention its symptoms.

You've probably had it yourself. After air travel across several time zones, you experienced attacks of intense sleepiness and fatigue. Perhaps, like some people, you felt nauseated or had other flu-like symptoms. But by the second day you began adjusting to the new time zone, and within a few days you felt just fine.

Most people find that time adjustment is faster and easier after flying westward than the reverse. Perhaps this is because the body's natural cycle is a little longer than 24 hours; perhaps it is because we can keep ourselves awake on the long trip home from

Europe, then crash for a truly splendid night's sleep. Studies have shown that adjustment to westward flights occurs at the rate of about 90 minutes per day, whereas adjustment to eastward flights is only about 1 hour per day. This is true regardless of which direction you fly when leaving home. Well, except north or south.

So, if (when) jet lag visits you, cope with it as you would with any other normal feature of contemporary life. You are in the remarkable situation of feeling ill without being sick.

Circadian Rhythm Sleep–Wake Disorder, Delayed Sleep Phase Type

Because they feel alert and active in the late evening, people with delayed sleep phase—variously called "owls" or "night people"—go to sleep late (sometimes progressively later each night) and awaken in late morning or afternoon. Left to their own devices, they feel just fine. But if they must arise early to attend class or get to work (or eat lunch), they feel drowsy and may even appear "sleep-drunk." Irregular sleep habits and the use of caffeine or other stimulants only worsen their plight.

Such people may account for up to 10% of sleep clinic patients who complain of chronic insomnia. The delayed sleep phase type is by far the most common type; it is especially common among teens and young adults. Delayed sleep phase is even estimated (telephone survey) to occur in about 3% of the older (ages 40–64) general population. A familial component can be identified in up to 40%.

Note that delayed sleep phase must be distinguished from the lifestyle issues of those who simply prefer going to bed late and sleeping in. Those people may feel quite comfortable with their eccentric schedules, which they don't make much effort to alter. People with the actual disorder complain of hypersomnolence and would like to change.

Circadian Rhythm Sleep–Wake Disorder, Advanced Sleep Phase Type

Patients with advanced sleep phase are the opposite of those just described; we might call this the "early to bed, early to rise" disorder. Their desired time to sleep is early rather than late, so they feel great in the morning but are sleepy in the late afternoon or early evening. Sometimes they're called "larks." Advanced sleep phase appears to be much less frequent even than delayed sleep phase, though this could be in part because it causes less discomfort and fewer social problems. It has been reported to occur more often with advancing age and to run in families.

Circadian Rhythm Sleep–Wake Disorder, Non-24-Hour Sleep-Wake Type

The non-24-hour type is also called the *free-running* type, and it occurs mainly in completely blind people, who of course have no light cues to entrain their biological clocks. (Up to 50% of blind people may be affected, beginning at the age total blindness begins; most of those with minimal light perception—even the equivalent of a single candle—remain normally entrained.) Sighted people who are affected tend to be mainly young (teens and 20s) and male; they often have other mental disorders. The 18-hour schedules that accompany life in a submarine can also lead to a free-running biological rhythm. Most sighted people who undergo a research protocol in which there are no visual time cues will ultimately develop non-24-hour sleep–wake type.

Circadian Rhythm Sleep–Wake Disorder, Irregular Sleep–Wake Type

The pattern here is . . . no pattern. The patients' total sleep duration may be normal, but they feel sleepy or insomniac at varying, and unpredictable, times of day. They may take naps, so it's important to rule out poor sleep hygiene. Irregular type may be encountered in various neurological conditions, including dementia, intellectual disability, and traumatic brain injury. The prevalence is unknown, but it's probably rare. As far as we know, this condition affects the sexes about equally. Age is a risk factor, mainly due to the late-life presence of medical disorders such as Alzheimer's disease.

Circadian Rhythm Sleep–Wake Disorder, Shift Work Type

When workers must change from one shift to another, especially when they must be active during their former sleep time, sleepiness sets in and performance declines. Sleep during the new sleep time is often disrupted and too brief. The symptoms, which can affect nearly a third of people doing shift work, are worst after a switch to night work, though people vary considerably in the time required for this adjustment. Additional factors include age, commuting distance, and whether the individual is naturally a "lark" or an "owl." Symptoms may last 3 weeks or longer, especially if workers try to resume their normal sleeping schedules on weekends or holidays.

Essential Features of **Circadian Rhythm Sleep–Wake Disorders**

A recurring mismatch between the patient's sleep–wake pattern and environmental demands causes insomnia or hypersomnolence.

The Fine Print

The D's: • Distress or disability (work/educational, social, or personal impairment) • Differential diagnosis (substance use disorders, other sleep disorders)

Coding Notes

Specify:

G47.21 [307.45] Delayed sleep phase type. The patient has trouble falling asleep and awakening on time.

G47.22 [307.45] Advanced sleep phase type. The patient has trouble remaining awake until the desired bedtime and awakens before time to arise.

G47.23 [307.45] Irregular sleep–wake type. The patient's sleep and wake periods vary irregularly throughout the 24-hour period.

G47.24 [307.45] Non-24-hour sleep–wake type. Times of sleep onset and wakefulness are not entrained to the 24-hour period, and each day gradually drifts (usually later).

G47.26 [307.45] Shift work type. Because of night shift work or frequently changing job shifts, during the main sleep period, the patient experiences hypersomnia during the major period of wakefulness or insomnia (or both).

G47.20 [307.45] Unspecified type.

Specify if:

Familial. Applies to both delayed and advanced sleep phase types.
Overlapping with non-24-hour sleep–wake type. Applies to delayed type.

Specify if:

Episodic. Symptoms last 1–3 months.
Persistent. Symptoms last 3+ months.
Recurrent. There are two or more episodes within 1 year.

Marcelle Klinger

Marcelle was a 60-year-old registered nurse, one of seven employed by her small community hospital in the northern California hills. The entire facility had only 32 beds, and although there were nursing aides and licensed practical nurses to assist, state law required a registered nurse always to be present in the facility. When the nurse who had worked the graveyard shift (11 P.M. to 7:30 A.M.) finally retired, the hospital administrator asked for a volunteer to fill that position.

"Nobody did," said Marcelle, "so some genius decided it was only fair that everyone take turns."

The result was 4-week shifts. In the course of a year, each nurse would work six of these shifts on days, four on evenings, and two on graveyard. Everyone grumbled, but Marcelle hated it the most. The switch from days to evenings wasn't too bad; she lived close by, so she could be home in bed by midnight. But the graveyard shift was a disaster.

"I'm the only registered nurse there, and I'm supposed to be awake and alert the whole time. Patients depend on me. But my eyes keep squeezing themselves shut, and my brain seems to hum, as if it's going to sleep. Part of the time I feel sick to my stomach. One time I did fall asleep at work, just for 10 minutes or so. When the phone rang, I woke up feeling hung over."

Marcelle's physical and mental health was excellent. She'd always been a light sleeper, so she found daytime sleeping nearly impossible. Heavy drapes could keep out most of the light, but traffic noise and the sounds from passersby on the sidewalk outside her bedroom frequently awakened her.

Moreover, the coffee Marcelle drank to keep awake at work prevented her from going to sleep as soon as she went to bed. It also got her up to the bathroom at least once or twice. By the time her husband came home in the afternoon from teaching school, she had seldom slept more than 3 or 4 hours. On weekends, she tried to resume a normal schedule so that she could be with her family, but that only made things worse. "I flew to Paris once and felt jet-lagged for a week. Now I'm sick that way for a whole month."

Evaluation of Marcelle Klinger

Several features of Marcelle's condition could have contributed to her discomfort:

1. Like many people who must work shifts (criterion A), she tried to *re*-readjust her sleep–wake schedule on the weekends.

2. Cues from outside her window served to arouse her when she tried to sleep.

3. She was 60; because of the physiology of their sleep, older people often have trouble making these adjustments.

4. She drank coffee to stay awake; the dual effects of the caffeine-induced stimulation and her need to get up to urinate interfered further with what sleep she could get. As a consequence, she suffered both from insomnia *and* hypersomnolence (B), with obvious attendant distress (C).

From her history, we learn that Marcelle had no **physical illness**, **substance use**, or **other mental disorder.** (Although patients with a psychosis such as **schizophrenia** are sometimes kept up progressively later at night by their hallucinations, **mood** and **anxiety disorders** generally produce only insomnia or hypersomnolence.) The vignette provides no evidence for any other sleep–wake disorder: When Marcelle napped, it was not refreshing (this would argue against **narcolepsy**). She had always been a light sleeper anyway, but light sleep per se is not considered a sleep disorder (except by some light sleepers).

The subtype is obvious; Marcelle's GAF score would be 65.

G47.26 [307.45]   Circadian rhythm sleep–wake disorder, shift work type, recurrent

Z56.9 [V62.29]   Varying work schedule

Fenton Schmidt

Remarkably, Fenton Schmidt had requested the earliest morning appointment he could get. As he explained to the sleep specialist, "It's partly because I knew I'd be at my worst. I thought you might get a better picture of what I'm up against." He rubbed his eyes, which were rimmed with dark circles. "I know, I look like a *Doonesbury* cartoon character."

Fenton's trouble had begun as long ago as high school. "I'd never have made those 8 o'clock classes if my mom hadn't been there for me." He rubbed his eyes again and yawned. "Well, at me. Couple of times, she dumped a pan of cold water on me. It did get me out of bed."

In college, Fenton had never scheduled a class before noon, when he could manage. That worked out pretty well because he was living with his father, who had kept the same schedule for 35 years as night shift manager at a convenience store. That was how he avoided the hung-over feeling of waking too early. "I saw him once when he got off an early plane. He was asleep on his feet. *His* dad was first-generation American, and the family still speaks a little German. He called it *Schlaftrunkenheit*—sleep drunkenness."

"'Early to bed, early to rise' must have been written by a sadist," Fenton commented. Several times over the years, he'd tried changing his own sleep schedule by going to bed earlier. After a few days, he'd always given it up. "Lifelong, if I hit the sack before 2 A.M., I just lie there, pissed off."

For a couple of years, Fenton had worked the swing shift for an electronics parts fabricator. "That strategy worked perfectly for me. When I got off at 11:30 at night, I could spend whatever time I needed at home, decompressing. I could go to bed when I wanted, and I only had to get up in time to start my shift at 4. That's P.M."

"So what is the problem now?" the clinician wanted to know.

Now Fenton had begun working at the pancake house run by the father of his fiancée, Jaylene. "Do you know what time people eat pancakes?" he asked. He and Jaylene both get up early to open up shop. "It works fine for her; she's a lark. But at 5 A.M., this owl doesn't give a hoot."

Evaluation of Fenton Schmidt

Fenton's problem is instantly apparent: His sleeping requirements just didn't jibe with those of his job and his social and personal life (criterion A). With no **physical illness** (such as traumatic brain injury) or **substance use problems** that would provide an alternative explanation, the resulting hypersomnolence (B) and distress (C) would complete the criteria for a circadian rhythm sleep–wake disorder. Of course, his clinician should carefully rule out **poor sleep hygiene.** The fact that he was genuinely troubled suggests that it was not simply a **lifestyle issue.**

Fenton's history provides ample evidence that, of the possible subtypes, his would be delayed sleep phase type. There was really no need for further verification by polysomnography. His GAF score would be 62.

G47.21 [307.45]   Circadian rhythm sleep–wake disorder, delayed sleep
                    phase type, familial
Z60.0 [V62.89]   Phase of life problem (impending wedding)
Z56.9 [V62.29]   Job change

Parasomnias

And here come those disorders where something abnormal happens during sleep—though the architecture (as the sleep people say) of sleep itself may be normal.

Non-Rapid Eye Movement Sleep Arousal Disorders

Although awakening to the jangle of a telephone in the dead of night can be a struggle, mostly it's a pretty straight shot from sleeping to fully awake. OK, we don't like it, feel unwell, curse the caller, and turn over to shut out the sound of the ring—but we're awake, all right, and we know it. For reasons largely unclear, however, it doesn't always work that way. For some people, a way station between being asleep and being awake causes reactions that range from bemusement to frank horror.

It all stems from the three possible states of the relationship of body and mind. During wakefulness, they both are working; in non-REM (deep) sleep, both are more or less idling. During REM (dreaming) sleep, though, the mind is at work but the body rests; in fact, our voluntary muscles are paralyzed, so that we cannot move. (The fourth conceivable combination, active body with sleeping mind, is the stuff of zombie films.) During non-REM sleep arousal disorders, patients experience simultaneous sleeping and waking EEG patterns; symptoms ensue.

Partial arousals that occur suddenly from non-REM sleep usually occur in the first hour or two of sleep, when slow-wave sleep is most prevalent. Though the behaviors sometimes overlap, there are three main types of abnormal arousal. I've listed them in order of increasing severity:

Confusional arousal < Sleepwalking < Sleep terror

In each of these, events tend to be poorly recalled. Each is more common in children, in whom they are considered generally benign, perhaps caused by a relatively immature nervous system. One of them, confusional arousal, didn't quite make it into the official DSM-5 pantheon (see sidebar, p. 335).

Some episodes occur spontaneously, but others follow apparent precipitants, which can include stress, irregular sleep, drugs, and sleep deprivation. Although family history is often positive, a genetic causation hasn't been nailed down.

Essential Features of **Non-Rapid Eye Movement Sleep Arousal Disorders**

The patient repeatedly awakens incompletely from sleep with sleepwalking or sleep terror (see Coding Notes). The attempts of others to communicate or console don't help much. The patient has little if any dream imagery at the time and tends not to remember the episode the next morning.

The Fine Print

The D's: • Distress or disability (work/educational, social, or personal impairment) • Differential diagnosis (substance use and physical disorders, anxiety and dissociative disorders, other sleep disorders)

Coding Notes

Specify:

> **F51.3 [307.46] Sleepwalking type.** Without awakening, the patient rises from bed and walks. The patient stares blankly, can be awakened only with difficulty, and responds poorly to others' attempts at communication.

> Specify if:
> **With sleep-related eating**
> **With sleep-related sexual behavior (sexsomnia)**

> **F51.4 [307.46] Sleep terror type.** Beginning with a scream of panic, the patient abruptly arouses from sleep and shows intense fear and signs of autonomic arousal, such as dilated pupils, rapid breathing, rapid heartbeat, and sweating.

Sleep paralysis isn't a disorder; it's a normal feature of sleep. But it can be frightening when it occurs right at the start (or conclusion) of sleep, when you're partly conscious. Lasting from mere seconds to several minutes, episodes may be accompanied by apparitions of being approached by some sort of "creature" that soon vanishes. Sleep paralysis when partly awake happens in around 8% of young adults. Its frequency is increased by all the usual suspects: sleep deprivation, stress, and keeping irregular hours (such as with shift work). Treatment, other than reassurance, is usually unnecessary.

Non-Rapid Eye Movement Sleep Arousal Disorder, Sleepwalking Type

Sleepwalking behavior tends to follow a fairly set pattern; it usually occurs during the first third of the night, when non-REM sleep is more prevalent. Sleepwalkers first sit up and make some sort of recurring movement (such as plucking at the bedclothes). More purposeful behavior may follow, perhaps dressing, eating, or using the toilet. The person's facial expression is usually blank and staring. If these individuals talk at all, it is usually garbled; speaking sentences is rare. Their movements tend to be poorly coordinated, sometimes resulting in considerable danger. Amnesia for the episode is usual, though this is variable.

Individual episodes last anywhere from a few seconds to 30 minutes, during which a person will often be hard to awaken, though spontaneous awakening may occur—usually to a brief period of disorientation. Some individuals simply return to bed without awakening. Occasionally a person who goes to sleep in one location will express surprise upon awakening elsewhere.

DSM-5 lists two subtypes of sleepwalking: with sleep-related eating, and with sleep-related sexual behavior (sexsomnia—yes, even DSM-5 actually calls it that). The former occurs mainly in women, and it's not the same as night eating syndrome, wherein the person is awake and remembers the next day. The latter, which includes masturbation and sometimes sexual behavior with other people, is more common in men and can have legal repercussions.

Sleepwalking may occur nightly, though the frequency is usually less. As with nightmares and sleep terrors, don't diagnose sleepwalking type unless the episodes are recurrent and cause impairment or distress. And, as with so many other sleep disorders, sleepwalking episodes are more likely when a person is tired or has been under stress. In adults, the condition appears to have familial and genetic components.

Perhaps 6% of all children sleepwalk; in them, it isn't considered pathological. It usually begins between the ages of 6 and 12 and lasts for several years, with most outgrowing it by age 15. Maybe 20% continue to sleepwalk into their adult lives; sleepwalking affects up to 4% of adult men and women, with a typical age of onset between 10 and 15. Then it tends to be chronic until the fourth decade of life. Although adults with sleepwalking type may have a personality disorder, sleepwalking in children has no prognostic significance.

Ross Josephson

"I brought along a video. I thought it might help to explain my problem." Ross Josephson handed a thumb drive to the clinician. Ross lived in a dormitory with two roommates, who had provided the video.

Ross walked in his sleep. He supposed it had started when he was quite young, though he hadn't fully realized it until one hot July dawn when he was 12 and had awakened in his pajamas, curled up on the porch swing. When he told his mother, she remarked that she and her two brothers had all walked in their sleep when they were young. She guessed that Ross would grow out of it, too.

Only he hadn't. A freshman in college now, Ross pursued his nocturnal strolls once or twice a month. At first his roommates had been amused; the video had been a hit at an impromptu party they had gotten up with some of the girls who lived downstairs. They had lain awake several nights until they caught the complete sequence. Ross had taken the joke well. In fact, he had been fascinated to see how he appeared when sleepwalking.

But last week his roommates had become alarmed when they caught him stepping through an open window onto the third-floor roof of their building. Other than a low rim around the edge, there was nothing to prevent a nasty 30-foot fall into the grape ivy below. Although they had pulled him back inside, it had not been without a struggle; clearly, the sleeping Ross had resisted guidance.

After an interview and physical exam by one of the consultants in the student health service, Ross had been pronounced healthy and referred to the campus mental health clinic.

The clinician and Ross watched the video together. The image was grainy and danced around a good deal, as if the cameraperson was trying to contain laughter. It showed a pajama-clad Ross sitting up in bed. Although his eyes were open, they didn't appear to be focused on anything, and his face registered no emotion. At first he only pulled—aimlessly, it seemed—at the sheet and blanket. Suddenly he swung his feet to the floor and stood up. He slipped off his pajama top and let it fall onto the bed. Then he walked out through the door into the hallway.

For 2 or 3 minutes, the camera followed Ross. He walked up and down the hall several times and finally disappeared into the bathroom, where the camera did not pursue. When he emerged, another young man ("That's Ted, one of my roommates," Ross explained) appeared on screen and tried to engage him in conversation. Ross responded with a few syllables, none of which was a recognizable word. Finally, he allowed Ted to guide him gently back to his bed. Almost as soon as he lay down, he appeared to be asleep. The entire video lasted perhaps 10 minutes.

"When they showed me this the next morning, I was amazed. I hadn't the slightest idea I'd done anything but sleep that night. I never do."

Evaluation of Ross Josephson

Although sleepwalking is not considered pathological in children, adults with the sleepwalking type of non-REM sleep arousal disorder may have a **personality disorder** or other psychopathology. They should be carefully investigated with a full interview (as should just about everyone who consults a mental health care provider). However, occasional sleepwalking is likely to be more annoying than pathological.

Let's quickly review Ross's relation to the criteria for non-REM sleep arousal disorder. His awakenings were incomplete (almost nonexistent, actually) and recurrent (criterion A1), during which he did sleepwalk, gazing with unseeing eyes. In the video, his roommate didn't exactly try to comfort him (college roommates tend more toward *Animal House* than *Terms of Endearment*), but he did try to engage Ross in conversation—to no avail. The vignette doesn't specify whether Ross had dream imagery (it should have; criterion B), but it does note that he never had any memory of the episodes the following day (C). Although Ross was himself not distressed, his roommates were: They didn't want to officiate as Ross plunged from a rooftop (D).

The differential diagnosis also includes **psychomotor epilepsy**, which can begin during sleep and present with sleepwalking. The dissociative condition known as the **fugue subtype of dissociative amnesia** may sometimes be confused with sleepwalking, but fugues last longer and involve complex behaviors, such as speaking complete sentences. Nighttime wandering can be found in **sleep apnea.** Ross had no evidence for **substance use** (F).

Other nighttime disturbances and sleep disorders can be associated with sleepwalking; these include nocturnal **enuresis, nightmare disorder**, and the **sleep terror type of non-REM sleep arousal disorder. Generalized anxiety disorder, posttraumatic stress disorder**, and **mood disorders** can also occur. However, none of these conditions is suggested in the vignette (F). Ross would have a GAF score of 75; his diagnosis would be as follows:

F51.3 [307.46]	Non-rapid eye movement sleep arousal disorder, sleepwalking type

---

In the hundreds of years that sleepwalking has been recognized, it has amassed an extensive, if inaccurate, mythology. Also known as *somnambulism* (which means—surprise!—"sleepwalking"), it has been a reliable device for playwrights (paging Mr. Shakespeare) and innumerable authors of mystery thrillers. One popular myth is that it is dangerous to awaken a sleepwalker. Perhaps this grew out of the observation that it is *difficult* to do so; in any event, I know of no evidence to support this belief.

Non-Rapid Eye Movement Sleep Arousal Disorder, Sleep Terror Type

Sleep terrors (also known as night terrors or pavor nocturnus) usually affect children, with a typical onset during ages 4–12. When they begin in adulthood, it is usually in the 20s or 30s—hardly ever after the age of 40. As is true of nightmares versus nightmare disorder (see p. 340), only events that are recurrent and produce distress or impairment qualify for a diagnosis of the sleep terror type of non-REM sleep arousal disorder.

A sleep terror attack begins with a loud cry or scream during a period of non-REM sleep, not long after the patient goes to bed. The person sits up, appears terrified, and seems to be awake but does not respond to attempts at soothing. There will be signs of sympathetic nervous system arousal, such as rapid heartbeat, sweating, and piloerection (hairs standing up on the skin). With deep breathing and dilated pupils, the person seems ready for fight or flight, aroused but not arousable. An attack usually lasts 5–15 minutes and terminates spontaneously with return to sleep. Most patients have no memory of the incident the following morning, though some adults may have fragmentary recall.

There is usually an interval of days to weeks between sleep terror attacks, though stress and fatigue may increase the frequency. In adults, the disorder is equally common in males and females.

With a peak at age 6, prevalence is around 3% in children—less than that for adults, but frequent enough not to be considered rare. In children, sleep terrors are not considered pathological. They almost invariably grow out of them and suffer no medical or psychological pathology later in life. The adult-onset type may be associated with some other mental condition such as an anxiety or personality disorder.

Bud Stanhope

Bud Stanhope and his wife, Harriette, had just begun marital counseling. They agreed on exactly one thing, which was that many of their problems could be traced to Bud's excessive need for support. They had married when each was on the rebound, soon after Bud's first wife divorced him. "I felt so uncomfortable being alone," said Bud.

His chronically low self-esteem meant that Bud couldn't so much as start a building project around the house without consulting Harriette. Once, when Harriette was out of town at a convention, he even called up his ex-wife for advice. And because he was afraid to disagree with Harriette, they never got anything resolved. "I don't even feel I can tell him how much it bugs me when he wakes me up with those night frights," she said.

"Night frights?" said Bud. "I thought those stopped months ago."

As Harriette described them, Bud's "frights" were always the same. An hour or so after they went to sleep, she'd awaken to his blood-curdling scream. Bud would be sitting bolt upright in bed, a look of stark terror on his face. His eyes wide open, he would be staring off into a corner or toward a wall. She was never sure if he was seeing something, because he never said much that was intelligible—only babble or the occasional random word. He would seem agitated, pluck at his bedclothes, and sometimes start to get out of bed.

"The hairs on his arms will be standing straight up. He's usually breathing fast and perspiring, even if it's cold in the room. Once when I put my hand on his chest, his heart seemed to be beating as fast as a rabbit's."

It would take Harriette 10 or 15 minutes to soothe Bud. He never fully awakened, but would eventually lie down. Then he would almost instantly fall fast asleep again, while she sometimes lay awake for hours. Bud would have one of these attacks every 2 or 3 weeks. Only once did it happen two nights running, and that was during one particularly bad period when he felt sure he was about to lose his job.

Evaluation of Bud Stanhope

Several features of Bud's attacks are distinctive for sleep terrors: the evidence of autonomic arousal (rapid heartbeat, sweating), occurrence soon after falling asleep, Harriette's inability to console him, his lack of full awakening, and his lack of recall the next day. Taken as a whole, this story is virtually diagnostic, but I'll list the important elements anyway. Bud's episodes of arousal were both incomplete and recurrent (criterion A). Harriet reported marked difficulty soothing him (A2). If he ever had dream imagery, he did not report it (B), and he had no recall (he was surprised he was still having the terror episodes; C). Without argument (certainly not from Bud or Harriet), they were distressing at the time (D). We'd have to enquire further to make sure that substance misuse played no role in his history (E). As an exercise, note how each of these features helps to differentiate this disorder from **nightmare disorder.**

Although this did not happen to Bud, **sleepwalking** (sometimes sleep running) occurs in many patients with sleep terrors. In adults, you may have to distinguish sleep terrors from **psychomotor epilepsy,** which can also produce sleepwalking. **Panic attacks** sometimes occur at night, but these patients awaken completely, without the disorientation and disorganized behavior of typical sleep terrors.

Bud also had significant personality problems. As noted in the vignette, he required a great deal of consultation and support (he even leaned on his ex-wife for advice when Harriette was out of town), and he had trouble disagreeing with others. His low self-confidence, discomfort at being alone, and rush into another marriage when the first one ended provide a strong basis for the diagnosis of **dependent personality disorder.** Other patients might qualify for **borderline personality disorder.** Bud's GAF score— 61—would be based more on the personality disorder than on the arousal disorder. Associated conditions in other patients can include **posttraumatic stress disorder** and **generalized anxiety disorder.**

Z63.0 [V61.10]	Partner relationship distress
F51.4 [307.46]	Non-rapid eye movement sleep arousal disorder, sleep terror type
F60.7 [301.6]	Dependent personality disorder

Confusional arousals occur during the transition from non-REM sleep to wakefulness. The person seems awake but is confused and disoriented, and may behave inappropriately (hence the term sometimes used, *sleep drunkenness*).

An episode may be set up by sleep deprivation or by bedtime use of alcohol or hypnotics. Sometimes triggered by a forced awakening, it may begin with physical movements and moaning, then progress to agitation during which the individual (with eyes open or closed) calls out and thrashes about, but cannot awaken. More complex behaviors may occur: sitting up, speaking incoherently, and performing actions that are purposeful though illogical (and, at times, dangerous).

Beginning over a century ago, various authors have published collections of violent crimes committed during states of confused arousal. These include at least a score of murders, mostly committed by persons who had had a personal (or, sometimes, family) history of sleep disorder. The lack of culpability of a sleeper who killed or wounded someone was noted as far back as 14th-century France; the principle was affirmed in subsequent centuries in Spain, the United Kingdom, and the United States.

Attempts at comfort are met with resistance and may even increase the person's agitation. The episode typically lasts 5–15 minutes, occasionally longer, before calm is restored and normal sleep returns. Amnesia for the event is typical; the individual usually doesn't even recall having a dream. When injury occurs, it may be because someone approached or attempted to interfere with a person who was asleep. It is also important— and reassuring—to note that, by a wide margin, most episodes of confusional arousal do not involve aggression or violence.

Although this relative newcomer (it was first noted in 1968) is said to occur mainly in infants and toddlers, it has also been self-reported in 3–4% of people age 15 and over. Males and females are represented about equally; shift and night workers may be especially vulnerable.

G25.81 [333.94] Restless Legs Syndrome

Restless legs syndrome (RLS) is an evil complaint that clinicians sometimes ignore because it seriously threatens no one; however, it inflicts exquisite torment upon its sufferers. Not usually painful, it's a nearly indescribable discomfort deep within the lower legs that's relieved only by movement, yielding an irresistible urge to shift leg positions every few seconds (trust me on this). Patients will tell you that the sensation feels like itching, tingling, creeping, or crawling, but none of these descriptors quite encapsulates a condition that confers seemingly inconsequential misery unimaginable by someone who's not afflicted.

With a tendency to begin before bedtime, this common disorder can delay onset of sleep; sometimes it awakens the patient during the night. It's associated with disturbed sleep and reduced sleep time. Relief can come in many guises—walking, pacing, stretching, rubbing, even riding a stationary bicycle. The trouble is that each of these stratagems increases wakefulness. Besides causing the person to feel tired the next day, RLS can lead to depression and anxiety. It tends to lessen throughout the night, allowing more refreshing sleep toward morning. Overall, it worsens with time, though it may wax and wane over a period of weeks. It's been associated with major depression, generalized anxiety disorder, posttraumatic stress disorder, and panic disorder.

Nobody's really sure why RLS occurs, though it may be related to the neurotransmitter dopamine. (It's often reported by patients with Parkinson's disease, whose basal ganglia are compromised.) One-quarter of pregnant women report it, especially in the third trimester. It's also found in neurological conditions such as neuropathy and multiple sclerosis, and in iron deficiency and renal failure. RLS can be exacerbated by medications, including antihistamines, antinausea preparations, mirtazapine (Remeron), and some other antidepressants. The effects of mild obstructive sleep apnea can sometimes look like periodic limb movements.

If asked, perhaps 2% of people in the general population will complain of RLS serious enough to cause impaired functioning (mostly disturbed sleep); it has even been reported by perhaps 1% of school-age children. It's more frequent in European Americans, and less so in people of Asian descent; the prevalence in women may be greater than in men. It tends to begin relatively early in life (the teens or 20s). Sometimes you'll find a family history positive for RLS; genetic markers have been identified. A simple interview is usually enough to make the diagnosis.

Especially alert readers may be asking themselves: Why is RLS even a sleep disorder? What does it have to do with sleep? First, RLS has a diurnal component to it, similar to the ebb and flow of other issues regarding sleep. Second, it can delay sleep onset; occasionally it even awakens patients during the night. Finally, RLS can result in daytime hypersomnolence—often a cause of distress or impaired functioning. If this logic doesn't appeal to you straight off, I suggest that you sleep on it.

Essential Features of **Restless Legs Syndrome**

Unpleasant leg sensations cause an impulse to move them, which tends to relieve the symptoms. Legs are most restless in the evening or later.

The Fine Print

The D's: • Duration (3+ times a week for 3+ months) • Distress or disability (work/ educational, social, or personal impairment) • Differential diagnosis (substance use and physical disorders)

Enoch Dimond

Now alone on the set, Enoch Dimond wiped at his makeup. He had twice viewed the digital replay of the 10 P.M. news, and had cringed at what he saw: a middle-aged anchorman whose Max Factor could barely conceal the deepening worry lines. His wandering gaze seemed to resist gazing directly at the camera; his hooded eyes betrayed trouble focusing on the script. He could almost visualize his feet tap-dancing nervously beneath the polished table that served as his on-camera desk.

In fact, concentration was a big problem: Enoch could so easily drift off into reverie, away from whatever was going on about him. Just last week, the floor director had said, "What's the matter, E? Lately you don't seem to be quite with the program—so to speak."

Well, true enough, he supposed. He'd been fine until the last 3 or 4 weeks, but lately he hadn't enough interest to sustain a run on a small bank. (His joke was an out-take from a special they'd recently aired on the financial system.) Always a conscientious performer, now he took no pleasure in his craft; indeed, he no longer felt good about much of anything. Even sex bored him.

Nothing had seemed to put Enoch off, just the gradual realization that his life wasn't moving in a positive direction; he'd began to feel uneasy, a sense that "something terrible was afoot."

Was he depressed? That's what his wife kept asking, but he didn't *feel* depressed. It's not that he went around crying all the time, for God's sake. He certainly didn't feel especially good. Food didn't taste right, so his appetite must have seemed a bit off. And he'd never considered doing himself in. From a network documentary he'd introduced a couple of months ago, he knew enough to pay attention to thoughts about dying and suicide. "Well, you sure look depressed to me!" was his wife's latest word on the subject. But not, he suspected, her last.

Enoch decided he just needed to be calm. He *was* calm, on camera. But whenever he started thinking about himself and his family, his insides roiled. He hoped that his public demeanor—artificial smiles and manufactured bonhomie—concealed the misery he felt.

No, what he felt was more like pepless. Fatigued. That was it. So tired he had trouble dragging himself out of bed, even after he'd slept his usual 8 hours. Maybe that could explain the peculiar sort of tension in his muscles, like his biceps were coiled springs that never, ever released. Probably because he was just too damned tired and he couldn't relax, even in his hot tub.

That tension was different from the peculiar sensation he'd had in his legs for a couple of years now. He could hardly sit still long enough to get through his half hour on camera. He had worried—could it indicate some weird form of cancer, buried deep within the calf of his leg? Legs, actually, for both of them gave him fits. Getting up and walking around, even for a moment, relieved the sensation completely, but he couldn't do that when he was broadcasting. At night in bed, he so often had to get up and walk that he felt wiped out the next day. But while working, even the relief of pacing was denied him. "I should have been a weatherman," he'd thought more than once. As it was, the only on-air relief from the jittery legs was to try to rub them together under the desk. It was worse when he was lying down, worst of all in the evening. ("Or do a morning show.")

Strangely (for him, because he wasn't really a worrywart), lately he kept thinking he'd be fired. Not that he had much reason to worry—he lived the risible cliché of being married to the boss's daughter. Of course, that wasn't doing him much good, either. They hadn't made love for a couple of months; he just didn't feel interested, in that or much of anything else. He felt ashamed of his physique, though Kristin said she loved the way he looked. Still, he had reflected more than once that someone born Oliver Schmick wasn't likely to find jobs thick on the ground.

Evaluation of Enoch Dimond

Enoch had two problems: one with his mood, one with his legs. The former was the more tendentious, so I'll save that discussion for later.

Enoch had all the important symptoms traditionally associated with RLS: the peculiar, uncontrollable sensation in both legs (criterion A), which led to the irresistible urge to seek relief in movement (A2), was present only when he was inactive or resting (A1), and was worse in the evening (A3). His sleep suffered and he often felt "wiped out" the following day (C), and its frequency and duration qualified for the diagnosis (B)—provided that no other diagnosis seemed more appropriate (D, E). To that end, his blood chemistries should be checked for iron deficiency anemia and renal failure.

And so we come to the matter of Enoch's mood. Here's the problem: He had several depressive symptoms (low interest, lack of pleasure, fatigue), but not enough for a **major depressive episode.** He also had a feeling of uneasy anticipation combined with tension and worry, though not enough of these to sustain a diagnosis of either **panic disorder** or **generalized anxiety disorder.** At one time, the authors of DSM-5 considered a diagnosis of mixed anxiety–depression (which would require a perhaps too-delicate balancing of criteria so as not to meet full criteria for any other mood or anxiety disorder). But that diagnosis was never adopted. Now, if we made any diagnosis at all, we'd have to say that Enoch had an unidentified form of depression, described in DSM-5 as other specified depressive disorder. If these symptoms later turned into major depression, we might add the specifier *with anxious distress.*

However, I'd be happy to wait a few days to see whether his depressive and anxiety symptoms would clear up spontaneously. Sometimes we're a tad too ready with a diagnosis when a tincture of time can sort things out. Being too quick off the mark can lead to diagnosis where none is justified and treatment where none is indicated.

Actually, the problem of separating out the symptoms of multiple diagnoses occurs pretty often and across every DSM-5 chapter. For example, how do we decide whether the peculiar sensation in Enoch's legs was due to agitated mood disorder or something else entirely? Two principles should guide us away from the former interpretation: (1) Enoch's motor activity was not generalized, but limited to his lower extremities; (2) and, more importantly, it preceded the other mood and anxiety symptoms by at least a year. All in all, I'd give Enoch Dimond only the one firm diagnosis, though we should realize that it is not at all a benign one: RLS can lead to insomnia and other complications. I'd also assign a GAF score of 61. If my record room demanded a coded diagnosis, I'd waffle a bit and use other specified depressive disorder, as you can see below. But I'd try to hold out for "wait and see."

F32.8 [311]	Other specified depressive disorder, depressive episode with insufficient symptoms
G25.81 [333.94]	Restless legs syndrome

F51.5 [307.47] Nightmare Disorder

Despite the name, nightmare disorder never had anything to do with lady horses; that historical mare, which dates at least to the 13th century, was a goblin that sat on your chest and caused awful dreams. Because most contemporary nightmares quickly bring us full awake, we tend to recall them vividly. They are usually about something that threatens either our safety or our self-esteem. When someone repeatedly has long, terrifying dreams of that sort, or suffers from daytime sleepiness, irritability, or loss of concentration, a diagnosis of nightmare disorder may be warranted.

Nightmares develop during REM sleep, most of which occurs toward the end of the night. (Onset early during the sleep period is noteworthy enough to earn a specifier.) They can be increased by withdrawal from REM-suppressing substances; these include antidepressants, barbiturates, and alcohol. Although some degree of rapid heartbeat is common, people with nightmares generally have fewer symptoms of sympathetic nervous system arousal (perspiration, rapid heartbeat, increased blood pressure) than do sufferers from the sleep terror type of non-REM sleep arousal disorder.

Childhood nightmares, especially those that occur in young children, have no pathological significance. About half of all adults report nightmares at some time or other. The number who have enough nightmares to be considered pathological is unknown, though perhaps 5% of adults claim to have frequent nightmares. They may be more common in women than in men. To some extent, the tendency to have nightmares may be inherited.

Although adults with frequent nightmares probably have a tendency to psychopathology, there is no consensus among sleep experts as to what that psychopathology might be. (When it is sorted out, it may turn out that the pathology has more to do with who complains than with the actual nightmare experience.) Vivid nightmares sometimes precede the onset of a psychosis. However, most nightmares may be an expected (and hence normal) reaction to stress; some clinicians believe that they help people to work through traumatic experiences.

At least half the population has had a nightmare at one time or another. So do all of these people (that is, do *we*) have a sleep–wake disorder? As with so many other conditions, making this decision is a matter of quantity (number of nightmare episodes) and of the reaction a patient has to the episodes. These factors must then be filtered through the judgment of the clinician. Sweet dreams.

Essential Features of **Nightmare Disorder**

The patient repeatedly awakens, instantly and completely, from terrible dreams that are recalled in frightening detail.

The Fine Print

The D's: • Distress or disability (work/educational, social, or personal impairment) • Differential diagnosis (substance use and physical disorders,; non-REM sleep arousal disorder, sleep terror type; REM sleep behavior disorder; other mental disorders)

Coding Notes

Specify if:

> **During sleep onset**

Specify if:

> **With associated non-sleep disorder**
> **With associated other medical condition**
> **With associated other sleep disorder**

Specify if:

> **Acute.** Has lasted less than 1 month.
> **Subacute.** Has lasted 1–6 months.
> **Persistent.** Has lasted 6+ months.

Specify severity:

> **Mild.** Less than once a week.
> **Moderate.** 1–6 episodes per week.
> **Severe.** Every night.

Keith Redding

"I wouldn't have come at all, but the other guys made me." Keith Redding twisted his garrison cap in his fingers and looked embarrassed. "Two of them are waiting out in the hallway, in case they're needed for information. I think they really stayed to make sure I kept the appointment."

After 6 months in the Army, Keith had just been promoted to private first class. He had enlisted right out of high school, thinking that he'd become a mechanic and learn a good trade. But his tests showed that he was gifted, so they plunked him into the medics and sent him to school after boot camp. Now he'd been at his new duty station in Texas for 2 weeks, living in comparative luxury in a barracks room with three roommates.

Having any roommates at all was a problem, because of his sleeping habits. "I have these nightmares," Keith explained. They didn't occur every night, but he did have them several nights a week. He usually awakened an hour or two before reveille, whimpering loudly enough to awaken the others. He'd been having this problem for several years, so he was more or less used to it. But, of course, his roommates objected. It had been worse in the last few months, with the stress of leaving home, moving around, and working at new jobs.

Although Keith's dreams varied, there were some common threads. In one of them he was in a group of people, buck naked. Recently it had been during inspection. All the other troops were lined up, looking smart in their Class A uniforms. He hadn't a stitch on, and he kept trying to cover himself, though no one seemed to notice. In another, he was the driver of an old "cracker-box" ambulance. For some reason, he had picked up a wounded gorilla. Maddened with pain, the gorilla was pulling itself forward and stretching out a hairy arm to wrap around him.

"Unfortunately, I have terrific recall. I come instantly awake, and every detail of the nightmare is just as sharp as if I'd seen it on TV. Then I'm awake for an hour or more, and so is everyone else."

The balance of Keith's history was unremarkable. He didn't use drugs and didn't drink; his health had been good, and he hadn't been especially depressed or anxious. He had never had blackouts or seizures, and he hadn't been taking medications. He loved his job in the dispensary and believed that his commanding officer found him to be alert and conscientious. He certainly wasn't falling asleep on the job.

"I've met some older guys who've had nightmares after being in combat," Keith said. "I can understand that. But about the worst thing that's ever happened to me since I enlisted has been a flat tire."

Evaluation of Keith Redding

Keith's nightmares didn't bother him much; he had grown used to them. It was his discomfort in regard to his roommates that would qualify his nightmares as sufficiently severe to warrant diagnosis (criterion C).

Three aspects of Keith's experience are typical of most nightmares: They occurred during the latter part of the night; he awakened fully and instantly (B); and he clearly recalled their content (typically threats to his safety or self-respect—A). Each of these features serves to differentiate nightmare disorder from **non-REM sleep arousal disorder, sleep terror type**: Sleep terrors occur early during non-REM sleep; they are poorly remembered; and the patient wakens only partially, if at all. Finally, although there may be some vocalization (for Keith, a suppressed whine) when the patient is about to awaken, the paralysis of muscles that normally occurs during REM sleep prevents the loud scream and physical movements that are typical of sleep terrors.

If the patient's complaint is of daytime sleepiness, other causes should be considered, such as some form of **sleep apnea.** Keith did not have daytime sleep attacks, though nightmares can be a feature of **narcolepsy.** Also consider the variety of other disorders in which nightmares can occur: **mood disorders**, **schizophrenia**, **anxiety disorders**, **somatic symptom disorder**, **adjustment disorder**, and **personality disorders** (E).

The fact that Keith had been taking no medications is also important to the differential diagnosis, because withdrawal from **REM-suppressing substances** such as tricyclic antidepressants, alcohol, or barbiturates can sometimes increase the tendency to nightmares (D). **Seizure disorders** (such as partial complex seizures) can occasionally present with bad dreams; abnormal movements noted by a bed partner during the time of the apparent nightmare could be an indication for EEG studies (E). As Keith himself noted, nightmares about a traumatic event are frequently encountered in patients who have **posttraumatic stress disorder** (these may occur in non-REM sleep, which is why patients with PTSD are more likely to scream).

Keith would qualify for a GAF score of 75. His full diagnosis would be simple:

F51.5 [307.47]   Nightmare disorder, persistent, moderate

G47.52 [327.42] Rapid Eye Movement Sleep Behavior Disorder

During normal REM sleep, our skeletal muscles are paralyzed, which protects us from injury while we're unconscious. But for people with REM sleep behavior disorder (RBD), that mechanism sometimes fails. Then dreams play out as activity, and mischief can ensue.

Although the motor behaviors in question may consist only of mild twitches, they can escalate to sudden, sometimes violent movements—by punching, kicking, or even biting, people can sometimes seriously harm themselves or a bed partner. Instead of gross motor behavior, or sometimes in addition to it, patients will sometimes whisper, talk, shout, swear, laugh, or cry. But the overall prevalence of injury to self or others is over 90%.

Usually these patients keep their eyes closed—another difference from sleepwalking—and it's rare that they get out of bed. Upon awakening, which they readily do, many patients with RBD report vivid dreams, often of being threatened or attacked by animals or people. Overt behavior may closely reflect their dream content, sometimes called "acting out their dreams." Occasionally, a funny dream can cause smiling or laughter. When severe, these behaviors occur as often as weekly or even greater.

Patients with RBD are overwhelmingly (80% or more) male. The usual onset is after age 50, so the typical patient is a middle-aged or older man. However, even children can be affected. Up to a third of patients are unaware of their symptoms, and perhaps half don't recall having unpleasant dreams. Overall, the condition affects less than 1% of the general adult population.

The initial diagnosis can be suspected from the observations of a bed partner; confirmation (with one exception) requires polysomnography. And here's the exception: The patient has symptoms that suggest RBD and a synucleinopathy condition such as Parkinson's disease and some others (see the sidebar below).

Of patients who present to sleep clinics with RBD, about half will have or develop one of these illnesses: Lewy body dementia, Parkinson's disease, or multiple-system atrophy. These are collectively referred to as *synucleinopathies*, because their underlying cause is abnormal intracellular masses of the protein α-synuclein. This is the only example I can think of where a mental health disorder is thought to powerfully predict a medical illness whose onset may lie far in the future. We can perhaps feel both encouraged and appalled.

Essential Features of **Rapid Eye Movement Sleep Behavior Disorder**

The patient has recurrent episodes of arousing from sleep accompanied by shouting or speech, or by physical actions that can injure the patient or bed partner. These symptoms often correlate with dream content. Subsequent awakenings tend to be complete. Because they occur during REM sleep, these episodes tend to take place after the person has been asleep quite a while, and not during naps.

The Fine Print

If the person has a typical history as described above, together with a synucleinopathy (such as Parkinson's disease or Lewy body dementia), no polysomnography is necessary. Without this history, there must be polysomnographic evidence of REM sleep with maintenance of muscle tone.

The D's: • Distress or disability (work/educational, social, or personal impairment) • Differential diagnosis (substance use and physical disorders, other sleep–wake disorders)

Jackson Rudy

Jackson Rudy attracted considerable clinical attention when he nearly died in the restraint he'd rigged for himself. One November dawn, his wife, Shawna, had had to call the paramedics.

For several years, Jackson explained later, he had had *really* vivid dreams. Usually these were benign, but once in a while "I'd dream I was being chased by big furry animals with slavering jaws. Then they'd turn from biting me to attack Shawna." In his sleep, he would lash out with fists and feet, but of course the only available target was his wife. "I thought I had to keep her safe—but I guess it was from me!"

As a boy, Jackson had lived on a ranch where wolves still roamed. Though he'd never seen one actually attack, more than once he had witnessed them prowling around the family's cattle.

Several months ago, when his nocturnal behavior was limited to yelling or sometimes jerking his arms and legs around, he had consulted his primary care provider. "She thought I could sleep in the guest room. Shawna and I both thought *that* was lame." So Jackson had dusted off the leatherworking skills from his ranch days and constructed a tether to restrain his movements. "It was supposed to loop around my arms and chest to keep me from slugging her," he said, "only I sort of got tangled up in it. It nearly hanged me."

With Jackson's permission, the clinician interviewed Shawna. She affirmed that his attacks came mostly in the predawn hours, and that when he awakened, he came instantly and completely alert. Had he been depressed? Did he drink or use drugs or medication? (Negatives all around.) Was his interest good in things generally? In sex?

Shawna smiled. "Even at 60, he's much better at lovemaking than at inventing."

Evaluation of Jackson Rudy

First, let's dispose of the criteria. We know from the history (including Shawna's helpful information) that Jackson's episodes were repeated and physical (criterion A), that they occurred while he was dreaming later in the night (not when first falling asleep—criterion B), and that they appeared to be a physical enactment of his dreams. He awakened right away (C), and hadn't been using drink, drugs, or medications that might cause similar behaviors (F). The arrival of the paramedics tells us that the behavior was dangerous and clinically important (E).

Polysomnography could also help with the differential diagnosis of some other disorders that entail violence during sleep: both the **sleepwalking** and **sleep terror types of non-REM sleep arousal disorder**, **nocturnal seizures**, and **obstructive sleep apnea hypopnea**. However, his history isn't strong for any of these disorders, and I feel comfortable putting them aside. There's no evidence for other medical or mental disorders (G).

The remaining criterion (D), verification by polysomnography, isn't quite as vital as DSM-5 might lead us to believe. Some experts state that we can omit it in relatively mild cases, where there's no significant worry about other disorders. But with the severity of Jackson's lashing out, safety is the better part of evaluation. Jackson probably wouldn't consider himself old yet, but still we need to know that he has none of the degenerative neurological disorders that can be the source of RBD: **Lewy body dementia** (about 70% of cases are associated with RBD), **Parkinson's disease** (50%), and **multiple-system atrophy** (upwards of 90%). RBD is also found in **strokes**, **tumors**, and some **medications** (beta blockers, some antidepressants), though it's rare in Alzheimer's disease.

Because of the circumstances in which Jackson nearly died, a few questions about paraphilias would be warranted, and his clinician would want to keep in mind the possibility of a suicide attempt—a red herring here, but something that we must always keep in mind.

Jackson Rudy's diagnosis is listed below. Although the paramedics were called, I'd say that any danger to himself was a one-off, unlikely to be repeated. I'd put his GAF score at a comfortable 70. His doctor should observe him carefully for development of an additional disorder (see the sidebar above).

G47.52 [327.42]   Rapid eye movement sleep behavior disorder

Other Sleep–Wake Disorders

Substance/Medication-Induced Sleep Disorder

As you might expect, substances of abuse can produce a variety of sleep disorders, most of which will be either insomnia or hypersomnolence. The specific problem with sleep can occur during either intoxication or withdrawal.

Alcohol. Heavy alcohol use (intoxication) can produce unrefreshing sleep with strong REM suppression and reduced total sleep time. Patients may experience terminal insomnia and sometimes hypersomnolence, and their sleep problems may persist for years. Alcohol withdrawal markedly increases sleep onset latency and produces restless sleep with frequent awakenings. Patients may experience delirium with tremor and (especially visual) hallucinations; this was formerly known as delirium tremens.

Sedatives, hypnotics, and anxiolytics. These include barbiturates, over-the-counter antihistamines and bromides, short-acting benzodiazepines, and high doses of long-acting benzodiazepines. Any of these substances may be used in the attempt to remedy insomnia of another origin. They can lead to sleep disorder during either intoxication or withdrawal.

Central nervous system stimulants. Amphetamines and other stimulants typically cause increased latency of sleep onset, decreased REM sleep, and more awakenings. Once the drug is discontinued, hypersomnolence with restlessness and REM rebound dreams may ensue.

Caffeine. This popular drug produces insomnia with intoxication and hypersomnolence upon withdrawal (no surprises here).

Other drugs. These include tricyclic antidepressants, neuroleptics, ACTH, anticonvulsants, thyroid medications, marijuana, cocaine, LSD, opioids, PCP, and methyldopa.

Essential Features of **Substance/Medication–Induced Sleep Disorder**

The use of some substance appears to have caused a patient to have a serious sleep problem.

The Fine Print

For tips on identifying substance-related causation, see sidebar, page 95.

The D's: • Distress or disability (work/educational, social, or personal impairment) • Differential diagnosis (physical disorders, delirium, other sleep disorders)

You'd only make this diagnosis when the symptoms are serious enough to warrant clinical attention *and* they are worse than you'd expect from ordinary intoxication or withdrawal.

Coding Notes

ICD-9 kept coding simple: 291.82 for alcohol, 292.85 for all other substances. Coding in ICD-10 depends on the substance used and on whether symptoms are met for an actual substance use disorder (and, if so, how severe the use disorder is). Refer to Table 15.2 in Chapter 15.

Specify:

> **With onset during {intoxication}{withdrawal}.** This gets tacked on at the end of your string of words.
> **With onset after medication use.** You can use this in addition to other specifiers. (See sidebar, p. 94.)

Specify:

> **Insomnia type**
> **Daytime sleepiness type**
> **Parasomnia type** (abnormal behavior when sleeping)
> **Mixed type**

Dave Kincaid

Dave Kincaid was a free-lance writer. As Dave explained it to his clinician, "free-lance" was the industry's way of saying that you were unemployed. He'd actually done reasonably well for himself, specializing in interviews with unimportant (but very interesting) people. Most of his work was published in small magazines and specialized reviews. His novel and a volume of travel essays had been remaindered early, with good reviews but disappointing sales.

When he had to, Dave supplemented his income by taking temporary jobs. To gather material for his writing, he tried to make his jobs as varied as possible. He had driven a taxi, been a bouncer at a bar, sold real estate, and (in his younger days) served as a guide on the Jungle River Cruise at Disneyland. Now 35, he had been supporting his third book, a murder mystery, for the last several weeks by working in a coffee roastery north of San Francisco. The job didn't pay much over minimum wage, but neither was it very demanding. Except for the busy 2 or 3 hours around noon, it left him with plenty of time for blocking out a section of his book to work on that night.

It also left Dave time to drink coffee. Besides grinding beans or selling them whole, the roastery served coffee by the cup. Employees could drink what they wanted. Dave was a coffee drinker, but he had always limited himself to three or four cups a day. "It sure isn't enough to explain the way I'm feeling now."

How he felt was, in a word, nervous. It was worst at night. "I have this uncomfortable, 'up' sort of feeling, and I want to write. But sometimes I just can't sit still at the word processor. I get that 'live flesh' sensation when your muscles twitch. And my heart beats fast and my gut seems to pour out water, so I have to spend a lot of time in the bathroom."

Dave seldom got to sleep before 2 A.M., sometimes after much tossing and turning. On Sundays he slept until noon, but on Monday through Saturday he awakened to his alarm, feeling hung over and in desperate need of a cup of coffee.

Dave's health had been excellent, which was a good thing because he'd seldom had a job with a health plan. Other than the mornings, his mood was good. He had tried marijuana in the past, but didn't like it. He confined his drinking to coffee, but "only three or four cups a day," he said again. He also denied drinking tea, cocoa, or cola beverages. After a moment he added, "Of course, there are the coffee beans."

When things were slow in the afternoon and Dave was thinking about his novel, he would dip into the supply of candy-coated coffee beans the roastery also sold (for $11.95 the half-pound). They came coated in white or dark chocolate; he preferred the dark. They also had decaffeinated beans, but these were dipped in yogurt, which he didn't care for at all.

"I don't keep track," said Dave, "but all in all, every afternoon I probably have a few handfuls. Or so."

Evaluation of Dave Kincaid

Although Dave drank fairly modest amounts of coffee, it was very strong and by itself probably contained more than the 250 mg or so usually required for caffeine intoxication. He also ate coffee beans; depending on the origin of the beans, it takes perhaps 70 beans to make a strong cup of brewed coffee, and he consumed chocolate-coated beans by the handful. That way, he may have eaten the equivalent of one or two additional cups of coffee per day. (In addition, chocolate contains theobromine, a xanthine with effects similar to caffeine.) No wonder he felt nervous. In its proper place (p. 417), I'll discuss Dave's symptoms of caffeinism.

In conjunction with his caffeine use, Dave noted increased latency of sleep onset. He felt tired when it was time to get up, and he had to use coffee to get going. Therefore, the basic criteria for substance-induced sleep disorder were all met: Use of a substance caused (criterion B1) a problem with sleep serious enough to require clinical attention (A, E). Of course, caffeine is famously associated with sleeplessness.

Sure, you could think up all manner of other sleep disorders that could cause Dave's symptoms (C, D)—but the rational course would be to eliminate (gradually!) the caffeine use, then reassess the patient's sleep. This was what Dave's clinician did. In some cases, there can be confusion as to the etiological contributions of physical illness and the medications that are used to treat it. At times, two diagnoses may be warranted.

With the subtype specifiers required in the criteria (and a GAF score of 65), Dave's diagnosis would be as follows:

| F15.929 [305.90] | Caffeine intoxication, moderate |
| F15.982 [292.85] | Caffeine-induced sleep disorder, insomnia type, with onset during intoxication |

The diagnosis of a substance-induced *anything* rests on deciding that the symptoms are more serious than you'd expect from ordinary substance intoxication or withdrawal. This is a judgment call. In the case of Dave Kincaid, the symptoms were sufficiently prominent to bring him for evaluation.

G47.09 [780.52] Other Specified Insomnia Disorder

DSM-5 gives these examples:

Brief insomnia disorder. Insomnia lasting less than 3 months.

Restricted to nonrestorative sleep. The person doesn't feel refreshed by sleep that is otherwise unremarkable.

G47.00 [780.52] Unspecified Insomnia Disorder

Use unspecified insomnia disorder when a patient's insomnia symptoms do not meet the full criteria for insomnia disorder (or any other sleep disorder) and you decide not to be specific about the reasons.

G47.19 [780.54] Other Specified Hypersomnolence Disorder

G47.10 [780.54] Unspecified Hypersomnolence Disorder

Use one of these categories when you've eliminated all other possibilities for a patient's hypersomnolence. The usual guidelines for choosing other specified versus unspecified apply.

G47.8 [780.59] Other Specified Sleep–Wake Disorder

G47.9 [780.59] Unspecified Sleep–Wake Disorder

By now, you know the drill.

CHAPTER 12

Sexual Dysfunctions

Quick Guide to the Sexual Dysfunctions

DSM-5 addresses three sorts of issues directly tied to sexual functioning. In DSM-IV and before, they were all included in the same chapter; now the sexual dysfunctions, gender dysphoria, and paraphilic disorders are spread out over three different chapters. As with most other diagnoses, patients can have problems in multiple areas, which can in turn coexist with other mental diagnoses.

With the exception of substance-induced sexual dysfunction, the sexual dysfunctions are gender-specific. DSM-5's organization is alphabetical; I've grouped these disorders by gender and stage in an act of sex at which the dysfunction occurs. The page number following each item indicates where a more detailed discussion begins.

Sexual Dysfunctions

Male hypoactive sexual desire disorder. The patient isn't much interested in sex, though his performance may be adequate once sexual activity has been initiated (p. 352).

Erectile disorder. A man's erection isn't sufficient to begin or complete sexual relations (p. 355).

Premature (early) ejaculation. A man experiences repeated instances of climax before, during, or just after penetration (p. 357).

Delayed ejaculation. Despite a normal period of sexual excitement, a man's climax is either delayed or does not occur at all (p. 359).

Female sexual interest/arousal disorder. A woman lacks interest in sex or does not become aroused enough (p. 362).

Genito-pelvic pain/penetration disorder. Genital pain occurs (only in women) during sexual intercourse, often during insertion (p. 364).

Female orgasmic disorder. Despite a normal period of sexual excitement, a woman's climax either is delayed or does not occur at all (p. 368).

Substance/medication-induced sexual dysfunction. Many of these problems can also be caused by intoxication or withdrawal from alcohol or other substances (p. 370).

Other specified, or unspecified, sexual dysfunction. These are catch-all categories for sexual problems that do not meet the criteria for any of the foregoing sexual dysfunctions (p. 371).

Other Causes of Sexual Difficulties

Paraphilic disorders. These include a variety of behaviors that most people regard as distasteful, unusual, or abnormal. Nearly all are practiced almost exclusively by males (p. 564).

Gender dysphoria. Some people strongly identify so strongly with the opposite gender that they are uncomfortable with their assigned gender roles (p. 372).

Nonsexual mental disorders. Many patients develop sexual dysfunctions as a result of other mental disorders. Lack of interest in sex may be encountered especially in somatic symptom disorder (p. 251), major depressive disorder (p. 122), and schizophrenia (p. 64).

Introduction

The sexual dysfunctions usually begin in early adulthood, though some may not appear until later in life—whenever the opportunity for sexual experience arises. Most of them are quite common. Any of them can be caused by psychological or biological factors or by a combination of these. Ordinarily, we wouldn't use one of these diagnoses if the behavior occurs only in the course of another mental disorder.

Also, any of these dysfunctions can be lifelong or acquired. *Lifelong* (also called *primary*) means that this dysfunction has been present since the beginning of active sexual functioning. *Acquired* means that at some time the patient has been able to have sex without that particular dysfunction. As you might imagine, lifelong dysfunctions are vastly more resistant to therapy.

Furthermore, most sexual dysfunctions may be either *generalized* or *situational* (that is, limited to specific situations). For example, a man may experience premature ejaculation with his wife but not with another woman. Some dysfunctions may not even require that the patient have a partner; they can occur during masturbation, for example. (Generalized and situational don't apply to genito-pelvic pain/penetration disorder.)

DSM-5 has tightened its advice on how much dysfunction is required for diagnosis. The patient must have the symptoms on the majority of occasions (in criteria sets, it is phrased as "almost all or all") of sexual activity over a 6-month period—and those phrases have been explicitly, and confusingly, defined as meaning 75% or more. However, the criteria also specify that they must cause "clinically significant distress," leaving some room for clinician judgment based on how long the problem has existed and the degree to which the problem affects patient and partner. This judgment will be influenced by the circumstances surrounding the particular sex activity—such as degree of sexual stimulation, the amount of that activity, and with whom it occurs. For example, female sexual interest/arousal disorder should not be diagnosed if it occurs only when intercourse is attempted after little or no foreplay.

In addition to these considerations, here are some additional factors to take into account. (Note that in DSM-IV they were subtypes that we added to the official title of each sexual disorder; DSM-5 has in essence demoted them to an advisory capacity.)

- Partner factors (such as partner's sexual problems or health status)

- Relationship factors (such as poor communication, relationship discord, discrepancies in desire for sexual activity)

- Individual vulnerability factors (such as a history of abuse or poor body image)

- Cultural/religious factors (for example, inhibitions related to prohibitions against sexual activity)

- Medical factors relevant to prognosis, course, or treatment (any chronic illness could be an example)

Although common, the sexual dysfunctions tend to be ignored by clinicians who don't specialize in their evaluation and treatment; too often, we simply fail to ask. An alert clinician may be able to make a diagnosis of one or more of these conditions in a patient who comes for consultation regarding unrelated mental health problems.

F52.0 [302.71] Male Hypoactive Sexual Desire Disorder

Relatively little is known about low sex interest and desire in men, compared to women. This has partly resulted from the unfounded assumption that it is uncommon. Yet, in a 1994 survey of over 1,400 men, 16% agreed that they had had a period of several months when they were not interested in sex (compared with 33% for women.) These men tended to be older, never married, not highly educated, black, and poor. Compared to other men, they were more likely to have been inappropriately "touched" before puberty, to have experienced homosexual activity at some time in their lives, and to use alcohol daily. Even a few percent of young men (in their 20s) will admit to relative lack of sexual desire, though it seldom rises to the level of male hypoactive sexual desire disorder (MHSDD).

MHSDD can be primary or acquired. The (relatively less common) primary type has been associated with some sort of sexual secret (such as shame about sexual orientation, past sexual trauma, perhaps a preference for masturbation over sex with a partner). Such a man's low sex desire may be masked by the effect of a new romance; this glow typically persists for only a matter of months before frustration and heartache (and more secrecy) set in, for patient and partner alike.

Acquired MHSDD is the more common pattern. It often develops as a consequence of dysfunctions of erection or ejaculation (early or delayed). These in turn can stem from a variety of causes: diabetes, hypertension, substance use, mood or anxiety disorders, sometimes a lack of intimacy with a partner. Whatever the origin, the man's confidence in his ability to achieve or maintain an erection (or to satisfy his partner) yields to a pattern of anticipatory anxiety and failure. He has trouble admitting that his sexual relationship is less than perfect, and so he retires from the fray, so to speak, defeated and uncommunicative.

Such a pattern can begin at almost any stage of life, though about two out of three couples stop having sex by their mid-70s. At any age, when this happens to heterosexual couples, it is overwhelmingly (90%) likely to be at the man's initiative.

Essential Features of **Male Hypoactive Sexual Desire Disorder**

A man lacks erotic thoughts or wishes for sexual activity.

The Fine Print

The clinician must judge the deficiency in light of age and other factors that can affect sexual function.

The D's: • Duration (6+ months) • Distress to the patient • Differential diagnosis (substance use and physical disorders, relationship problems, other mental disorders)

Coding Notes

Specify:

> {Lifelong}{Acquired}
> {Generalized}{Situational}

Specify severity of distress over the symptoms: {Mild}{Moderate}{Severe}

Nigel O'Neil

"She's not your typical trophy wife," Nigel O'Neil told the therapist in confidence. "I love Gemma because she's so competent, so organized—and such a nice person," he added, almost as an afterthought. "But she just doesn't turn me on the way Bea used to."

At age 53, Nigel was well into his second marriage, solemnized 3 years after his first wife died of malignant melanoma. For several years, Gemma had been his personal assistant in the office where he worked for a large publisher. Around the time of

Bea's death, he had turned to her for more than his morning mug of Darjeeling. During his first session, he admitted that he still felt guilty about that.

Born in London, Nigel had been reared a strict Catholic. "That operationalized to the fact that, before we were married, Bea and I hadn't done much more than a little fooling around. We were very young and inexperienced." Afterwards, he had been able to obtain and maintain an erection satisfactory for intercourse "most of the time, though even then we had our problems, Bea and I." He declined to elaborate, stating only that they seemed minor in comparison.

Gemma was 15 years younger than Nigel. For several months, they had pursued an active sex life—"something else she organized." At the office, he had appreciated the way she managed his schedule. "At home, not so much." In the last 6 months, when she approached him for sex, he usually fobbed her off with the excuse that he was too tired or preoccupied. On the few occasions she could persuade him to try, he couldn't maintain an erection long enough to achieve penetration. The one time they did have intercourse, his attention had "wandered off to the office," and he withdrew before either of them climaxed.

Nigel's internist had checked his testosterone level, which was within normal range. On his second visit, Gemma tagged along. She and Nigel agreed that they drank little and had never used drugs or tobacco. Gemma added that a few months earlier, in desperation, she had subscribed to *Playboy* for him. "He's the only man I know who really does just read the articles," she commented.

Nigel hadn't seen other women; he didn't even masturbate. "For months, the magazine's the only thing I've put to bed. I don't even have randy fantasies any more." The issue didn't distress Nigel for himself ("It's just not something I ever think about!"), but he became almost tearful as he talked about how deeply he cared for Gemma, how he longed that she be happy—that she not abandon him for someone else.

One session when Nigel was in the room, Gemma explained, "Besides books and magazines, our company makes films, mostly about love and lovemaking. Nigel thinks that's a total irony, but I don't think we've finished shooting yet."

Evaluation of Nigel O'Neil

Nigel's history is loaded with indicators of a persistent sexual disorder, including multiple failures of his erection, his interest, his response (to invitations from Gemma), and even his fantasy life (criterion A). His interest in work was good and he denied feeling depressed, so a **mood disorder** seems unlikely (D), but a thorough review to identify any possible **anxiety disorder** would seem a good idea. The history appears to rule out an etiological role for **drugs** or **alcohol** (also D); there wasn't any apparent relationship distress—yet, at any rate. The duration met the 6-month requirement (B), and Nigel's distress was palpable (C).

In addition, Nigel would probably qualify for the diagnosis of **erectile disorder**. If so, it should also be made (other sexual disorders can coexist with MHSDD). It's just one more issue he and his clinician would need to explore.

Once the principal diagnosis was nailed down, the clinician's real work would begin—examining the possible causes of Nigel's lack of sexual interest. Each of these could indicate a therapeutic avenue to explore. Multiple possible contributing factors must be considered:

Relationship factors—did Nigel resent Gemma's overmanagement of their lives?

Medical factors—did Nigel have, say, diabetes or a cardiovascular condition? (If medical factors were the exclusive cause of Nigel's current sexual problems, we wouldn't make this diagnosis at all; see criterion D.)

Cultural/religious concerns—sex with Gemma while Nigel was still married to Bea could play a role.

Though there's no information for partner factors or for any individual vulnerability factors such as depression, further exploratory interviews of both Nigel and Gemma would clearly be in order.

Nigel's still unelaborated sexual problems with Bea even make us wonder whether his problem could have been lifelong, rather than acquired. Had his sex interest been on the low side with her, too? Had she complained? Did he fantasize about other women? Men? How affectionate were they as a couple?

In its bare-bones form, Nigel's diagnosis would read as given below, but there's much more work to be done. Despite his difficulties with sex, I'd put his GAF score at a relatively healthy 70.

F52.0 [302.71]   Male hypoactive sexual desire disorder, acquired, generalized, severe

F52.21 [302.72] Erectile Disorder

Erectile disorder (ED), otherwise known as impotence, can be partial or complete. In either case, the erection is inadequate for satisfactory sex. Impotence can also be situational, in which case the patient can achieve an erection only under certain circumstances (for example, with prostitutes). ED is probably the most prevalent male sexual disorder, occurring at least occasionally in perhaps 2% of *young* men; that number does not improve with age. Of all the sexual dysfunctions, this is the one most likely to occur for the first time later in life.

A variety of emotions can play a role in the development or maintenance of ED. These include fear, anxiety, anger, guilt, and distrust of the sexual partner. Any of these feelings can so preoccupy a man's attention that he cannot focus adequately on feeling sexual pleasure. Even a single failure may lead to anticipatory anxiety, which then precipitates another round in the circle of failure. The prominent sex researchers Masters and Johnson also talked about a factor they called *spectatoring*, in which the patient evaluates his performance so constantly that he cannot concentrate on the enjoyment of sex. Such a patient might have an erection with foreplay but lose it upon penetration.

ED should not be diagnosed if biological factors are the principal or only cause. This is unlikely if erections occur spontaneously, with masturbation, or with other partners. Some authorities now estimate that half or more of patients who complain of impotence have a biological cause for it, such as prostatectomy for cancer. When psychological factors are judged to be a part of the cause, as is often the case, the diagnosis can be made.

Like the other sexual dysfunctions, ED can be either lifelong or acquired; the former is rare and hard to treat.

Essential Features of **Erectile Disorder**

The patient almost always has marked trouble achieving or maintaining an erection adequate to consummate sex.

The Fine Print

The D's: • Duration (6+ months) • Distress to the patient • Differential diagnosis (substance use and physical disorders, relationship problems, other mental disorders)

Coding Notes

Specify:

    {Lifelong}{Acquired}
    {Generalized}{Situational}

Specify severity of distress over the symptoms: **{Mild}{Moderate}{Severe}**

Parker Flynn

"I think I must be over the hill."

If you didn't count the three counseling sessions he had had while sifting through the wreckage of his first marriage, this was Parker Flynn's first visit ever to a mental health professional. At age 45 he had been a bridegroom for only 7 months, and he was afraid he was losing his sexual potency.

Everything had been fine before the wedding, but the first evening of their honeymoon, Parker had been unable to get enough of an erection to do either him or his wife much good. He supposed he'd had too much champagne—normally he didn't touch alcohol. His wife had also been married before and knew a thing or two about men. She hadn't criticized; she'd even said it would be all right. But she was attractive and 10 years younger than Parker, and he was worried: Most of the time since, he'd been unable to perform.

"Some of the guys warned me, it's what happens when you get older," Parker insisted. "That which should be easy is hard, and that which should be hard isn't."

Before he popped the question, he had undergone a complete physical examination. Other than being a few pounds overweight—Parker was devoted to chocolate ice cream—he was given a clean bill of health. Besides the ice cream, he denied any other addictions, including alcohol, drugs, and tobacco.

"I get so nervous when it's time to make love," Parker explained. "I can get a pretty good erection when we're fooling around, but when it's time to get serious, I lose it. Her first husband was something of a stud, and I keep wondering how my performance measures up to his."

Evaluation of Parker Flynn

Parker's interest in sex seemed to be just fine; he gave every indication (normal erections) that there was nothing wrong with the excitatory phase. But because he worried about maintaining his erection, he did have difficulty maintaining an erection (criterion A2) stressful enough that he sought care (C). His problem was exacerbated by the phenomenon of spectatoring (see above), in which his performance was affected by wondering how well he was doing while he was doing it. His problem had been present for 7 months—just qualifying for the DSM-5 time requirement (B, though in obvious cases I'd be a little relaxed about this requirement; it does say "approximately," after all).

Parker's physical condition was good, pretty much ruling out a causative **physical illness** (D). Some patients with impotence may suffer from **sleep apnea**; of course, it is vital to explore this possibility, because of the potentially lethal nature of that disorder. He had no previous mental health problems that would preclude the diagnosis of ED. His difficulty may have begun with an alcohol-related incident, but from his history, substance use played no role in its maintenance. Also note that, as they age, men may require more stimulation to achieve erection than they did when they were younger; such a physiological change should not constitute evidence of ED. **Sporadic erectile problems** that don't cause important distress also should not be given this diagnosis.

Parker's problem was not lifelong but acquired; the vignette provides no evidence that it applied only in specific situations, so neither situational nor generalized type would be specified. With no other obvious specifiers to note (and a GAF score of 70), his diagnosis would read:

F52.21 [302.72]   Erectile disorder, acquired

F52.4 [302.75] Premature (Early) Ejaculation

As the disorder's name implies, the man climaxes before he wants to—sometimes just as he and his partner reach the point of insertion. However, different studies use widely varying standards of how many minutes actually constitutes *early*: Is it 7 minutes? Is it 1? Both standards have been proposed. Whatever the duration, the climax yields disappointment and a sense of failure for both partners; secondary impotence sometimes follows. Stress in a relationship can exacerbate the condition, which of course promotes even greater loss of control. However, some women may value premature ejaculation (PE) because it decreases their exposure to unwanted sexual activity or pregnancy.

PE is a commonplace disorder; it accounts for nearly half the men treated for sexual disorders. It is especially frequent among men with more education—presumably because their social group is especially sensitive to the issue of partner satisfaction. Whereas anxiety is often a factor, physical illness or abnormalities rarely cause this problem.

Essential Features of **Premature (Early) Ejaculation**

The patient almost always ejaculates before he wants to, within moments of penetration.

The Fine Print

The D's: • Duration (6+ months) • Distress to the patient • Differential diagnosis (substance use and physical disorders)

Coding Notes

Specify:

> {Lifelong}{Acquired}
> {Generalized}{Situational}

Specify severity:

> **Mild.** The patient ejaculates 30–60 seconds after penetration.
> **Moderate.** 15–30 seconds after penetration.
> **Severe.** 15 seconds after penetration or less (perhaps before penetration).

Let's be practical. And honest. The official criteria state two time standards for the patient with premature ejaculation, which boil down to "about a minute" and "too early." DSM-5 claims that men can pretty accurately estimate time as long as it's a minute or less, and in the heat of the moment, it seems unlikely in the extreme that anyone is going to clap a stopwatch on the activity. Therefore, for the vast majority of our patients, we will eschew the clock and accept the statement that "I just flat-out come too soon."

Claude Campbell

Claude Campbell could remember, in embarrassing detail, the first time it ever happened. He had been a very young Marine second lieutenant stationed in Vietnam in the last year of the war. Suddenly granted leave to go to town, he had had to borrow a pair of Class A uniform trousers from the battalion chaplain.

Claude and two friends were seated at a sidewalk table, drinking a mixture that the military called a "Bombs Away," when a prostitute sat down next to him. When she set to work warming her hand between his thighs, it only took a few moments before Claude felt himself lose control. A crimson blush spread across his face as a stain darkened the front of the chaplain's khaki trousers.

"That was one of the worst times, but it sure wasn't the last," said Claude. After he left the Marines, he finished college and got a job selling computers. He soon married a girl he had dated during high school. Their wedding night, and most of their other nights, were never quite the disaster of the Vietnam bar, but he could never last longer than a minute or so after insertion."

"Not that it bothered her," commented Claude ruefully. "She never enjoyed sex much, anyway. She was always glad to get it over with in a hurry. I know now why she insisted on 'saving it' for after we were married. She never wanted to spend it in the first place."

Claude always hoped that his problems had been largely due to his first wife's prudery and disapproval, but several months into his new marriage, things hadn't improved much. "She's being very patient," he said, "but we're both beginning to get desperate."

Evaluation of Claude Campbell

Claude's difficulty had been with him ever since his sex life began, and it occurred every time (criterion B). Although a few such incidents might be dismissed in a youngster or in any man with a new partner, in a mature adult (we don't know Claude's age at evaluation) who has been in a lasting relationship with frequent sexual activity, it must be considered pathological (A). Claude's difficulty was clearly causing him distress (C); we'd have to enquire further about substance use (D). As noted earlier, **physical illness** does not play a significant role in the development of PE.

Claude's problem was not situational (it had occurred with both of his wives and with the prostitute). As far as we're aware, he'd had it forever. I'd place his GAF score at 70.

F52.4 [302.75]   Premature ejaculation, generalized, lifelong, moderate

F52.32 [302.74] Delayed Ejaculation

Men with delayed ejaculation (DE) achieve erection without difficulty, but have problems reaching orgasm. Some only take a long time; others may not be able to ejaculate into a partner at all. Prolonged friction may cause the partners of these patients to complain of soreness. Anxiety about performance may cause secondary impotence in the patients themselves.

Even when it has been present lifelong, a man can usually ejaculate by masturbating (alone or with the help of his sex partner). The personalities of patients with lifelong DE have been described as rigid and puritanical; some seem to equate sex with sin. Or the disorder may be acquired from interpersonal difficulties, fear of pregnancy, or a partner's lack of sexual allure. DE is somewhat more common in patients with anxiety disorders.

DE is probably uncommon. When men do have problems with delayed (or absent) climax, there is often a medical cause; examples include hyperglycemia, prostatectomy, abdominal aortic surgery, Parkinson's disease, and spinal cord tumors. Some men have a physical abnormality that, upon orgasm, causes semen to be expelled into the urinary bladder (retrograde ejaculation). Drugs like alphamethyldopa (an antihypertensive) and thioridazine (a neuroleptic), as well as alcohol, have also been implicated. If any of these factors is the *sole* cause, it cannot be regarded as an example of DE.

The drug thioridazine, which can inhibit a man's ability to have orgasm, is sometimes used to treat patients with premature ejaculation (see the previous diagnosis).

Essential Features of **Delayed Ejaculation**

The man experiences pronounced delay or infrequency of climax.

The Fine Print

The D's: • Duration (6+ months) • Distress to the patient • Differential diagnosis (substance use and physical disorders, relationship problems)

Coding Notes

Specify:

> {Lifelong}{Acquired}
> {Generalized}{Situational}

Specify severity: {Mild}{Moderate}{Severe}

Rodney Stensrud

Rodney Stensrud and his girlfriend, Frannie, had come to the clinic seeking relief for Rodney's "performance problem." They had been together for nearly a year, and they disagreed as to the extent of the problem.

Rodney was frankly worried. It had always taken him a long time to have a climax, and now, after 40 minutes or so of vigorous intercourse, he sometimes found himself wilting under pressure. Frannie was more sanguine. Her previous boyfriend had never been able to last longer than 5 minutes, and that often left her feeling frustrated.

"Now I almost always come more than once," she said with an air of satisfaction. Recently Rodney had been taking even longer, and she admitted that she was getting pretty sore. "Maybe if we could get it back down to about half an hour," she suggested.

Rodney's parents had reared him strictly. Throughout his childhood, he had attended parochial school, so that he was "pretty clear on the concept of good versus evil." He admitted that he felt guilty that he and Frannie were living together without benefit of clergy, but she wasn't ready to take that step yet. She used to laugh and tell him that she wanted to "save something for after the baby came."

Before meeting Frannie, Rodney's only experience had been with two prostitutes he had encountered while he was in the Navy. It had taken him hardly any time at all with either of them. In fact, he felt that the one with the mouth had rather shortchanged him. "There sure wasn't any delay involved," he said. Neither had he experienced any particular problem masturbating, either when he was an adolescent or more recently when Frannie was gone on an extended business trip.

Rodney had been referred by a urologist, who had found nothing physically wrong. The couple's only drinking was an occasional glass of white wine. At one time Rodney had occasionally used marijuana at parties, but Frannie was death on drugs, so he had given it up a year ago.

Evaluation of Rodney Stensrud

After apparently normal desire and excitation phases, Rodney always took an inordinately long time to reach climax (criterion A1). From the vignette, this does not appear to have been a lifelong problem, though it had now lasted for many months (B). The problem was causing him enough distress to seek help (C); already he seemed headed down the road to secondary impotence.

Rodney's problem was situational; he had experienced no ejaculatory delay when with a prostitute or when masturbating. His referring physician had noted no **physical illnesses** that might account for his disorder, and there was no significant **substance use;** with no evidence of any **other mental disorder** that might be diagnosed instead, we've exhausted the possibilities of criterion D. His upbringing was puritanical, reinforcing the impression that the basis of his disorder was psychological, not physical.

Frannie's reaction to Rodney's disorder was perhaps somewhat atypical. Female partners sometimes complain of discomfort from prolonged intercourse necessary to achieve climax. Would the fact that Frannie found value in Rodney's disorder present a possible problem for therapy? When working with the couple, Rodney's clinician should keep this factor in mind—along with the possibility that he could have an anxiety disorder.

Rodney's GAF score would be about 70. His diagnosis would be as follows:

F52.32 [302.74]   Delayed ejaculation, acquired, situational, moderate

F52.22 [302.72] Female Sexual Interest/Arousal Disorder

Female sexual interest/arousal disorder (FSIAD) represents the fusion of two older diagnoses: hypoactive sexual desire disorder and female sexual arousal disorder. DSM-5 has combined them for several reasons. Especially in women, there is a high overlap between desire and arousal; some authorities think of desire as just the cognitive component of arousal. Moreover, one phase doesn't always precede the other; their relationship really depends on the individual. And treating low desire also improves arousal.

Sexual desire depends upon a number of factors, including the patient's inherent drive and self-esteem, previous sexual satisfaction, an available partner, and a good relationship with the partner in areas other than sex. Sexual desire may be suppressed by long abstinence. It may present as infrequent sexual activity, or as a perception that the partner is unattractive. Some patients actually become averse to sex, expressing loathing of any genital contact or of aspects of genital sexual contact.

Lack of interest in sex is the most common complaint of women coming to treatment. About 30% of women ages 18–59 will admit to having a period of at least several months when they've lacked sexual desire. As a result, perhaps half feel distress, which can affect the individuals or their relationships. Low desire is greater for women who are postmenopausal (either naturally or after surgery). There may be a history of painful intercourse, feelings of guilt, or rape or other sexual trauma occurring in childhood or in a patient's earlier sexual life.

Don't diagnose FSIAD if the problem occurs only in the context of another mental condition, such as major depressive disorder or a substance use disorder. (Among the medications that can contribute are antihistamines and anticholinergics.) Also note that postmenopausal females may need more foreplay to lubricate to the same degree than they did when they were younger. However, FSIAD often coexists with another sexual condition, such as female orgasmic disorder. A woman who doesn't express interest in sex but does respond to sexual activity with excitement would not qualify for a diagnosis of FSIAD. Neither would someone who identifies herself as having been "asexual" her whole life.

Essential Features of **Female Sexual Interest/Arousal Disorder**

A woman's low sexual interest or arousal is indicated by minimal interest in sexual activity, erotic thoughts, response to partner overtures, and enjoyment during sex. She will generally not initiate sexual activity and doesn't "turn on" to erotic literature, movies, and the like.

The Fine Print

The D's: • Duration (6+ months) • Distress to the patient • Differential diagnosis (substance use and physical disorders, relationship problems)

Coding Notes

Specify:

{Lifelong}{Acquired}
{Generalized}{Situational}

Specify severity: {Mild}{Moderate}{Severe}

Ernestine Paget

"She hardly ever wants to do it," James Paget told the marriage therapist.

"That's not quite accurate," Ernestine responded. "The truth is, I never want to do it. It's disgusting."

When they got married 3 years earlier, Ernestine had been uninterested in sex, though receptive to the idea of it. "It seemed to mean a lot to him, so I put up with it," she explained. "But he was never satisfied. No matter how often we made love, a few days later there he was, wanting more. It got old fast."

"It is the usual expectation," her husband remarked dryly, "and it's not my fault how she was brought up."

In Ernestine's family, sex was never discussed and nudity wasn't allowed. Ernestine could never remember having much curiosity about sex, let alone interest. She had been an only child. "I assume her parents only did it once," offered James.

For the first few months, Ernestine would simply lie still and think about other things, enduring what was for her a basically boring activity because it was important to her new husband. Her gynecologist had assured her that as far as her anatomy and hormones were concerned, she was completely normal. Unless she was figuring out whether it was time to start taking her new prescription of birth control pills, she never thought about sex.

"God knows, I never dream about it," Ernestine said. "Maybe if he'd led up to it more, it would have helped. His idea of foreplay is half an hour of David Letterman and a slap on the butt." She had once tried to explain this to James, but he had only called her "frigid." That was the last word they had exchanged on the subject until now.

Now James pretty much ignored Ernestine. She undressed in the closet; they slept on the two edges of their king-sized bed. She didn't know where he was getting his sex these days, but it wasn't at home and she said she didn't care.

"At least he doesn't have to worry that I'd try to cut it off, like that Bobbitt woman," Ernestine said. "I don't even like to look at it, let alone touch it with a 10-inch knife."

Evaluation of Ernestine Paget

Ernestine's low sex interest was shown not just by absent interest (criterion A1); she denied even fantasizing (A2) about what was for her a boring activity (A4). This is an important point: Some patients may reject the idea of sex with a current (or with any) partner, yet may still harbor an abstract interest in sex or in sex with some hypothetical person. When Ernestine began her sexual life with her husband 3 years earlier (B), she was merely uninterested in sex. It was only with experience that she became intolerant of the very idea of sexual contact, from which we can infer criterion A3. (Three of the six criterion A requirements for FSIAD must be met.) Although she could face the prospect of no sex with equanimity, her husband couldn't, and that disparity was causing distress for them both; criterion C was thus satisfied.

Ernestine's clinician needed to ascertain that she had no other major disorder—such as **major depressive disorder, somatic symptom disorder**, or **obsessive–compulsive disorder**—that could explain her antipathy to sex (D). In the presence of any of these, she'd only receive the additional diagnosis of FSIAD if her sexual symptoms remained once the other pathology had been eliminated. Similar arguments would hold for substance use or another medical condition.

The Pagets were also having severe problems with other aspects of their marriage—enough to warrant mention as a spousal relationship problem. Her abhorrence of sexual contact could also meet the criteria for **specific phobia**; under the circumstances, however, no such additional diagnosis is necessary. In DSM-IV, Ernestine would have qualified for a diagnosis of sexual aversion disorder, but DSM-5 has eliminated it.

Ernestine's condition appears to have lasted throughout her sexual life. With our current information, we couldn't determine whether her disorder was generalized or situational. Although we suspect that something in her upbringing may lie at its roots, in DSM-5 we have no way to code this putative etiology. With a current GAF score of 61, her diagnosis would be as follows:

F52.22 [302.72]   Female sexual interest/arousal disorder, lifelong, severe
Z63.0 [V61.10]   Relationship distress with husband (emotional withdrawal)

Disorders of female sexual arousal and orgasm are often highly correlated. Among health care clinicians, you may encounter less than slavish adherence to the criteria used for these disorders.

F52.6 [302.76] Genito-Pelvic Pain/Penetration Disorder

Genito-pelvic pain/penetration disorder (GPD), new in DSM-5, subsumes the DSM-IV categories of dyspareunia and vaginismus, which were combined because they couldn't be discriminated reliably. The old terms will probably retain some currency as descriptors of particular types of discomfort.

Some women experience marked discomfort when attempting to have sexual intercourse. The pain may be experienced as a cramping contraction of the vaginal muscles (vaginismus) that may be described as an ache, a twinge, or a sharp pain. Anxiety can produce tension in the pelvic floor, with resulting pain severe enough to prevent consummation of a relationship (sometimes for years). Soon anxiety comes to replace sexual enjoyment. Some patients can't even use a tampon; a vaginal exam may require anesthesia.

Nearly a third of women who have had gynecological surgery will experience some degree of pain with intercourse. Infections, scars, and pelvic inflammatory disease have also been reported as causes. Don't diagnose GPD when pain is only a symptom of another medical condition or is due to substance misuse. What percentage of women will qualify for GPD remains unknown.

Two examples of this somewhat clumsily named condition follow.

Essential Features of **Genito-Pelvic Pain/Penetration Disorder**

A patient has major, repeated pain or other problems with efforts at vaginal intercourse; she may experience anxiety, fear, or pelvic muscle tension.

The Fine Print

The D's: • Duration (6+ months) • Distress to the patient • Differential diagnosis (substance use and physical disorders, relationship problems)

Coding Notes

Specify:

> {Lifelong}{Acquired}
> {Generalized}{Situational}

Specify severity: {Mild}{Moderate}{Severe}

Mildred Frank

Mildred Frank and her twin sister, Maxine Whalen (see next vignette), had been having problems with pain during intercourse. Their symptoms were different and quite personal, but they had always discussed everything with each other. Now they had made the joint decision to seek help. The gynecologist had referred them both to the mental health clinic.

"It's sort of a burning," was how Mildred described her difficulty. "When it's bad, it feels like your hands do if you're sliding down a rope. It's awful! Even if I use Vaseline, it still bothers me."

The referral letter noted that she'd had surgery for a prolapsed uterus but was otherwise healthy. "I could have told you that," she said. "I've never even been to a doctor, except to have my babies."

On close questioning, Mildred admitted that the pain didn't occur often. But during the past year or two she had always been afraid it would hurt, and that made her invariably tense up when she was having intercourse with her husband. She'd had some vaginal infections, but these had been largely under control during the last few months; the gynecologist didn't think that they caused the pain she complained of. The letter also noted that her physical exam had been completed easily, with no evidence of vaginal spasm.

"Maybe I do overreact," she said. "At least that's what my husband tells me. He says I'm too excitable, that I should just relax."

Evaluation of Mildred Frank

Many women have **sporadic pain with intercourse**, in which case diagnosis is usually not warranted. But for a couple of years (criterion B) Mildred had experienced pain, tensing, and fear; each was enough to qualify her for the form of GPD that was once known as dyspareunia (A2, A4, A3). Her distress was evident (C); as ever, the real problem is to rule out other causes first.

Mildred described herself as otherwise healthy, and her gynecologist made no mention of other **medical problems**. Although she had had some vaginal infections, the doctor felt that they couldn't completely account for her pain. Her clinician would have to determine that there was no **substance-induced disorder**, though this would seem unlikely. Sexual dysfunctions can be expected with a number of mental conditions (**anxiety, mood,** and **psychotic disorders**), but her history supports none of them as a possible cause. Painful intercourse famously occurs in patients with **somatic symptom disorder,** but Mildred claimed that she was otherwise healthy, which would greatly reduce the likelihood of this diagnosis. All of the foregoing factors should lay to rest our concern about other causes (D).

Although Mildred's pain with intercourse was acquired fairly recently and only occurred occasionally, it did cause her to seek treatment. She had had no partners other than her husband, though nothing in the vignette suggests that she would have fared better with someone else. Although insufficient symptoms were noted to warrant a **personality disorder**, her clinician should note in the chart any behaviors that seem to justify further investigation. I'd give her GAF score as 71.

F52.6 [302.76]   Genito-pelvic pain/penetration disorder, acquired, mild to moderate

---

In men, the symptom of painful intercourse is rare and almost always associated with some physical illnesses, such as Peyronie's disease (a lateral bend in an erect penis), prostatitis, or infections (for example, gonorrhea and herpes). It can cause an inability to complete penetration during sex—or fear that pain will occur. However, at least one study has reported that, contrary to expectation, men with a pelvic pain syndrome experience minimal impact on their interpersonal relationships; indeed, pain levels and good relationship adjustment were directly proportional. Such a situation would obviate a diagnosis of GPD, even if DSM-5 had been disposed to allow it in a man.

Maxine Whalen

Maxine Whalen and her twin sister, Mildred Frank (see preceding vignette), had both been having problems with pain during intercourse; as noted above, they made a joint decision to seek help. Finding no anatomical causes for either of them, the gynecologist had referred both to the mental health clinic.

Maxine wasn't married yet, and she didn't think she wanted to be. "It's not that I don't get horny," she explained. "And I love foreplay. I could do it all night. But every time a man has tried to enter me, something inside me clamps down like a trap. I couldn't even get a pencil inside, let alone a penis. I can't even use a tampon."

Maxine usually relieved her frustration by masturbating, which reliably produced a climax. Oral sex had also worked. "Not many men are likely to be satisfied with that for long," she remarked. "It makes me feel like a freak."

The spasms that contracted Maxine's vaginal muscles produced severe, cramping pain. They were so extreme that her gynecologist had to insert the speculum under general anesthesia. The exam revealed no physical abnormalities.

On her second visit, Maxine remembered something that Mildred apparently hadn't known. When the girls were 4, they had been molested in some way. Even Maxine wasn't sure exactly what had happened. She only knew that some man—she thought it might be the Uncle Max for whom she had been named—had taken the girls to a tavern, stood them on the bar, and allowed the other patrons to "play" with them.

Evaluation of Maxine Whalen

Maxine's lifelong (criterion B) history of severe pain and obstructed penetration (A1, A2—only one required) suggests the diagnosis. The fact that the spasm was reproduced by the attempted introduction of the gynecologist's speculum was diagnostic. Unless a patient is both unattached and content to refrain from intercourse, it is axiomatic that vaginal spasms will produce distress or interpersonal difficulty (C).

Maxine's history did not indicate that there had ever been a time since she became sexually active when she was free of vaginal spasm (B); therefore, we'd call it lifelong. It also occurred in a variety of contexts, so it was generalized rather than situational. Her gynecologist found no physical cause (no surprise there, since none are usually reported—D). Her GAF score would be 65.

In DSM-IV-TR, Maxine's diagnosis would have been vaginismus.

F52.6 [302.76]   Genito-pelvic pain/penetration disorder, lifelong, generalized, severe

F52.31 [302.73] Female Orgasmic Disorder

Achieving climax is a problem for a lot of women, though studies have been persistently inconsistent as to just what that means. Perhaps 30% of women report significant difficulties; 10% never learn the trick. A few physical illnesses, including hypothyroidism, diabetes, and structural damage to the vagina, can contribute to the condition; if judged to be exclusively the cause, they obviate the diagnosis of female orgasmic disorder (FOD). Orgasm can also be inhibited by medications such as antihypertensives, central nervous system stimulants, tricyclic antidepressants, and monoamine oxidase inhibitors. Possible psychological factors include fear of pregnancy, hostility of the patient toward her partner, and feeling guilty about sex in general. Age, previous sexual experience, and the adequacy of foreplay must also be considered in diagnosing FOD.

Once learned, a woman's ability to achieve orgasm persists, often improving throughout life. But women just don't complain of having premature orgasms, the way men do. Although it occurs (shown by surveys), it often doesn't pose a problem. Many women are able to enjoy sex without experiencing climax on a frequent basis. FOD is often comorbid with other sexual dysfunctions, especially female sexual interest/arousal disorder.

Essential Features of **Female Orgasmic Disorder**

A woman has been troubled by orgasms that are too slow, too rare, or too weak.

The Fine Print

For tips on identifying substance-related causation, see sidebar (p. 95).

The D's: • Duration (6+ months) • Distress to the patient • Differential diagnosis (substance use and physical disorders, problems in partner relationship)

Coding Notes

Specify if: **Never experienced an orgasm under any situation**

Specify:

   {Lifelong}{Acquired}
   {Generalized}{Situational}

Specify severity: {Mild}{Moderate}{Severe}

Rachel Atkins

"I don't think anyone has quite the understanding of *frustrating* that I do," Rachel Atkins said to her gynecologist.

Her early history was "a sociological nightmare." She was born to a 16-year-old high school dropout who had gone on to a lifetime of serial marriages and alcoholism. Beginning when she was in middle school, a series of stepfathers had molested Rachel until, when *she* was 16, she'd bolted—into prostitution.

"How ironic is that, escaping from sex by going on the game?" she asked. But she was lucky enough to avoid AIDS and, when she was 22, smart enough to jump at a chance at college, financed by a conscience-stricken former client.

As a sex worker, Rachel had experienced hundreds of men. "It wasn't as bad as you might think," she explained. "I could pick my own johns, and some of them I rather liked—not at all like Mom's collection of rats." One possible victim of her experiences was her orgasm, which had always been missing in action. "I always figured it'd be there when I really wanted it. Only it never was."

Now a university graduate solidly planted in the academic world (she taught anthropology at a college in her community), Rachel was nearing 30 and had a boyfriend who wanted to marry her. "He knows all about my past, and he's OK with it. But he wants me to come when we have sex. I think it would reassure him that he's different from all those others. I desperately want to please him, but there's just something missing in me. It's beyond distressing!"

Rachel loved the closeness she felt with Henry, and she lubricated well. "I just never quite get over the top. It's like when you think you're going to sneeze, you know? And instead, it just dissolves in your nose." She'd tried mood music, alcohol, marijuana, erotic literature, and clitoral stimulation. "But I could be digging pottery shards, for all the good any of it does."

Apart from the usual teenage experimentation and the brief "therapeutic" flirtation with white wine and marijuana, Rachel had used no drugs. Her general health was excellent, she said.

"I promised Henry I'd always be truthful with him, and I intend to keep that promise. So I refuse to fake it. I could, though—I've sure had practice!"

Just why women have orgasms isn't actually known. Of course, the reason for the male counterpart is obvious: Its absence would leave us bereft of males *or* females. One of the more popular theories is that it developed in parallel with the male orgasm, and there's just been no evolutionary pressure for it to go away. The author of *that* theory must have been a guy.

Discussion of Rachel Atkins

Rachel's problem wasn't lack of interest in sex—she looked forward to it with her boyfriend, and she lubricated normally during foreplay. Her difficulty was solely her inability to climax—ever (criterion B). If she had had occasional orgasms, or if she climaxed only with masturbation, she could still receive this diagnosis, according to DSM-5's criterion A1; low intensity of orgasm would also qualify (A2). There was no evidence that **other medical** or **mental conditions** or **substance use** contributed in the slightest (D). What she did have in abundance was distress (C).

Because she'd never experienced a climax, we should add that verbiage to her diagnosis (which obviates the other possible specifiers). Her GAF score would be rated very high (95) for any patient, because of her overall excellent adjustment. I would rate the severity of her FOD as only moderate, largely because of the composure and well-balanced approach to her life she showed during the discussion with her clinician.

F52.31 [302.73]   Female orgasmic disorder, never experienced an orgasm under any situation, moderate

Substance/Medication-Induced Sexual Dysfunction

As with physical illness, a variety of psychoactive substances can affect the sexual abilities of men and women. Note that you would substitute the diagnosis of substance/medication-induced sexual dysfunction for a specific substance intoxication diagnosis only when the patient's problems in that area exceed those you would expect in the usual course of substance intoxication.

On average, perhaps half of patients taking antipsychotic and antidepressant drugs will report sexual side effects, though these will not always reach the level of clinical significance. Users of street drugs also often have sexual side effects, though they may complain less, since they may value their drug of choice more highly than sex.

The vast number of possible expressions has persuaded me not to include a vignette for this section.

Essential Features of **Substance/Medication-Induced Sexual Dysfunction**

Substance use appears to have caused sexual dysfunction.

The Fine Print

The D's: • Distress to the patient • Differential diagnosis (physical disorders, delirium, primary sexual disorders)

You'd only make this diagnosis when the symptoms are serious enough to warrant clinical attention *and* they are worse than you'd expect from ordinary intoxication or withdrawal.

Coding Notes

When writing down the diagnosis, use the exact substance in the title: For example, alcohol-induced sexual dysfunction.

ICD-9 kept coding simple: 292.89 for alcohol, 292.89 for all other substances. For coding in ICD-10, refer to Table 15.2 in Chapter 15.

Specify if:

With onset during {intoxication}{withdrawal}. This gets tacked on at the end of your string of words.
With onset after medication use. You can use this in addition to other specifiers.

Specify severity:

Mild. Dysfunction in 25–50% of sexual encounters.
Moderate. 50–75% of encounters.
Severe. 75% or more.

F52.8 [302.79] Other Specified Sexual Dysfunction

F52.9 [302.70] Unspecified Sexual Dysfunction

Use one or the other of these categories for patients whose sexual dysfunctions don't qualify for any of the specific sets of criteria spelled out above. Such conditions would include those for whom you conclude that there is a sexual problem, but one of the following obtains:

Atypical symptoms. The symptoms are mixed, atypical, or below threshold for a defined sexual disorder.

Uncertain cause.

Insufficient information.

As usual, the other specified designation should be used in cases where you choose to state the reasons for not assigning one of the other diagnoses described in this chapter; the unspecified designation should be used when you do not so choose.

CHAPTER 13

Gender Dysphoria

Quick Guide to Gender Dysphoria

As in earlier chapters, the page number following each item indicates where a more detailed discussion begins.

Primary Gender Dysphoria

Gender dysphoria in adolescents or adults. Patients strongly identify with the gender other than their own assigned gender role, with which they are uncomfortable. Some request sex reassignment surgery to relieve this discomfort (p. 372).

Gender dysphoria in children. Children as young as 3 or 4 years can be dissatisfied with their assigned gender (p. 374).

Other specified, or unspecified, gender dysphoria. Use one of these categories for gender dysphoria symptoms that do not meet full diagnostic criteria (p. 377).

Other Causes of Transgender Dissatisfaction or Behavior

Schizophrenia. Some patients with schizophrenia will express the delusion of being the other gender (p. 64).

Transvestic disorder. These people have sexual urges related to cross-dressing, but do not wish to be of the other gender (p. 583).

F64.1 [302.85] Gender Dysphoria in Adolescents and Adults

Adult patients with gender dysphoria (GD) feel intensely uncomfortable with their own assigned gender (sometimes called *natal gender*). Some actually detest their own genitalia. They wish to live as members of the other gender, and many of them do adopt opposite-gender dress and mannerisms. Cross-dressing (though not for sexual stimulation) is a common first step toward a complete gender change. Next, they may request to take hormones to stop menstruation, enlarge their breasts, suppress male characteristics, or otherwise change their body appearance or functioning.

A few persons with GD feel so uncomfortable with their nominal, assigned gender that they request hormone treatment or reassignment surgery. Although many patients who have such surgery are reportedly satisfied and live contentedly in their new gender, some ultimately request to change back. A few genetic males retain their genitals but have their breasts augmented chemically or through surgery.

GD, popularly still referred to as *transsexualism* (though far from all patients with GD desire sex reassignment measures), is one of the more recently described disorders in DSM-5. Until the 1950s, clinicians did not even recognize the existence of people with GD. It was through the widespread publicity that occurred in 1952, after Christine Jorgensen received sex reassignment surgeries in Denmark and emerged as a woman, that this disorder became generally acknowledged. Even now, GD is relatively infrequent (around 1% for natal males and perhaps one-third that for females). It begins in early childhood (typically, preschool) and appears to be chronic. Causation isn't known for sure. However, there is evidence support at least a weak genetic component.

Many natal males with GD have low sex drive; if they engage in sex at all, most prefer men. Nearly all affected women are sexually attracted to women.

Posttransition Specifier

The *posttransition* specifier indicates that the patient now lives exclusively as a person of the desired gender and has undergone (or is undergoing) one or more cross-sex medical procedures. These would include regimens such as regular cross-sex hormone treatments and gender reassignment surgery to the desired gender. Surgery would entail orchiectomy, penectomy, and vaginoplasty in a genetic male, mastectomy and phalloplasty in a genetic female.

Army Private First Class Bradley Manning was convicted in 2013 of the WikiLeaks publication of 700,000 documents. The day after he was sentenced to 35 years in prison, he announced that he wanted hormone therapy and wished to live the rest of his life as a female, Chelsea Manning.

Michelle Kosilek has languished for the past 20 years in a Massachusetts prison, sentenced for killing her wife during a domestic dispute (despite nearly life-long gender dysphoric issues, when married, Michelle still occupied her natal gender). Five specialists have recommended sex change surgery.

The lives of these two people highlight how far we have come in recognizing this fraught condition, and how far we have yet to go.

F64.2 [302.6] Gender Dysphoria in Children

In the general population, a small percentage of boys (1–2%)—and a smaller still percentage of girls—want to be of the other gender. It's mainly boys who are ever referred for clinical evaluation, probably because parents worry more about an effeminate son than about a tomboy daughter. Although cross-gender behaviors often begin by age 3, the typical child isn't referred until years later.

Exactly what behaviors are we talking about? From a very young age, these children know they are different. Boys prefer playing with dolls, assuming a female role in play, cross-dressing, and especially associating with a peer group of girls. Girls with GD take the male role in family games and strongly reject female activities such as playing with dolls. Of course, all such children, boys particularly, risk teasing, bullying, and other forms of peer rejection. The 2011 book *Transition*, which describes the childhood struggle with his own gender identity, recounts Chaz (née Chastity) Bono's anguish when the development of breasts and onset of menses during puberty caused both physical and emotional torment.

Of course, GD isn't the only possible explanation for behavior that is "different": some boys just don't like sports or rough games, and some girls, perceiving social advantages in being male, prefer boys' clothing. And, sure enough, follow-up studies of children who had been clinically referred for GD behavior find that, by their late teenage years, most will no longer qualify for a formal diagnosis. On average, those who still are affected (*persisters*, as they are sometimes termed) had had as children a greater degree of GD. Girls are somewhat more likely than boys to remain dysphoric.

It is far more common for boys with GD to grow up to become gay men than to have GD; a minority become normally heterosexual; perhaps a few have GD as adults (though the studies vary tremendously as regards percentage). The rate of persisters among natal females is higher, but still well under 50%. Ultimate diagnosis in children or adolescents may require prolonged evaluation.

The case vignette of Billie Worth below contains a lot of information that illustrates GD, both in children and in adults.

Essential Features of **Gender Dysphoria**

In Adolescents or Adults

There is a marked disparity between nominal (natal) gender and what the patient experiences as a sense of self. This can be expressed as a rejection or wish not to have one's own sex characteristics or to have those of the other gender. The patient might also express the desire to belong to the other gender and to be treated as though that were the case. Some patients believe that their responses are typical of the other gender.

In Children

The characteristics of GD in children are similar to those in adults, but manifest themselves in age-appropriate ways. So, in their powerful longing to be the opposite gender, kids may insist that's what they *are*; they prefer clothing, toys, games, playmates, and fantasy roles of the other gender while rejecting their own; and they may say that they hate their own genitalia and want that which they don't have. Note that in children, the number of criteria required (six out of eight) is far greater than for adults (two of six); this is a protective device for persons who have not yet fully matured.

The Fine Print

The D's: • Duration (6+ months, regardless of age) • Distress or disability (work/educational, social, or personal impairment) • Differential diagnosis (substance use and physical disorders, psychotic disorders, body dysmorphic disorder, and [in adolescents/adults] transvestic disorder)

Coding Notes

Specify if:

With a disorder of sex development (and code the actual congenital developmental disorder)

Posttransition (for adolescents/adults). The patient is living in the desired gender and has had at least one cross-gender surgical procedure or medical treatment (such as a hormone regimen).

The addition of the posttransition specifier addresses the fact that patients who have undergone procedures to achieve their desired gender will no longer meet the criteria for GD; yet they continue to pursue psychotherapy, hormonal treatment, or other remedies for the condition with which they were once diagnosed.

Billie Worth

"I just want to get rid of it. All of it." For the third time that day, Billie Worth explained his feelings. He wasn't depressed or melodramatic. Patiently, quietly, he stated the facts.

One of his earliest memories was of watching an actress on TV. When she walked, she brushed her hand against her skirt, so it appeared to dance. He had tried to imitate that walk, to the delight and applause of his mother. His father had for years been imprisoned for forgery.

When he was 6, Billie discovered that playing with cap pistols and spaceships like the other boys gave him a violent headache. He preferred a Barbie doll that another child had discarded in a dumpster, and he chose his playmates, insofar as he was able, from neighborhood girls who were his age. When playing house, he would insist that one of them be "the dad."

When he was a baby, his 6-year-old sister, Marsha, had died of meningitis. Billie's mother had kept Marsha's room just as it had been when she died. Some of his happiest childhood afternoons were spent donning Marsha's dresses and sitting on her bed with Barbie. Sometimes, wishing he were a girl, he pretended to be Marsha. He continued to wedge his feet into her black patent leather shoes until long after he had grown too big for them.

In his early teens, about the age that adolescents begin to think seriously about themselves, he realized that in fact he *was* a girl. "It suddenly struck me that the only masculine thing about me was these revolting things between my legs," he much later told one of his clinicians. Claiming to have chronic asthma, he persuaded a physician to excuse him from gym class throughout his 4 years of high school. Although he was a good swimmer, his abhorrence of the locker room prevented him from trying out for the team. He took shorthand and home economics (four semesters of each). He did join the science club, which was about as asexual a club as he could find. One year he entered a project in the science fair on the use of various yeasts in baking bread.

When Billie was 16, he bought his first bra and panties with money he had earned babysitting. When he put them on for the first time, he could feel some of the tension drain out of him. Although he sometimes wore his lingerie to school, he didn't begin cross-dressing in earnest until he started college. Because he lived off campus, he had the privacy in which to experiment with skirts, blouses, and makeup. A sympathetic physician provided him with estrogens, and in his junior year he changed the spelling of his name and began to live as a woman.

Two years out of college, Billie requested sex reassignment surgery. She had had several gay male lovers—unsatisfying experiences, because she did not consider herself to be homosexual. "I'm not a gay man; I feel that I'm a straight woman." By now, thanks to hormones, she had small though well-developed breasts; her penis and testicles "just get in the way." She wanted to be rid of them, and told the examining clinician that if necessary, she would have the job done in Mexico.

Evaluation of Billie Worth

Billie's early realization that he somehow didn't fit in with the other boys is typical of children with GD. He showed this by several sorts of behaviors, which constitute the principal childhood indicators of this diagnosis when it is made in children: Pretending to be Marsha, he wished he were a girl (criterion A1). He preferred wearing his sister's dress and shoes (A2). Preferring a cross-gender role for himself, he assigned girls to play the dad (A3) He rejected boys' games (A6) and preferred girls' play (A4), and he preferred playing with girls (A5).

As an adult, he met several of the DSM-5 symptomatic criteria. He voiced a profound incongruence between his natal and preferred gender (A1), a desire to be a woman (A4) and be rid of his genitalia (A2), a wish to have breasts and a vagina (A3), and the conviction that he had the characteristics of a straight woman (A6). He needed only two of these to fulfill the DSM-5 criteria.

Billie's full realization that he had been born the wrong sex didn't come until adolescence. At about that time, he began a progression—first dressing as a female, then living as a female and taking hormones—culminating in the request for sex reassignment surgery. Although the vignette does not specify that no intersex condition was present, neither does it contain any information that would suggest such a condition. (Not that it matters: DSM-5 allows patients with a disorder of sex development to be diagnosed with GD. Such a person would receive an additional specifier.) Throughout his childhood, adolescence, and into his adult life, Billie's distress was way beyond "clinical significance."

The differential diagnosis of GD includes **schizophrenia**, in which the patient may occasionally have delusions of being the opposite sex. Billie showed no evidence of delusions, hallucinations, or any other typical symptoms. The absence of sexual excitement as a reaction to cross-dressing would rule out **transvestic disorder**, though some patients with GD initially have this paraphilia.

Many (perhaps most) patients with GD also have an associated personality disorder, such as **borderline** or **narcissistic personality disorder**. (This may be less often true of natal female patients with GD.) No evidence of any personality disorder is presented in the vignette, though Billie's clinician should search diligently for such pathology, which can strongly influence the management and outcome of this condition. A note in the summary would be an important reminder not to forget this step. As you might expect, **anxiety** and **mood disorders** are also common associated features. **Use of substances** (alcohol and/or street drugs) may also be a factor, especially in natal female patients.

Billie's diagnosis at the time of evaluation (GAF score of 71) would read as follows:

F64.1 [302.85]   Gender dysphoria in an adult

Had he been interviewed as a child, he would have fully met even the rather restrictive DSM-5 criteria for children:

F64.2 [302.6]   Gender dysphoria in children

F64.8 [302.6] Other Specified Gender Dysphoria

Here you could include a patient who has met GD criteria for less than the 6-month minimum.

F64.9 [302.6] Unspecified Gender Dysphoria

Use unspecified GD for cases of GD symptoms that do not meet full diagnostic criteria and about which you do not wish to be more specific.

CHAPTER 14

Disruptive, Impulse-Control, and Conduct Disorders

Quick Guide to the Disruptive, Impulse-Control, and Conduct Disorders

As usual, the page number following each item indicates where a more detailed discussion begins.

Primary Disruptive, Impulse-Control, and Conduct Disorders

Conduct disorder. A child persistently violates rules or the rights of others (p. 381).

Conduct disorder, with limited prosocial emotions. Use the *with limited prosocial emotions* specifier for children whose disordered conduct is callous and disruptive, showing no remorse and no regard for the feelings of others (p. 383).

Oppositional defiant disorder. Multiple examples of negativistic behavior persist for at least 6 months (p. 380).

Intermittent explosive disorder. With no other demonstrable pathology (psychological or general medical), these patients have episodes during which they act out aggressively. As a result, they physically harm others or destroy property (p. 384).

Kleptomania. An irresistible urge to steal things they don't need causes these patients to do so repeatedly. The phrase "tension and release" characterizes this behavior (p. 390).

Pyromania. Fire setters feel "tension and release" in regard to the behavior of starting fires (p. 387).

Antisocial personality disorder. The irresponsible, often criminal behavior of people with antisocial personality disorder (ASPD) begins in childhood or early adolescence with truancy, running away, cruelty, fighting, destructiveness, lying, and theft. In addition to criminal behavior, as adults they may default on debts, or otherwise show irresponsibility; act recklessly or impulsively; and show no remorse for their behavior. DSM-5 actually includes ASPD in this chapter, though it gives the symptoms in detail with those of the other personality disorders (p. 541).

Other specified, or unspecified, disruptive, impulse-control, and conduct disorder. Use one of these categories for disturbances of conduct or oppositional behaviors that do not meet the criteria for other disorders covered in this group (p. 392).

Other Disorders Associated with Disruptive or Impulsive Behavior

Trichotillomania (hair-pulling disorder). Pulling hair from various parts of the body is often accompanied by feelings of "tension and release" (p. 210).

Paraphilic disorders. Some people (nearly always males) have recurrent sexual urges involving a variety of behaviors that are objectionable to others. They may act upon these urges in order to obtain pleasure (p. 564).

Substance-related disorders. There is often an impulsive component to the misuse of various substances (p. 396).

Bipolar I disorder. Patients with bipolar I may steal, gamble, act out violently, and engage in other socially undesirable behaviors, though this happens only during an acute manic episode (p. 129).

Schizophrenia. In response to hallucinations or delusions, patients with schizophrenia may impulsively engage in a variety of illegal or otherwise ill-advised behaviors (p. 64).

Disruptive mood dysregulation disorder. A child's mood is persistently negative between frequent, severe explosions of temper (p. 149).

Child or adolescent antisocial behavior. This code (Z72.810 [V71.02]) can be useful when antisocial behavior in a young person cannot be ascribed to a mental disorder such as oppositional defiant disorder or conduct disorder (p. 593).

Adult antisocial behavior. This code (Z72.811 [V71.01]) is used to describe activities by an adult that are illegal, but do not occur in the context of mental disorder (p. 593).

Introduction

This section considers conditions that in other professions might elicit a value judgment of "bad behavior." Fortunately, we have the luxury of not having to judge them; rather, we can study them from the standpoints of understanding why they occur and learning how to ameliorate them.

These disorders entail problems with the regulation of behavior and emotions. The behaviors in question may occur on the spur of the moment, or they may be planned; some are accompanied by efforts to resist. The acts themselves are often illegal, with consequent injury to the perpetrator or to others.

Each disorder in its own way brings the patient into conflict with what we understand as social norms. In each, males predominate; all typically start in childhood or adolescence. Sometimes there is a progression—for instance, from oppositional defiant disorder (ODD) to conduct disorder (CD) to ASPD. However, we must not draw the mistaken conclusion that having one foot on the pathway means eventual arrival at the end of the trail. In fact, the majority of patients with ODD do not go on to develop CD, just as most patients with CD do not progress to ASPD. Still, in an important minority of patients, there is that developmental arc.

I usually put child diagnoses toward the end of each chapter. Here I'm going to break my rule, in order to underscore the (occasional) march from one disorder to the next.

F91.3 [313.81] Oppositional Defiant Disorder

ODD ushers in a triad of disorders spanning a spectrum of behavior from resistance that is barely outside the expected to acts that are execrable. ODD itself can be relatively mild, with symptoms of negativism and defiance that seem to grow out of any child's normal quest for independence. On the one hand, they are distinguished from normal opposition by severity and duration; on the other, they are distinguished from the more problematic CD by the fact that children with ODD don't violate the basic rights of others or age-appropriate societal rules.

The symptoms of ODD first show up around age 3 or 4; diagnosis is typically made a few years later. Younger children will show oppositional behavior almost every day, whereas for older children the frequency tends to decline. The effects are worst at home, though relationships with teachers and peers can also be affected. Younger age and more severe symptoms at onset predict a worse outcome. DSM-5 does caution us to consider possible modifying factors such as developmental age, culture, and gender; it notes that symptoms *must* occur with people other than siblings.

Though ODD runs in families, genetic relationships are not certain. Some authorities attribute ODD to discipline that is harsh and inconsistent, others to imitation of parental behavior. Low socioeconomic status may contribute through the stress of living at or near the poverty line.

Along with CD, ODD is among the most common reasons for referral to mental health professionals. It affects about 3% of all children (boys predominate), with a broad range, depending on the study, of 1–16%. When it does occur in girls, its expression may be at once more verbal and less obvious; predictions made from its diagnosis may be less robust than for boys.

Over half of those who initially meet ODD criteria will not do so several years later. However, CD will develop later in about a third of patients, especially those whose ODD begins early and coexists with attention-deficit/hyperactivity disorder (ADHD; these diagnoses are strongly comorbid). Perhaps 10% will eventually be diagnosed with ASPD. The irritable mood symptoms of ODD predict later anxiety and depression; defiance symptoms point toward CD.

ODD can be diagnosed in an adult, and sometimes it is: It has been reported in 12–50% of adults with ADHD. However, in adults the symptoms of ODD may be obscured by other disorders, or they may appear to constitute a personality disorder.

Essential Features of **Oppositional Defiant Disorder**

These patients are often angry and irritable, tending toward touchiness and hair-trigger temper. They will disobey authority figures or argue with them, and they may refuse to cooperate or follow rules—if only to annoy. They sometimes accuse others of their own misdeeds; some appear malicious.

The Fine Print

The D's: • Duration and demographics (6+ months—more or less daily for age 5 and under; weekly for older children) • Distress (patient or others) or disability (educational/work, social, or personal impairment) • Differential diagnosis (substance use disorders, ADHD, psychotic or mood disorders, disruptive mood dysregulation disorder, ordinary childhood growth and development)

Coding Notes

Specify severity:

> **Mild.** Symptoms occur in only 1 location (home, school, with friends).
> **Moderate.** Some symptoms in 2+ locations.
> **Severe.** Symptoms in 3+ locations.

Conduct Disorder

From as early as 2 years of age, boys normally display more aggressive behavior than do girls. Even beyond this, however, aggressive breaking of rules dominates the behavior of a substantial minority of children. For some patients, the symptoms of CD may represent only an extreme expression of normal efforts to differentiate themselves from their parents. But note that most CD symptoms, whether they occur in the juvenile years or later, are quite serious and can lead to arrest or other legal consequences. CD is defined in part by the degree to which a child's family, social, or scholastic life becomes affected by such behavior. That can happen as early as age 5 or 6.

DSM-5's 15 listed behaviors constitute four categories: (1) aggression, (2) destruction, (3) lying and theft, and (4) rule violation. Just 3 of the 15 symptoms suffice for diagnosis (they need not be spread across multiple categories). With these criteria, 6–16% of boys will score positive for CD; for girls, prevalence is perhaps half that. Imputed causes include the environment (large families, neglect, abuse) and genetics (substance use, CD, ADHD, psychosis).

About 80% of children diagnosed as having CD have previously had ODD. (In fact, some writers question whether ODD and CD are two disorders or one.) But what we really want to know is this: To what degree will such behavior persist into adolescence and beyond?

Children who are highly aggressive by age 7 or 8 are at risk for a serious and constant antisocial/aggressive lifestyle. They are three times as likely as other children to have police records as adults. Indeed, the age of onset—before versus at or after age 10 years—confers enough predictive power that we are encouraged to state it as a specifier. Those with earlier onset (mostly boys) are more likely to be aggressive; half of them will progress to a diagnosis of ASPD. Later onset predicts an outcome less fraught. Girls with early-onset CD are less likely than boys to develop ASPD; rather, they may develop somatic symptom disorder, suicidal behavior, social and occupational problems, or other emotional disorders.

What about CD in adults? As with ODD, the diagnosis is at least theoretically possible, but it is far more likely that an adult will have some other disorder that will obscure the CD symptoms.

Milo Tark's early history (p. 543) illustrates some of the symptoms of CD; Dudley Langenegger's early history (p. 437) included a few of its elements.

Essential Features of **Conduct Disorder**

In various ways, these people chronically disrespect rules and other people's rights. Most egregiously, they use aggression against their peers (and sometimes elders)—bullying, starting fights, using dangerous weapons, showing cruelty to people or animals, even sexual abuse. They may intentionally set fires or otherwise destroy property; breaking and entering, lying, and theft are well within their repertoires. Truancy, repeated runaways, and refusal against a parent's wishes to come home at night round out their bag of tricks.

The Fine Print

The D's: • Duration (symptoms occurring within 1 year, with 1+ symptoms in past 6 months) • Disability (educational/work, social, or personal impairment) • Differential diagnosis (ADHD, ODD, mood disorders, ordinary childhood growth and development, ASPD, intermittent explosive disorder)

Coding Notes

Based on age of onset, specify:

> **F91.1 [312.81] Childhood-onset type.** At least one problem with conduct begins before age 10.
> **F91.2 [312.82] Adolescent-onset type.** No problems with conduct before age 10.
> **F91.9 [312.89] Unspecified onset.** Insufficient information.

Specify severity:

> **Mild.** Has sufficient, but not a lot of symptoms, and harm to others is minimal.
> **Moderate.** Symptoms and harm to others are intermediate.
> **Severe.** Many symptoms, much harm to others.

Specify if:

> **With limited prosocial emotions.** See separate discussion below.

With Limited Prosocial Emotions Specifier for Conduct Disorder

The above-described criteria for CD address the behavior of these patients. The specifier *with limited prosocial emotions* asks us to engage with the emotional underpinnings of—or reactions to—that behavior.

CD behavior can take either of two forms. In one, the patient has trouble regulating powerful, angry, hostile emotions. These children tend to come from dysfunctional families that are prone to physical abuse. They are likely to be rejected by their peers, leading to aggression, playing truant, and associating with delinquents.

Rather than possessing emotions such as anger and hostility, a minority of patients with CD lack something—empathy and guilt. These children tend to use others for their own gain. With low anxiety levels and the tendency to become easily bored, they prefer activities that are novel, exciting, even dangerous. As a result, they typically report the four symptoms mentioned in the specifier *with limited prosocial emotions*.

That is, they *might* report the four specifier symptoms. However, candor isn't necessarily the strong suit of these young people, who are loath to reveal personal feelings (and much about behavior). So it's more important than ever to seek collateral sources of information.

Reading the prototype, you can see why this is sometimes called the *callous unemotional* type of CD, from which the specifier was renamed because the older label sounded so pejorative. (Use of the CD diagnosis has fallen off in recent years, anyway, partly because *it* is stigmatizing.) Call it what you will, this subtype of CD predicts an adolescence with more severe, persistent problems of conduct.

Essential Features of **With Limited Prosocial Emotions Specifier for Conduct Disorder**

Such patients lack important emotional underpinnings. They have a callous absence of empathy (that is, they are without concern for the emotions or suffering of others). They tend to have limited affect and little remorse or guilt (other than regret if caught). They are indifferent to the quality of their own performance.

The Fine Print

To receive the specifier, these symptoms must be experienced within the past year.

With DSM-5 criteria, you can't code a patient with CD as ***without*** *limited prosocial emotions.* I think this is a mistake—one that clinicians can, and should, correct. There's no special code number attached to the *with limited prosocial emotions* designation. It's only verbiage you tack onto the diagnosis. So for any patient with CD, you can add "With limited prosocial emotions" or "Without limited prosocial emotions." The double negative conveys valuable information about the patient, whatever the severity status. (Well, I'm assuming that everyone knows what *prosocial* signifies, or even means.)

F60.2 [301.7] Antisocial Personality Disorder

Last on the path that often connects with ODD and CD comes ASPD, which is more or less the culmination of aggressive, destructive behavior that sets all of society against such patients—whom we soon begin to call *perpetrators*. However, I'll follow DSM-5's lead and defer presentation to its *other* proper place—along with the other personality disorders in Chapter 17 (p. 541).

F63.81 [312.34] Intermittent Explosive Disorder

Whatever you might think of intermittent explosive disorder (IED), it is a condition with a long pedigree. Although it wasn't listed per se in the first DSM (published in 1952), the concept was there all right, hiding in plain sight on page 36. There it masqueraded as *passive–aggressive personality, aggressive type*, whose symptoms were "persistent reaction to frustration with irritability, temper tantrums, and destructive behavior…" In DSM-II it was called *explosive personality*, which by DSM-III in 1980 had morphed into the familiar IED.

With such a long history, it is surprising that proper investigation has taken so long to begin. It's enough to make a person angry. Really, really angry.

People with IED have periods of aggression that begin suddenly (the classic "hair-trigger temper") on little or no provocation. The stimulus may be quite benign—an off-hand comment from a friend, an accidental bump from a passerby on the sidewalk—and all hell breaks loose. The form the particular hell takes may be only verbal, but actual physical violence is a possibility. In either case, the situation may rapidly escalate, sometimes to the point where the individual completely loses control. The whole episode rarely lasts longer than half an hour, and may end with the person's expressing remorse. Or posting bail.

Patients with IED are mostly young males, and many are relatively undereducated (less than a high school diploma). The condition affects as many as 7% of Americans lifetime (2% in the previous month); the figures are higher for young people and for those whose education stopped with high school. Reported rates are considerably lower in other countries.

Up to a third of first-degree relatives also have IED; some authorities suggest a strong genetic component. But a history of childhood trauma is also higher in patients with IED than in comparison groups.

IED comes attended by other mental conditions, including substance use, mood, and anxiety disorders. The IED usually begins first, by a substantial number of years. (Clinicians note that in the case of patients with bipolar I disorder, it is important to make the IED diagnosis only when the patient is not in an episode of mania.) What's important about this is that we should vigorously attempt to rule out all other possible causes of explosive episodes before diagnosing this disorder.

Essential Features of **Intermittent Explosive Disorder**

The patient has frequent, repeated, spontaneous outbursts of aggression (verbal or physical without damage) *or* less frequent physical eruptions with harm to people, property, or animals. These outbursts are unplanned, have no goal, and are excessive for the provocation.

The Fine Print

The D's: • Duration (aggression without harm 2 times a week for 3 months, *or* aggression with harm 3 times in past year) • Demographics (the patient is 6+ years old, or the developmental equivalent) • Distress or disability (work/educational, social, or personal impairment) • Differential diagnosis (substance use and physical disorders, cognitive disorders, mood disorders, personality disorders, ordinary anger; adjustment disorder for children under age 18; disruptive mood dysregulation disorder)

The use of dual tickets of admission for IED (relatively benign "aggression" twice a week for 3 months vs. harmful "assault" three times in a year) is something new in DSM-5 for this disorder. In fact, it's something new in any DSM for *any* disorder—no other condition features intensity-based versus frequency-based dual qualifiers. Of course, the criteria for nearly every disorder allow for differing degrees of severity, but then they are stated in terms of numbers of criteria met, or the quality or frequency or duration of criteria that are demonstrated. The way it's stated here, IED occupies a niche unique in the diagnostic spectrum.

The justification for this duality is the observation that there are basically two patterns of outbursts (high-intensity/low-frequency and the reverse), and that limiting the definition to one group omits from consideration a considerable proportion of patients who repeatedly have problems related to their aggressive impulses. In actuality, patients with IED may mix the two patterns of behavior.

DSM-5 assures us that, regardless of which pattern a patient shows at intake, outcome and response to treatment will be roughly the same. Isn't it odd, though, that we aren't encouraged to add some sort of specifier that would tell the world just which bar the patient cleared to gain admittance? Frankly, I think it's another bull's-eye for prototypes, another black eye for fussy criteria.

Liam O'Brian

From the time he was a teenager, Liam O'Brian had had a flash-point temper. He had been suspended from 10th grade for using a pair of scissors to assault a classmate who had teased him about wearing the wrong colors on "Clash Day." The following year the police had visited him for breaking a headlamp on the car belonging to the baseball coach, who had called him "out" in a close play at home plate. After he paid for the headlamp, charges were dropped; the coach noted that Liam was "basically a good kid with too much red hair." That year a neurologist reported that his physical exam, EEG, and MRI were all normal.

During his first few years of school, Liam had had difficulty sitting still in class and concentrating on his schoolwork. By the time he entered junior high, these behaviors were no longer a problem. In fact, he earned mostly B's and A's, and in the 2- to 4-month intervals between explosive episodes he was "no more trouble than the average kid," as Liam himself reported to the interviewer.

Following Liam's graduation from high school, his pattern of periodic temper flareups continued pretty much unchanged. After he was fired from two successive jobs for fighting with coworkers, he joined the Army. Within 6 weeks he had received a badconduct discharge for assaulting his first sergeant with a bayonet. Each of these incidents had been triggered by a trivial disagreement or an exchange of words that could hardly be called provocation. Liam said afterwards that he felt bad about his behavior; even the targets of his attacks usually agreed that he "wasn't mean, only touchy."

Liam was now 25, and his most recent evaluation had been ordered by a judge.

Liam had been arrested by an off-duty policewoman in a supermarket. He had pushed her after she dumped 15 cans of tuna onto the carousel in the express checkout line. The usual examinations, X-rays, and EEG (this time with esophageal leads and sleep recordings) revealed no pathology. He denied ever having delusions or hallucinations. His father, he said, used to rough up his mother when he was drinking, so Liam had always been afraid to try alcohol or drugs himself.

Liam denied ever having extreme swings of mood, but he did express regret for his unpredictable, explosive behavior. "I just want to get a handle on it," he said. "I'm afraid I just might kill someone, and I'm not mad at anyone."

Evaluation of Liam O'Brian

Liam had a history of many outbursts over a period of at least 10 years (criterion A2). The facts of his behavior would not be the issue here; he easily met the requirements for age (E), frequency, disproportionate rage (B), consequences (marked distress, D) and lack of premeditation (C). Rather, a clinician evaluating Liam should carefully search for evidence of other diagnoses that might merit precedence for treatment (F).

Liam's mood showed no evidence of either mania or depression, effectively ruling out temper flare-ups that could be associated with a **mood disorder**. At wide intervals he had had two neurological evaluations, neither of which revealed evidence for **seizures**. He never touched **drugs** or **alcohol**, and he denied symptoms of **psychosis**. The presence of any such underlying medical disorder might suggest a **personality change due to another medical condition**, but there was no evidence of this, either.

Patients with **antisocial personality disorder** will often act out violently and unpredictably, but, unlike Liam, they do not feel remorse afterwards. Neither did he show the manipulation, deceit, and callousness that are required by DSM-5 for ASPD. Patients with **borderline personality disorder** will sometimes have temper outbursts and engage in fights, but the generic criteria for personality disorder (p. 531) urge us first to rule out other mental disorders. I'd give Liam a GAF score of 51 and this diagnosis:

F63.81 [312.34]   Intermittent explosive disorder

F63.1 [312.33] Pyromania

As with the relationship of kleptomania to shoplifting, pyromania accounts for only a small minority of fire setters. Only when there is a typical history of yielding with relief to an irresistible impulse can the diagnosis be sustained.

At least 80% of these people are male; often the behavior begins in childhood. With their interest in various aspects of fire, they will turn in false alarms, appear as spectators at fires, or collect the apparatus used by firefighters. They may even serve as volunteer firefighters, thereby becoming their own best customers.

Although pyromania is classified as an impulse-control disorder, these patients may make advance preparations, such as searching out a site and collecting combustibles. They may also leave clues, almost as if they want to be identified and apprehended. Fire setters may have low self-esteem and reportedly often have problems getting along with peers. Look for coexisting CD, ASPD, substance misuse, and anxiety disorders in these people.

As a free-standing diagnosis, pyromania is probably rare, with (again) more instances reported in males.

Essential Features of **Pyromania**

These patients deliberately set multiple fires, but without motivation for profit, revenge, an act of terrorism, or other gain. Rather, theirs is a general interest in fire and its appurtenances (fire trucks, the exciting aftermath). Such patients feel tense or excited before starting the fire, and experience a sense of release or pleasure afterwards.

The Fine Print

The D's: • Differential diagnosis (mood and psychotic disorders, CD, delirium or dementia, intellectual disability, ordinary criminal behavior)

Elwood Telfer

Elwood Telfer's earliest childhood memory was of a candle burning on the kitchen table. He would kneel on a chair as his mother sat in the dark and waited for his father to come home. His father drank, so they often waited a very long time. Periodically, she would put a strand of her own hair into the flame, sending a curl of acrid smoke spiraling toward the ceiling.

"Maybe it's why I've always been fascinated by fire," Elwood told a forensic examiner when he was 27. "I even have a big collection of firefighting memorabilia—old helmets, a badge from an 1896 fire brigade, and so on. I get them at antique shows."

Elwood had set his first fire when he was only 7. He had found an old Zippo lighter that still had enough flint, and he used it on an oily rag that was lying in a hay field. About a quarter-acre burned in the 20 exhilarating minutes before the fire trucks arrived to put it out. He always remembered the day's excitement as being well worth the beating his father had administered, once he'd sobered up.

Elwood set most of his fires in fields or vacant lots. Once or twice he had torched an abandoned house, after first making sure that no one, not even a transient, could be inside. "I never wanted to hurt anyone," he told the examiner. "It's the warmth and the color of the flame and the excitement I like. I'm not mad at anybody."

Elwood had hardly ever had friends. When he entered high school, he was over-joyed to learn that there was a club called the Fire Squad. When he inquired about joining, two upperclassmen laughed and told him that it was an honorary group you could only belong to if you had lettered in football. Elwood felt almost sick with disap-pointment. That evening he started a small brush fire that consumed a neighbor's tool shed. It was the first time he noticed the healing effect of fire.

Months might go by when he was inactive and calm. Then he would spot a field or empty building that seemed right, and the tension would begin to mount. He might deliberately let it build over several days, to enhance the feeling of release that was almost orgasmic. But he indignantly denied that he ever masturbated at a fire scene. "I'm no pervert," he said.

After he graduated from high school, Elwood took enough accountancy courses to obtain a job as bookkeeper for a security alarm company. He had worked steadily at that job until the present time. He had never married, hadn't even dated, and had no close friends. In fact, he actually felt uncomfortable around other people. The forensic clinician noted no abnormalities of mood, cognition, or content of thought.

Elwood's only arrest ever, which was the reason for the forensic evaluation, came about because of a change in the weather. It was summertime, and all week the wind had been blowing steadily off the ocean. Elwood had located a promising field of dry grass and manzanita. On Saturday morning he was off work, and the wind still held. With almost uncontrollable excitement, he used a tin of gasoline to start the fire. He reacted with horror and panic when the wind suddenly began to blow toward the ocean; the fire jumped the small service road he had driven in on, and gobbled up his car and several beach dwellings. Firefighters and police found him sitting on the stony beach, crying quietly.

When the police searched Elwood's apartment, they found a huge collection of videos depicting newscasts of wildfires.

Evaluation of Elwood Telfer

The phenomenon of "tension and release" required for a diagnosis of pyromania (criteria B, D) is well detailed in the vignette. And there's also not much argument that Elwood deliberately set fires (A) and was fascinated by them and the trappings of firefighting (C). His clinician's task would be to sort through the differential diagnosis, which is not unlike that for kleptomania. Patients with **ASPD** or **other personality disorders** will sometimes set fires for either profit or revenge. But Elwood had worked at one job for a decade, and his legal difficulties were restricted to fire setting. Patients with **cogni-tive disorders** will sometimes set their clothing or kitchens ablaze through inattention. However, Elwood had symptoms of none of these conditions (F).

Patients with **schizophrenia**, a **manic episode**, or other severe mental conditions may sometimes set fires to communicate their desires (for example, to be released from jail, to be returned to a former place of residence). This behavior has been termed *com-*

municative arson. Another item to consider in the differential diagnosis is **arson with a purpose**: fires set as a matter of political protest or sabotage, or fires set for profit (E), none of which applied to Elwood.

Although Elwood had a great deal of difficulty relating to other people, this vignette includes insufficient evidence to support a diagnosis of **avoidant personality disorder**. This is not to say that it might not be warranted, only that more information would be needed. I'd make a note that he had "avoidant personality features." A very low GAF score (20) would be given because of Elwood's potential for harming others with his behavior.

F63.1 [312.33]   Pyromania

Among other things, two "manias" are included in this chapter. (Another, trichotillomania, has been moved to the new DSM-5 section on obsessive–compulsive and related disorders; see Chapter 5.) In these disorders, the term is not used by itself in the sense of having a manic episode. Rather, as a suffix, it means having a passion or enthusiasm ("madness" in Greek) for something.

F63.2 [312.32] Kleptomania

In kleptomania, stealing occurs not as the result of need, or even necessarily of desire. When caught, these patients typically have enough money with them to pay for whatever they have taken. Once they have left the scene undetected, they may give away or discard their loot. These people recognize that their behavior is wrong, but they cannot resist. Fear (of apprehension), guilt, and depression are frequent accompaniments.

OK, many otherwise normal people have stolen something—over a quarter of college students in one study admitted to it—but fewer than 0.5% met criteria for kleptomania. (The diagnosis is much more common, up to 8%, in inpatient samples.) It's especially common among younger people; indeed, it typically begins in adolescence. Women outnumber men by perhaps 2:1. Once it begins, often in childhood, it tends to be chronic.

Dating back over 200 years, kleptomania is one of the oldest named disorders in the diagnostic manuals. It is probably also highly overused. Although fewer than 1 in 20 shoplifters can be accurately diagnosed with this disorder, many try to avoid prosecution when they are caught by claiming that they were driven by an irresistible impulse. Look for substance misuse and depression as comorbid diagnoses.

Essential Features of **Kleptomania**

Patients repeatedly act on the impulse to steal objects they don't really need. Before the actual theft, they experience mounting tension, which yields to a sense of release when the theft takes place.

The Fine Print

The D's: • Differential diagnosis (mood and psychotic disorders, personality and conduct disorders, ordinary criminal activity, revenge or anger)

Roseanne Straub

"Fifteen years!" It was how long Roseanne Straub had been shoplifting, but from the expression on her tear-streaked face, it might have been the length of her sentence.

Roseanne was 27, and this was her second arrest, if you didn't count the one time as a juvenile. Three years earlier, she had been arrested, booked, and released on her own recognizance for walking out of a boutique with a silk blouse worth $150. Fortunately for her, 2 weeks later the shop fell victim to a recession; the owner, otherwise preoccupied, did not follow through with prosecution. Badly frightened, she had resisted the temptation to shoplift for several months afterwards.

Roseanne was married and had a 4-year-old daughter. Her husband worked as a paralegal. After her previous arrest, he had threatened to divorce her and obtain custody of their child if she did it again. She worked as a research assistant for a civilian contractor to the military, and a conviction would also doom her security clearance and her job.

"I don't know why I do it. I've asked myself that question a thousand times." Aside from the stealing, Roseanne considered herself a pretty normal person. She had lots of friends and no enemies; most of the time she was quite happy. In every other respect she was law-abiding; she wouldn't even let her husband cheat when he prepared their taxes.

The first time Roseanne had ever stolen from a store was when she was 6 or 7, but that was on a dare from two school friends. When her mother found the candy she had taken from the convenience store, she had gone with Roseanne and made her return it to the store manager. It was years before she was again tempted to steal something.

In junior high, she noticed that periodically a certain tension would build up inside her. It felt as if something was itching deep within her pelvis where she couldn't scratch. For several days she would feel increasingly restless, but with an excited sense of anticipation. Finally she would dart into whatever store she happened to be passing, whisk some article under her coat or into her handbag, and walk out, flooded with relief. For a time it seemed to be associated with her menstrual periods, but by the time she was 17 her episodes had become completely random events.

"I don't know why I do it," Roseanne said again. "Of course, I don't like being caught. But I deserve to be. I've ruined my life and the lives of my family. It's not as if I needed another compact—I must have 15 of them at home."

Evaluation of Roseanne Straub

Ordinary shoplifters plan their thefts and profit from them (criterion A); they do not have the buildup of tension (with subsequent release) that characterized Roseanne's shoplifting episodes (B, C). People with **ASPD** or **other personality disorders** may steal impulsively, but they will also have histories of committing many other antisocial acts. When criminals falsely claim to have symptoms of kleptomania, **malingering** may be diagnosed instead. Patients with **schizophrenia** or **manic episodes** will sometimes have hallucinations that order them to steal things.

Anxiety, guilt, and depression are often found in patients with this disorder. Therefore, watch for diagnoses such as **generalized anxiety disorder**, **persistent depressive disorder (dysthymia)**, and **major depressive disorder**. Kleptomania may also be associated with the eating disorders, especially **bulimia nervosa**. Patients with **substance use disorder** may steal in order to support a drug habit. None of these, however, applied to Roseanne. With her GAF score of 65, her diagnosis would be as follows:

F63.2 [312.32]   Kleptomania

Tension and release (or *relief*) is a phrase that describes several DSM-5 conditions. Among them are pyromania and kleptomania, but it can also be found in trichotillomania in Chapter 5 (though it no longer serves as a criterion for that disorder). It expresses the typical buildup of anxiety or tension, sometimes for a day or more, until the impulse to act becomes overwhelming. Once the action has been taken, the person experiences a sense of release that may be perceived as relief or pleasure. However, remorse or regret may later come to dominate the emotional landscape.

F91.8 [312.89] Other Specified Disruptive, Impulse-Control, and Conduct Disorder

F91.9 [312.9] Unspecified Disruptive, Impulse-Control, and Conduct Disorder

Use one of these two categories to code any problems with the control of impulses or conduct that do not meet the criteria for the disorders described above or elsewhere in DSM-5. As usual, the other specified category should be used when you wish to be specific about a particular presentation; the unspecified category should be used when you do not wish to be specific.

CHAPTER 15

Substance-Related and Addictive Disorders

Quick Guide to the Substance-Related and Addictive Disorders

Mind-altering substances all yield three basic types of disorders: substance intoxication, substance withdrawal, and what we now call substance use disorder (formerly substance dependence and substance abuse). Most of these DSM-5 terms apply to nearly all of the substances discussed; I'll note exceptions as they occur. In addition, because its diagnostic features and some of its physiological features are nearly identical to those of substance use, gambling disorder has been moved into this chapter.

Basic Substance-Related Categories

Substance use disorder. A user has taken a substance frequently enough to produce clinically important distress or impaired functioning, and to result in certain behavioral characteristics. Found in connection with all classes of drugs but caffeine, substance use disorder can even develop accidentally, especially from the use of medicine to treat chronic pain. The discussion, in which alcohol use disorder serves as a model, begins on page 396.

Substance intoxication. This acute clinical condition results from recent overuse of a substance. Anyone can become intoxicated; this is the only substance-related diagnosis likely to apply to a person who uses a substance only once. All drugs but nicotine have a specific syndrome of intoxication. The symptoms of these syndromes can be found summarized later in Table 15.1. Using alcohol as the model, a general discussion of substance intoxication begins on page 411.

Substance withdrawal. This collection of symptoms, specific for the class of substance, develops when a person who has frequently used a substance discontinues it or markedly reduces the amount used. All substances except phencyclidine (PCP), the other hallucinogens, and the inhalants have an officially recognized withdrawal syndrome; see Table 15.1. Again using alcohol as the model, a discussion of substance withdrawal begins on page 402.

Specific Classes of Substances

For quick reference, here are the substances you'll find discussed in the following pages.

Alcohol (p. 397).

Amphetamines and other stimulants (including cocaine) (p. 450).

Caffeine (p. 416).

Cannabis (p. 420).

Hallucinogens (including PCP) (p. 426).

Inhalants (p. 435).

Opioids (p. 439).

Sedative, hypnotic, or anxiolytic drugs (p. 445).

Tobacco (p. 461).

Other or unknown substances (p. 463).

Other Substance-Induced Disorders

Most DSM-5 chapters include disorders associated with substance use; every class of substance is represented except nicotine. They can be experienced during intoxication, during withdrawal, or as consequences of the substance use that endure long after misuse and withdrawal symptoms have ended. They include **substance/medication-induced**:

Psychotic disorder (p. 93).

Mood (bipolar or depressive) disorder (p. 151).

Anxiety disorder (p. 193).

Obsessive–compulsive and related disorder (p. 214).

Sleep–wake disorder (p. 346).

Sexual dysfunction (p. 370).

Delirium (p. 483).

Neurocognitive disorder, major or mild (p. 522).

Non-Substance-Related Disorder

Gambling disorder. These patients repeatedly gamble, often until they lose money, jobs, and friends (p. 470).

Introduction

We of the 21st century have access to a growing variety of mind-altering substances, but using these substances can lead to basic behavioral, cognitive, and physiological problems. These substances, all of which affect the central nervous system, include medications, toxic chemicals, and illegal drugs. Several substances. however, can be obtained legally without a prescription: alcohol, caffeine, and tobacco, as well as some of the inhalants.

DSM-5 lists just over 300 numbered (in ICD-10) substance-related disorders. When all the subcodes and qualifiers are taken into account, there are hundreds more ways to code a patient with a substance-related disorder. For any of these, the clinician must specify the substance(s) responsible, the type of problem, and in some cases the time relationship of substance use to the onset of the problem behavior.

DSM-5 uses nine major groupings, plus the catch-all *other (or unknown)*, to categorize substances. These groupings are all artificial, however, and among them we can identify certain similarities:

- Central nervous system depressants (alcohol and the sedatives, hypnotics, and anxiolytics)

- Central nervous system stimulants (cocaine, amphetamines, and caffeine)

- Perception-distorting drugs (inhalants, cannabis, hallucinogens, and phencyclidine [PCP])

- Narcotics (opioids)

- Nicotine

- Other (corticosteroids and other medications)

The terminology keeps changing, but the basic problem remains the same: the fact that people misuse alcohol and drugs. One of the problems with substance use disorders has been that because they have been so variously defined—by different writers, for different substances, in different eras (and in different DSMs)—there has been substantial disagreement as to exactly what they are and who engages in them.

DSM-5 continues the DSM-IV tradition of defining the disorders related to all the substances in terms that are more or less uniform. The trouble is that the uniform keeps getting redesigned. The definitions now in use replace older words such as *alcoholism*, *problem drinking*, *episodic excessive drinking*, *addiction*, *habituation*, *dependence*, *abuse*, and other (often pejorative) terms applied over the years to people who use mind-altering substances.

Of course, most adults use some substances; however, most of us don't use them pathologically. But what is *pathological use*? Let's define it as use beyond which the negative effects outweigh any positive effects. Often this point comes up fast—with first exposure, for some patients and substances. Usually the use is frequent, heavy, or both, and it always involves symptoms and maladaptive changes in behavior.

Note also that none of the symptoms of substance use explain why users like their chosen substances. In an effort to be objective and consistent, the DSM-5 criteria ignore many of the nuances of addiction to specific substances. Gone, for example, is the descriptive richness of the stages of alcoholism. You should consult mental health textbooks, scientific articles, and even literary works to supplement these criteria.

One last note: For several months now, I've been searching for a noun describing substance use disorder that fits comfortably into the new nomenclature. I've finally decided to throw caution to the winds and call it *addiction*. A lot of the substance use experts bemoan its loss, and it seems to describe the behavior well and succinctly.

The Basic Substance-Related Categories, Illustrated by Alcohol-Related Disorders

My approach in this part of the chapter differs somewhat from the DSM-5 format. I'll present the Essential Features of substance use disorder, intoxication, and withdrawal, using the example of alcohol for each of these categories. Later in the chapter, I discuss whatever intoxication and/or withdrawal syndromes apply to each of the other substance groupings. I also briefly mention other disorders related to each substance, as well as other substances that may be used in conjunction with each substance.

Substance Use Disorder

As I have noted in the sidebar above, clinicians and researchers have argued for years about the definitions of addiction. The DSM-5 approach is to define substance use disorder as the core behavior of those who misuse substances. These criteria specify a type of addiction that includes behavioral, physiological, and cognitive symptoms. As an exercise, let's dissect the language concerning the diagnosis of alcohol (indeed, any substance) use disorder:

1. The use is problematic. Though it is perhaps begun to cope with other problems, it only makes things worse for the user, as well as for the user's relatives and associates.

2. There is a pattern to the use. The repetition of this use forms a predictable habit pattern.

3. The effects are clinically important. This usage pattern either has come to the attention of professionals or warrants such attention. (Actually, the official DSM-5 language reads "clinically significant." However, the word "significant"

has statistical implications that cannot be sustained in clinical practice. I think *important* works better here. In this text, I have sometimes substituted the adjective *material*.)

4. The use causes distress or impairment. This says that the substance use must be serious enough to interfere in some way with the patient's life. Substance use disorder is thereby defined in terms similar to those employed for many non-substance-related mental disorders.

5. The interference in the patient's life must be shown by at least 2 symptoms from a list of 11: more use than intended; attempts to reduce usage; much time spent getting or using; craving; shirking obligations; social problems; reduced activities; use despite its physical danger; use despite physical or psychological disorder; tolerance; and withdrawal symptoms. Severity is judged by counting up the number of these symptoms that are checked off (but see my caveat in a sidebar, p. 402).

Finally, in diagnosing substance use disorder, intoxication, and withdrawal, remember that rapidity of onset and rapidity of elimination affect the likelihood that a patient will have problems with any given substance. Rapid absorption of a substance (by smoking, snorting, or injection) favors quicker onset of action, shorter duration of action, and greater likelihood of a substance use disorder. A longer half-life (the time it takes the body to eliminate half the remaining substance) reduces the likelihood of withdrawal symptoms but extends the period during which the user could experience them.

Whatever happened to *polysubstance dependence*? DSM-IV used this term to indicate a situation in which a patient used two or more substances, but didn't have enough problems to warrant a diagnosis of addiction to any of them—and yet, in aggregate, had enough symptoms from substance use to fulfill a "group" diagnosis of an addiction. That definition was a little complicated and tended to be seldom used. There is also precious little research to indicate that it ever predicted much of anything for anyone.

In DSM-5, any patient who would meet the somewhat byzantine criteria just mentioned would have to be diagnosed as having an unspecified or other specified substance-related disorder for each substance involved. Perhaps someone can persuade me there's a payoff in *that*.

Alcohol Use Disorder

Although nearly half of all adult Americans at least once in their lives have had some sort of problem with alcohol (driving while intoxicated, missing work due to a hang-over), far fewer (about 10%) have had problems sufficient to qualify for a diagnosis of alcohol use disorder. Note that the criteria are the same as for any other substance use disorder, which I've stated below in generic form.

Alcoholism is extremely common. More than 10% of the population of the United States have had the problem at one time or another; a man's risk is at least twice as great as a woman's. Onset tends to be in the teen years, though older age groups are not immune. Physiological complications such as withdrawal are likely to appear much later in the disease.

Alcoholism is highly heritable; first-degree relatives have several times the risk of the general population. It has many comorbidities, especially with mood disorders and antisocial personality disorder.

Essential Features of **Substance Use Disorder**

These patients use enough of their chosen substance to cause chronic or repeated problems in different areas of their lives:

- *Personal and interpersonal life.* They neglect family life (duties to spouse/partner, dependents) and even favorite leisure activities in favor of using their substance of choice; they fight (physically or verbally) with those they care about; and they continue to use despite the realization that it causes interpersonal problems.
- *Employment.* Effort formerly devoted to work (or other important activities) now goes to getting the substance, consuming it, and then recuperating from its use. Result: These people are repeatedly absent or get fired.
- *Control.* They often use more of the substance or for longer than they intended; they (unsuccessfully) attempt to eliminate or reduce the usage. Through it all, they desperately crave more.
- *Health and safety.* Users engage in behavior that is physically dangerous (most often, operating a motor vehicle); legal issues can ensue. They continue to use despite knowing that it causes health problems such as cirrhosis or hepatitis C.
- *Physiological sequels.* Tolerance develops: The substance produces less effect, so the patient must use more. And once they stop using, patients suffer symptoms of withdrawal characteristic of that substance.

The Fine Print

Tolerance isn't a factor with most hallucinogens, though users may develop tolerance to the stimulant effects of PCP.

Withdrawal isn't a factor with PCP, other hallucinogens, or inhalants.

Don't count tolerance or withdrawal that's caused by taking medication as prescribed.

The D's: • Duration (the symptoms you count must have occurred within the past 12 months) • Differential diagnosis (physical disorders, primary disorders from nearly every other DSM-5 chapter, *truly* recreational use)

Coding Notes

Apply course modifiers from page 409.
    See Tables 15.2 and 15.3, near the end of this chapter, for codes.

Quentin McCarthy

"I can get off it, but I can't stay off it." Quentin McCarthy was 43, and he was talking about alcohol. He liked to say that throughout his adult life he had been successful at two things—drinking and selling insurance. Now he was having trouble with both.

Quentin was the second of three sons born to parents both of whom were attorneys. His brothers had been excellent students. Quentin was bright, but he had been hyperactive and the class clown. In school, he had never been able to focus his attention well enough to excel at anything but physical education.

To please his parents, after high school Quentin tried a semester of junior college. It was worse than high school; the only thing that kept him going was guilt. Whereas his older brother was admitted to law school (with honors at entrance), and his younger brother mopped up the prizes at the state science fair, Quentin felt almost joyful when his birthday was that year's fourth pick in the national draft lottery. The following day he enlisted in the Army.

Somewhere in his schooling Quentin had learned to type, so he was assigned to his battalion's administrative section. He liked to say that throughout 4 years in the military, he never fired his weapon in anger. By comparison with some of the older men's alcohol use, his drinking was moderate. Although he had about the usual number of fights, he managed to avoid serious trouble. When he left the service at age 22, he had held onto his sergeant's stripes through two tours of duty in Vietnam.

After that, life suddenly got serious. Working part-time after hours in the post exchange, Quentin had discovered that he was a natural salesman. So it had seemed a logical move to take a job selling life insurance. It also seemed sensible to marry the boss's daughter. When 2 years later his father-in-law died suddenly, Quentin became sole proprietor of the agency.

"The business made me, and it ruined me," he said. "I made a lot of money having lunch with people and selling them large policies. I told myself that I had to drink with them in order to make a sale, but I suppose that was just rationalization."

As time went on, Quentin's two-martini lunches turned into four-martini lunches. By the time he was 31, he was skipping lunch completely and nipping throughout the afternoon to "keep a glow on." At the end of the day, he was sometimes surprised to see how much had disappeared from the bottle he kept in his desk drawer.

The past year had brought Quentin two unpleasant surprises. The first came when his doctor informed him that the nagging pain just above his navel was an ulcer; for the sake of his health, he would have to stop drinking. The second, which in a way seemed worse because it injured his pride, occurred one afternoon over lunch. A long-time client of the agency apologetically said that he would be taking his substantial business elsewhere; his wife didn't feel comfortable that he was "doing business with a lush." Thinking back, Quentin realized that there had been several other, less blatant instances of customers departing the fold.

The result had been his resolve to quit, or at least to reduce the amount of his drinking. ("Quitting is easy," he remarked ruefully. "I did it twice in 1 month.") At first he promised himself he wouldn't drink before 5 P.M.; that proved impractical, and he later amended it to "around lunchtime." With the level in his desk drawer bottle receding as fast as ever, Quentin decided he would try Alcoholics Anonymous. "That was worse than useless," he explained. "The stories I heard from some of those people made me feel like a teetotaler."

A comment made by his wife eventually brought him in for evaluation. "You used to drink to have a good time," she told him. "Now you drink because you need it."

Evaluation of Quentin McCarthy

The Essential Features of substance use disorder (see above) are not especially complicated, just tedious. Quentin's history of alcohol use illustrates many of them. At least two are needed to qualify for the diagnosis, and they must occur within a 1-year period. This is not to say that they must have begun within the year prior to evaluation, only that the problems must have been present within a relatively compact time frame. Note that some patients may sporadically present new symptoms and abandon old ones.

- *Using more.* Many patients start out consuming relatively small amounts ("just a nip before dinner"), but end up skipping dinner and just nipping. As a result, they use more of their substance of choice than they intend. Quentin was sometimes surprised how much the level in his bottle had gone down by day's end (criterion A1).

- *Control issues.* The person wants to control use or repeatedly fails in attempts at control. Quentin tried to quit by setting rules and attending Alcoholics Anonymous (A2). Others, for whom quitting completely may seem too drastic and frightening, may instead try to reduce the amount they use.

- *Time investment.* This symptom is especially characteristic of those who use substances other than alcohol. (Alcohol users often carry on with other activities, drunk or sober.) And like tobacco, alcohol is legal and hence easy to obtain. Quentin spent a good deal of time drinking, which would probably qualify him on this criterion (A3), even though he kept right on working. Other patients, especially those who use drugs other than alcohol, may spend a great deal of time ensuring the continuity of their supply. For example, see the vignette of Kirk Aufderheide (p. 447).

- *Craving* (A4). This is the only completely new criterion in DSM-5—one that many authorities had complained was missing from previous editions. It has been linked to dopamine release in substance use and other behaviors such as gambling. We didn't note it in Quentin's vignette, but then perhaps the interviewer forgot to ask.

- *Obligations shirked* (A5). Many patients with alcohol use disorder abandon their roles at home, in the community, or at work in favor of drinking. Quentin gets a pass on this one.

- *Worsening interpersonal/social relations*. The patient continues to use, though it causes fights or arguments with close associates. You could argue (I would) that Quentin's customers' taking their business elsewhere was such an example (A6).

- *Reduction of other activities* (A7). Patients with substance use disorders commonly ignore work and social activities. This was not the case with Quentin, who devoted the necessary time to work (though some clients objected to his drinking).

- *Physical dangers ignored* (A8). Driving while under the influence is by far the most common, but many others, such as operating heavy machinery, can also occur. The vignette doesn't indict Quentin on physical danger.

- *Psychological/medical warnings ignored*. Quentin drank despite the danger from ulcers (A9). Other patients may ignore physician warnings about liver disease (cirrhosis or hepatitis) or esophageal varicose veins, which can rupture after prolonged retching. Those who use drugs intravenously often continue to share needles, despite the well-known risks of HIV and hepatitis. Most substances can also exacerbate suicidal ideas, mood disorders, and psychoses—which are likewise ignored.

- *Tolerance*. When a substance has been used so extensively that the user's body has grown accustomed to the chemical effects, we say that tolerance has developed. This is especially apparent as regards alcohol, opioids, and sedatives, but it can be found in all other substance groups, with the possible exception of hallucinogens. With tolerance, the patient either requires more of the substance to obtain the same effect or feels less effect from the same dose. Quentin experienced some of this when he began drinking throughout the afternoon to keep his "glow" on (A10).

- *Withdrawal* (A11). This criterion can show up either as a symptom picture that is characteristic for the class of substance, or as use of the substance to avert or treat these symptoms. I've discussed substance withdrawal further on page 402.

Quentin showed at least 5, possibly 6, of the 11 criteria for alcohol use disorder. The next vignette will reveal whether he also met the criteria for alcohol withdrawal.

DSM-5 is the first manual to include severity criteria specific for substance use disorders. In part, that was necessitated by the deletion of the substance abuse category—a staple of previous DSMs since 1980, and misunderstood by many clinicians as a sort of "substance use lite." Numerous studies determined over the years that the substance abuse criteria failed in regard to both validity and reliability. The diagnosis of alcohol abuse, when made at all, was usually based on one criterion, driving while intoxicated—a behavior that, while in itself dangerous, is a weak reed on which to prop a diagnosis. But most of all, the abuse diagnosis simply didn't predict enough to make it worthwhile.

The idea of severity criteria is a good one, but its implementation does sow the seeds of discontent, partly because we determine severity simply by totaling the number of criteria met. Here's the seed: Not all criteria are created equal. Some imply far more disability and distress than others. For example, either tolerance or withdrawal suggests that the individual has been using heavily and for a very long time (in most cases, many months, and probably for years).

Other criteria may have far less serious import. Arguments with a spouse or partner, while not trivial (as most of us can testify), depend not only on the person's actual use, but on the other person's perception of use and, yes, tolerance for the behavior. Craving may be found even in individuals who don't meet other criteria for a substance use disorder. Fortunately, these are issues that are solvable with more research and experience. Maybe in DSM-5.1.

Substance Withdrawal

Withdrawal symptoms develop as the concentration of a substance decreases in the brain of a frequent user. The generic criteria for substance withdrawal are simple: They require only that the patient experience specific symptoms after quitting a substance that has been used heavily for a specified time. Stress or impairment must result, and no physical illness or other mental disorder must better explain the symptoms.

The symptoms that develop during substance withdrawal are specific to the substance used and are described in the relevant sections of this chapter. However, certain symptoms are found in withdrawal from many substances:

- Alteration in mood (anxiety, irritability, depression)

- Abnormal motor activity (restlessness, immobility)

- Sleep disturbance (insomnia or hypersomnia)

- Other physical problems (fatigue, changes in appetite)

See Table 15.1 for a more complete listing.

For a substance to cause withdrawal symptoms, patients must first become tolerant to it. This requires frequent use for a period of time that depends on the specific sub-

TABLE 15.1. Symptoms of Substance Intoxication and Withdrawal

		Substance intoxication								Substance withdrawal					
		Alcohol/sedatives[a]	Cannabis	Stimulants[b]	Caffeine	Hallucinogens	Inhalants	Opioids	PCP	Alcohol/sedatives[a]	Cannabis	Stimulants[b]	Caffeine	Tobacco	Opioids
Social	Impaired social functioning			×											
	Inappropriate sexuality	×													
	Social withdrawal		×												
	Interpersonal sensitivity			×											
Mood	Labile mood	×													
	Anxiety		×	×		×				×	×			×	
	Euphoria		×	×			×	×							
	Blunted affect, apathy			×			×	×							
	Anger			×							×			×	
	Dysphoria, depression					×		×		×	×	×	×	×	×
	Irritability										×		×	×	
Judgment	Impaired judgment	×	×	×		×	×	×	×						
	Assaultiveness, belligerence						×		×						
	Impulsivity								×						
Sleep	Insomnia, sleeplessness				×					×	×	×		×	×
	Bad dreams									×	×				
	Hypersomnia											×			
Activity level	Aggression	×								×					
	Agitation, increased activity			×	×		×	×	×	×		×			
	Tirelessness				×										
	Restlessness				×						×			×	
	Decreased activity, retardation			×			×	×				×			
Alertness	Reduced attention	×						×							
	Hypervigilance			×											
	Stupor or coma	×		×			×	×	×						
	Time seems slowed		×												
	Poor concentration												×	×	

(cont.)

[a]This grouping also includes hypnotics and anxiolytics.

[b]Cocaine and amphetamines

TABLE 15.1 (cont.)

		Substance intoxication								Substance withdrawal					
		Alcohol/sedatives[a]	Cannabis	Stimulants[b]	Caffeine	Hallucinogens	Inhalants	Opioids	PCP	Alcohol/sedatives[a]	Cannabis	Stimulants[b]	Caffeine	Tobacco	Opioids
	Confusion			×											
	Drowsiness							×					×		
Perception	Ideas of reference					×									
	Fears of insanity					×									
	Persecutory ideas					×									
	Perceptual changes					×									
	Brief hallucinations/illusions					×				×					
	Depersonalization/derealization					×									
Autonomic	Dry mouth		×												
	Constricted pupils							×							
	Dilated pupils			×		×									×
	Sweating			×		×				×	×				×
	Piloerection														×
Muscle	Muscle weakness			×			×								
	Muscle twitching				×										
	Muscle aches												×		×
	Muscle rigidity								×						
Neurological	Dystonia, dyskinesia			×											
	Nystagmus	×					×		×						
	Tremors				×		×			×	×				
	Blurred vision				×		×								
	Double vision						×								
	Impaired reflexes						×								
	Seizures			×					×	×					
	Numbness								×						
	Headache										×		×		
Gastrointestinal	GI upset, diarrhea				×										×
	Nausea, vomiting			×						×			×		×
	Abdominal pain										×				

404

		Substance intoxication								Substance withdrawal					
		Alcohol/sedatives[a]	Cannabis	Stimulants[b]	Caffeine	Hallucinogens	Inhalants	Opioids	PCP	Alcohol/sedatives[a]	Cannabis	Stimulants[b]	Caffeine	Tobacco	Opioids
	Increased appetite/weight gain		×									×		×	
	Decreased appetite/weight loss			×							×				
Motor	Incoordination	×	×			×	×								
	Unsteady gait	×					×								
	Stereotypies			×											
	Trouble walking								×						
	Lethargy						×								
	Trouble speaking								×						
	Slurred speech	×					×	×							
Cardiovascular	Chest pain			×											
	Irregular heartbeat			×	×	×									
	Slow heart rate			×											
	Rapid heart rate		×	×	×	×			×	×					
	Blood pressure up or down			×					×						
General	Depressed breathing			×											
	Dizziness						×								
	Red eyes		×												
	Chills			×							×				
	Fever										×				×
	Reduced memory	×						×							
	Nervous, excited				×						×				
	Rambling speech				×										
	Hyperacute hearing								×						
	Red face				×										
	Increased urination				×										
	Fatigue											×	×		
	Tearing, runny nose														×
	Yawning														×

405

stance. Heroin may require only a few injections, whereas for alcohol, weeks of heavy drinking are usually needed to produce clinically important tolerance. Most patients who are dependent on a substance will experience withdrawal if it is suddenly denied them.

Some substances do *not* produce withdrawal. Hallucinogens, for example, can induce an addiction, yet no withdrawal syndrome has been reported. On the other hand, DSM-IV listed no caffeine withdrawal syndrome—a serious gaffe, as any coffee drinker who switches suddenly to decaf will testify. Fortunately, DSM-5 has put that one right.

The time course of withdrawal depends on the drug's *half-life*—the time it takes for the body to eliminate one-half of the substance. Usually withdrawal symptoms begin within 12–24 hours after the last dose is consumed, and persist no longer than a few days. A powerful urge to resume use of the substance often accompanies the withdrawal symptoms.

Analysis of blood, breath, or urine can attest to the patient's substance use, but more often evidence is obtained from history. Denial may color self-report, so histories are often more reliable if a relative or friend—anyone other than the patient—augments the information. As a rule of thumb, many clinicians mentally double the amount of a substance a patient claims to have used.

Essential Features of **Substance Withdrawal**

After using a substance heavily and at length, the patient suddenly stops or markedly reduces intake. This yields a substance-specific syndrome that causes problems.

The Fine Print

The D's: • Duration to symptom onset (generally hours to days) • Differential diagnosis (physical disorders, primary mental disorders)
    You can find the specifics of each substance withdrawal syndrome in Table 15.1.

Alcohol Withdrawal

Heavy drinking for days or longer is required to produce alcohol withdrawal. (Drinkers can tolerate greatly varying amounts of alcohol, so it's hard to be more precise.) Symptoms begin a few hours after drinking stops and coincide with a rapidly declining blood alcohol level. Nearly all patients will show evidence of central nervous system overactivity, such as sweating, racing pulse, or heightened reflexes (see sidebar below). The most common symptom is tremor; nausea and vomiting may also occur. Some patients may have brief hallucinations that last 12–24 hours. After 2 or 3 days, a few may even have seizures.

Sometimes this common syndrome is called *uncomplicated withdrawal*. It is usually brief, lasting but a few days and peaking on the second. However, the accompanying anxiety, irritability, and sleeplessness may persist a good deal longer.

The heavier the drinking has been, the more likely it is that symptoms will be severe, so "uncomplicated" withdrawal shades into other, more serious syndromes. The best known of these is delirium, which affects only about 5% of those hospitalized for withdrawal. When delirium occurs during the course of severe alcohol withdrawal, it is commonly called *delirium tremens* (DTs). When a patient has both seizures and delirium, the seizures almost invariably come first. Rodney Partridge, a patient with alcohol withdrawal delirium, is described later (see p. 483).

Another alcohol withdrawal syndrome is alcohol-induced psychotic disorder with hallucinations. Formerly known as *alcoholic auditory hallucinosis*, it is an uncommon (though not rare) disorder whose symptoms can almost exactly mimic schizophrenia. Danny Finch, a patient with this disorder, is described in Chapter 2 (see p. 95).

The number 100 serves as a useful reminder when looking for physiological signs of alcohol withdrawal: pulse over 100 beats per minute; temperature over 100°F; diastolic blood pressure approaching 100 mm Hg. Rapid respirations—though nowhere close to 100 per minute—may serve as another sign.

Essential Features of **Alcohol Withdrawal**

After heavy, long-lasting use of alcohol, the patient suddenly stops or markedly reduces intake. Within hours to days, this yields symptoms of increased nervous system and motor activity such as trembling, sweating, nausea, rapid heartbeat, high blood pressure, agitation, headache, insomnia, weakness, short-lived hallucinations/ illusions, and/or convulsions.

The Fine Print

The D's: • Duration to onset (a few hours to a day or more) • Distress or disability (work/ educational, social, or personal impairment) • Differential diagnosis (physical illness; psychotic, mood, and anxiety disorders; withdrawal from sedatives and other substances)
    You can find the specifics of alcohol withdrawal in Table 15.1.

Coding Notes

Specify if: **With perceptual disturbances.** The patient has altered perceptions: auditory, tactile, or visual illusions or hallucinations with intact insight (that is, realization that the perceptual symptoms are unreal, caused by the substance use).
    Coding in ICD-10 depends on the presence of perceptual disturbances; see Table 15.2 (p. 465).

Quentin McCarthy Again

By the time Quentin sought help, he was drinking the equivalent of nearly a pint of hard liquor per day. He declined the offer of a brief hospitalization to detoxify, and instead began an outpatient withdrawal regimen of decreasing doses of a benzodiazepine. He was asked to return in 3 days.

On Quentin's next visit, he looked gray and unhappy. He signed in at the registration desk with a wobbly scrawl, and his hand shook as he reached out an arm to have his blood pressure and pulse taken. Each of these vital signs was elevated.

For 3 days Quentin had drunk no alcohol at all. Beginning the second morning, he had felt increasingly anxious—a sensation reminding him of his first night in Vietnam, when he had awakened to the booming of howitzers. His anxiety grew throughout the day. Although he was exhausted by bedtime, he hardly slept at all. When he arrived 4 hours early for his clinic appointment, he admitted that he had taken none of the medicine he had been given. "I wanted to do it myself," he explained.

Over the next several days, Quentin's withdrawal symptoms abated. Within 2 weeks, he no longer needed the medication. However, because he felt strongly tempted to drink when he was having lunch with clients, he requested disulfiram (Antabuse) therapy.

Three months later, Quentin was still taking disulfiram and still hadn't touched alcohol. He attended at least one Alcoholics Anonymous meeting each day. He had rescued his insurance business from the doldrums and had even persuaded two of his former clients to return with their business. However, he admitted that he occasionally felt acute episodes of anger when he wanted a drink.

Further Evaluation of Quentin McCarthy

When he stopped using alcohol (alcohol withdrawal criterion A), Quentin developed typical alcohol withdrawal symptoms (see Table 15.1). They included rapid pulse, insomnia, anxiety, and tremor (criteria B1, B3, B7, and B2—though only two of these are required), all of which made him so uncomfortable that he hurried back to the mental health clinic (C). Going longer without medication might have put him at serious risk for withdrawal seizures or perceptual disturbances such as auditory or visual hallucinations. Then he might have qualified for other diagnoses—for example, **alcohol-induced delirium** or **alcohol-induced psychotic disorder with hallucinations.** Of course, Quentin's withdrawal symptoms further substantiated his primary diagnosis of **alcohol use disorder.**

Could any physical or other mental disorder have caused these symptoms (D)? The differential diagnosis for withdrawal symptoms is long and substance-specific. For opioid withdrawal, it includes **flu-like syndromes.** Patients withdrawing from cocaine and amphetamines typically have symptoms of **depression.** But both Quentin's history and symptoms were so typical for alcohol withdrawal that other diagnoses would seem highly unlikely.

Before coding Quentin's diagnosis, however, we must consider the matter of course modifiers for substance use disorder.

> Can someone go into substance withdrawal without having substance use disorder? If you scrutinize the criteria and do the math, it's theoretically possible. The criteria don't say it couldn't happen, but, aside from patients who are medically addicted (not to alcohol, we'll stipulate), it must be a rare event.

Course Modifiers for Substance Use Disorder

After at least 3 months with no substance-related symptoms other than craving, the patient can be considered for a course modifier of *early remission* or *sustained remission*. The standard for early remission is 3 months to 1 year; for sustained remission, it is 1 year or longer. To either time period can be added a further specifier: *in a controlled environment*, if the patient is living in a facility that prevents access to substances. Such an environment would include jails and prisons (well, some of them), locked hospital wards, and therapeutic communities.

Essential Features of **Substance Use Disorder Course Modifiers**

These designations are pretty straightforward and self-explanatory. They do suggest a caveat, however, which I've addressed in a sidebar just below.

Remission

Remissions are divided into early versus sustained. Until a patient has been clean (or sober) for 90 days, no designation of remission is possible.

  In early remission. *Early remission* begins after 3 months clean and sober for that substance (and without any of the substance use disorder symptoms—with one allowed exception: craving) and lasts until the person has been so for 1 year. (Patients are especially vulnerable to relapse during the first year of sobriety.)

  In sustained remission. After the first year, *sustained remission* begins.

In a Controlled Environment

Someone who is in early or sustained remission and lives in an environment that restricts access to the substance may be given this modifier. Good control of contraband would characterize such an environment—a well-run jail, therapeutic community, or locked hospital ward.

In a controlled environment can apply to these classes of substance use: alcohol; cannabis; hallucinogens; inhalants; opioids; sedatives, hypnotics, or anxiolytics; stimulants; other (or unknown); tobacco.

On Maintenance Therapy

A patient who is taking a medication designed to reduce the effects of a substance may be described as *on maintenance therapy*. It is listed as a specifier for either opioids or tobacco, when there are currently *no* symptoms of the substance use disorder. Why not alcohol, for which there's Antabuse? (Good question. See sidebar below.)

Severity

Mild. Presence of 2–3 criteria substance use disorder criteria.
Moderate. Presence of 4–5 criteria.
Severe. Presence of 6+ criteria.

There's a very good question implied in the statement concerning the specifier *on maintenance therapy*: Why does it apply *only* to tobacco and opioids? Why not to alcohol (Antabuse)? Or anything else for which an effective maintenance treatment is devised? Of course, this statement is only a set of words, so you can apply it wherever you like. If your patient is doing well on Antabuse, say so.

Evaluation of Course Modifiers for Quentin McCarthy

When he first came to the clinic, Quentin had been alcohol-free for only a few hours; at this point, his diagnosis of alcohol use disorder would have qualified for no course modifier other than severity (which was indeed *severe*—we've counted 5 or 6 criteria). On his return to the clinic after 3 days, moreover, he would also have qualified for a diagnosis of alcohol withdrawal. But at his reevaluation, 3 months into recovery, he had no symptoms of alcohol use disorder (other than perhaps craving); his withdrawal symptoms had abated; and he was still taking disulfiram. (The occasional episodes of anger, when a patient would like a drink, are pretty typical for alcoholism recovery; patients themselves sometimes refer to them as "dry drunk" experiences.)

According to Table 15.2 (which accompanies the discussion of coding toward the end of this chapter), Quentin's diagnosis (finally!) at 3 months would thus read as given below. His GAF score on admission would be 40; his 3-month GAF would be 70. I tacked on the "on disulfiram," though the official manual doesn't say I can do so. So far, no one's complained.

F10.20 [303.90]   Severe alcohol use disorder, early remission, on disulfiram

Substance Intoxication

Anyone can get drunk. Anyone can inhale toxic fumes. Although most people who become intoxicated do so voluntarily, people can also be affected accidentally (for example, through exposure to industrial chemicals or drinking doctored punch). Regardless of intent, for a diagnosis of substance intoxication to be appropriate, the central nervous system effects of the substance must cause psychological changes or behaviors that don't work well for the individual. Note that substance intoxication is almost always reversible. When there are permanent effects of substance use, look instead to another diagnosis (for example, substance-induced cognitive disorder).

The behavior of an intoxicated person changes in disadvantageous ways; that is, the changes are problematic. (DSM-IV called them *maladaptive*, which I think is a useful term.) These include work/educational or social problems, abnormally labile (unstable) mood, impaired thinking, defective judgment, and belligerence. This criterion is important because it helps to discriminate patients who are only intoxicated in the physiological sense (excessive digitalis, for example) from those whose behavior impairs functioning. A person who drinks a 6-pack of beer and then goes quietly to bed without disturbing anyone may well be intoxicated in the physiological sense, but has not earned the mental health diagnosis of alcohol intoxication. (Going to bed is a behavioral change, but not usually maladaptive. Quite the reverse, actually.) To diagnose someone as having substance intoxication requires both hurtful behavioral changes and physiological symptoms and signs.

As for the signs of physiological impairment that will be noted, these tend to be substance-specific, but there are certain common themes:

- Motor coordination loss or agitation

- Loss of ability to sustain attention

- Impaired memory

- Reduced alertness (drowsiness, stupor)

- Effects on the autonomic nervous system (dry mouth, heart palpitations, gastrointestinal symptoms, changes in blood pressure)

- Mood changes (depression, euphoria, anxiety, and others)

You'll find more in Table 15.1.

Then there remains the ubiquitous requirement that all physical illnesses and other mental disorders must be ruled out. As a general rule, symptoms of intoxication (or withdrawal) that last longer than about 4 weeks may point to another mental or physical disorder. For example, a drinker who still has depressive symptoms a month after drying out should be evaluated for major depressive episode.

Essential Features of **Substance Intoxication**

Shortly after using a substance that can affect the central nervous system, the patient develops characteristic physical symptoms and clinically important behavioral or psychological changes that are maladaptive.

The Fine Print

The D's: • Duration to symptom onset (shortly after) • Differential diagnosis (physical disorders, intoxication from other substances, other mental disorders)

You can find the specifics of each substance intoxication syndrome in Table 15.1.

Alcohol Intoxication

The picture of acute alcohol intoxication is so familiar that it seems almost unnecessary to describe it again here. However, we should make several observations.

There is a great deal of variability in the blood levels of alcohol different people can tolerate without appearing drunk. The range may be as great as fivefold (from 0.3 to 1.5 mg/ml), despite the fact that many jurisdictions now set the sobriety level for driving at 0.8 mg/ml and will be setting it even lower in the future. Furthermore, the symptoms of alcohol intoxication are usually more prominent when the blood level is rising (during the early part of the drinking period) than when it is falling and the person is sobering up. Levels of alcohol in the body can be measured in urine, blood, breath, or even saliva.

Alcohol intoxication should only be diagnosed when there is evidence (usually historical) that the patient has drunk enough, rapidly enough, to intoxicate most people. In borderline cases, this may mean factoring in the drinker's weight, age, and general state of health. Someone who becomes markedly intoxicated after drinking a small amount of alcohol would be assigned the code for unspecified alcohol-related disorder (see p. 415).

We need to consider briefly a little semantic issue. That's the fact that the word *intoxication* doesn't always means a substance intoxication, as we're using the term here. In the broad sense, *intoxication* just means that there has been a psychological or physiological change that may or may not have caused problems. For example, a person whose coffee drinking causes insomnia is technically intoxicated, but if that's the only issue, then it isn't problematic in a clinical sense.

(By the way, this is a definitional quibble that is peculiar to clinicians and pharmacologists—you won't find it in the dictionary. Not any of mine, anyway.)

Essential Features of **Alcohol Intoxication**

Shortly after drinking alcohol, the patient becomes disinhibited (argues; is aggressive; has rapid mood shifts or impairment of attention, judgment, or personal functioning). There is also evidence of neurological impairment (imbalance or wobbly gait, unclear speech, poor coordination, jerking eye movements called nystagmus, reduced level of consciousness).

The Fine Print

The D's: • Differential diagnosis (physical disorders, intoxication from sedatives or other substances, other mental disorders)

You can find the specifics of alcohol intoxication in Table 15.1.

Coding Notes

See Tables 15.2 and 15.3, toward the end of this chapter, for codes.

Dolores McCarthy

In one of Dolores McCarthy's earliest memories, she was 4 years old and sitting on her grandfather's lap. She would rest her head against his soft old cotton sweater. He would wrap his arms securely around her, and she would cling to his neck. Also clinging to him was a particular smell that she always associated with her grandfather. It wasn't until she was a teenager that she realized what it was: beer.

By the time Dolores was 10, she had watched in horror as the old man died by degrees of cirrhosis. Then, in her teens, she saw how her father's drinking wrecked her parents' marriage. In college, when she discovered that two glasses of wine would ease her chronic sense of tension, she promised herself that she would use alcohol and never let it use her.

Accordingly, she had evolved a set of rules to limit her consumption. She allowed herself only one drink before dinner, and never more than three in a day (except on weekends and vacations, when she could have four). From her father's unfortunate example, she had learned: Regardless of the occasion, never drink during work and never allow "extras." Even on her 22nd birthday—which was also the day she married Quentin, the young salesman in her father's office—she had only four glasses of champagne (just enough to maintain her customary comfortable glow).

Despite her control, Dolores had had two lapses. The first had occurred 12 months earlier, when she became pregnant for the first and only time. Although she wanted a child, she took the precaution of having an amniocentesis. When it revealed that she was carrying a baby with Down syndrome, she gulped several extra drinks and drove around while deciding what to do. A Breathalyzer-measured blood alcohol level of 1.2 landed her in traffic court just 1 week after the abortion.

Her second arrest for driving while intoxicated had occurred 6 months later, when she lost her self-control once again after her mother died of Alzheimer's disease. The day Quentin entered treatment was therefore only the third time he had ever known his wife to be drunk.

Dolores accompanied her husband to his second clinic appointment. She had been worried about Quentin for several months, and when his agitation kept them both awake most of that night, she had gone down to the kitchen and poured them each a drink. When he refused his, she drank it for him. Then she lost count and had a couple more.

"Anything was besher—was better than what he was going through," Dolores told the clinician that morning. After correcting herself, she spoke slowly and deliberately.

On the spur of the moment, Dolores had decided that she should accompany Quentin to his appointment, to be sure he didn't get into trouble. They had taken her car, and she had insisted on driving. Quentin hadn't dared remind her what had happened on the other occasions she had driven after drinking. Fortunately, traffic was light, and her only difficulty was that she needed two extra tries when parking in an unusually long space at the curb.

As Dolores entered the clinic building, however, she stumbled and might have fallen if someone had not grabbed her elbow and steadied her as she wobbled into the waiting room. She fumbled with the large buttons of her coat until her husband undid them for her. She then slumped into a chair where, with her coat thrown over her, she dozed until they were called into the clinician's office.

Evaluation of Dolores McCarthy

We'll first address the question of alcohol use disorder. Although Dolores drank more than the average American, she had had few problems from her alcohol use, because of her vigilance and the unfortunate examples of the men in her family. She had never drunk enough to develop tolerance or withdrawal symptoms, and her control had been almost unwaveringly iron-fisted. When it slipped, however, she'd had legal problems: two arrests for driving under the influence of alcohol within a 12-month period. Drunk driving qualifies for using alcohol when it's dangerous to do so (criterion A8 for alcohol use disorder). In other patients, such evidence might include fights or arguments with family or friends, lapses in business judgment, or embarrassing behavior (such as making sexually inappropriate remarks).

That's one criterion met for alcohol use disorder, but a patient needs two to qualify, even minimally. As we scan the list, we see that Dolores's qualifications were not impressive. She certainly had never shown tolerance or withdrawal, and there was no evidence of interference with her work and personal life. You might think that all her efforts at control would qualify her, but they were almost completely *successful*. OK, so we'll agree she had a persistent strong desire to use (A4), which would barely gain her admittance to the alcohol use disorder ballpark. Still, she would have a severity rating of only *mild*.

However, Dolores could claim several criterion C symptoms of alcohol intoxication, any one of which would qualify her for that diagnosis. Shortly after drinking (A), her judgment was impaired (she drove—B). She slurred her words, walked unsteadily, and had difficulty even *un*buttoning her coat (C1, C3, C2). When she finally got into the office, she lapsed into a doze, but that's hardly a (C6) coma, is it?

A clinician attending Dolores would have to consider whether a history, physical exam, or laboratory data would be needed to be sure her symptoms were not due to **another medical condition** (D). However, her typical symptoms and history of recent alcohol use make that seem unnecessary. A diagnosis of **alcohol-induced delirium** would not be warranted in Dolores's case: Although her reduced attention span and lowered state of consciousness had come on quickly, the vignette contains no evidence of cognitive changes such as disorientation, memory loss, perceptual disturbance, or language problems (though her speech was slurred, her thought processes seemed intact).

The generic criteria for substance intoxication specify, as noted earlier, that the syndrome must be reversible. Of course, the question of reversibility could not be answered for several hours, until the symptoms had had a chance to wear off. Until then, the diagnosis could be made only on a presumptive basis. Although Dolores had had an abortion and experienced the death of her mother, neither of these events had happened recently, and so seemed unlikely to affect the course of her treatment; we don't need to give them a Z-code/V-code. With a GAF score of 75, Dolores' diagnosis would be as below. But to get the code, we have to make use of Table 15.2 and pinpoint intoxication with mild use disorder.

F10.129 [305.00, 303.00]   Mild alcohol use disorder, with alcohol intoxication

Other Alcohol-Induced Disorders

Toward the end of the chapter, Table 15.2 lists and gives the codes for other alcohol-induced disorders. Additional alcohol-related vignettes are provided elsewhere: Danny Finch (p. 95), Barney Gorse (p. 221), Rodney Partridge (p. 483), Mark Culpepper (p. 522), Charles Jackson (p. 524), Jack Weiblich (p. 554), and at least one patient in Chapter 20.

F10.99 [291.9] Unspecified Alcohol-Related Disorder

Use unspecified alcohol-related disorder to describe any alcohol-related symptoms that cause clinically important impairment or distress but do not meet full criteria for any of the disorders described above. One example would be *alcohol idiosyncratic intoxication*. Some people react strongly to a very small amount of alcohol (too little for most people to appear intoxicated). For instance, a person who is usually withdrawn and unassuming may become hostile and belligerent after a single glass of wine. This condition occurs within minutes of the drinking, and lasts a few hours at most. Predisposing factors may be advancing age, fatigue, and brain injury, such as that which might result from trauma or infection. This phenomenon has also been called *pathological intoxication*; in DSM-III-R, it had a code number of its own. In DSM-5, assuming it is serious enough to cause problems, code it here.

Caffeine-Related Disorders

Caffeine, the most widely used psychoactive substance in the world, is present in coffee, cola beverages, tea, chocolate, and a variety of prescription and over-the-counter drugs. Perhaps two-thirds to three-quarters of adults frequently consume at least one of these. Although tolerance and some degree of withdrawal are undeniably associated with caffeine, few people would ever experience enough social problems to qualify for caffeine use disorder; in any case, DSM-5 provides no such criteria set. Caffeine is the only psychoactive drug in the manual that carries no legal restrictions whatsoever on its use.

Black coffee has long been used as a folk remedy to sober up people who have drunk too much alcohol. However, caffeine does nothing to relieve their symptoms. Rather, it only adds agitation to the mix for someone who was formerly "only" inebriated.

F15.929 [305.90] Caffeine Intoxication

The symptoms caused by "Mr. Coffee Nerves" (the now-retired star of advertisements for Postum, a hot drink alternative to coffee) may seem too familiar to rate much space. However, it has been estimated that as many as 10% of adults may at some time have symptoms of caffeine intoxication, also known as *caffeinism*. The symptoms are much like those of generalized anxiety disorder (p. 191). The patient feels "wired," excessively energetic, excitable, and driven. Loud speech, irritability, and jitteriness are also commonly associated with caffeine intoxication.

The effects are determined by several factors. Of course, the individual degree of tolerance is important, but so is the amount ingested. A naïve user might experience symptoms from as little as 250 mg of caffeine—just a couple of cups of strong brew. However, even an experienced coffee drinker who takes in more than 500 mg per day risks intoxication. Other individual characteristics, such as age, fatigue, physical condition, and expectations, can also play a role. A diagnosis of caffeine intoxication is usually not made in people who are younger than 35; perhaps it takes years to develop awareness that there is even a problem.

Although I have not included a separate vignette in this section, the case of Dave Kincaid, described in Chapter 11 for substance-induced sleep disorder, illustrates caffeine intoxication as well. (For Dave's full case vignette, see p. 347.) I evaluate Dave's caffeinism below.

Readers who are wide awake (my diagnosis: too much coffee) may have noticed something funny about the ICD-9 number for caffeine intoxication. The humor is this: 305.90 has already been assigned—to three *mild use disorders*: inhalant, PCP, and other (or unknown). What's going on?

As this book goes to press, that excellent question still doesn't have a good answer. To be consistent, the assigned number for any intoxication other than alcohol should be 292.89, but consistency didn't win the battle here. ICD-9 code numbers seem to be have been assigned via roughly the same process as that involved in making sausages and laws, and I'm guessing that we don't truly want to know the details.

Here's the punch line: After October 1, 2014, ICD-9 will be history and no one will care.

Essential Features of **Caffeine Intoxication**

Shortly after consuming caffeine, the patient develops symptoms of increased nervous system and motor activity, such as fidgeting, increased energy, insomnia, rapid heartbeat, twitching muscles, intestinal upset, excess urination, red face, rambling speech.

The Fine Print

The D's: • Duration to symptom onset (recent) • Distress or disability (work/educational, social, or personal impairment) • Differential diagnosis (physical disorders, intoxication from other substances, other mental disorders)

You can find the specifics of caffeine intoxication in Table 15.1.

Evaluation of Dave Kincaid's Caffeinism

Dave Kincaid worked at a coffee-roasting store while he was writing his novel. He had free access to the rich, thick coffee they served there. He also snacked on quite a few chocolate-covered coffee beans. In all, he probably consumed over 1,000 mg of caffeine per day (criterion A for caffeine intoxication), so he had reason to feel "up" (B3). He couldn't sit still when he was trying to type (B1), and at night he lay awake with insomnia (B4). Rapid heartbeat, abdominal upset, and nervousness (B10, B7, B2) are also fairly typical symptoms that can be encountered even with relatively mild caffeinism (which Dave's was not).

Most of the DSM-5 symptoms can be found after as few as two cups of coffee, though perhaps not in full concert, as with Dave. Muscle twitching ("live flesh," as Dave called it—B8), agitation, and periods of tirelessness require caffeine intake substantially greater (1 gram of caffeine or more per day). He had in all at least six symptoms; only five are required by the DSM-5 criteria. No wonder he was distressed (C).

Because its symptoms are sometimes confused with other mental disorders, it is important to keep caffeine intoxication in mind. If we assume that Dave included his mental health when he said that he had been well, he probably would not have had a previous history of disorders such as anxiety disorders (especially **generalized anxiety disorder** and **panic disorder**), mood disorders (especially with **manic** or **hypomanic episodes**), and various **sleep disorders.** He had once smoked a little **marijuana**, but he had never used other substances whose effects might be confused with caffeinism. These would especially include the central nervous system stimulants: **cocaine, amphetamines, and related substances.**

Ruling in or out caffeine-induced anxiety disorder and caffeine-induced sleep disorder requires some clinical judgment. For these disorders, the symptoms must be more severe than are usually found in plain caffeine intoxication, and they must be serious enough to need independent clinical attention.

The rest of Dave's history (and diagnosis) can be found on page 347.

F15.93 [292.0] Caffeine Withdrawal

In *DSM-IV Made Easy*, I noted that caffeine withdrawal wasn't an official DSM diagnosis, but that it should be. A lot of other clinicians apparently had the same idea, for the clamor to move it into The Good Book began years ago.

Caffeine withdrawal may be especially likely during changes in a person's social schedule, as during vacations, over weekends, and the like. Then that person is likely to encounter fatigue, headache, and sleepiness. Somewhat less frequent symptoms include impairment of concentration and motor performance. DSM-5 notes that migraine and viral illness are examples of possible physical disorders to rule out.

Essential Features of **Caffeine Withdrawal**

The patient suddenly stops or markedly reduces the extended, heavy intake of caffeine, yielding symptoms suggesting flu (headache, nausea, muscle pain) and central nervous system depression (fatigue, dysphoria, poor concentration).

The Fine Print

The D's: • Duration to symptom onset (3+ symptoms within 1 day) • Distress or disability (work, social, or personal impairment) • Differential diagnosis (physical disorders, other substances, other mental disorders)

You can find the specifics of caffeine withdrawal in Table 15.1.

You

How many coffee drinkers have had an experience like this one? You have come to stay with a friend who, you realize upon awakening the first morning, eschews coffee and hasn't so much as a bean in the house. After frantic, futile foraging for even a jar of instant, you decide, "This isn't worth the effort. I'll get along without it for a change."

And for the first few hours, you do just fine. But as lunchtime inches around, you find you aren't feeling quite so well. Last night you were eager to see old friends and new places; today you've only the strength to crawl back into the old sack. Because your stomach is fomenting revolution, you wonder, "What that's intestinal could I have been exposed to on the plane?" As your headache, which for a couple of hours has been hanging back at the edge of your skull, now asserts itself, you can only growl when your hosts suggest it's a lovely day.

Finally, in desperation, you make your painful way to the nearest Starbuck's. An espresso and a double latte later, your headache scurries for the exit, the day brightens, and you depart renewed, leaving a generous tip for the barista.

Evaluation of You

Look, this isn't astrophysics. You've suddenly been cut off from your quotidian coffee fix (criterion A), whereupon you develop classic symptoms of caffeine withdrawal: headache, fatigue, irritability, and physical complaints that resemble the flu (B1, B2, B3, B5; only three symptoms from criterion B are required). You feel so lousy you'd risk the distress and social embarrassment of alienating good friends you see too rarely (certainly not recently enough to remember that they don't stock your beverage of choice—C).

Of course, you might have the flu or **another medical condition**, or maybe it's jet lag. Yes, you'd need to rule out other, competing causes for your symptoms (D), but this shouldn't prove too onerous: With your GAF score of 85, You hardly need a physical exam; rapid improvement with a shot of the Elixir of Life confirms that the diagnosis for You is:

F15.93 [292.0]   Caffeine withdrawal

I have an ulterior motive for choosing *You* as an example of caffeine withdrawal: It demonstrates how easily just about anyone can sneak into the DSM.

Many books and articles comment on the countless Americans (and, by extension, perhaps billions of ordinary people the world over) who could eventually be diagnosed with a mental or behavioral disorder. Even a decade ago, 46% of Americans were diagnosable by DSM-IV criteria.

If I sound preachy here, I apologize—without feeling especially sorry—but I do want to underscore the extent to which we've pathologized some of our most cherished behaviors. For if even *You* can inhabit the pages of DSM-5, who can't?

Other Caffeine-Induced Disorders

Caffeine use disorder has been included in Section III of DSM-5 as a subject for further study. That's partly because quite a few long-time caffeine users develop symptoms of a substance use disorder. These especially include making multiple attempts to stop using and continuing to use despite knowing that it is creating medical problems for them—and withdrawal symptoms. You will find a complete listing of caffeine-induced disorders in Table 15.2.

F15.99 [292.9] Unspecified Caffeine-Related Disorder

Cannabis-Related Disorders

Cannabis is the generic name of the hemp plant, *Cannabis sativa*, whose active ingredient is tetrahydrocannabinol (THC). Depending on the variety of hemp and the place where it is grown, the leaves and tops may contain anywhere from 1% to about 10% THC, a figure that has been rising for several decades. (In some California locales, careful nurturing of selected cultivars has produced the latter figure and higher— a dubious triumph of U.S. agriculture.) Hashish, which is a resin produced from the leaves of the hemp plant, contains about 10% THC.

Cannabis is the most widely used illicit substance in the United States, and indeed in the world. As many as 4% of all American adults may at some time qualify for a cannabis-related disorder. Since 2007, its popularity appears once again to be on the rise. Unsurprisingly, it is more common among younger people, especially men. The extent of the effect that the legalization of marijuana in certain jurisdictions of the United States will have remains, at this time, unclear.

Use of cannabis more often than weekly increases the likelihood of addiction. People who suddenly quit after heavy use may experience mild physiological symptoms that can last several weeks; these include anxiety, sleeplessness, and other symptoms similar to sedative withdrawal. The serious behavioral and psychological consequences seen in those withdrawing from other substances (cocaine, opioids, alcohol, and the like) are less problematic with cannabis. Therefore, it wasn't until DSM-5 that criteria for cannabis withdrawal were included in a DSM. Heavy users may learn with surprise that they have developed tolerance. Relative to other substance use disorders, the development of cannabis use disorder can take a long time. It tends to occur in the context of social use, which may be more common than with other drugs of abuse. Eventually, the familiar symptoms of substance use disorder emerge.

Flashbacks are rare. So is depression, which, when present, is usually temporary and mild. Some patients experience paranoia that can last as long as several days. Using cannabis may worsen the psychosis of someone who already has schizophrenia.

Cannabis may be one of the most difficult substances for some patients to stop using, simply because it causes relatively few of the medical complications that can motivate the cessation of other, more dangerous substances. Although cannabis is usually smoked, THC can be absorbed from the gastrointestinal tract—hence the stories you hear about marijuana brownies. Because absorption can be erratic, THC that has been swallowed is especially dangerous.

Some clinicians believe that there is also a syndrome of chronic cannabis use. Though variable, the symptoms are said to include mild depression, reduced drive, and decreased interest in ordinary activities. Adolescents are especially likely to experience cognitive effects from heavy use. These include decreased memory, attention, and thinking, which can persist beyond the period of acute intoxication and worsen with long years of habitual use.

Cannabis Use Disorder

The characteristics of cannabis use disorder are similar to those of nearly every other specific substance use disorder. The criteria are identical to those for a generic substance use disorder (p. 396). For coding, see Tables 15.2 and 15.3.

Cannabis Intoxication

Devotees of cannabis value it for the relaxation and elevation of mood it confers. It causes their perceptions to seem more acute; colors may seem brighter. Adults seem to see the world afresh, much the way a child does. Their appreciation for music and art is enhanced. Their ideas flow rapidly; they may find their own conversation especially witty.

The effects of cannabis are many and varied, with both negative and positive reactions strongly influenced by setting and frame of mind. Time sense often changes—a few minutes may seem like an hour. Users may become passive and drowsy; mood drifts into apathy. Motor performance suffers (cannabis notoriously impairs driving performance). Usually cannabis also produces red eyes and a rapid heartbeat.

Often a user will appear more or less normal, even when highly intoxicated. Illusions may occur, but hallucinations are rare. Users generally retain insight; they remain unconvinced by their own misperceptions, and may even laugh about them.

Especially in first-time users, intoxication often begins with anxiety, which can progress to panic. In fact, the most common untoward reaction to cannabis is an anxiety disorder. Some patients fear that body distortions mean impending death.

Essential Features of **Cannabis Intoxication**

Shortly after using cannabis, the patient develops symptoms of motor incoordination or altered cognition (anxiety or exhilaration, poor judgment, isolation from friends, a sense of slowed time) plus telltale red eyes, dry mouth, rapid heart rate, and hunger.

The Fine Print

The D's: • Duration to symptom onset (minutes to hours, depending on route of administration) • Differential diagnosis (intoxication from hallucinogens and other substances)

You can find the specifics of cannabis intoxication in Table 15.1.

Coding Notes

Specify if: **With perceptual disturbances.** The patient has altered perceptions: illusions of vision, hearing, or touch, or hallucinations with intact insight (the patient recognizes that the symptoms are unreal, caused by the substance use). Hallucinations without this insight suggest a diagnosis of cannabis-induced psychotic disorder.

Coding in ICD-10 depends on the presence of perceptual disturbances; see Table 15.2.

As with intoxication due to any substance, the criteria for cannabis intoxication require that recent use produce clinically important, troublesome psychological or behavioral changes. It would be hard to argue that social withdrawal and defective judgment are anything but clinically significant, but euphoria? Suppose a person reports feeling really, really happy and nothing comes of it? Then is that person not intoxicated? Some diagnostic criteria work better than others. Some still leave much to the interpretation of the individual clinician.

Russell Zahn

"You got a candy bar on you?" Russell Zahn shambled into the interviewer's office and slumped onto the sofa. He flicked a lock of hair back across one shoulder of his torn denim jacket. "I know it's only an hour since breakfast, but I'm really hungry."

At age 27, Russell lived on general relief and was often homeless. In the hills of northern California where he grew up, the principal cash crop was marijuana. For the first several years since leaving high school, he had worked at its cultivation and marketing; more recently, he had been more or less exclusively a consumer. Now he had been referred to the mental health clinic by a judge who had grown weary of his repeated courtroom appearances for possession of small amounts of marijuana. Russell volunteered that he had enjoyed a joint in the alley outside, just before coming in for his appointment.

Russell wasn't especially unhappy about being evaluated; he just didn't see much need for it. He required very little to live on. Whatever his relief check didn't cover, he earned by begging. He had his own corner in the business section of town, where for 6 hours a day he lounged behind a sign requesting contributions. Every couple of hours he would walk back to the alley and sneak a toke. "I don't smoke on duty," he said. "It's bad for business."

All in all, life seemed a lot better now than when he was a kid. Both of Russell's parents had died in an automobile accident when he was 6. For 2 years after that, he had been passed around among grandparents, aunts and uncles, and a cousin. No one really wanted him, and he had terminated a 6-year tour of various foster homes by running away when he was 14.

The alternative lifestyle of the northern California marijuana industry had suited Russell just fine, until he discovered that no industry at all suited him even better. It had been years since he had worked at anything, and he supposed he never would again. His mood was always good. He had never had to see a doctor. He had tried all the other drugs ("except smack"), but he didn't really care for any of them.

Russell stood and stretched. He rubbed his already brick-red eyes. "Well, thanks for listening."

The interviewer asked where he was going and pointed out that his appointment wasn't over. "You've only been here about 20 minutes."

"Really?" Russell slouched back into his chair. "It seemed more like an hour. I've always had a lousy sense of time."

Evaluation of Russell Zahn

According to DSM-5, Russell's time distortion (typically, time seems to crawl) would fulfill the requirement for a maladaptive behavior (criterion B for cannabis intoxication) due to recent cannabis use (A). It is not clear how clinically important this was for Russell, but the interviewer certainly noticed. Red eyes (C1) and heightened appetite (suggested by his desire for a midmorning candy bar—C2) provided the two physical indicators necessary to make the diagnosis. For coding purposes, note that he had no evidence of disturbed perception (such as illusions or hallucinations).

Of course, possible use of other substances (notably **alcohol** and **hallucinogens**, if perceptual problems are noted) should be considered in the differential diagnosis of cannabis intoxication. History and the odor of alcohol can be important to this differentiation and to ruling out mental disorders such as **anxiety** and **mood disorders** (D).

Did Russell have a cannabis use disorder? He had smoked it for a number of years. Although he might have greater tolerance to the drug than the average user (substance use disorder criterion A10), there was no evidence that he used more than he intended or that he had ever tried to exercise control. In DSM-5, there is at last a withdrawal syndrome for cannabis; stay tuned for more of Russell's history (below). Russell did spend considerable time procuring and using marijuana (A3), and his homeless, aimless life could have been due in part to the use of the drug (A4). (Alternatively, you could argue that a personality disorder caused these problems *and* the cannabis use.) The vignette does not suggest any physical or psychological problem caused by the cannabis. Still, considering the low quality of Russell's work ethic, the time he spent using, and his probable tolerance to the drug, a diagnosis of cannabis use disorder seems warranted.

In any event, with no evidence of perceptual changes such as hallucinations or illusions, we can use Table 15.2 to arrive at a preliminary diagnosis. (ICD-10 gives us different numbers to use, depending on the presence of perceptual disturbances.) Note also that ICD-9 requires separate numbers for intoxication and the use disorder (see Table 15.3).

F12.229 [304.30, 292.89]   Moderate cannabis use disorder, with intoxication, without perceptual disturbances

Cannabis Withdrawal

As recently as the debut of DSM-IV, some researchers still wondered whether cannabis withdrawal even existed. Perhaps it simply took time to emerge from the haze created by a relatively weak available drug combined with relatively few truly heavy users. In the past decade or so, however, much evidence has accumulated that cannabis withdrawal is real—that, indeed, perhaps a third of users experience this debilitating state at one time or another. It needs to be repeated that, as for certain other drug classes, withdrawal that stems from medical use should not be counted as a criterion for cannabis use disorder. This is becoming ever more relevant in our era of medical availability of marijuana in so many jurisdictions, and legal recreational pot in a few.

Half or more of those who experience withdrawal mention craving the drug, with dysphoria and restlessness. Some report vivid, often unpleasant dreams or nightmares. Symptoms can be about as severe as for nicotine withdrawal; in fact, some users substitute tobacco (or alcohol) to combat their withdrawal symptoms. Symptoms last for a few days to a couple of weeks; physical symptoms decrease sooner than do psychological symptoms. In several studies, withdrawal symptoms were a strong predictor of relapse.

Essential Features of **Cannabis Withdrawal**

After stopping major, long-lasting cannabis use, the patient experiences symptoms of dysphoria and central nervous system overactivity, along with troubled sleep, poor appetite, depression, anxiety, restlessness, and physical discomfort from shakiness, sweating, chills/fever, headache, or abdominal pain.

The Fine Print

The D's: • Duration (heavy, daily use for months; onset within a few days of reduction) • Distress or disability (work/educational, social, or personal impairment) • Differential diagnosis (physical disorders, other substance or mental disorders)

You can find the specifics of cannabis withdrawal in Table 15.1.

Coding Note

Coding is given in Tables 15.2 and 15.3, but note that ICD-10 (Table 15.2) allows only one code for withdrawal (there must be a use disorder, and it can only be moderate or severe).

Russell Zahn Again

Russell was taken into custody after his evaluation. A bored judge quickly agreed that he should remain incarcerated, then departed for the long Labor Day weekend.

Russell's first few hours in jail weren't too bad. That day and the next, he talked to a friendly guard and played cribbage with his cellmate. But he slept fitfully, and by Sunday he was boisterous and agitated, hitting the bars of his cell with a spoon—which was the only good he got from his dinner tray. "I'm just not hungry, OK?" he snapped, as the guard removed the untouched meatloaf.

Russell lay awake practically the whole night. He felt sweaty and had chills (but no fever), headache, and a cramping pain in his stomach that doubled him over on his bunk. "It was like the worst flu you ever imagined," he whined to the nurse practitioner making rounds, even though it was a weekend.

The NP found nothing physically wrong and told the guard, "Just a pothead coming unglued. A couple of weeks will put him right."

Further Evaluation of Russell Zahn

Can we stipulate that Russell's experience with cannabis was both long-lasting and heavy (criterion A for cannabis withdrawal)? Abruptly deprived of weed, Russell experienced nearly every criterion in the cannabis withdrawal list, including anger (B1), anxiety (B2), insomnia (B3), anorexia (B4), agitation (B5), and abdominal pain (B7)—certainly enough to provoke the distress required for diagnosis (C). We'll take the NP's word that they weren't due to the flu or **some other physical ailment** (D).

The symptoms for cannabis withdrawal are a lot like those of **withdrawal from other substances (alcohol, sedatives, stimulants,** and **tobacco)**, each of which we'd have to place on our list of differential diagnoses. But the history makes Russell's diagnosis crystal clear; to his previous use disorder symptoms, we would just append withdrawal. With all that we've now learned, I'd upgrade his cannabis use disorder to a level of severe, regardless of how many symptoms we can enumerate.

Russell's GAF score would be 50 (about his highest level in the past year). Using Table 15.2, we'd give Russell (no longer intoxicated) a diagnosis reflecting withdrawal and his use disorder. And somewhere in the summary I wrote up, I'd want to stress the importance of investigating further for the possibility of a personality disorder. Right now, there's too little information and too much pot to allow any sort of personality assessment.

F12.288 [304.30, 292.0]   Severe cannabis use disorder, with withdrawal
Z59.0 [V60.0]   Homeless
Z56.9 [V62.29]   Unemployed
Z65.3 [V62.5]   Repeated arrests

Other Cannabis-Induced Disorders

You will find a complete listing of cannabis-induced disorders in Tables 15.2 and 15.3. Two possibilities deserve special mention:

Cannabis-induced psychotic disorder, with delusions. This disorder involves delusions that are usually persecutory. It lasts only a day, or several days at the most. In the United States, it is rare and most often seen in juveniles. But in other countries and cultures (for example, Gambia), it may be more common. Most U.S. patients who have delusions associated with cannabis probably have other diagnoses as well, such as schizophrenia and drug–drug interactions.

Cannabis-induced anxiety disorder. The case of Bonita Ramirez, a college student who had cannabis-induced anxiety disorder, is given in Chapter 4 (see p. 194).

F12.99 [292.9] Unspecified Cannabis-Related Disorder

Hallucinogen-Related Disorders

Also called *psychedelic* and *psychotomimetic* drugs, hallucinogens as a rule produce illusions, not hallucinations. Two such drugs that occur naturally are psilocybin (obtained from certain mushrooms) and peyote (cactus, though probably not the one sitting on a shelf in your kitchen). However, phencyclidine (PCP) is a manufactured hallucinogen that has very similar toxic effects. I also discuss lysergic acid diethylamide (LSD) and other hallucinogens. (A withdrawal syndrome hasn't been established for this drug class, so the substance use criteria include only 10 criteria, not the customary 11.)

Phencyclidine

In DSM-IV, PCP was listed in its own separate section; in DSM-5, reason has prevailed, and it is now bundled in with the other hallucinogens—though the respective criteria for use disorder and intoxication remain distinct. Called *angel dust* on the street, PCP is a hallucinogen with both stimulant and depressant qualities. In its typical street dose of 5 mg, this highly potent drug can produce psychotic symptoms so convincing that you sometimes cannot distinguish them from schizophrenia. A person with a genetic predisposition to schizophrenia who takes it risks activating serious pathology.

PCP was originally developed as an anesthetic agent; harmful side effects caused it to be scrapped for human use in the mid-20th century, and even its use in veterinary medicine has been halted. Its less potent analogue, ketamine, is still used as an anesthetic agent in both human and veterinary medicine. However, because PCP is cheap and easy to produce (it can be mixed up almost literally in a bathtub), it is still sometimes used by young men who value it for the euphoria it produces.

Despite lack of a withdrawal syndrome in humans, PCP's addictive potential is pronounced—as dangerous as that of cocaine and heroin, some say. When it is swallowed, symptoms begin within an hour; if it is smoked, they begin within a few minutes. A high lasts from 4 to 6 hours and can be repeated in runs lasting several days. The use of PCP is seemingly limited only by the user's imagination—by snorting, by swallowing, or by injection. It can even be absorbed vaginally. Now it is usually smoked in cigarettes, which are preferred because the effects from smoking occur so quickly that the user can titrate them with some precision, perhaps averting emergency room visits for overdose.

PCP and ketamine are both used by relatively small numbers of individuals, especially males in their teens and 20s.

LSD and Other Hallucinogens

The prototype of the manufactured hallucinogens is LSD, which in the 1960s was embraced as the first new mind-altering substance to be developed in generations. In the United States, legal manufacture of LSD has long since vanished; all supplies currently come from illicit labs, largely in northern California. Newer synthetics—MDA, MDMA, and others—continue to turn up. These are sometimes called "designer drugs" because they resemble the pharmacological properties of known hallucinogens while escaping (at first) their illegal status. Then there are the venerable natural substances—mescaline, psilocybin, and lysergic acid amide, similar to LSD and found in morning glory seeds—each of which is generally a less potent hallucinogen than LSD or PCP.

During the past 20 years or so, LSD appears to have fallen out of fashion; it is now used by under 1% of college students. However, designer drugs (especially MDMA, which combines hallucinogenic and stimulant qualities; see sidebar, p. 451) may have increased in popularity. Most users consume other drugs, too. In many cases, drugs sold on the street are quite different from what is promised. Lacking a quality control ethic, vendors freely substitute cheap for dear, available for rare. Thus, for example, so-called "psilocybin" may in fact be ordinary mushrooms onto which some entrepreneur has sprayed LSD or PCP.

Tolerance to LSD occurs so rapidly that an individual will rarely use it more than once a week. More frequent use simply doesn't produce an effect worth the trouble. No withdrawal syndrome from LSD or other hallucinogens is defined, though some people reportedly crave them after stopping.

Because one hallmark of successive DSMs has been renaming disorders in the interests of greater descriptive accuracy, it is astonishing that the hallucinogens *still* retain their mendacious label. (I emphasize *still* because I was similarly appalled two decades ago, at DSM-IV.) Typically, they do not produce hallucinations at all, but illusions; some writers have referred to them as *illusionogens*. Now there's a movement afoot to replace the term *psychedelic* ("mind-manifesting") with *entheogen*, used to denote a substance that evokes a religious or spiritual effect. I don't think it has a prayer.

Phencyclidine Use Disorder and Other Hallucinogen Use Disorder

The characteristics of the use disorder for both PCP and other hallucinogens are similar to those of nearly every other substance use disorder in the manual. Except for the symptom of withdrawal, which doesn't appear to occur with most hallucinogens, the criteria are a straightforward adaptation of those for a generic substance use disorder (p. 396). I discuss them as they apply to the two vignettes that follow. Code numbers are given in Tables 15.2 and 15.3.

Phencyclidine Intoxication

With much variability, the effects of PCP are related to dose. Besides euphoria, PCP can produce lethargy, anxiety, depression, delirium, and behavioral problems that include agitation, impulsivity, and assault. Even catatonic symptoms and suicide have been reported. Some users experience violent, exaggerated, unpredictable responses to light or sound; as a result, clinicians may recommend sensory restriction for intoxicated patients. Physical symptoms include high fever, muscle rigidity, muteness, and hypertension. Heavy doses can result in coma, convulsions, and death from respiratory arrest.

Essential Features of **Phencyclidine Intoxication**

Shortly after using PCP, the patient develops serious, sometimes lethal symptoms of behavioral disinhibition—unpredictable impulsivity, aggression, poor judgment. With it, there are signs of neurological impairment and muscle dyscontrol: jerking eye movements called nystagmus, trouble walking or speaking, stiff muscles, numbness, coma, or seizures. Heartbeat or blood pressure can be high, and sometimes hearing seems abnormally acute.

The Fine Print

The D's: • Duration to onset of symptoms (within 1–2 hours) • Differential diagnosis

(physical disorders; intoxication from hallucinogens and other substances; other mental disorders, especially psychotic disorders)

You can find the specifics of phencyclidine intoxication in Table 15.1.

Coding Notes

See Tables 15.2 and 15.3 for codes.

Jennie Meyerson

At age 24, Jennie Meyerson had been troubled half her life. When she was 12, her father had walked out on the family in the midst of the worst argument she could remember between her warring parents. The divorce had preoccupied her mother and driven her older sister from home, leaving Jennie pretty much on her own.

By the time she was 14, she had begun smoking marijuana after school and sometimes between classes. Within a year, she was smoking instead of going to classes. On her 18th birthday, her mother kicked her out of the house. She lived with a succession of boyfriends, each of whom introduced her to a new recreational drug. She had been in and out of mental hospitals and was a double alumna of the local Betty Ford clinic.

Jennie's last interviewer was Patrolman Reggie Polansky, a young police officer. One Saturday afternoon, he was called to the sixth floor of a run-down apartment building, where a young woman was sitting on a ledge high above the street. The sweetish smell of marijuana smoke enveloped Polansky as he walked through the room to the window.

The ledge just outside the window was perhaps 10 inches wide. About a yard to his left sat Jennie, barefoot and bare-legged, wearing a cotton blouse and a thin dress. She sat quietly, her face tilted up to the late summer sunshine. On the pavement 80 feet below, a crowd had gathered.

Gripping the window sill, Polansky poked his head out. "What are you doing out there?"

"Just ress—jes' res-ting." With an effort, she finally pronounced the word. She didn't open her eyes or turn her head. "I'm gonna fly."

"You don't want to do that. Come on back in here."

"You c'mon out—here. I'm Amelia Earhart. We can both fly." Jennie giggled, and they talked for several minutes. OK, she was joking about being Amelia Earhart, but she did think she could learn to fly. It had come to her in a flash this morning, after she "got dusted." She'd been using angel dust off and on for the past several months.

Patrolman Polansky pointed to her hand. The webbed space between her thumb and finger was bleeding. "You've cut yourself."

Jennie said she must have done it on the jagged window cornice as she was climbing out. Perhaps it was a message from God. That must be it, she said, because she hadn't felt it at all. It was like God's wounds. Instead, she felt happy, strong, and light. She felt like practicing for the Labor Day air show on Monday.

"Look how close the ground is," she said. "It seems like I can just step down there."

She stood, raised both arms until they extended straight out from her shoulders, and stepped lightly forward onto the wind.

Evaluation of Jennie Meyerson

Jennie's recent use of angel dust and badly affected judgment amply met criteria A and B for phencyclidine intoxication. Of the criterion D physical symptoms required, two are documented in the vignette: trouble speaking (her speech was slurred—C5) and reduced pain perception (she hadn't noticed that she had torn the skin of her hand while climbing out the window—C3). Two are what's required.

Jennie also had an illusion (the ground looked close to her, rather than six stories down). Such perceptual distortions can also be the work of **intoxication** with other drugs, including **stimulants, opioids**, and **cannabis.** The odor in the room suggested to Patrolman Polansky that marijuana had been used, but PCP users often spray their drug onto something they can smoke (usually marijuana or tobacco, sometimes parsley). When reliable information is lacking, a definitive diagnosis often depends on a toxicology report.

The vignette gives no information as to the extent of Jennie's problem with PCP, so we couldn't confirm a diagnosis of phencyclidine use disorder. The vignette clearly indicates that Jennie had had, at a minimum, previous occupational (school) problems resulting from her use of a variety of substances. Further diagnosis would depend on additional information about her usage patterns. All things considered, a *provisional* diagnosis of moderate to severe phencyclidine use disorder seems justified. Considering the outcome, I think that the severity code I've given is justified, regardless of how many symptoms we can conjure.

Jennie's statements that she could fly and that she had stigmata ("God's wounds") were not firmly held, and therefore not delusional. This would rule out **schizophrenia** and any other psychosis. There was no evidence that her disorder was due to a physical illness (D). In other patients, rapid resolution (often without treatment) may help differentiate intoxication due to hallucinogens from other mental disorders such as mood and anxiety disorders. Hallucinogen users should also be evaluated for personality disorders and the use of other mind-altering substances.

Jennie's postmortem diagnosis would be as below. Of course, her GAF was nil, and we'll never have the chance to explore her for possible personality disorder.

F16.229 [304.60, 292.89]   Severe phencyclidine use disorder (provisional), with phencyclidine intoxication

Other Hallucinogen Intoxication

The first symptoms of other hallucinogen intoxication are usually somatic. Patients may mention dizziness, tremor, weakness, or numbness and tingling of extremities. Perceptual changes (usually illusions) include the apparent amplification of sounds and visual distortions (such as of body image), as well as *synesthesias* (in which one type of sensory experience produces the sensation of another—for example, a professor I knew of saw red, white, and blue upon hearing a C-E-G chord played on the piano).

Hallucinations, if they occur at all, may be of vivid geometric forms or colors. Auditory hallucinations can also occur. Many people experience intense euphoria, depersonalization (that is, a sense of detachment from oneself), derealization (a sense of unreality in one's perceptions), dream-like states, or the sense that time speeds up or slows down. Attention may be impaired, though most users retain insight.

The specific features are greatly influenced by setting and by a person's expectations. Some users find the experience pleasant; others become extraordinarily anxious. A "bad trip" usually includes feelings of anxiety and depression; panic attacks may occur. These reactions will occasionally be prolonged, characterized by fears of becoming psychotic. Usually, acutely negative reactions subside within 24 hours—the time it takes to excrete all of the drug.

LSD is an extremely potent agent; just a few micrograms (an amount that can be soaked onto a postage stamp) can produce significant symptoms. It is absorbed from the gut, and action usually begins within an hour. The effects tend to peak at 2–4 hours, and may last half a day. Like PCP, LSD and other hallucinogens can be lethal.

Essential Features of **Other Hallucinogen Intoxication**

Shortly after using a non-PCP hallucinogen, the patient develops symptoms of dysphoria, misperception, or poor judgment, plus autonomic overactivity: dilated pupils and blurred vision, sweating, rapid or irregular heartbeat, trembling, reduced muscle coordination.

The Fine Print

The D's: Duration until onset of symptoms (usually 1 hour or less) • Differential diagnosis (other substances, other mental disorders, other medical conditions)
     You can find the specifics of other hallucinogen intoxication in Table 15.1.

Coding Notes

In recording your diagnosis, use the specific name, rather than *other hallucinogen*.
     See Tables 15.2 and 15.3 for codes.

Wanda Pittsinger

Though she was 26, Wanda Pittsinger still worked at the cinema. She had started this job on a part-time basis as a high school senior; after graduation, she had moved to full-time and stayed on. The pay was entry-level, but making change and popcorn was undemanding, and she got to see a lot of first-run movies (though not necessarily in start-to-finish order).

Wanda's job had lasted longer than her marriage. The year she was 22, she had been married to Randy for almost 10 months. Other than a pregnancy (which she'd also terminated), the main thing she got out of the relationship was an introduction to LSD. She still saw Randy occasionally, but by this time they were not much more than friends; about the only activity they pursued together was tripping, which almost invariably wiped out their sex drive.

Wanda had tried other drugs. Marijuana gave her headaches; cocaine made her nervous. The one time she had snorted heroin, she threw up. But acid was just about right. It always raised her spirits and made her feel giddy. Sometimes, if she was looking into a mirror, she seemed to see herself melting. This didn't bother her; you expected weird things to happen when you dropped acid. Besides the usual colored diamonds, triangles, and squares, she thought that LSD could reveal new meanings or insights. She valued that sensation of thinking deeply. The experience was almost always worth the palpitations and blurred vision that were her only side effects.

Acid even gave Wanda a better feeling about Randy. Occasionally she'd still trip with him on a day off, and he continued to supply her with the little squares of blotting paper impregnated with LSD. As a present, he had once given her two movie tickets that had been soaked in LSD. She'd kept them tucked into the corner of her dresser mirror.

Evaluation of Wanda Pittsinger

Wanda's psychological and behavioral changes while taking LSD were minor, and the pluses and minuses were pretty much a wash. They helped her tolerate Randy, but she lost interest in sex. One could argue whether these were clinically important—they weren't enough to get her into treatment, as a "bad trip" might (criterion B). But she had additional symptoms of other hallucinogen intoxication: She noted the usual side effects of blurred vision and palpitations of her heart (D5, D4). She also had some typical perceptual changes: illusions of lights, patterns, and shapes (C), and the sensation of having special insight. Moreover, she felt euphoric—another common experience with this drug.

The differential diagnosis of other hallucinogen intoxication includes **delirium**, **dementia**, **epilepsy**, and **schizophrenia.** Beyond her illusions, Wanda had symptoms suggestive of none of these disorders. However, her clinician would have to do a complete workup, including a mental status evaluation, to rule out other disorders completely. **Hypnopompic imagery** (visual imagery experienced between the sleeping and waking states) can take on the aspect of a flashback, but Wanda's illusory experiences occurred at times other than when she was waking up.

DSM-5 allows a diagnosis of other hallucinogen use disorder, but it is probably rare. Like Wanda, most users take LSD infrequently; rapid tolerance (loss of effect) results from use more often than once or twice a week. There was no evidence presented that she had lost control over the use of this substance or that its use altered the way she approached her job or social life.

OK, it's problematic whether Wanda could qualify for a diagnosis of other hallucinogen intoxication (F16.929 [292.89]). I'll give a fuller diagnosis a bit later.

F16.983 [292.89] Hallucinogen Persisting Perception Disorder

When a patient reexperiences some of the same symptoms that occurred during intoxication, but in the absence of the hallucinogen, a *flashback* is said to occur. Symptoms of flashbacks can include seeing faces, geometric forms, flashes of color, trails, afterimages, or halos; *micropsia* (in which things look small); and *macropsia* (in which things look huge). Diminished sex interest may be a feature. The patient usually has insight into what is happening.

Flashbacks may be triggered by stress, by entering a dark room, or by using marijuana or phenothiazines. Although brief flashbacks, lasting perhaps a few seconds, are common—over half of hallucinogen users have them—only a small percentage report enough of these symptoms to be distressing or to interfere with their activities. These experiences usually decrease with time; however, they can occur weeks or months after use and persist for years.

Essential Features of **Hallucinogen Persisting Perception Disorder**

After stopping the use of a hallucinogen, the patient again experiences at least one of the misperceptions that occurred during intoxication.

The Fine Print

The D's: • Duration to symptom onset (variable) • Distress or disability (work/educational, social, or personal impairment) • Differential diagnosis (physical disorders, delirium, other mental disorders, hypnopompic imagery)

You can find the specifics of hallucinogen intoxication in Table 15.1.

Coding Notes

See Tables 15.2 (especially footnote *d*) and 15.3 for codes.

Wanda Pittsinger Again

Wanda came for help because she sometimes found herself tripping when she hadn't dropped acid for several days.

"I noticed it one night at work when I walked into the auditorium just before the main feature. I saw myself on the screen, first all in green, and then sort of sparkly.

Then my image seemed to sort of dissolve, and I saw that it was only a trailer for a Woody Allen film that would be playing in 2 weeks."

When Wanda told Randy about this the next day, he called it a flashback and said that it was "cool." Despite Randy's reassurance, these experiences worried her. She stayed home from work for a day or two, because she felt she couldn't cope with the flashbacks at work. She had never used drugs of any sort since.

In the nearly 2 months since she had last used LSD, Wanda had experienced a number of flashbacks. Mostly she saw "trails"—ghostly afterimages of people or objects that had traversed her field of vision. A couple of times she had seen Randy's face on the ceiling of her bedroom. Once the kitchen table seemed to grow in size to the point that she thought that she would never be able to reach it to eat her breakfast. But she never again experienced her own image on the silver screen.

Further Evaluation of Wanda Pittsinger

Though the details had changed, when Wanda walked into the darkened theater on the occasion that eventually triggered her clinic visit, she experienced a recurrence of the illusions she had had during LSD intoxication (criterion A). Flashbacks of some degree or other are common; perhaps one-quarter of LSD users have them. Wanda's wouldn't qualify for a diagnosis at all if they hadn't so upset her (B).

As in hallucinogen intoxication, Wanda's clinician would have to rule out **delirium**, **dementia**, **schizophrenia**, **epilepsy**, and **space-occupying lesions in the brain** (C). She would not qualify for a diagnosis of **hallucinogen-induced psychotic disorder** because she had insight that her misperceptions were caused by substance use. The previous history of LSD use and the typical presentation would make her current diagnosis secure. Her GAF score would be 70.

F16.983 [292.89]   Hallucinogen persisting perception disorder

> Note that the description of hallucinogen persisting perception disorder doesn't distinguish it all that sharply from substance-induced psychotic disorder. Indeed, the principal bulwark separating the two is the verbiage asserting that flashbacks must not be due to another medical condition and must not be better explainable by another mental disorder. The requirement, like so many others, invokes your judgment as the clinician; your decision must rest on the patient's degree of insight and the history of substance use. The criteria won't help you a lot here; it's better to depend on the logic of your evaluation.

Other Phencyclidine-Induced or Hallucinogen-Induced Disorders

You will find a listing of PCP-induced and other hallucinogen-induced disorders in Table 15.2. Here are several that merit special mention:

Hallucinogen-induced mood disorder. Depression or anxiety is relatively common; euphoria is rare. Sleep is often decreased. Patients may be restless and experience feelings of guilt. They may express fear that they have destroyed their brains or gone crazy. Hallucinogen-induced mood disorder may last relatively briefly, or it may endure for months.

Hallucinogen-induced personality change. Chronic or one-time use may lead to character change, such as the development of magical thinking or a basic change in attitude.

Hallucinogen-induced persisting psychosis. Occasionally a hallucinogen seems to trigger a psychosis that may last a long time, perhaps forever. There has been a good deal of controversy as to whether this is "only" an underlying psychosis that might eventually have developed, even if the patient had never used drugs.

F16.99 [292.9] Unspecified Phencyclidine-Related or Hallucinogen-Related Disorder

Inhalant-Related Disorders

Accidentally inhaled, a volatile substance is called a *toxin*; if it is used on purpose to produce intoxication, it is called an *inhalant*. Intentional users will breathe almost anything that evaporates or can be sprayed from a container. Inhalants include glue and gasoline (which are perhaps the most popular), solvents, thinners, various aerosols, correction fluid, and refrigerants. Preference may be guided more by availability than by effect.

Users value inhalants for a number of reasons. They relieve boredom and alleviate concern. They alter ideas, moods, the sense of time, and perceptions (producing changes in color, size, or shape of objects, and sometimes frank hallucinations). Inhalants are also cheap and, like everything else that is absorbed through the lungs, quick to take effect.

Neurological damage from prolonged use of inhalants can be quite variable. Encephalopathy and peripheral neuropathy are widely experienced. Also, there can be ataxia, symptoms of parkinsonism, loss of vision, and involvement of the fifth and seventh cranial nerves, producing numbness and paralysis of the face. Chronic users may experience weight loss, weakness, disorientation, inattentiveness, and loss of coordination. Death, while rare, usually results when a patient uses a bag or mask that excludes oxygen from the mixture being breathed. Fetal malformation is another untoward complication of use.

Three groups of patients use inhalants. Boys and girls experiment with them, often as a group activity; the incidence peaks at around age 14, though popularity has been declining through the first years of the 21st century. Adults (mostly males) can become dependent on them. Finally, they are used by individuals who are also chronic users of other drugs. Many inhalant users come from underprivileged minorities. Personality disorders, especially antisocial personality disorder, are common among inhalant users.

Inhalant Use Disorder

The characteristics of inhalant use disorder are similar to those of nearly every other substance use disorder. They are identical to the generic criteria (p. 396), except that, as with the hallucinogens, you won't find withdrawal among the symptoms of inhalant use disorder. (OK, there may be some mild withdrawal symptoms, but DSM-5 doesn't consider them serious enough to list withdrawal as a criterion.) Score according to the usual rules (see Table 15.2).

DSM-5 notes that it's often not possible to determine exactly what volatile hydrocarbon is responsible for inhalant use disorder, and recommends using the general term *inhalant use disorder* whenever you aren't certain. Of course, if the principal component of, say, glue is toluene, then you'd go with *toluene use disorder*. Nitrous oxide and any of the nitrites (amyl, butyl, isobutyl) are considered to be other (or unknown) substances, and a use disorder involving any of these is coded accordingly.

Inhalant use disorder is pretty uncommon, even among the primary user group: teenage boys. It tends to remit spontaneously, giving way to other substances and various other mental disorders. Of course, for some, the end stage is death from various breathing-related catastrophes.

Inhalant Intoxication

People with inhalant intoxication are rarely encountered in emergency rooms or medical offices (though they're occasionally found in morgues). Many of their symptoms are similar to those of people with alcohol intoxication. Early symptoms include drowsiness, agitation, lightheadedness, and disinhibition. Later on, they may develop ataxia, disorientation, and dizziness. More severe intoxication produces insomnia, weakness, trouble speaking, disruptive behavior, and occasionally hallucinations. After a period of sleep, a user will often be lethargic and feel hung over.

Toluene, a widely used solvent, is a principal component of many of the substances abused. It is associated with headache, high mood, giddiness, and cerebellar ataxia (irregular, uncoordinated movements often accompanied by poor balance, walking with feet wide apart, and staggering). With smaller doses, there may be fatigue, headache, inhibited reflexes, and tingling sensations.

Inhalants are usually absorbed by *bagging* or by *huffing*. When bagging, people spray, squeeze, or pour the contents into a plastic bag and then inhale from the bag. They huff by placing substance-soaked rags into their mouths and inhaling. Either method can sustain a high that lasts for hours.

When you are evaluating someone you suspect of using inhalants, be sure to ask carefully about all other substance classes. The use of multiple substances is common in these patients, whose symptoms may be due in part to the use of alcohol, cannabis, hallucinogens, or tobacco. The only sure way to determine what a patient has been using is chemical analysis for substances in the patient's blood or urine.

Essential Features of **Inhalant Intoxication**

Upon inhaling a chemical substance, the patient experiences poor judgment, aggression, or other behavior changes, plus various symptoms of neuromuscular incoordination: trouble walking, lightheadedness, slow reflexes, trembling, weakness, blurred or double vision, drowsiness, jerking eye movements called nystagmus, unclear speech.

The Fine Print

The D's: • Duration to onset (within moments) • Differential diagnosis (physical disorders, other mental disorders)

You can find the specifics of inhalant intoxication in Table 15.1.

Coding Notes

See Tables 15.2 and 15.3 for codes.

Dudley Langenegger

Since he was 12, Dudley Langenegger had been in trouble for running away, for breaking and entering, and for something he didn't understand they called "incorrigibility." Days before his 18th birthday, the judge had given him a choice: "Jail or the military."

Now he'd been in the Army for 6 months, just long enough to finish basic training. Even when he was clean and sober, which wasn't often, Dudley hadn't been an especially good soldier. Often insolent, he was only compliant enough to spend most of his weekends confined to base rather than the stockade. When his unit boarded a ship for its joint operation with the Navy, Dudley went along.

So, apparently, did several tubes of model airplane cement. At least that was what Dudley said he had been huffing in the galley at midnight. As he told his story, he required several sharp commands and at least one good shaking from the first sergeant to keep him from wandering off the subject or falling asleep. His breath smelled like a paint shop.

Dudley had been inhaling various vapors, mainly organic solvents, for about 3 years. Where he grew up, a lot of the guys did this; the stuff was easy to get, cheap, even legal. He admitted that the issue of legality didn't weigh heavily upon him, but cost and ease of acquisition were important.

Airplane glue produced a quick, reliable high. Dudley liked it because it raised his mood and made long hours seem to flash by. Tonight he'd had his own private party. Everyone else had gone to bed, and he wanted to boost himself out of the low mood he had been in. It had worked so well that he had thought that it might be a good idea to throw pots and pans around in the galley, which was how the military police had found him.

The sea was calm when Dudley was escorted to the brig, but he stumbled, swayed, and almost fell onto the bunk. He rubbed his eyes, which were already brick-red, and seemed to be trying to determine where he was. "It couldn't be the barracks," he said with a giggle, "there's no Playmate posters on the wall."

"I never use it more than once or twice a week," he said with another giggle. "Too musha stays vits s'posed, uh, bad for your brain."

Evaluation of Dudley Langenegger

As a result of sniffing glue, Dudley had the bad judgment (criterion B) to throw things in the galley; the giggling suggested maladaptive emotional changes. In addition to the obvious ill timing of his drug use, he had a number of the physical symptoms of inhalant intoxication. These included slurred speech (C4), lethargy (his first sergeant had to keep him awake during the interview—C6), and poor coordination (C3). The giggling would suggest euphoria (C13), but we'd want a direct question about his mood to be sure. His eyes were irritated, and he had the odor of solvents on his breath. (A physical examination might well have revealed nystagmus and depressed reflexes as well; however, only two of these numerous symptoms are required for a diagnosis.)

The differential diagnosis would include use of other drugs such as **alcohol**; the history is usually sufficient to discriminate these causes, and the odor of airplane glue on the patient's breath can be a dead giveaway. Various neurological conditions (such as **multiple sclerosis**) must also be ruled out (D).

Dudley came close to fulfilling criteria for **inhalant intoxication delirium.** When apprehended and interviewed, he was obviously less than fully alert and could not sustain attention without a lot of direction from his first sergeant. He was also disoriented (he didn't know where he was), and he couldn't speak clearly. However, we'd only diagnose delirium if his impairment lasted longer than expected for an intoxication and if it independently required clinical attention.

Would Dudley qualify for a diagnosis of **inhalant use disorder**? That judgment would require some extrapolation on the part of his clinician. Huffing had certainly interfered with Dudley's work (substance use disorder criterion A4), but there is little direct evidence that other criteria had been met. His problems with fights, poor work performance, and the legal system might be related to his use of inhalants, but they could also be attributed to a personality disorder. (There isn't enough information for one of those diagnoses, either. This should be explored later.) No one seems to have thought to ask him whether he craved inhalants. Though we might infer a strong desire to use them from his behavior, it would remain just that: an inference. Although he continued to use these drugs despite evidence of psychological or physical problems, did he *know* this? Again, we could only infer, as we would with the question of how much time he spent obtaining and using inhalants.

All in all, the farthest I'd go is to call Dudley's a provisional case of inhalant use disorder. After all, the criteria are meant to guide, not impede us as we navigate the diagnostic shoals. Dudley's 3-year history, with attendant difficulties, would seem enough to sustain the diagnosis. With too few definite criteria nailed down, however, I'd call it of moderate intensity—and interview him hard, when he had improved, for more information. I'd note in the case summary that I could make no diagnosis of a personality disorder, but that he had antisocial personality traits. He'd also had some symptoms suggestive of conduct disorder, but they'd require further exploration to make a retrospective diagnosis.

If we knew that toluene, for example, was the solvent used in the airplane glue, we'd use that word in the diagnosis (toluene intoxication). We don't, so Dudley's complete diagnosis (with a GAF score of 40) would be as follows:

F18.229 [304.60, 292.89]	Moderate inhalant use disorder (provisional), with inhalant intoxication
Z65.3 [V62.5]	Arrested by MPs

Other Inhalant-Induced Disorders

You will find a complete listing of inhalant-induced disorders in Tables 15.2 and 15.3.

F18.99 [292.9] Unspecified Inhalant-Related Disorder

Opioid-Related Disorders

Years ago, opioids were the most feared of the mind-altering substances. (Cocaine has long since assumed that distinction.) In terms of human wastage and criminal activity, however, opioids are still among the most costly of illegal drugs. Users can spend several hundred dollars a day on their habits, mostly obtained through criminal activity. Of the opioid drugs, heroin remains the worst of a bad lot—far ahead of any other substance in terms of both physical harm and addictive potential.

Opioid users value their drugs because of the high, which they experience as euphoria and diminished concern for the present. Heroin has several times the power of morphine to produce euphoria and to blunt the perception of pain, to the point that users become indifferent to pain. First-time opioid users, on the other hand, often experience vomiting and dysphoria.

Some users, especially those who are middle-class and middle-aged, may start to abuse opioids during the course of medical treatment. Ready access to drugs places health care professionals at special risk for opioid use. However, most users begin in their teens or 20s as a result of peer pressure. Opioid use is generally preceded by the use of other drugs, such as alcohol or marijuana. In this group, risk factors for opioid use include low socioeconomic status, residence in an urban area, divorced parents, and relatives who abuse alcohol.

Some degree of tolerance to any opioid drug develops within the first few doses; then the lives of users quickly become dominated by the pursuit and consumption of the drug. However, it remains unclear why some people exposed to narcotics become addicted and others do not. Once hooked, users go to nearly any length to obtain drugs. They will plead, steal, lie, and promise you just about anything in the world.

Overall, there is under a half percent lifetime prevalence of severe opioid use in the adult population, with rates falling off in older age cohorts. Males outnumber females by about 3:2. Even after detoxification, once opioid users return to familiar environments, many begin to use again; usually this occurs within 3 months. But of those who live long enough, a substantial number eventually shake off their addiction.

Most users of heroin inject the drug intravenously, and half or more of these users test positive for HIV or hepatitis C. These are important considerations for clinicians who work with this population. Needle marks indicate the injection of heroin or "speedballs" (mixed heroin and cocaine). From all sources (overdose, violence, and associated illness), the overall mortality among active heroin users approaches 2% per year.

Some writers interpret the fact that users of "hard" drugs often begin with alcohol and marijuana as denoting what they call a "gateway effect," meaning that the latter drugs lead to opioid addiction. That conclusion could be correct, but after years of research, no one yet is sure whether it is. It is still entirely possible that some hereditary or environmental precursor leads to a variety of behaviors, including the use of alcohol, marijuana, and opioids.

Opioid Use Disorder

The characteristics of this disorder are similar to those of all other specific substance use disorders. The features are those for a generic substance use disorder (p. 396); coding is given in detail in Tables 15.2 and 15.3.

Opioid Intoxication

When an opioid drug is injected, its effects are felt almost immediately. This "rush," which has been compared to an orgasm, is rapidly followed (depending on the individual) by euphoria, drowsiness, the perception of warmth, dry mouth, and heaviness in the extremities. Some users experience a flushed face and itching nose. In contrast to cocaine intoxication, violence is rare during opioid intoxication.

Opioid intoxication can sometimes be confused with sedative or alcohol intoxication. The typical presence of extremely constricted (pinpoint) pupils can help make the distinction; however, pupils can dilate in severe overdose. Once again, a urine or blood test may be necessary to differentiate among the various possible causes of an individual's symptoms.

Although opioid users often become tolerant to enormous quantities, overdose with opioids is always a medical emergency. It can produce clouding of consciousness (including coma), severe respiratory depression, shock, and ultimately death from anoxia. Opioid overdose is treated intravenously with naloxone, a potent opioid antagonist.

Patients who use opioid drugs often wear dark glasses. Sometimes this is the fashion of their culture; sometimes they do it to hide their pupils. When you interview opioid users, ask them to remove dark glasses. Other physical stigmata of opioid use include scarring of the arms and of just about any other location where veins are prominent enough to inject drugs. The subcutaneous route of administration, called "skin popping," is a last resort for those who have already destroyed their accessible veins by years of needle use.

Essential Features of **Opioid Intoxication**

Shortly after using an opioid, the patient experiences mood changes (first elation, later apathy), increased or reduced psychomotor activity, or poor judgment. Then come constricted "pinpoint" pupils (or dilated pupils, in overdose) along with evidence of depressed neurological functioning: lethargy, unclear speech, wandering attention, or poor memory.

The Fine Print

The D's: • Differential diagnosis (physical illness, other mental disorders)
You can find the specifics of opioid intoxication in Table 15.1.

Coding Notes

Specify if: **With perceptual disturbances.** The patient experiences hallucinations during which insight is retained. This unusual state must be discriminated from delirium.
Coding in ICD-10 depends on the presence of perceptual disturbances; see Table 15.2.

Herm Cry

Herm Cry was admitted to the detox unit 24 hours after he last shot up. The junk had been good-quality—he knew, because afterwards he had slept for nearly 8 hours. But then he awakened to the all-too-familiar aching muscles and runny nose that told him it was time to go out and earn his next fix. He had had no regular job for at least a year, but he knew some ways of getting money that didn't involve waiting for a paycheck.

At a young age, Herm had become familiar with the symptoms of withdrawal. His father's drinking was well known in their working-class St. Louis neighborhood. By the time he was 10, Herm had watched his father suffer through at least two episodes of DTs. Alcohol had never done much for Herm. He didn't care for the taste, and he certainly didn't need the hangover. His mother, a public health nurse, had her own problems with Demerol.

Off and on since he was 12, Herm had smoked marijuana. But it wasn't until a neighborhood block party the night he turned 16 that he first snorted heroin. "All of a sudden," he told his most recent clinician, "I knew I'd found the way."

Within a few minutes, Herm had felt happier than ever before in his life. It was as if a warm bath had leached out all the anger, depression, and anxiety he had ever contained. For a few hours, he even forgot how much he hated his old man. All he had left was an overwhelming sense of tranquility that gradually gave way to drowsy apathy.

The following day, using a sterile syringe he stole from his mother, Herm injected heroin for the first time. Almost immediately, he vomited; this was followed at once by a sense of pleasure that seemed to race outward to the tips of his fingers and toes. Rubbing his itching nose, he fell asleep. When he aroused himself, several hours had passed. He injected again, using a smaller quantity of the drug (all he had left). When he awakened this time, he briefly considered stopping. His next thought was the realization that, more than anything else he could remember, he wanted to use heroin again.

Evaluation of Herm Cry

The sense of tranquility and peace that Herm experienced (criterion B) after injecting heroin (A) is what causes people to return to the drug after the first time, even if it has made them sick. Of course, after they have used it for a few days, they no longer need a positive reason; simply avoiding the curse of withdrawal is enough motivation to continue.

Herm also had at least one typical symptom of opioid intoxication: profound drowsiness that lasted for several hours after injecting (intoxication—C1). (The runny nose and aching muscles are symptoms of the impending withdrawal. See the next vignette, which continues Herm's story.)

Criterion C also requires that the patient have pinpoint pupils. These are sometimes so pronounced that the user cannot see clearly. Patients are unlikely to complain about this feature, so the diagnosis of opioid intoxication requires us to observe it. Assuming that Herm had constricted pupils and that no other **mental disorder** or **physical illness** better explained his symptoms (D), criteria for opioid intoxication would be fulfilled.

Most opioid users meet criteria for a comorbid mental disorder. These include **mood disorders** (up to 75%), **alcohol-related disorders** (about 30%), **antisocial personality disorder** (25%), and the **anxiety disorders** (12%). Up to 13% of opioid users attempt suicide—small wonder, considering their situation.

Because there is very little material in this first vignette pertaining to the issue of personality disorder, we'd have to defer that diagnosis for Herm. I'd phrase my note in the summary so as to alert future clinicians to the possibility, without prejudicing them as to its nature. He would also seem a likely candidate for problems with the legal system, but the first vignette includes no such evidence.

Although we already have evidence of craving, much of the material that would qualify Herm for a diagnosis of opioid use disorder is contained in the next vignette. So at this point, for coding purposes, we'll pretend he has no use disorder. With no perceptual disturbances (see Table 15.2), his diagnosis would be simply this:

F11.929 [292.89]   Opioid intoxication

Opioid Withdrawal

Although some symptoms of opioid withdrawal may appear after a very few doses, it takes a week or two of continuous use to produce the typical withdrawal syndrome. Opioid withdrawal strongly resembles a flu-like viral illness: nausea and vomiting, dysphoria, muscle aches and pains, watery eyes and runny nose, fever, and diarrhea. Another symptom of autonomic nervous system activation that occurs during withdrawal is *piloerection*: Small hairs stand up, producing "goose flesh." (This is the origin of the term "going cold turkey.") How rapidly symptoms of withdrawal appear depends principally on which drug is used; consult a reference on opioids (or search the Internet) for information about the half-lives of specific drugs. Even after most of the symptoms have abated, some patients may suffer a protracted abstinence syndrome, characterized by anxiety and low self-esteem, that can last as long as 5 or 6 months.

Essential Features of **Opioid Withdrawal**

After cutting back from several weeks of heavy opioid use, the patient develops characteristic symptoms of rebound excitation—dysphoria, nausea, diarrhea, muscle aches, tearing (runny nose), yawning, sleeplessness, and autonomic symptoms such as dilated pupils, hairs standing up, and sweating.

The Fine Print

If withdrawal is induced by administering an opioid antagonist such as naloxone, signs and symptoms will begin within minutes.

The D's: • Duration to symptom onset (within several days) • Distress or disability (work, social, or personal impairment) • Differential diagnosis (physical illness, other mental disorders)

You can find the specifics of opioid withdrawal in Table 15.1.

Coding Notes

See Tables 15.2 and 15.3 for codes.

Herm Cry Again

Sixteen hours after his last fix, Herm still hadn't scored. His usual suppliers had refused to extend him credit. He had tried to borrow money from his mother, but she had refused, and the earrings he'd stolen from her dresser top had proven worthless. Although the abdominal cramps were worsening and he felt nauseated, he managed to make it to the apartment of a former girlfriend for whom he had briefly pimped. But she had just shot up the last of her own stash and was asleep. He appropriated her used syringe for his own use later, in case he scored.

Ducking into a restroom in the bus station, Herm narrowly averted the disastrous consequences from a bout of explosive diarrhea. As he was about to emerge from the stall, he suddenly retched into the grimy toilet bowl. He sat down on the cool tile floor and tried to rub away the goose flesh on his arm. He dabbed at his runny nose with a bit of toilet paper. He was too weak, he realized, to hustle. He would have to enter detox for a few days and get his strength back.

Then he could go out and get what he really needed to make him well.

Further Evaluation of Herm Cry

Earlier, Herm had awakened to muscle cramps and a runny nose—typical early symptoms (criteria B3, B4) of opioid withdrawal. As the day went on and he could not obtain more heroin (A1), he developed gastrointestinal symptoms of nausea, vomiting, and diarrhea (B2, B6). He had goose flesh (B5), and by the time he was admitted, a clinician would also probably find dilated pupils. (Just three symptoms from criterion B are needed for a diagnosis of withdrawal.)

On the basis of the symptoms related in the two vignettes, we should also give Herm a diagnosis of opioid use disorder. Of course, he suffered from withdrawal (substance use disorder criterion A11). Herm's most notable behavioral symptom was the impairment in his normal functioning (for a year or more, he had forsaken work for criminal activities—A7). He spent a great deal of time trying to obtain heroin (A3), and he had had no job for a year or more (A6), in part because his drug habit fully occupied his time. Craving for the drug is almost universal in addicted individuals who have, like Herm, suddenly stopped using (A4); we've noted it in the first vignette. He probably met other criteria for opioid use disorder as well, such as tolerance and attempts to quit, but these are not addressed in the vignette. Even so, we can agree that Herm was probably severely dependent. Table 15.2 spells out the coding for ICD-10. For ICD-9, see Table 15.3. Because it was the main reason for Herm's entering treatment, opioid withdrawal is listed first in his diagnostic summary.

Herm's personality diagnosis would not change. He had several characteristics (thievery and pimping) of **antisocial personality disorder**, but we don't know that these ever occurred outside the context of his substance use. That personality disorder is certainly well represented among other users of opioids, however. I'd give him a GAF score of 55.

F11.23 [304.00, 292.0]   Severe opioid use disorder, with withdrawal

Other Opioid-Induced Disorders

You will find a complete listing of opioid-related disorders in Tables 15.2 and 15.3.

Sedative-, Hypnotic-, or Anxiolytic-Related Disorders

Sedatives, hypnotics, and anxiolytics are used for different purposes but share many features. Those most relevant to mental health are the symptoms of intoxication and withdrawal they have in common. The terms applied to these substances are somewhat confusing, and not always precisely used. A *sedative* is anything that reduces excitement and induces quiet without producing drowsiness. A *hypnotic* helps the patient get to sleep and stay there. And an *anxiolytic* is one that, well, reduces anxiety. Depending on dose, however, most of the drugs discussed in this section can have any of these actions.

The major drug classes covered in this section are the benzodiazepines, such as diazepam (Valium) and alprazolam (Xanax), and the barbiturates, such as pentobarbital (Nembutal); other classes include the carbamates (such as meprobamate, or Miltown) and the barbiturate-like hypnotics. Users value the barbiturates and benzodiazepines for the disinhibition they produce, which means that they induce euphoria, reduce anxiety and guilt, and boost self-confidence and energy. There are two main patterns of abuse, which can be summarized roughly as follows.

Some people get started with a prescription, usually obtained to combat the effects of insomnia or anxiety. Then, to varying degrees, they increase the dose. Although they would probably have withdrawal symptoms if they abruptly stopped using the drug, many of these people would never meet the behavioral criteria for a generic substance use disorder (p. 396). They may not even recognize, or admit to, cravings.

A more frequent route to misuse occurs when (mainly young) people employ these drugs to produce euphoria. This is the history we classically associate with the misuse of most of the substances described in DSM-5. In the past, this has been especially true of the use of barbiturates and specialty drugs such as methaqualone and glutethimide. In recent years, however, the legitimate manufacture of these drugs has been either greatly curtailed (barbiturates) or banned altogether (methaqualone). Physicians' prescribing practices have also changed. Government regulation has been an important catalyst for these changes.

Only infrequently are benzodiazepines the primary substances misused, but they are often employed to mitigate the undesired effects of other drugs—for example, to calm the jitters induced by central nervous system stimulants. Benzodiazepines are also sometimes used to boost the high of methadone or to ease the symptoms of heroin withdrawal. In the early 2000s, use during the previous year of sedatives and tranquilizers ranged from 0.3% (for teenagers) downward (for older people). The benzodiazepines preferred by users are diazepam, alprazolam, and lorazepam; users will pay premium prices to be sure they are getting the real thing. Other than those with substance use disorder, mental health patients have a very low rate of abusing, say, benzodiazepines.

Sedative, Hypnotic, or Anxiolytic Use Disorder

The characteristics of this disorder are similar to those of nearly every other specific substance use disorder. The criteria are those for a generic substance use disorder (p. 396). Note, however, that when a drug is prescribed for medical purposes, tolerance and withdrawal are not to be used as symptoms of a use disorder. See Tables 15.2 and 15.3 for coding.

Sedative, Hypnotic, or Anxiolytic Intoxication

As with most drugs, the effects achieved through the use of sedatives, hypnotics, or anxiolytics depend strongly on the setting where they are consumed and the expectations of those who use them. Mood is often labile, with case reports ranging from euphoria to hostility and depression. Loss of memory similar to that occurring in heavy alcohol consumption has also been reported, notoriously with flunitrazepam (Rohypnol), the so-called "date rape" drug. Other common effects include unsteady gait, slurred speech, nystagmus, poor judgment, and drowsiness. In very high doses, these drugs produce respiratory depression, coma, and death, though these outcomes are far more likely with barbiturates than with the benzodiazepines. The DSM-5 criteria for this category are identical to those for alcohol intoxication.

Essential Features of **Sedative, Hypnotic, or Anxiolytic Intoxication**

Shortly after using a sedative, hypnotic, or anxiolytic drug, the patient becomes disinhibited (argues; is aggressive; has rapid mood shifts or impairment of attention, judgment, or personal functioning). There is also evidence of neurological impairment (imbalance or wobbly gait, unclear speech, poor coordination, jerking eye movements called nystagmus, reduced level of consciousness).

The Fine Print

The D's: • Differential diagnosis (physical illness, alcohol intoxication, other mental disorders)

You can find the specifics of sedative, hypnotic, or anxiolytic intoxication in Table 15.1.

Coding Notes

See Tables 15.2 and 15.3 for codes.

Kirk Aufderheide

When the forklift load of galvanized iron pipe crushed his pelvis, Kirk Aufderheide promised himself that he would never complain about anything else again, if only he could regain the use of his legs. Four months later, on the day he hobbled out of the hospital using an aluminum walker, he began trying to fulfill that promise. What he hadn't reckoned on were the muscle spasms.

Kirk was 35 when the warehouse accident happened. Despite the insulin-dependent diabetes he'd had for 15 years, he considered himself healthy. His only previous hospitalization had been for febrile convulsions as a child. The combination of his diabetes and a strict religious upbringing had caused him to avoid street drugs, alcohol, and tobacco. Until his accident, he had prided himself on never taking so much as an aspirin tablet.

But the muscle spasms changed all that. They had probably been there ever since the accident, though Kirk didn't notice them until the first day he was allowed out of bed. Thereafter, any time he was up and about, he was likely to be seized with excruciating cramps in the muscles of his lower back. Reluctantly, he accepted a prescription for diazepam. A 5-mg tablet four times a day, his doctor assured him, would help relax his muscles.

Miraculously, it worked. For nearly 2 weeks Kirk was able to move around comfortably, if not pain-free. When the spasms returned and his doctor told him that 20 mg per day was the maximum dose he should take, he sought the advice of another doctor.

Within a few months, Kirk was seeing four physicians and taking between 60 and 80 mg of diazepam every day. He saw one doctor under an assumed name (in the state where Kirk lived, the prescription of benzodiazepines was tightly controlled). The other two physicians he consulted worked across the state line, just a few miles from his house. A fifth doctor had noticed his low mood and warned him not to take too much of the drug; he had never returned to see that physician again.

What with waiting for his appointments and driving to distant pharmacies, Kirk needed several hours each week just to obtain his supply. Much of the rest of his time— he hadn't yet been able to return to work, so he stayed home and kept house for his wife and two daughters—he spent in front of the television set, recalling little of what he watched. His wife complained that he had changed; he had become moody and he seemed to have trouble following the thread of a conversation.

Evaluation of Kirk Aufderheide

Kirk's wife described him as moody, which is the sort of psychological change you'd expect from diazepam intoxication (criterion B). He had an unsteady gait and poor memory (for the TV he watched), two of the specific symptoms for intoxication (C3, C5). He only needed one for the diagnosis.

Although the present criteria are exactly the same as for alcohol intoxication, historical information and the smell of alcohol on the breath should allow ready discrimination (D). In Kirk's case, there was no history to implicate alcohol. However, for another patient a blood test may be needed to identify use of both.

Would Kirk qualify for a diagnosis of diazepam use disorder? He had developed a degree of tolerance (substance use disorder criterion B9) that caused him to take four times the maximum dose recommended—far more than any one of his physicians would prescribe. He spent considerable time going to four different doctors and pharmacies to obtain his supply (B3). He also continued to use diazepam, even though one physician told him that high doses could harm him (B8).

With a GAF score of 2.5, Kirk's diagnosis at this point would be as follows:

F13.229 [304.10, 292.89]	Moderate diazepam use disorder, with intoxication
Z87.828 [V15.59]	Fracture (crush) of pelvis, healed
E10.9 [250.01]	Type 1 diabetes without complications
Z56.9 [V62.29]	Unemployed

Sedative, Hypnotic, or Anxiolytic Withdrawal

When a patient stops using (or markedly reduces a high dose of) a sedative/hypnotic drug, the result is much like the abrupt cessation of alcohol use; the criteria for withdrawal are identical. (In this context, a high dose means several times the therapeutic dose—for example, 60 mg or more of diazepam.) However, the time course varies with the half-life of the drug. As in the case of the opioids, consult a reference on these drugs for information about a specific drug's half-life.

One diagnostic challenge is to distinguish withdrawal symptoms from the reemergence of those symptoms that led to treatment in the first place (anxiety, agitation, and insomnia play a prominent role in both). The time course can help: Any symptoms that remain (or appear) 2–3 weeks after the drug has been discontinued are probably old symptoms reemerging.

Essential Features of Sedative, Hypnotic, or Anxiolytic Withdrawal

After heavy, long-lasting use of a sedative, hypnotic, or anxiolytic drug, the patient suddenly stops or markedly reduces intake. Within hours to days, this yields symptoms of increased nervous system and motor activity such as trembling, sweating, nausea, rapid heartbeat, high blood pressure, agitation, headache, sleeplessness, weakness, short-lived hallucinations or illusions, convulsions.

The Fine Print

The D's: • Duration to onset (a few hours to several days) • Distress or disability (work/educational, social, or personal impairment) • Differential diagnosis (physical illness; psychotic, mood, and anxiety disorders; withdrawal from alcohol; delirium)

You can find the specifics of sedative, hypnotic, or anxiolytic withdrawal in Table 15.1.

Coding Notes

Specify if: **With perceptual disturbances.** The patient has altered perceptions: auditory, tactile, or visual illusions or hallucinations with intact insight (the patient recognizes that the symptoms are unreal, caused by the substance use).

Coding in ICD-10 depends on the presence of perceptual disturbances; see Table 15.2.

Kirk Aufderheide Again

Four days short of the first anniversary of his accident, Kirk's wife received notice that she was being transferred to a branch office in the interior of the state. The transfer forced the family to move. At their new location, Kirk encountered tighter controls on the prescription of benzodiazepines, together with far fewer physicians and pharmacies. Once they had settled into their new home, he realized that he had no choice but to reduce his dose of diazepam.

Although Kirk intended to taper his usage, he put it off until he was nearly out of medication. So on a warm summer morning he found himself suddenly facing the prospect of taking only 4 tablets, whereas the day before he had had 16. At first, he was surprised at how little it bothered him. For several days he experienced insomnia, but he had expected that. (With no work to go to, he had had time to read some magazine articles about the effects of substance use.)

But at 4 A.M. of the third day, Kirk awakened to a sense of anxiety that bordered on panic. He felt nauseated and noticed that his pulse was racing. For 2 days his agitation mounted, to such an extent that he had difficulty sitting still long enough to eat the supper he had prepared. On the fifth day, his wife arrived home to find him having a grand mal seizure.

Further Evaluation of Kirk Aufderheide

When he drastically decreased his intake of diazepam (criterion A), Kirk noted some of the classic symptoms (two are required) of withdrawal: racing pulse, insomnia, and nausea (B1, B3, B4). (Diazepam's relatively long half-life meant that it took quite some time for withdrawal symptoms to develop.) Childhood febrile seizures might have made him more susceptible to withdrawal seizures; Kirk's occurred within a few days (B8)—the fate of perhaps one-fourth of people who abruptly withdraw from these substances. His impairment could go without saying (C).

Anxiety and panic attacks commonly occur as rebound phenomena; therefore, **anxiety disorders** form an important part of the differential diagnosis (D). When hallucinations occur during withdrawal, they can be mistaken for a **manic episode** or various **psychotic disorders. Delirium** is also a relatively common complication. **Antisocial personality disorder** is often encountered among patients who obtain these medications illegally.

Kirk had had no illusions or hallucinations to qualify for the specifier of *with perceptual disturbances*. Because the seizure was the focus of treatment on admission, I've listed it first. The rest of his diagnosis remains as it was before.

R56.9 [780.39]	Withdrawal seizure
F13.239 [304.10, 292.0]	Moderate diazepam use disorder, with withdrawal

Other Sedative-, Hypnotic-, or Anxiolytic-Induced Disorders

You will find a complete listing of these disorders in Tables 15.2 and 15.3. I'll briefly mention one of these:

> **Sedative, hypnotic, or anxiolytic withdrawal delirium.** When delirium occurs, it is almost always within a week of the patient's discontinuing a drug. Like delirium due to other causes, it features reduced attention span and problems with orientation, memory, perception (visual, auditory, or tactile hallucinations or illusions) or language disturbance. It is usually preceded by insomnia.

F13.99 [292.9] Unspecified Sedative-, Hypnotic-, or Anxiolytic-Related Disorder

Stimulant-Related Disorders

Stimulants (sometimes called psychostimulants) affect mental or physical functioning, or both. For example, these drugs typically improve—at least for a time—alertness, mood, and activity levels. Worldwide, some stimulants are used by prescription to ameliorate the effects of both mental and physical disorders. In addition, many are used, and misused, recreationally. Although caffeine is also a stimulant, it occupies its own niche among psychoactive drugs.

DSM-5 mentions two main types of stimulants: amphetamines and cocaine. In previous editions, though the symptoms for intoxication and withdrawal are identical for these two drug classes, they occupied separate sections. Now, with commendable logic, they have been combined. Still, their patterns of use are different enough that I've continued to provide two sets of vignettes as illustrations.

Amphetamines and Related Compounds

Abusers value amphetamines (the international spelling is *amfetamines*) for the euphoria, appetite suppression, and increase in energy they provide. Although many people begin amphetamine use by snorting, blood vessel constriction in the nose makes absorption unpredictable, so other routes are sought. Smoking or injection produces a rapid effect, such that binge users take the drug repeatedly for half a day to 2–3 days. Effects of the drug fall off rapidly as tolerance develops. It is almost inevitable that a period of nonuse will occur, but users remember how "wonderful" the drug was (that's the euphoria talking) and want more. This institutes a cycle of use and withdrawal that usually lasts about 10 days.

Amphetamine users tend to look sleep-deprived and anorectic. Physical signs include circles under the eyes, poor hygiene, and dry, itchy skin that is prone to acne-like lesions. Users who inject can get vasoconstriction at the site, with necrosis of skin. Those who inhale may develop nosebleeds, even perforated nasal septum. Toxic symptoms include chest pain, palpitations, and shortness of breath.

When they were first synthesized in 1887, no regulations limited amphetamine use. Through the middle years of the 20th century, it was commonplace to use them for weight control, depression, and nasal stuffiness; they were widely abused in the 1960s and into the 1970s. Since then, however, tight controls and changing prescription practices have greatly reduced their availability. Virtually their only legitimate uses now are to treat obesity, narcolepsy, some depressive disorders, and attention-deficit/hyperactivity disorder.

Amphetamines may be taken intermittently at relatively modest doses by truckers, students, and others (most are young men) who want something beyond caffeine to keep them awake. Some users take these drugs to produce euphoria, often leading to "speed runs" that can last for weeks. There may be episodes of delirium during these runs and "crashes" when the supply runs out. Others use stimulants to counterbalance the effects of sedatives and other drugs of abuse.

Only about 2% of emergency room drug-related visits are due to amphetamines and their related substances. The prevalence among high-school age youngsters is around 2 per 1,000, pretty close to that for cocaine. Some data suggest that those dependent on amphetamines may stop using them after a decade or so. The substances related to amphetamine that are available by prescription include methamphetamine (Desoxyn), dextroamphetamine (Dexedrine), amphetamine combinations (Adderall), diethylopropion (Tenuate), and methylphenidate (Ritalin). Illicit methamphetamine can be synthesized in small batches, but much of the product available in the United States is made in laboratories, either domestic or Mexican.

Ecstasy (MDMA) has structural similarities to both amphetamines and mescaline, one of the hallucinogens, and its effects are both stimulant and mildly psychedelic. It's been around for a hundred years; nearly 4% of Americans have tried it. It is rarely used every day; rather, its typical use occurs at "raves" and in other social situations. Although it has a terrible reputation for causing physical harm and addiction, it rates somewhere near the lower end of the scale, according to a study published in *The Lancet* in 2007.

Cocaine

Cocaine has filled a good part of the niche once occupied by amphetamines. (The effects of cocaine are nearly identical to those of amphetamines, but half-life in the body is much briefer. This may explain cocaine's greater addicting powers—and appeal.)

With a short half-life, cocaine creates powerful craving, and users will use it more frequently than is the case for amphetamines. Also, toxic symptoms are briefer than for amphetamines. Severe intoxication includes convulsions, heartbeat irregularities, high fever, and death. Paranoid thinking can increase as the binge goes on. Delusions (often of plots or attack on the user) are usually self-limited and brief (a matter of hours). Perceptual distortions occur; hallucinations are rare.

Long out of fashion after a brief spurt of popularity in the early 1900s, cocaine enjoyed a resurgence when the U.S. government clamped down on the manufacture and distribution of amphetamines during the 1970s. Since then, plummeting cost and skyrocketing availability have made it the second most frequently used illicit drug (behind marijuana) in the United States and worldwide. In recent years, about a quarter of drug-related visits to emergency rooms have been due to cocaine. Concentrated among younger adults (age 15–34), men more than women tend to be afflicted by this scourge. Those who use have 4–8 times the expected mortality of their nonusing peers.

Cocaine that has been heated with bicarbonate yields a white lump that is not destroyed by heating. It produces a popping sound when smoked; hence the name *crack*. The availability of crack accounted for much of the rise in cocaine use during the latter part of the 20th century; however, the number of users may have declined somewhat during the first decade of the 21st century.

Most users of cocaine begin by taking it intermittently, but will rapidly progress to "runs" similar to those of amphetamine users. Addiction to crack cocaine usually occurs after only a few weeks of use. Because almost no tolerance to cocaine develops, runs can continue for several days, though a day or less is more usual.

Note that the cross-sectional evaluation may not adequately discriminate patients who use cocaine from those who use amphetamines or related drugs. Even history can be unreliable: What is sold on the streets doesn't always match what's advertised. Even the more reliable purveyors have little control over impurities or contaminants. The only sure way to determine what substance a patient is using is to obtain a urine or blood specimen for toxicology.

Khat

An African plant called khat contains an alkaloid, cathinone, which breaks down into ephedrine. Indigenous people (in Yemen, for example) chew the leaves for the effect of euphoria and excitement, similar to a strong brew of coffee. A mild withdrawal syndrome can occur. It ranks near the bottom of the stimulants for physical harm and addiction potential, though mild psychoses and hypomanic states have been reported.

"Bath Salts"

Relatively new are so-called "bath salts," often marketed "not for human consumption" in an effort to evade state and federal drug laws. These compounds, variously named and sold online or in head shops as an alternative to cocaine, usually contain a version of cathinone (the alkaloid in khat) that's been fiddled with chemically. The powerful inhibition of monoamine reuptake leads to a variety of physical and mental symptoms—delirium, hallucinations, paranoid delusions, agitation, rapid heartbeat, blood pressure elevation, fever, and seizures. Withdrawal can lead to profound craving; overdose can mean death. Users tend to be male and relatively young (20s). Since 2011, bath salts have been illegal in the United States.

Stimulant Use Disorder

The characteristics of stimulant use disorder are similar to those of nearly every other specific substance use disorder. The criteria are those for a generic substance use disorder (p. 396). I've listed the coding stuff in Tables 15.2 and 15.3. But you probably know that by now.

Stimulant Intoxication

DSM-5 has mashed together amphetamine and cocaine use syndromes, but there are enough differences that they deserve to be discussed separately anyway. The Essential Features of intoxication and withdrawal are the same for both, however.

Essential Features of **Stimulant Intoxication**

Shortly after using a stimulant drug, the patient exhibits changes of mood/affect, as well as impaired judgment or psychosocial functioning. In addition, there will be physical indicators of neurological excitation: lowered or raised blood pressure, heart rate, and motor activity; dilated pupils; sweating or chills; nausea; anorexia; and weakness, chest pain, respiratory depression, or irregular heartbeat. Very ill patients may experience seizures, coma, or perplexity.

The Fine Print

The D's: • Duration to onset of symptoms (within minutes) • Differential diagnosis (physical illness, other mental disorders)

You can find the specifics of stimulant intoxication in Table 15.1.

> ## Coding Notes
>
> Specify if: **With perceptual disturbances.** The patient has altered perceptions: auditory, tactile, or visual illusions or hallucinations with intact insight (the patient recognizes that the symptoms are unreal, caused by the substance use). Hallucinations without this insight suggest a diagnosis of stimulant-induced psychotic disorder.
>
> When recording, specify the stimulant by name.
>
> Coding in ICD-10 depends on the presence of perceptual disturbances; see Table 15.2.

Amphetamine Intoxication

If an amphetamine is injected, feelings of euphoria, confidence, and well-being begin quickly. Users experience a "rush" of energy and euphoria; they find their own thoughts profound, and their sexual interest picks up. But they pay the price of anorexia and agitation. When the intoxication is severe, they become confused and their speech rambles.

With longer use, the person may begin to withdraw from other people and focus more or less exclusively on obtaining and using drugs. Hallucinations (such as bugs crawling on the skin) or paranoid ideas can develop. Delirium may be accompanied by violence. Some people adopt stereotyped behaviors: ritualistic reenactments of things they normally like to do (such as assembling and dismantling electronic equipment). Any of these syndromes can resemble schizophrenia, but the alert clinician will focus on the longitudinal history as obtained from informants. Laboratory studies help confirm the toxic origins of the behavior.

Freeman Cooke

"I was hyperactive when I was a child," said Freeman Cooke to the interviewer. "My mother used to give me coffee to slow me down."

Moving restlessly around the office, Freeman looked as if he'd just had several cups too many. He had already twice excused himself to the bathroom, where he nearly threw up. The nurse who checked him had noted that his blood pressure was up, and that his pulse was racing along at 132 beats per minute. He admitted that he had snorted a half gram of "crystal meth" not long before coming to the office.

Freeman was the oldest of four children. His mother had been an unhappy, nervous woman who always seemed unwell. His father made good money as a finish carpenter, but his appetite for vodka grew as his family increased. When still a child, Freeman had promised himself that he would avoid alcohol and treat his wife, if he ever had one, with more respect than his father had done. He managed to keep half his promise.

After completing high school, Freeman got married and obtained a job as a helper with a long-distance moving company. The pay was good, but the hours were awful.

When he and his boss were on the road, they sometimes worked 18 hours straight. Like most of the other truckers, he used dextroamphetamine to pep him up and keep him awake. At first, he took them only when he was working. When he came home from a 10-day trip, he would "crash and burn," sometimes sleeping as long as 20 hours at a stretch. But by the time he had enough seniority and experience to buy his own truck, he was using amphetamines recreationally, too.

Freeman had started to snort powdered methamphetamine ("meth"), but he rapidly switched to smoking because it gave him a better "flash." When he was high, he felt insanely happy, tireless, and powerful. "Like I could lift a grand piano, all by myself," he explained. He also developed the tendency to argue, and would sometimes keep his wife up late at night with a tirade about matters that the next day even he found trivial. After a few hours, as the effect of the high began to wear off and only the memory of the flash remained, he felt driven to smoke up again and again. But with each use during a run, it took more of the drug to produce the flash. Eventually, either his supply or his constitution would give out, and he would once again crash and burn. When he struggled back to consciousness, he was often astonished at how much of the stuff he had consumed.

When Freeman awakened after an unusually memorable 2-day run, he found a note saying that his wife was leaving him. For the first time, he realized how exactly like his father he had become.

Evaluation of Freeman Cooke

Like all other types of substance intoxication, stimulant intoxication must be documented with marked, detrimental behavioral or psychological changes (criterion B). For Freeman, that would be easy: His recent use (A) had led to arguments with his wife, which culminated in her departure. Of the physical signs and symptoms (two required), he had elevated pulse and blood pressure (C1, C3) as well as agitation and nausea (C7, C5). At evaluation, he had no hallucinations or illusions that would qualify for the perceptual disturbances specifier.

Freeman also qualified for a diagnosis of amphetamine use disorder. Requiring more of the drug to achieve a high on successive occasions of use, he clearly experienced tolerance (A10). He sometimes used more methamphetamine than he intended (A1), and he spent a great deal of time and energy in using it and recovering from the effects (A3). The judgment that his use pattern was severe is based in part on evidence of amphetamine withdrawal (A11), discussed below, though I would also claim clinician's privilege in asserting that he was seriously dependent. I'd give him a GAF score of 55.

F15.229 [304.40, 292.89]	Severe methamphetamine use disorder, with intoxication
Z63.0 [V61.10]	Separated from wife

Cocaine Intoxication

Cocaine is probably the strongest pharmacological reinforcer ever devised. Laboratory animals will choose it in preference to food, water, and sex; given free access, they will use it again and again until they die.

Humans use it by snorting, injecting, or smoking. Smoking crack can produce a rush of euphoria and a feeling of well-being that begins within seconds. The user feels alert and self-confident, and has increased sexual desire. These positive feelings last for a few minutes, then give way to dysphoria and an intense craving for more of the drug. With continuing use, the euphoric effects lessen and the dysphoria (anxiety, depression, fatigue) takes over. Motivation is bent to a single goal: obtaining more cocaine.

Behavioral changes associated with cocaine intoxication include aggression and agitation, often leading to fighting and hypervigilance. Cocaine postpones fatigue, and the resulting increase in energy breeds impaired judgment and an increased willingness to take risks. Violence and crime are frequent products of the cocaine-intoxicated state.

Cognitive symptoms include delusions, feelings of omnipotence, ideas of reference (beliefs that external events have a special meaning unique to oneself), and haptic (tactile) hallucinations. Other symptoms include irritability, increased sensory awareness, anorexia, insomnia, and spontaneous ejaculation. If the intoxication is severe, there may be rambling speech, perplexity, anxiety, headache, and palpitations of the heart.

Amanda Brandt

Since her graduation from college at age 22, Amanda Brandt had worked as a futures trader on the Chicago Stock Exchange. It was a fast-paced, high-pressured life, and she loved it. "I was an economics major in college," she explained, "and what can you do with that? Teach?"

Futures trading exactly suited Amanda's temperament. Since early high school, she had been energetic and outgoing. Her job introduced her to a lot of young people who were as bright and well paid as she.

Amanda's father was a Baptist minister; he and her mother were both teetotalers. Though both of her grandfathers were long dead, Amanda thought that they had suffered from alcoholism. She supposed that this might have had something to do with her parents' attitude toward alcohol. "I'm sure they never dreamed I smoked pot in college," she said. "But it never seemed to bother me, and it was the social thing to do."

What was social in her corner of the Exchange, she soon discovered, was cocaine. She and her fellow traders made more than enough money to afford quantities of the powdery stuff, though not as much as they actually used. With the advent of crack, the price decreased, and Amanda's use soared. She had always hated the pain of needles, so instead of snorting, she learned to smoke it.

"Within a few seconds of lighting up, you felt wonderful. It was like a total body climax," she said. "I felt like even my lungs were coming."

The rush of the intense high blasted her with a pleasure that obliterated any concern she might have had about the pounding heartbeat and the feelings of agitation. For 15 minutes or so she felt incalculably witty; she loved and controlled the world. While she orbited, she didn't need sex, people, food, water, or even air. For that quarter of an hour, she felt she could live forever.

Evaluation of Amanda Brandt

Amanda's use of cocaine produced profound behavioral and psychological changes, including alterations in her judgment and social life (criterion B). She thought that the pleasure produced by the drug was worth the side effects it caused—in her case, rapid heartbeat and a sense of agitation (C1, C7). An outside observer would probably have noticed other symptoms of acute intoxication mentioned in the criteria, but two suffice for diagnosis. Her subjective feelings give some inkling of why people become addicted to cocaine.

Besides **amphetamine intoxication** (the symptoms are of course exactly the same), some of the other mental disorders that feature hyperactivity or mood instability should be considered. These would include **bipolar disorders. Physical illnesses** such as hyperthyroidism should also be considered. **Phencyclidine intoxication** can have perceptual distortions similar to cocaine intoxication. Patients who become psychotic or delirious when intoxicated must be discriminated from those with **schizophrenia** and other psychotic disorders, and from **delirium due to another medical condition** (D).

A fuller diagnosis is provided later, but from the information given in this vignette, Amanda's principal diagnosis at this point would be as given below.

F14.929 [292.89]   Cocaine intoxication

Stimulant Withdrawal

As with intoxication, the Essential Features of amphetamine and cocaine withdrawal are identical, so I've given them only once.

Essential Features of **Stimulant Withdrawal**

After heavy, long-lasting use of a stimulant, the patient suddenly stops or markedly reduces the intake. This yields symptoms of dysphoria plus evidence of nervous system stimulation or exhaustion: intense dreams, reduced (sometimes increased) sleep or motor activity; feelings of hunger.

The Fine Print

The D's: • Duration to onset of symptoms (hours to days) • Distress or disability (work/

educational, social, or personal impairment) • Differential diagnosis (physical illness, other mental disorders)

You can find the specifics of stimulant withdrawal in Table 15.1.

Coding Notes

List the specific stimulant responsible for the withdrawal when you code the patient. See Tables 15.2 and 15.3 for codes.

Amphetamine Withdrawal

A few hours after the last use of amphetamines, there comes the crash: agitation, anxiety, depression, and exhaustion. The user experiences an intense craving that may later wane in the face of oncoming depression, fatigue, and insomnia (which is accompanied by a paradoxical craving for sleep). Still later, voracious appetite may develop. The fatigue and apathy worsen in the half day to 4 days following the crash; acute withdrawal lasts 7–10 days. Suicide attempts may result. In short, the user becomes a patient.

Freeman Cooke Again

When he checked into detox, Freeman was still wired from the last half gram of meth he had smoked that morning. Coming off a 2-day binge, he knew from past experience that if he was going to do something about his habit, he had to take the plunge when he was still intoxicated. If he waited until he crashed, he wouldn't do anything except sleep. Then he'd start looking for drugs.

Freeman had declined lunch and was playing cards with three other patients at a table in the corner of the day room when he felt himself begin to slip. He noted almost with amusement that he felt like a wind-up turntable, running slower every moment. With each hand, it seemed harder to play the cards; they might have been made of lead. Suddenly, he was overwhelmed with depression so profound that, tired as he was, he had to try to escape. His body ached for some speed.

Back in his room, he started to pack the few things he had brought in. When the gym bag was half full, he put it aside and collapsed onto the bed. He realized that he utterly lacked the energy to go out and hustle. The drug craving was gradually giving way to the need for sleep, but his eyes remained resolutely open. He was doomed to lie there for hours, paralyzed by fatigue but locked in wakefulness. It was going to be a long night.

Further Evaluation of Freeman Cooke

After he stopped using amphetamines (criterion A), Freeman rapidly became depressed (B). He also suffered from fatigue (B1), psychomotor slowing (B5), and insomnia (B3)—even though he badly wanted to sleep—more than fulfilling the (two) symptoms required. His typical, profound craving for speed is not a criterion for stimulant withdrawal, though it is for stimulant use disorder. The misery these symptoms caused him (C), together with the lack of any other disorder that could better explain them (D), qualify him for the diagnosis of stimulant withdrawal.

The differential diagnosis of Freeman's condition would include **bipolar I disorder** (because of his fluctuating moods) and other substance-induced disorders, such as **cocaine withdrawal** and **phencyclidine intoxication.** Patients who develop psychosis during intoxication may be mistakenly diagnosed as having **schizophreniform disorder** or other psychotic disorders.

Even after most of the acute effects of withdrawal have dissipated, mood symptoms can last for weeks or months. If that happened to Freeman, I'd consider a diagnosis of methamphetamine-induced mood disorder—later.

Now we'd exchange Freeman's diagnosis above for the following:

F15.23 [292.0]   Severe methamphetamine use disorder, with amphetamine withdrawal

Cocaine Withdrawal

After the acute intoxication phase, blood cocaine levels drop rapidly. Unless more drug is immediately consumed, a rapid crash into depression occurs. The patient may also experience irritability, suicidal ideas, fatigue, loss of interest, and a decreased ability to experience pleasure. Panic attacks are common; the need for cocaine is intense. Most of these symptoms tend to increase for 2–4 days and then abate, but depression can linger for months. Suicide attempts are fairly common; sometimes they succeed.

About half of all those who have problems with cocaine use also have mood disorders, often bipolar or cyclothymic. This sets them quite apart from individuals with opioid-related disorders.

Amanda Brandt Again

In the aftermath of her intoxication, Amanda died—or so it would seem, as she'd feel suddenly, incurably depressed. The supreme self-confidence of moments before would be shoved aside by an anxious uncertainty that over the next day or two would gradually overwhelm her. The only remedy was to smoke another lump of crack, and then another and another, until her supply ran out. Then she would be left sleepless and exhausted, while every cell in her body remembered exactly how exhilarating it felt to be high, and craved to experience it again.

By her fourth year on the Exchange, Amanda's life had begun to unravel. Compared to the importance of using cocaine, work now seemed irrelevant. For days in a row, she would call in sick; when she did go in, her mind was focused on when and how she would score her next vial of crack. When she was finally fired, she moved to a smaller apartment and sold her BMW. Now that she could devote all of her time to obtaining and using crack, it took just 2 months to smoke up her life savings and the proceeds from her car.

It was her final binge that brought Amanda in for treatment. After smoking her last pipeful, she roamed the hallway in her apartment building, weeping and knocking on doors. When anyone answered, she tried to push her way in. Someone called the police, who took her to the emergency room. There she became enraged and lashed out with her fists. Ultimately, she was restrained and admitted to a mental health inpatient unit.

Further Evaluation of Amanda Brandt

Amanda's history makes it painfully clear that cocaine was the source of her disorder. When she ran out of it (criterion A), she showed (by weeping and anxiety) the requisite dysphoria and several of the physical symptoms listed in the criteria: insomnia, fatigue, and speeded-up psychomotor activity (B3, B1, B5). For any withdrawal syndrome to be diagnosed by DSM-5 criteria, it must cause marked distress or greatly affect the patient's life (C); Amanda conformed. Not included in the criteria, but typical nonetheless, were her eidetic memory for the experience of using crack and her crushing desire for more.

At this point, we have enough information to give Amanda another substance-related diagnosis: cocaine use disorder. She spent nearly all of her time (substance use disorder criterion A3) satisfying her craving (A4) for crack cocaine, which had consumed her car and her job (A7). Already tolerant (A10), she finally developed withdrawal symptoms (A11).

A number of other cocaine-related disorders are listed in DSM-5, some of which are encountered more frequently than others. If Amanda's depression persisted substantially longer than the period of withdrawal, **cocaine-induced mood disorder** might be added to her list.

Other patients may have associated mental conditions, such as **gambling disorder**, **antisocial personality disorder**, and **posttraumatic stress disorder.** With a GAF score of 35 and her extensive history, I'm going to rate Amanda as severely ill, and *you* can count symptoms—if you wish.

F14.23 [304.20, 292.0]	Severe cocaine use disorder, with withdrawal
Z56.9 [V62.29]	Unemployed

Other Stimulant-Induced Disorders

You will find a complete listing of amphetamine-related disorders in Tables 15.2 and 15.3. Some are described more fully at other points in this book. I'm briefly mentioning three here:

Stimulant-induced psychotic disorder, with delusions. These patients often, though not always, develop paranoia with ideas of reference and well-formed delusions. Their awareness of the environment is accentuated. They may watch other people very carefully and later become "aware" that others are watching them. They may also overreact to any perception of movement; some actually hallucinate. The delusions can last a week or longer. When well developed, this disorder may resemble schizophrenia in all but the time course.

Stimulant-induced psychotic disorder, with hallucinations. Patients with this type of psychotic disorder may scratch excessively if they think they see bugs crawling on their skin.

Stimulant intoxication delirium. Some patients experience an agitated delirium associated with intoxication. They may perform remarkable feats of strength, and their wild, irrational behavior occasionally results in someone's death.

F15.99 or F14.99 [292.9] Unspecified Stimulant-Related Disorder

The coding depends on whether the substance is related to amphetamines (or similar drugs, F15) or to cocaine (F14).

Tobacco-Related Disorders

Because tens of millions of Americans are dependent on tobacco, the potential for withdrawal problems is enormous. Owing in part to the intense craving tobacco induces, it has been called the most widely used addictive drug in the United States. (And percentage-wise, fewer Americans—about one-fifth of adults—smoke than is the case for citizens of most other countries.) Men and women are affected at more or less equal rates. Each year, tobacco is responsible for 5 million deaths worldwide; that's at least 60 times greater than for heroin.

It is hard to find clear evidence of primary reinforcers in tobacco. That is, its chemical effects do not include the direct production of euphoria, elevated self-esteem, or the enhancement of energy—the effects so valued by those who use, say, cocaine or opioids. Rather, tobacco produces nausea, vomiting, and anxiety, especially in the novice smoker. (Although it has been reported to reduce anxiety, this is probably the effect of "curing" the user's tobacco withdrawal.) So why do people smoke? In a nutshell, social factors get them started, and then they are hooked.

In 2013 it was reported that people with mental illness are 70% more likely to smoke than are those without. There is a strong positive correlation between addiction to tobacco and alcoholism, schizophrenia, and other mental disorders. When you are interviewing mental health patients, always ask about tobacco use.

Like caffeine, tobacco is legal, easy to obtain, and cheap (well, relative to heroin). Most people can use it without interfering in any material way with their other, non-substance-related pursuits. But in the course of a single year, they may repeatedly try to stop, suffer from withdrawal symptoms, and eventually return to smoking despite the knowledge that they are courting a cardiovascular catastrophe.

Tobacco Use Disorder

The characteristics of tobacco use disorder are similar to those of nearly every other specific substance use disorder. The criteria are those for a generic substance use disorder (p. 396), and coding is given in Tables 15.2 and 15.3.

F17.203 [292.0] Tobacco Withdrawal

A patient who is withdrawing from tobacco often complains most bitterly not of the specific symptoms listed in these criteria, but of yearning for a cigarette. This persistent craving can overwhelm the ability to focus on other, more substantive (but less pressing) issues. The result is a moody, anxious person who sleeps poorly and eats too much, knowing that everything could be fixed by one dose of a perfectly legal substance that is being used every day by over a billion people worldwide. No wonder these folks are irritable! Onset of withdrawal symptoms occurs within a day of last use, and is often detectable within a few hours. Withdrawal will occur in about half of those who stop using.

I've provided no separate case vignette for tobacco withdrawal. However, Hoyle Garner had a sleep disorder due to chronic obstructive pulmonary disease that was caused by smoking; his story begins on page 302. He was also diagnosed as having tobacco use disorder, and had at one time experienced tobacco withdrawal.

Essential Features of **Tobacco Withdrawal**

The patient suddenly stops or markedly reduces regular, prolonged tobacco use. Within a day, this yields multiple symptoms of dysphoria (irritability, depression, anxiety), restlessness, trouble concentrating, insomnia, and hunger.

The Fine Print

The D's: • Duration to onset of symptoms (within 24 hours) • Distress or disability (work/educational, social, or personal impairment) • Differential diagnosis (physical illness, other mental disorders)

You can find the specifics of tobacco withdrawal in Table 15.1.

Other Tobacco-Induced Disorders

The other tobacco-induced disorders are listed in Tables 15.2 and 15.3.

F17.209 [292.9] Unspecified Tobacco-Related Disorder

Other (or Unknown) Substance-Related Disorders

The category of other (or unknown) substance-related disorders covers disorders linked to substances not included in the categories listed in Tables 15.2 and 15.3 and already described in this chapter. The generic criteria for substance use disorder (p. 396), substance intoxication (p. 411), and substance withdrawal (p. 402) given earlier, or the criteria for substance-induced disorders described in other chapters (for example, substance-induced bipolar disorder), are applied here when appropriate.

Here are some examples of the substances that could be included in this category:

Anabolic steroids. The value to users of the anabolic steroids derives from enhanced physical attractiveness and athletic ability. For body builders and other athletes, this desire can be a powerful motivator to use these drugs. Besides the obvious effects on the physique, users report euphoria, increased libido, and at times aggression (so-called "'roid rage"). Steroid use has been implicated in the killing of 16 civilian Afghanis by U.S. Army Sergeant Robert Bales in 2012—but then, so has the antimalaria drug mefloquine.

Anabolic steroids are often used in a social context, and this use may continue unabated for months or years. Similar to other substances of misuse, people take them longer than initially desired, cannot stop, spend excessive time using or trying to get them, and use them even though they know they cause harm. Cessation can also cause withdrawal symptoms, such as include depression, fatigue, restlessness, insomnia, loss of appetite, and reduced interest in sex. Some users develop an intense drug craving.

Nitrous oxide. Nitrous oxide is an anesthetic inhalant that produces lightheadedness and mild euphoria; hence its nickname, "laughing gas." It is used as a propellant in cans of whipped cream and cooking sprays—except when it is used to produce a high. Then it can result in a degree of depersonalization/derealization and dizziness, with some distortion of sound. First used recreationally late in the 18th century, it may be the world's oldest artificially produced substance of abuse.

Over-the-counter/prescription drugs. Over-the-counter and prescription drugs that can result in addiction include antiparkinsonian drugs, cortisone and its derivatives, antihistamines, and others.

Betel nut. People in many cultures chew betel nut to achieve a mild high or sensation of floating.

Kava. Made from a pepper plant that grows in the South Pacific, kava causes sedation and loss of coordination and weight.

Other (or Unknown) Substance Use Disorder

Symptoms of other (or unknown) substance use disorder are identical to the generic disorder symptoms (see p. 396). Coding is given in Tables 15.2 and 15.3.

Other (or Unknown) Substance Intoxication

The symptoms of other (or unknown) substance intoxication are identical to those in the generic substance use intoxication criteria (p. 411). Their coding is given in Tables 15.2 and 15.3.

Other (or Unknown) Substance Withdrawal

The symptoms of other (or unknown) substance withdrawal are identical to those of the generic substance use withdrawal criteria (p. 402). Their coding is given in Tables 15.2 and 15.3.

Recording and Coding Substance-Related Disorders

Use Tables 15.2 and 15.3 to code four classes of problems: substance use disorder, substance intoxication, or substance withdrawal (or a combination of these), or a substance-induced mental disorder. The table for ICD-9 codes (Table 15.3) is pretty self-evident (and, as of October 2014, will no longer be necessary), so I won't elaborate further on its use. For ICD-10 codes (Table 15.2), however, read on.

If your patient has substance use disorder, intoxication, or withdrawal, but no additional substance-induced mental disorder, use the three columns ("Just use," "Intoxication," and "Withdrawal") under "Substance use/intoxication/withdrawal" in Table 15.2 as follows:

A. Determine the substance, and write down the "F" number. For alcohol (as an example), that would be F10.

B. If substance use has been extensive enough to qualify as a substance use disorder, decide whether it is mild or moderate/severe in intensity. If there is no current intoxication or withdrawal and no associated mental disorder, read across to the "Just use" column, note down the decimal and trailing digits—and you are done. For alcohol (indeed, for all substances), that would be either .10 or .20.

C. If the patient has intoxication or withdrawal, read across to the appropriate column, and write down decimal and number. (By definition, you cannot diagnose withdrawal if the patient's substance use disorder is only mild.) For alcohol, you would record F10.129 for mild use disorder with intoxication, F10.229 if use

TABLE 15.2. ICD-10-CM Code Numbers for Substance Intoxication, Substance Withdrawal, Substance Use Disorder, and Substance-Induced Mental Disorders

Substance and use disorder (or not)	Just use	Intoxication	Withdrawal	Psychotic	Mood	Anxiety	OCD	Sleep	Sex	Delirium I	Delirium W	NCD major	NCD mild	Unspecified
Alcohol F10				I/W[a]	I/W	I/W		I/W	I/W	I	W			.99
w/mild use dis.	.10	.129		.159	.14	.180		.182	.181	.121	.121			
w/mod./severe use dis.	.20	.229	.239 (.232)[b]	.259	.24	.280		.282	.281	.221	.231	.27 (.26)[c]	.288	
No use disorder		.929	.93	.959	.94	.980		.982	.981	.921	.921	.97 (.96)[c]	.988	
Caffeine F15						I		I/W						.99
w/mild use dis.						.180		.182						
w/mod./severe use dis.						.280		.282						
No use disorder		.929				.980		.982						
Cannabis F12				I		I		I/W						.99
w/mild use dis.	.10	.129 (.122)[b]		.159		.180		.188		.121				
w/mod./severe use dis.	.20	.229 (.222)[b]		.259		.280		.288		.221				
No use disorder		.929 (.922)[b]		.959		.980		.988		.921				

(cont.)

Note. OK, I confess: This table's *really* fussy. You can just accept the fuss, or you could try to understand the original DSM-5 explanations. That way lies madness. Abbreviations in column heads: OCD, obsessive–compulsive and related disorder; Sleep, sleep disorder; Sex, sexual dysfunction; Delirium I, intoxication delirium; Delirium W, withdrawal delirium; NCD, neurocognitive disorder.

[a] I, occurs during intoxication; W, occurs during withdrawal; I/W, either.
[b] Two numbers in a cell indicate separate codes for intoxication or withdrawal without (or with) perceptual disturbances.
[c] Alcohol-induced NCD can occur without or with confabulation and amnestic syndrome. The number in parentheses is for amnestic–confabulatory type.

TABLE 15.2 (cont.)

Substance and use disorder (or not)	Substance use/intoxication/withdrawal			Substance-induced disorders										
	Just use	Intoxication	Withdrawal	Psychotic	Mood	Anxiety	OCD	Sleep	Sex	Delirium I	Delirium W	NCD major	NCD mild	Unspecified
Phencyclidine F16				I	I	I								
w/mild use dis.	.10	.129		.159	.14	.180				.121				.99
w/mod./severe use dis.	.20	.229		.259	.24	.280				.221				
No use disorder		.929		.959	.94	.980				.921				
Other hallucinogens F16			.983[d]	I	I	I								.99
w/mild use dis.	.10	.129		.159	.14	.180				.121				
w/mod./severe use dis.	.20	.229		.259	.24	.280				.221				
No use disorder		.929		.959	.94	.980				.921				
Inhalants F18				I	I	I								
w/mild use dis.	.10	.129		.159	.14[e]	.180				.121		.17	.188	.99
w/mod./severe use dis.	.20	.229		.259	.24[e]	.280				.221		.27	.288	
No use disorder		.929		.959	.94[e]	.980				.921		.97	.988	
Opioids F11					I	W		I/W	I/W					
w/mild use dis.	.10	.129 (.122)[b]			.14[e]	.188		.182	.181	.121	.121			
w/mod./severe use dis.	.20	.229 (.222)[b]	.23		.24[e]	.288		.282	.281	.221	.23[f]			
No use disorder		.929 (.922)[b]			.94[e]	.988		.982	.981	.921	.921	.97	.988	.99
Sed./hyp./anx. F13				I/W	I/W	W		I/W	I/W					.99
w/mild use dis.	.10	.129		.159	.14	.180		.182	.181	.121	.121			

w/mod./severe use dis.	.20	.229	.239 (.232)b	.259	.24	.280	.288	.282	.281	.221	.231	.27	.288	
No use disorder		.929		.959	.94	.980	.988	.982	.981	.921	.921	.97	.988	.99
Amphetamines/other stimulants F15				I	I/W	I/W	I							.99
w/mild use dis.	.10	.129 (.122)b		.159	.14	.180	.188	.182	.181	.121				
w/mod./severe use dis.	.20	.229 (.222)b	.23	.259	.24	.280	.288	.282	.281	.221				
No use disorder		.929 (.922)b		.959	.94	.980	.988	.982	.981	.921				
Cocaine F14				I	I/W	I/W	I							.99
w/mild use dis.	.10	.129 (.122)b		.159	.14	.180	.188	.182	.181	.121				
w/mod./severe use dis.	.20	.229 (.222)b	.23	.259	.24	.280	.288	.282	.281	.221				
No use disorder		.929 (.922)b		.959	.94	.980	.988	.982	.981	.921				
Tobacco F17							W							.209
w/mild use dis.	Z72.0					I/W								
w/mod./severe use dis.	.200		.203			.208								
No use disorder														
Other (unknown) F19				I/W	I/W	I	I/W	I/W						.99
w/mild use dis.	.10	.129		.159	.14	.180	.188	.182	.181	.121	.121	.17	.188	
w/mod./severe use dis.	.20	.229	.239	.259	.24	.280	.288	.282	.281	.221	.231	.27	.288	
No use disorder		.929		.959	.94	.980	.988	.982	.981	.921	.921	.97	.988	

b Two numbers in a cell indicate separate codes for intoxication or withdrawal without (or with) perceptual disturbances.

d This code is for hallucinogen persisting perception disorder (see p. 433); I couldn't find any better place to put it. Tables are great, but they do have limitations.

e For inhalants and opioids, you can only have depressive mood disorder, not bipolar ones.

f Yes, I realize that opioid withdrawal delirium has only two numbers after the decimal. Deal with it.

TABLE 15.3. ICD-9-CM Code Numbers for Substance-Related Mental Disorders

	Use mild	Use mod./severe	Intox.	Withdr.	Psychotic	Depr.	Bipol.	Anxiety	OCD	Sleep	Sex	Del./I	Del./W	NCD[a]	Unspec.
Alcohol	305.00	303.90	303.00	291.81	291.9	291.89	291.89	291.89		291.82	291.89	291.0	291.0	291.2/291.1/291.89	291.9
Caffeine			305.90	292.0				292.89		292.85					292.9
Cannabis	305.20	304.30	292.89	292.0	292.9			292.89		292.85		292.81			292.9
Phen-cyclidine	305.90	304.60	292.89		292.9	292.84	292.84	292.89				292.81			292.9
Other halluc.	305.30	304.50	292.89	292.89[b]	292.9	292.84	292.84	292.89				292.81			292.9
Inhalants	305.90	304.60	292.89		292.9	292.84		292.89				292.81		292.82/292.89	292.9
Opioids	305.50	304.00	292.89	292.0		292.84		292.89		292.85		292.81	292.0		292.9
Sed./hyp./anx.	305.40	304.10	292.89	292.0	292.9	292.84	292.84	292.89		292.85		292.81	292.0	292.82/292.89	292.9
Stimulants (amph./other)	305.70	304.40	292.89	292.0	292.9	292.84	292.84	292.89	292.89	292.85	292.89	292.81			292.9
Stimulants (cocaine)	305.60	304.20	292.89	292.0	292.9	292.84	292.84	292.89	292.89	292.85	292.89	292.81			292.9
Tobacco	305.1	305.1		292.0						292.85					292.9
Other	305.90	304.90	292.89	292.0	292.9	292.84	292.84	292.89	292.89	292.85	292.89	292.81	292.0	292.82/292.89	292.9

[a]Alcohol-induced NCD has three sets of numbers. The first is for major NCD, nonamnestic–confabulatory type; the second is for major NCD, amnestic–confabulatory type; third is for mild NCD. Also, NCD induced by inhalants, sedatives/hypnotics/anxiolytics, or other has two sets of numbers. The first is for major NCD; the second is for mild NCD.

[b]Here, the number refers to hallucinogen persisting perception disorder, which is not strictly a withdrawal phenomenon but occurs after use. See text.

disorder is moderate or severe, and F10.929 if there is intoxication but no use disorder at all.

D. If there's only intoxication or withdrawal, and no use disorder, read across the row "No use disorder" for that substance. Record decimal and number from the column for the intoxication or withdrawal. Combine the F-number with the decimal to create the whole code. For caffeine, that would be F15.929 and F15.93.

E. In some instances, intoxication or withdrawal can occur with perceptual disturbances. If this is the case, at step D, use the number in parentheses. In any case, you will have coded the patient for both substance use disorder and substance intoxication or withdrawal.

If your patient has a substance-induced mental disorder, use the 11 columns under the "Substance-induced disorders" heading in Table 15.2 as follows:

F. Determine the F-number for the substance.

G. Determine whether there is a use disorder. If so, is it mild or moderate/severe?

H. If there's no use disorder, read across the row "No use disorder" for that substance. Record decimal and number from the column for the appropriate substance-induced mental disorder. Combine the F-number with the decimal to create the whole code.

I. If there is a use disorder, select the line for either mild or moderate/severe use disorder, and read across to the appropriate substance-induced disorder column.

J. For a disorder (mood, delirium, anxiety, etc.) caused by a medication taken as prescribed, code as you would for "No use disorder." So, for a substance-induced mood disorder, opioid would be F11.94, sedative/hypnotic/anxiolytic would be F13.94, and so forth. Note that you have to specify intoxication delirium or withdrawal delirium, inasmuch as the codes are mostly the same.

K. Beyond the numbering, there's a prescribed order for how you should lay down the words involved in a substance-related illness. Rather than a template, I've provided some ICD-10 examples:

F10.929 Alcohol intoxication
F10.232 Severe alcohol use disorder with alcohol withdrawal, with perceptual disturbance
F10.14 Mild alcohol use disorder with alcohol-induced bipolar disorder, with onset during intoxication

F10.121 Mild alcohol use disorder with alcohol-induced intoxication delirium, acute, with mixed level of activity

F10.26 Severe alcohol use disorder with alcohol-induced major neurocognitive disorder, persistent, amnestic–confabulatory type, with behavioral
disturbance

And it's conceivable that a patient could have both intoxication (or withdrawal)
and a substance-induced mental disorder. Then you'd end up with two sets of codes,
each of which indicates the substance use disorder status. This won't happen often.

F19.99 [292.9] Unspecified Other (or Unknown) Substance-Related Disorder

Non-Substance-Related Disorder

F63.0 [312.31] Gambling Disorder

Gambling is extremely common behavior that, like so much else in life, becomes a
disorder only when carried to such excess that it causes problems. There are striking
similarities between pathological gambling and the use of substances, not least of which
is that it, like substance use, activates reward centers (ventral striatum) of the brain
(dopamine is implicated). This helps explain why DSM-5 has moved gambling disorder
to its current location.

During an episode, most gamblers report feeling high or aroused—behavior that
usually takes several years to become pathological. Initially, success leads to increased
gambling; at some point, "the big win" of an amount that may exceed the gambler's
usual yearly earnings produces overconfidence and risk taking. From here on, because
all games of chance are weighted toward the house, it is an easy (if painful) spiral into
crushing loss, desperate attempts to get even, broken ties of family and friendship, and
eventual ruin. In fact, attempts at suicide are a frequent complication.

In the United States, gambling disorder affects about 1 adult in 200. Prevalence
estimates range between 1 and 3 million individuals in the United States. Males outnumber females by about 2:1; women develop gambling problems later than men and
seek treatment earlier. Some people only become symptomatic at certain times, such
as when their sport of choice is being played. So a person who quite literally bets the
farm on college football during the fall of each year may have few, if any, problems with
gambling at other times of the year. Others, with broader interests, may be affected
more or less chronically. Some gamblers will eventually cast off their addiction and go
into remission.

Clinicians need to be sensitive to the broad range of gambling activities, from
convenience store scratch tickets to bingo to casual sports, slot machines, poker, dice,
dogs, and the ponies.

Essential Features of **Gambling Disorder**

Gambling so takes over the lives of these patients that they will borrow, lie, and otherwise jeopardize important relationships or opportunities. As they try to recoup their losses, they may risk more money; repeated (and futile) efforts at control yield irritability and restlessness. Some gamble as a way of coping with stress. Some borrow or steal from others to relieve their increasingly desperate financial straits.

The Fine Print

The D's: • Duration (a year or more) • Distress or disability • Differential diagnosis (substance use disorders, manic episode, professional gambling, social betting)

Coding Notes

Specify if course is:

> **Episodic**
> **Persistent**

Specify if: **In {early}{sustained} remission.** No criteria for gambling disorder are met for {3–12 months}{over 1 year}.

Specify severity:

> **Mild.** Meets 4–5 criteria
> **Moderate.** Meets 6–7 criteria.
> **Severe.** Meets 8–9.

Randy Porter

The Christmas he was 12, Randy Porter's parents gave him a roulette wheel. It was handmade from shiny ebony, and it had mother-of-pearl inlaid numbers. The layout was printed on green felt, and the ball was ivory. "Best quality you'll find outside of Monte Carlo," his father bragged when Randy opened it. Throughout high school, Randy loved operating a casino for his friends. Once or twice some adults drifted in from his parents' bingo night; then they played for real money.

Now Randy was 25, divorced, and broke. He'd had a good job managing a restaurant near the Las Vegas strip. He couldn't honestly say he had taken his job to be near the action, but it had seemed a godsend after he'd flunked out of college because of too many all-night bridge sessions (penny a point). It was an easy 5-minute walk to two of the most glittering casinos in town—a walk that Randy used to take frequently on his lunch hour. "I knew everybody there," he reported. "I used to have accounts all over town. But nobody's let me run a tab for years."

Randy's early encounters with a real roulette table had been harmless enough. At noon, he would stroll over to watch the action and place the odd bet. He won a few dollars and lost a few more. All in all, he found that he could take it or leave it, mostly take it—he relished the surge of adrenaline when he had money in play. He could afford modest losses; by then, he was married and his wife was making good money dealing blackjack at another casino. Then one Saturday afternoon when his wife had to work, black came up seven times in a row, and he walked away from the table with over $55,000 in his pocket. Later he said, "It was maybe the unluckiest day of my entire life."

In subsequent weeks, Randy lost himself (not to mention the $55,000) in gambling fever. His lunch hour soon stretched to two as he returned to the table again and again in an effort to recoup his losses. After he was caught "borrowing" from his employer, he tried Gamblers Anonymous; he quit because he "didn't believe in a higher power." Over the next 2 years he became "totally obsessed," as his wife put it on more than one occasion, with the idea of scoring another big win so that he could quit ahead. Tired of being ignored and lied to about their finances, she finally left him.

"She said she might as well be married to a one-armed bandit," Randy sadly remarked.

Attentive and pleasant, Randy sat quietly throughout his interview. Though he expressed remorse for the difficulties he had caused himself and others, he described his mood as neither depressed nor ecstatic, but "in the middle." His speech was clear and goal-directed. His cognition and reasoning were excellent.

Before his wife left, Randy had pleaded with her to stay. He promised to reform. "I wouldn't bet on it," she'd told him.

Evaluation of Randy Porter

Like many other nascent gamblers, Randy got his start as an adolescent through gambling activities in his home. In the course of a few years, he became thoroughly preoccupied with gambling (criterion A4); unsuccessfully tried to control it (A3); chased his losses with more betting (A6); and lied, stole, and eventually lost his wife and his job (A7, A9, A8). He would therefore amply meet the symptomatic criteria (only four are required) for gambling disorder, provided that his behavior was not better accounted for by a **manic episode** (B). However, Randy showed no symptoms of mania, no depression, and no evidence of periodicity in his gambling behavior—so we can safely rule that out. **Social gamblers** set limits on their losses and gamble in the company of friends; **professional gamblers** respect the odds and maintain strict self-discipline. Randy's behavior fit neither pattern.

The real challenge in evaluating any patient who gambles excessively is to determine whether there is an associated mental disorder. Commonly associated conditions include **mood disorders**, **panic disorder**, **obsessive–compulsive disorder**, and **agoraphobia**. Also look for problems with **substance use** (which can precede or accompany gambling behavior) and **suicide attempts** (which may result from it). When present, any comorbid mental disorder is likely to have begun first.

Of course, people with **antisocial personality disorder** can become heavily involved in gambling, and research has also identified **borderline personality disorder** in such a population. However, Randy showed none of the behaviors that would be diagnostic of those personality disorders. Neither had he demonstrated any evidence that his behavior was episodic, and he certainly wasn't in remission (the other possible specifier, other than severity), so his full diagnosis would be—

Uh, wait a minute. Let's talk about severity. According to the DSM-5 criteria, Randy barely qualifies for a severity level of moderate. But here's a fellow whose addiction (I'm not afraid to call it that) had essentially ruined his life. I don't know where he's working now, but I doubt that it's for his original employer, and he's probably sleeping in his car. I'd give him a relatively low GAF score of 55, and I don't call any of this a moderate *anything*. Once again, I'm going to assert clinician's prerogative and say that his level of severity would be—severe.

F63.0 [312.31]	Gambling disorder, severe, persistent
Z63.5 [V61.03]	Divorced

CHAPTER 16

Cognitive Disorders

Here's why I'm departing from the DSM-5 name for this chapter:

When I was re-reading this chapter prior to publication, I noticed that *I* was growing confused. The new name for dementia is *major neurocognitive disorder*, whereas the new name for the collected cognitive disorders is *neurocognitive disorders*. In some passages, I wasn't sure myself exactly what I had meant—one disorder or the whole collection! If it gave me trouble, surely it would other readers, too. So, after much thought and consultation, I decided to stick with the DSM-IV title for the chapter, and reserve *neuro*cognitive disorder (NCD) for the conditions we used to call dementia.

Quick Guide to the Cognitive Disorders

With a structure simplified in DSM-5, classification of the cognitive disorders is logical, though the details can be pretty darned complex.

Delirium

A *delirium* is a rapidly developing, fluctuating state of reduced awareness in which the following are true:

- The patient has trouble with awareness (operationally defined as orientation) and shifting or focusing of attention, *and*
- The patient has at least one defect of memory, orientation, perception, visuospatial skills, or language, *and*
- The symptoms are not better explained by coma or another cognitive disorder.

One of the following causes can be identified (here and throughout, the page number in each case indicates where a more detailed discussion begins):

Delirium due to another medical condition. Delirium can be caused by trauma to the brain, infections, epilepsy, endocrine disorders, toxicity from medications, poisons, and various other diseases affecting almost any part of the body (p. 480). I have listed many of these conditions in the "Physical Disorders That Affect Mental Diagnosis" table in the Appendix. Occasionally more than one cause for delirium will be identified in the same patient.

Substance intoxication delirium, substance withdrawal delirium, and medication-induced delirium. Alcohol and other sedative drugs of abuse, as well as nearly every class of street drug, can cause delirium in both intoxication and withdrawal. Medications can also be implicated (p. 483).

Delirium due to multiple etiologies. Delirium can have multiple causes in the same patient (p. 486).

Other specified, and unspecified, delirium. Use one of these categories when you don't know the cause of a patient's delirium or when it doesn't fully meet diagnostic criteria (p. 487).

Major and Mild Neurocognitive Disorders

A major or mild neurocognitive disorder (NCD) differs from delirium in several ways:

- The time course is relatively slow. Delirium develops across hours or days, an NCD across weeks and months.
- Although patients with NCDs can have impaired ability to focus or shift attention, it isn't prominent.
- The cause of an NCD can usually be found within the central nervous system; the cause of delirium is often elsewhere in the body.
- Some patients recover from an NCD, but this isn't the usual course.

DSM-5 now distinguishes between major NCD (which was called dementia in previous DSMs) and mild NCD. In mild NCD, any of the etiologies listed below can be implicated in relatively mild effects on a person's ability to function independently. Discerning the boundaries between major and mild NCD can be problematic, however.

One of the following types of NCD will be identified:

Major or mild NCD due to Alzheimer's disease. This is the most common cause of NCD. It begins gradually and usually progresses inexorably. A bit more than half of all major NCDs are of the Alzheimer's type (p. 498).

Major or mild vascular NCD. Due to vascular brain disease, these patients experience loss of memory and other cognitive abilities. Often this is a stepwise process, with relatively sudden onset and a fluctuating course. Some 10–20% of major NCDs are vascular (p. 516).

Major or mild NCD due to other medical conditions, A large number of medical conditions can cause NCDs (again, see "Physical Disorders . . . " in the Appendix). Some of the most noteworthy (pp. 504ff) include brain tumor, Creutzfeldt–Jakob disease (infection by a slow virus, or prion disease), traumatic brain injury, human immunodeficiency virus (HIV) disease, Huntington's disease, Parkinson's disease, and frontotemporal NCD (formerly Pick's disease). The most common toxins causing NCDs are those resulting from kidney and liver failure.

Substance/medication-induced major or mild NCD. Some 5–10% of NCDs are related to prolonged use of alcohol, inhalants, or sedatives (p. 522).

Major or mild NCD due to multiple etiologies. Like a delirium, an NCD can have multiple causes in the same patient (p. 526).

Unspecified NCD. This category is useful when you know the patient's cognitive status is impaired, but you don't know why (p. 527).

Other Causes of Cognitive Symptoms

Dissociative disorders. Profound, temporary loss of memory may occur in persons who suffer from dissociative amnesia (p. 239) or dissociative identity disorder (p. 245).

Pseudodementia. From their apathy and slowed responses, some patients often look as if they have the severe memory loss and other symptoms of major NCD (dementia). But careful clinical evaluation and psychological testing reveal severe major depressive disorder (p. 122) and cognitive functioning that is relatively intact, though they may have problems with attention and concentration. Pseudodementia accounts for about 5% of elderly patients referred for a dementia workup. Pseudodementia is a useful term DSM-5 doesn't use.

Malingering. Some patients will intentionally exaggerate or falsify cognitive symptoms to obtain funds (insurance, workers' compensation) or to avoid punishment or military service (p. 599).

Factitious disorder imposed on self. Some patients may feign cognitive symptoms, but not for direct gain (such as gaining money or avoiding punishment). Their motive often appears to be hospitalized or otherwise cared for (p. 268).

Whatever happened to age-related cognitive decline? This DSM-IV diagnosis referred to the fact that older patients often report trouble remembering names, telephone numbers, or places where they put things. On testing, they tend to look pretty normal. However, DSM-5 just considers it a part of what's normal, deserving of no special coding. It takes objective evidence of impairment in at least one cognitive domain to cause DSM-5 to sit up and take notice.

Introduction

Cognition refers to the mental processing of information—more specifically, memory and thinking in the storage, retrieval, and manipulation of information to achieve knowledge. A clinician obtains information about these processes by observation during an interview and by asking the patient to perform certain tasks during the mental status evaluation.

The cognitive disorders (major, mild, and delirium) are abnormalities of these mental processes that are associated with temporary or permanent brain dysfunction. Their main symptoms include problems with memory, orientation, language, information processing, and the ability to focus and sustain attention on a task. A cognitive disorder is caused by a medical condition or substance use that leads to defects of brain structure, chemistry, or physiology. However, the underlying causative agent cannot always be defined.

With early recognition and adequate treatment, many cognitive disorders (especially deliriums) are reversible; ignored, they will sometimes spontaneously improve, but often they cause permanent disability. Moreover, though the criteria are relatively simple, their associated symptoms can cause cognitive disorders to mimic virtually any other mental condition. For example, delirium can present with symptoms of depression and anxiety; major neurocognitive disorder (dementia) can present with psychosis. Whatever your patient's history or symptoms, it is therefore vital to consider neurocognitive etiologies near the top of your differential diagnosis. If you forget about cognitive disorders, emotional symptoms can all too easily obscure an underlying delirium, or you might diagnose a psychotic disorder when your patient actually has a dementia.

Depending on the underlying cause, cognitive disorders can begin at any age. They are extremely common, especially in a hospital setting. They may constitute up to one in five of all mental health admissions.

Delirium

Although the brain itself can be involved directly (as with a brain tumor or seizure disorder), most deliriums are caused by disease processes that begin outside the central nervous system. These include endocrine disorders, infections, drug toxicity or withdrawal, vitamin deficiency, fever, liver and kidney disease, poisons, and the effects of surgical operations. (A more complete listing is given in the "Physical Disorders . . ." table in the Appendix.)

We can easily state the basic symptoms of delirium:

- In just hours to several days, the patient develops . . .
- *Reduction in awareness and attention*, accompanied by . . .

- Some sort of additional *cognitive deficit,* such as problems with orientation, memory, language, perception, or visuospatial capability.

- The intensity of these symptoms tends to fluctuate during the course of a day.

Inattention is often the first symptom you might notice. During an interview, you identify difficulty focusing on the topic at hand; the patient may experience it as drowsiness or somnolence. Thought processes slow down and appear vague; you may detect trouble with reasoning and solving problems. You may have to ask questions several times before the patient responds. On the other hand, inattention may show up instead as a hyperalert distractibility, with rapid shifting from one focus to another.

Any of several areas can constitute the additional cognitive deficit; two or more may occur at the same time.

Language. You will recognize problems with language in speech that is rambling, disjointed, pressured, or incoherent, or speech that leaps from one topic to another. Some patients will have trouble writing or naming things. Speech that is merely slurred, without demonstrating incoherent thoughts, suggests intoxication, not delirium.

Memory. Delirious patients nearly always have trouble remembering things. Recent events are always affected first; older memories (especially those from childhood) are usually the last to go.

Executive functioning. The person has difficulty in planning, organizing, sequencing, or abstracting information. In practice, the person has trouble making decisions, taking steps that break a habit pattern, correcting errors, or searching for the source of a problem (troubleshooting). Obviously, novel or complicated situations will be fraught for these people.

Orientation. Many patients will be disoriented, sometimes so severely that you cannot examine them adequately. Disorientation is most likely to be for time (date, day, month, year); next comes disorientation for place; last, patients fail to recognize relatives and friends (disorientation for person). Only the most severely ill patients are unsure of their own identities.

Perception. Patients with even mild or early delirium don't perceive their surroundings as clearly as usual: Boundaries are fuzzy, colors are abnormally bright, images distorted. Some patients misidentify what they see (illusions), whereas others experience false perceptions (hallucinations are especially likely to be visual). If they later experience false beliefs or ideas (delusions) grafted onto their hallucinations, these delusions are usually incomplete, changing, or poorly organized. Confronted by visual misperceptions, patients may not be able to tell whether they are dreaming or awake. Those who accept their hallucinations as reality may feel quite anxious or fearful.

Other areas often revealing disturbance in delirium include the following:

Sleep–wake cycle. A change in a patient's normal sleep cycle (insomnia, day–night reversal, vivid dreams, nightmares) almost invariably occurs.

Psychomotor activity and behavior. Sometimes physical movements may be slowed, especially if the delirium is due to metabolic problems; these patients appear retarded and sluggish. Others may experience increased motor activity (agitated behavior, picking at bedclothes). A flapping tremor of the hands is common. So are vocalizations, which are sometimes no more than muttering or moans, though some patients may weep or call out. Those who feel threatened may strike out or attempt to escape.

Mood. Depression and fear are common emotional reactions to the experiences mentioned above; mood often becomes unstable, perceived by others as lability of affect. (Dysphoria can sometimes be the presenting symptom in delirium; then there is a danger of misdiagnosing the patient as having a major depressive disorder.) Some patients will only react with perplexity; still others will exhibit bland, calm acceptance, or perhaps even intense anger or euphoria.

Delirium usually begins suddenly, and its intensity often fluctuates. Most patients will be more lucid in the morning and worse at night—a transient phenomenon called *sundowning*. When you suspect delirium, try to interview the patient in sessions several hours apart. Because the symptoms of delirium so often fluctuate with time of day, normal or marginal findings at noon may give way to clear evidence of illness in the evening. If multiple visits are not practical, nursing staff (or chart notes) may provide the needed information.

Though symptoms may persist for days to weeks, most deliriums last a week or less and then resolve, once the underlying condition has been relieved. Some, however, will evolve into dementia. After delirium resolves, most patients recall the experiences incompletely; they may have amnesia for certain (or all) aspects, and that which is recalled may seem like a dream. Delirium is common on medical wards, where it may be mistaken for other mental disorders, including psychosis, depression, mania, "hysteria," or personality disorder.

Delirium has the overall highest incidence of all mental disorders. By some estimates, up to half of hospitalized elderly patients become delirious. It is more common in children and the elderly than in young and middle-aged adults.

Delirium has many aliases. Neurologists and internists call it *acute confusional state*. Other terms sometimes used for delirium include *toxic psychosis*, *acute brain syndrome*, and *metabolic encephalopathy*. These terms are useful to know when you are discussing a delirious patient with clinicians who do not specialize in mental health.

Some clinicians regard delirium as a state of agitated mental confusion during which the patient experiences visual hallucinations that are unusually vivid. This would be the case for delirium tremens. However, DSM-5 uses the term *delirium* in a much broader sense, to encompass conditions with the more varied symptoms mentioned in the Essential Features.

Essential Features of **Delirium**

Over a short time, the patient develops problems with attention that wanders and with orientation (especially to the environment); additional cognitive changes (memory, use of language, disorientation in other spheres, perception, visuomotor capability) set in. Severity fluctuates during the day. The cause can be pinned on a physical condition, substance use, toxicity, or some combination.

The Fine Print

For tips on identifying substance-related causation, see sidebar, page 95.

The D's: • Duration of onset (hours to days; generally brief, though it can endure) • Differential diagnosis (major neurocognitive disorder, coma, psychotic disorders)

Coding Notes

Specify if:

Hyperactive. Agitation or otherwise increased level of activity.
Hypoactive. Reduced level of activity.
Mixed level of activity. Normal or fluctuating activity levels.

Specify duration:

Acute. Lasts hours to a few days.
Persistent. Lasts weeks or longer.

Code numbers for substance- (and medication-)caused delirium are given in Chapter 15, Tables 15.2 and 15.3. ICD-10 prescribes the order as to how you lay down the words when a delirium has been caused by substance use; see the footnotes to Table 15.2.

F05 [293.0] Delirium Due to Another Medical Condition

Delirium can have many causes, related in part to the patient's age group. In children, fever and infection are the most common causes; in young adults, drugs; in middle-aged adults, withdrawal from alcohol and head injury; in the elderly, metabolic issues, cardiovascular failure, and excessive medications. Often delirium in an older patient will have multiple causes (see p. 486).

Because it may be caused by a disease that can lead to dementia or even kill outright, any delirium is a true emergency. When you suspect one, immediately obtain appropriate medical consultation or testing; often evaluation by a neurologist will be required. However, formal (neuropsychological) testing can be difficult in patients who cannot adequately sustain attention on a task. Therefore, the diagnosis of delirium may sometimes depend on a bedside evaluation.

Again, the "Physical Disorders . . . " table in the Appendix lists some of the more frequently encountered medical causes of delirium.

Harold Hoyt

After rheumatic heart disease had led to years of gradually worsening fatigue and shortness of breath, Harold Hoyt, a 48-year-old bricklayer, finally consented to a mitral valve replacement. Warning him that open heart surgery could cause delirium, his surgeon had recommended mental health consultation as a preventive measure.

"I ain't crazy," Harold replied by way of refusal.

The procedure went well, but the recovery room staff noticed right away that Harold seemed withdrawn and uncommunicative. He ignored his wife and daughter during their brief hourly visits. When he spoke or wrote notes, it was usually to complain about the tube in his nose or about his inability to sleep in the brightly lighted intensive care unit.

On the third postoperative day, Harold became increasingly restless. After he pulled out his nasogastric tube, he was quieter for a time, but in the evening he was found crying and trying to get out of bed. He asked a nurse why he was there, and was incredulous when told that he had had open heart surgery. As they spoke, his voice trailed off, and he seemed to forget that anyone was there. When he spoke again, he asked about a football game that had been played the week before.

The following morning Harold carried on a routine, though brief, conversation with the dietary aide who brought breakfast. But by nightfall he was again talking to himself and had to be restrained from pulling out his IV. He was able to give the date accurately, however.

A mental health consultant diagnosed a "classic postcardiotomy delirium" and recommended that family members sit with Harold to provide stimulation and reality checks. Within 36 hours he was fully oriented and conversing normally with his family, and his improved physical condition allowed him to be moved to a bed on the ward. He remembered nothing of his behavior of the previous 2 days and seemed surprised that he had required restraints.

Evaluation of Harold Hoyt

In the hours after surgery, Harold's problem with attention caused him to have difficulty even expressing a thought (his voice trailed off in midsentence, and he veered off into a discussion of football); the fact that he was also unaware of his surroundings completes the requirement for delirium criterion A. His cognitive problems had developed rapidly and fluctuated with time of day, increasing in the evening and at night (sundowning—criterion B). He had further problems with short-term memory (among other things, he forgot that he had had surgery), and on at least one occasion he was disoriented to time (either of these issues would pass muster for criterion C). He wasn't comatose, and he'd had no preexisting **neurocognitive disorder** that would better explain his symptoms (D). His recent history of heart surgery provides evidence of a direct link to his delirium; indeed, his surgeon had warned him it might happen (E).

We need to consider a differential diagnosis, even though the criteria do not describe one beyond a cognitive disorder. When his delirium was first developing, Harold was withdrawn and seemed irritable. These features suggest a **depressive disorder**, which is only one of many mental disorders sometimes confused with the cognitive disorders. Because hallucinations are so common, **schizophrenia** and other **psychotic disorders** also appear in the differential diagnosis, though the history of an operation and rapid fluctuations in cognition are pretty reliable (but hardly infallible) giveaways. Occasionally a patient (especially one who has a background in health care) will feign the symptoms of delirium to obtain money or some other material benefit. This sort of deception can be difficult to detect; when it is found, **malingering** is the usual designation (though I tend to be *really* parsimonious with this Z-code). When the motive behind such deception is only to be a patient, consider **factitious disorder imposed on self.** Harold became somewhat agitated and tried to get out of bed; perhaps this was due to **anxiety** at finding himself in a strange place without knowing why. But there are plenty of people who have anxiety symptoms without having an **anxiety disorder.**

The variety of potential causes of delirium is vast; although many of them are included in the "Physical Disorders . . ." table in the Appendix, the list there is by no means comprehensive. As Harold's consultant noted, cardiotomy is a classical precipitant of delirium (experienced by about 25% of patients after open heart surgery). Somewhat ironically for Harold, the strongest preventative measure against postcardiotomy delirium is a mental health consultation before surgery.

When you are coding a delirium, be sure to include the medical condition(s) responsible. Harold's GAF score at consultation was a low 40; by discharge, it had improved to a relatively robust 71.

Z95.2 [V43.3]	Prosthetic heart valve
F05 [293.0]	Delirium due to chest surgery, acute, hyperactive

---

"Delirium Due to Medical Cause Often Misdiagnosed." That headline in an online report described a paper recently presented at a geriatric psychiatry meeting. Of 112 consecutive patients admitted with the diagnosis of a mental health disorder, 27—nearly one-quarter—were ultimately found to be suffering from a delirium due to some underlying medical disorder. The most frequent diagnosis was a urinary tract infection. Other conditions affecting more than a single patient included drug usage and poor control of blood sugar. Mostly, the patients were at first diagnosed as having a different cognitive disorder, but psychoses and mood disorders were also prevalent.

Substance Intoxication Delirium, Substance Withdrawal Delirium, and Medication-Induced Delirium

People who abuse street drugs or alcohol are at serious risk for developing a delirium. Many drugs can produce intoxication delirium, but abrupt cessation of heavy use of other sedative drugs, such as alcohol and barbiturates, are notorious for causing withdrawal delirium. The most commonly known is alcohol withdrawal delirium (popularly called delirium tremens, or DTs). Its hallmarks are agitation, tremor, disorientation, and vivid hallucinations. In someone who has suddenly stopped after many weeks of heavy drinking, DTs can occur within a few days. DTs can also be precipitated when a substance-misusing patient develops a medical illness (such as liver failure, head trauma, pneumonia, or pancreatitis); alcohol users are at special risk for each of these conditions. Alcohol withdrawal delirium isn't especially common, even among the heaviest users of alcohol. But it is so severe that if it goes untreated, up to 15% die. This makes it an extremely important mental health event.

Delirium—especially intoxication delirium, but also the withdrawal type—can also be caused by prescribed medications, which don't necessarily have to be present in high concentrations. In combination with other drugs or illnesses, low doses can cause delirium, especially in older people. Drugs with anticholinergic effects (such as antiparkinsonian agents and antidepressants) are probably the most likely to produce delirium. Although intoxication delirium can occur within minutes of taking cocaine or hallucinogens, for many other substances it will occur only after drug levels have built up over several days or longer.

Rodney Partridge

A barroom knife fight had left Rodney Partridge with a severed artery in his arm that required 2 hours in the operating room and several units of whole blood. But apart from a slight tremor, when Rodney awakened from the anesthesia late Sunday morning, he felt almost as good as new. By evening he was eating voraciously and enjoying the attentions of the nursing staff. On Monday, however, when the surgeon came around to make sure the dressing was still dry, the head nurse confided in a worried whisper: "He's been awake most of the night, demanding to be released. The last hour or two, he's been trying to pick things off his sheets."

When the mental health consultant appeared in his doorway, Rodney was propped up in bed; he was restrained by a canvas halter around his chest and by leather cuffs around his ankles and left wrist. His free hand trembled and roamed the bedclothes, pausing occasionally to pinch up a bit of air and fling it to the floor. Then Rodney threw a triangle of toast at the curtain rod over his window.

"Got him! Cheeky bugger."

"Got who?" the consultant wanted to know.

"Oh, my God!" Startled, Rodney lurched against his chest restraints and dropped a second piece of toast onto the sheet. Leaving the toast where it lay, he returned to plucking at his bedclothes.

"Got who?" repeated the consultant.

Rodney's gaze returned to the curtain rod. "It was those guys up there. One of them mooned me."

The guys were about 4 inches tall and wore short pants, green jackets, and pointed caps. For half an hour they had been parading around on top of the curtain rod, making obscene gestures and throwing multicolored caterpillars onto Rodney's bed. Whenever a caterpillar landed, it would begin crawling toward him, munching a swath across the sheet as it came.

Although he wasn't exactly frightened, Rodney was far from placid. With his gaze constantly darting around the room, he seemed to be watching for other predators. He insisted that the guys and caterpillars were real, but he had no idea why they were there. He was also vague about his orientation. He knew he was in a hospital whose name he had "never been told," thought he had been admitted a week earlier, and missed the date by nearly 5 months. When Rodney was asked to subtract sevens from 100, he responded: "Ah, 93 . . . 80 . . . um . . . there's a purple one."

With a little urging and a lot of Librium for sedation, Rodney admitted that he had been a heavy drinker most of his adult life. Too many vodka sours had landed him currently between jobs (and wives), and for the last 3 months he had spent most of his waking hours consuming a quart or more of hard liquor per day. Although his morning shakes often required "a hair of the dog," he had never before had hallucinations. He agreed that he was "probably an alcoholic"—in fact, he'd started with Alcoholics Anonymous several times, but had never been able to stay the course.

Evaluation of Rodney Partridge

Several points in Rodney's history suggest some sort of cognitive disorder. First, his orientation was poor (he was unclear about the date and had no idea what hospital he was in). The second tipoff to delirium was his reduced attention span (he had difficulty focusing on his conversation with the mental health consultant). Together, these two features constitute criterion A for a delirium. The symptoms had begun rapidly and appeared to be a change for Rodney (B); it is only with time that we would know the extent to which they would fluctuate, and Rodney's consultant intervened with treatment first.

Rodney also had rather dramatic hallucinations (perceptual changes, one of the several alternative additional disturbances required by criterion C). The hallucinations of alcohol withdrawal and other withdrawal deliriums are classically visual, but they can be auditory or tactile. If delusions occur, their content is often related to the hallucinations.

Rodney had several other symptoms typically associated with delirium. He had become so hyperactive (increased startle response, trying to get out of bed) and agitated that he had to be restrained. His tremor was evident. Although Rodney was only bemused, many patients are badly frightened by hallucinations, which can be grotesque beyond belief. His symptoms were clearly more severe than you'd encounter in simple alcohol withdrawal; by themselves they would warrant clinical attention.

Hallucinations could suggest **schizophrenia**, a mistake careful clinicians avoid by asking informants how long the patient has had psychotic symptoms. (See the sidebar below for some points that discriminate causes of psychosis.) As with any delirium, other conditions to rule out include other **psychotic disorders**, **malingering**, and **factitious disorder.** In Rodney's case, history provided ample evidence for a causal relationship between his drinking and his symptoms (E).

Although Rodney Partridge would meet the criteria for alcohol withdrawal (p. 406), this diagnosis is superseded by alcohol withdrawal delirium. We need to choose between the specifiers for acuteness and activity level. And here's another point: Because they occurred only during a delirium, we don't make a separate diagnosis for his psychosis. That's a general point that has applicability for problems with mood, anxiety, sleep, and sex, any of which can become problematic during a delirium.

Of course, Rodney would also qualify for a diagnosis of alcohol use disorder (see p. 397): In addition to the symptoms of withdrawal, he had tried Alcoholics Anonymous without success, and he preferred drinking to working. Although the number of substance use symptoms mentioned here isn't high by actual count, I'd still code as *severe* just about any patient who has had DTs. In any event, the presence of alcohol use disorder helps determine his two mental health diagnoses. In coding Rodney's disorders, I have referred to Tables 15.2 and 15.3 in Chapter 15. His GAF score on admission would be a strikingly low 30.

F10.231 [303.90, 291.0]	Severe alcohol use disorder, with acute alcohol withdrawal delirium, hyperactive
S45.119A [903.1]	Laceration of brachial artery
Z56.9 [V62.29]	Unemployed
Z63.5 [V61.03]	Divorced

When psychotic symptoms turn up in patients with major neurocognitive disorder (dementia), delirium may be the cause. Of course, it's important to know when that is the case, because treatment of the delirium can greatly ameliorate the discomfort (to all) of the hallucinations and, sometimes, delusions. But studies show that delirium is often underdiagnosed in patients with dementia, and that the two disorders often occur together. Here are a few differences:

Delusions. In dementia, they are typically of being robbed or abandoned. In delirium, they more likely to concern dangers in the immediate environment.

Hallucinations. In delirium, visual hallucinations and illusions are common. In

Alzheimer's dementia, they are not so common (but they are more common in Lewy body dementia).

Flow of thought. Delirious people are likely to have thought processes that are illogical, perhaps with derailment. In dementia, poverty of thought is more likely.

Attention. It's affected in delirium, though relatively spared in Alzheimer's dementia (however, it is deeply affected in Lewy body dementia).

F05 [293.0] Delirium Due to Multiple Etiologies

Probably more patients than are ever recognized have multiple causes for delirium. Many such diagnoses are undoubtedly missed because the clinician is aware of one cause and fails to identify the others. The signs and symptoms do not differ from those in the foregoing examples, but of course, successful treatment can hinge heavily upon accurate identification of all contributing factors.

Delirium due to multiple etiologies is not really a single diagnosis—it is a collection of two or more diagnoses occurring in a single patient. I include it here as a reminder of its importance: Treatment is hard when you don't know all of the causes. It is especially common among older people, who are likely to have numerous medical problems.

Emil Brion

At age 72, Emil Brion already had such severe emphysema that he required oxygen day and night. "I always warned him about smoking, but he was actually proud of being a three-pack-a-day man," said his wife. "Now, if he takes the oxygen off to smoke, he gets goofy and scared."

She meant that Emil would see things: A light cord would become a snake; a pile of clothes on the chair looked for an instant like a lion ready to spring. He might wake up whimpering from a nightmare. Sometimes he seemed so distracted that she could hardly persuade him to put the oxygen back on. But all things considered, he was doing pretty well. He could even drive a little, as long as he used his oxygen.

That lasted until the Fourth of July, when Emil strolled barefoot into the back yard and sliced the outer sole of his heel on a broken piece of glass. The cut didn't hurt much, so he forgot to clean it up when he went back inside. It was several days before either he or his wife noticed how red and swollen the injured area had become. By that time, according to the specialist in infectious diseases who admitted him to the hospital, he had developed a severe septicemia.

Despite continuous IV antibiotics, for 3 days Emil's temperature hovered above 102 degrees. Even with nasal oxygen running, his arterial oxygen saturation was low. During much of the day he slept; at night he was awake, mumbling to himself and groaning. When he spoke clearly enough to be understood, he complained that he was a miserable old man and wished he were dead.

On Emil's seventh hospital day, his fever finally broke. He removed the oxygen tube and told the nurse, "Wheel me outside so I can have a smoke."

Evaluation of Emil Brion

Emil's wife noted that when he went without his oxygen, he was sometimes so distracted that he couldn't even focus on restarting his oxygen. When a second disorder (systemic infection) was added to the anoxia, he rapidly (delirium criterion B) became somnolent (A). His other cognitive difficulties (C) included illusions (the light-cord snake) and nightmares, and he began to mumble (language difficulties).

Several other symptoms typically associated with delirium were also apparent. He had a change in his sleep pattern (drowsy during the day, awake at night). He became depressed and even wished himself dead; perhaps at times he recognized how desperately ill he was. As to preexisting cognitive conditions (D), the only one would be the possibility of another delirium.

Even before the infection set in, Emil had fluctuating states of consciousness and attention with occasional hallucinations, suggesting a persistent delirium caused by anoxia. But his mental condition had more than one cause, as shown by the fact that the infection made him sicker, even when nasal oxygen was running. That either could cause delirium satisfies criterion E. Once the infection in his bloodstream was resolved and his fever broke, his cognition suddenly improved. However, a complete evaluation of his mental status would be needed to be sure there were no residual symptoms of dementia or a depressive disorder. We wouldn't confuse his perceptual problems with **schizophrenia** because they developed so rapidly.

Note that in the coding of Emil's delirium, a separate code for each specific cause is indicated by a separate line, though in his case the numbers remain the same. His GAF score on admission was only 25; it was 80 at discharge.

J43.9 [492.8]	Emphysema
A41.9 [038.9]	Septicemia
F05 [293.0]	Delirium due to anoxia, persistent, hypoactive
	Delirium due to septicemia, acute, hypoactive

R41.0 [780.09] Other Specified Delirium

R41.0 [780.09] Unspecified Delirium

Use other specified or unspecified delirium as a catch-all category for any delirium that does not meet the criteria for one of the previously described types. For other specified delirium, DSM-5 specifically mentions the following:

> **Attenuated delirium syndrome.** The symptoms of delirium are not severe enough for a more specific diagnosis.

Symptom Domains

Although we can organize our thinking about them in different ways, over the years some consensus has developed of what constitutes the domains important for the study of what DSM-5 now calls major and mild neurocognitive disorders (NCDs). Here are descriptions of those that DSM-5 considers central to the understanding of all cognitive disorders, but especially to major NCD (dementia).

Those who write (and do research) about cognitive matters often refer to neurocognitive domains. However, they never quite define just what they mean by *domain*. DSM-5 has carried that tradition forward, even to the extent of ignoring it in its own glossary; I will now attempt to break it. The *Oxford English Dictionary* says that a domain is "a sphere of thought or action," a dimension of thought or a field of knowledge. Therefore, we can regard a neurocognitive domain as a group of functions that pertains to one aspect of thinking, perception, or memory.

And, wouldn't you know, even domains can have domains (well, sometimes DSM-5 calls them *facets*). For example, the domain of language includes naming, grammar, receptive language, fluency, and word finding. And just where DSM-5's facets belong is also a bit fraught. Depending on the expert you consult, you can find working memory located as an aspect of memory and learning, a component of complex attention, or a subdivision of executive functioning. Good luck.

Complex Attention

Complex attention means the ability to focus on tasks in such a way that their completion isn't derailed by distractions. It is more than the simple attention span you evaluate when you ask a patient to repeat a string of digits or spell *world* backwards. It also involves processing speed, holding information in mind, and being able to attend (more or less) to more than one thing at once, like writing a grocery list while listening to the radio. In mild NCD, a patient may be able to perform tasks when a lot is going on, but it will take extra effort.

Pauline has begun to have trouble using her computer. If a phone call interrupts her, she may spend minutes trying to determine where she left off. She used to read the newspaper and write email online; now she must limit herself, so as not to become confused.

Jason's daughter-in-law complained (for him) that in the past several months, he'd had increasing difficulty dressing himself. "If I'm talking to him, he gets distracted and is likely to leave a shoe untied. A year ago, he'd be able to listen and talk and dress, but there might be some hesitation. It was as though he needed to restart himself between tasks. Now, *I* have to restart him."

Jason's attention span and processing capability (together, these are sometimes called *working memory*; see the sidebar above) were no longer up to the task of coping with the need for divided attention. A year ago, Jason could complete his task by putting forth some extra effort, compatible with a diagnosis (then) of *mild* NCD. Now, of course, his cognition had fallen further behind and he was operating at the level of an actual dementia—*major* NCD.

Learning and Memory

Memory exists in many variations. Just a few years ago (it seems), we spoke mainly of long- and short-term memory. Now there's a congeries of terms that we must, um, remember. A good, simple categorization is summed up by the mnemonic PEWS:

- *Procedural memory.* That's the sort of memory we need for skills such as typing and playing the flute (ahem!) and riding a bicycle. It allows us to learn a sequence of behaviors and repeat them, without having to expend conscious effort.

- *Episodic memory.* This is the memory for events the individual has experienced as personal history—the night Mom died, where you went on your last vacation, your dessert choice at supper yesterday. Episodic memory always takes our personal point of view; it is often visual.

- *Working memory.* By this we mean the very short-term storing of data that we are actively processing. We test it by asking the patient to do mental arithmetic or spell words backwards. It is often regarded as synonymous with immediate memory and regarded as an executive function.

- *Semantic memory.* This is the type of memory we mean when we speak of general knowledge—in short, facts and figures. This is where most of what we learn ends up, because we no longer associate it with anything concrete in our lives, such as where we were when the learning took place.

In each division except working memory, memories tend to endure for up to many years—though episodic tends to be shorter than semantic. Working memory, however, is brief (spanning but a few minutes, if that).

As memory deteriorates, the time it takes to process information increases. So a person might have trouble performing mental arithmetic or repeating back a story name that was just related, or holding in mind a telephone number long enough to dial it. With advancing dementia, the little assists that once helped out lose their punch.

Just before Christmas, 74-year-old Sarah had spent 2 days searching the house for the presents she had hidden. She and her son, Jon, finally found them in the storage shed, but her problems were only just beginning. She had always prided herself on her ability to remember telephone numbers, but in February, when Jon was assigned a new extension number at work, she could never seem to recall what it was or where she had written it down. After several days of frustration, Jon finally pasted the new number onto the base of both of their telephones. However, it was the two fires she started while cooking that led to an evaluation. When asked to name the president of the United States, she said, "That's what you should know for yourself. I don't feel like helping you any more."

By the time Audrey turned 80, she had trouble remembering where her room was; some days, she didn't recognize her daughter when she came to call. But she could still play her favorite songs on the piano.

Perceptual–Motor Ability

Perceptual–motor ability is one's ability to assimilate visual and other sensory information and use it. The use is usually motor, though also included would be facial recognition, which lacks a motor component. Note that the sensory abilities themselves are just fine: The person can actually see things about as well as average, but has difficulty navigating the immediate environment, especially when perceptual cues are reduced (as at twilight or nighttime). Handwork and crafts take extra effort; copying a design onto a sheet of paper could be a real problem. As with other attributes of cognitive functioning, problems in this domain exist on a continuum from nil to mild to major.

When Jeanne moved into her senior living apartment three years ago, she relied on the sign on her door—"Jeanne's Room"—to tell her where to point her walker. Now, however, she shuffles right on past the sign, unless someone is there to direct her.

Agnes has an agnosia: She cannot recognize or identify familiar objects (such as the parts of a ballpoint pen), even though her sensory functioning is intact.

Perceptual–motor ability requires contributions from other domains—executive functioning, for example—so that there is a great deal of confusion, even among researchers who study the subject, as to exactly what domain is meant. Overlearned motor behaviors such as the use of a fork and knife are usually preserved until late in the course of a dementia.

Many different tests have been recommended, each of which is subject to various interpretations, depending on the expert you consult. Copying a simple design is one just about everyone accepts.

Executive Functioning

Executive functioning is the set of mechanisms people use to organize simple ideas and bits of behavior into more complex ones on the way to a goal, such as dressing or finding their way around town. When executive functioning is affected, patients have trouble interpreting new information and adapting to new situations. Planning and decision making become difficult. As mental flexibility is lost, behavior becomes driven by habit rather than by reason and feedback error correction.

> Sarah looks a good 10 years younger than her stated age of 75, but once again she's misbuttoned her silk blouse. She's trying to sort the laundry, but several times she just picks up an item and moves it to a different countertop.

> Marcus has always done the cooking in his household. (His wife is an attorney who still earns most of the money.) At age 67, he is having more and more trouble in the kitchen. He used to plan a different menu for each day of the week, but now he sticks pretty much to mac and cheese. Even so, he sometimes leaves out the salt. Twice last month he forgot the pan on the cooktop and started a small fire.

Language

The *language* domain includes both receptive language (understanding) and expressive language. The latter includes naming (the ability to state the name of an object such as a fountain pen), fluency, grammar, and syntax (structure) of language. Some patients may use circumlocutions to get around words they can't remember. Increasingly, they may come to depend on clichés; they may become vague, circumstantial, or (in the end) completely mute.

> In her last years, Marcelle developed a naming aphasia: She said the word "thingy" for an increasing variety of objects she encountered.

> Several years into his dementia, Jerome now mixes up words such as *table* and *chair.*

Social Cognition

Social cognition refers to the processes that help us recognize the emotions of other people and respond to them appropriately. It includes decision making, empathy, moral judgment, knowledge of social norms, emotional processing, and *theory of mind*—the ability to imagine that other people have beliefs and desires, and to recognize that others may have ideas different from our own. A person with defects in social cognition may have difficulty recognizing the emotion portrayed in a scowling (or smiling) face.

These people, who have damage to the amygdala, may be overly friendly toward others. Some, however, don't adhere to accepted standards of propriety or conventional social interaction.

> To their faces, Eileen has begun to criticize the morals of her two grandkids; they just roll their eyes and ignore her. She has distanced herself from others in her large extended family, and carries many of her meals into her bedroom to eat there alone. The others laugh and say she's had a "personality transplant."

> A lifelong atheist, Harold loudly utters blasphemies even when passing a church on Sunday. He may greet parishioners with an open fly, because he often neglects to zip up.

Confusion is a term often used to describe slowed thinking, loss of memory, perplexity, or disorientation in patients with NCDs. Of course you're familiar with it, because other health care providers (neurologists and internists), as well as patients and the general public, use it. DSM-5 even sneaks it in, once in a while. However, the term is inexact and, well, confusing; in all my writing, I've avoided it whenever possible. Unless I get confused.

Major and Mild Neurocognitive Disorders

Whatever the underlying etiology, patients with NCD share a number of features that serve as criteria for diagnosis. Then the difference between the major and mild forms of NCD boils down to severity of the symptoms. Before getting into the criteria, let us review these several important points.

Decline

NCD implies loss; there is always a decline from a previous level in one or more areas of functioning. Patients who have always functioned at a low level (individuals with intellectual disability) do not necessarily have an NCD. However, like anyone else, such a person can develop an NCD. In fact, many patients with Down syndrome eventually do develop an Alzheimer's type of NCD. Even a child who suffers a decline, perhaps due the lasting effects of a traumatic brain injury, may be said to have suffered NCD.

Every patient with an NCD will have a deficit in at least one of the cognitive domains discussed just above. Most patients, however, especially early in the course of a disease, won't have them all. Whereas loss of memory is paramount in Alzheimer's and some of the other degenerative disorders, it may be less prominent in patients whose underlying condition is vascular disease. Other patients may first develop problems with language, executive functioning, perceptual–motor functions, or social cognition. But there's always decline.

Overall prevalence ranges for NCD depend on exact definition and the particular study quoted. As of 2013, they ranged from about 2% at age 65 to the neighborhood of 5–10% at age 75 to 15–30% at age 80 and above. (Actually, a Rand study in 2013 reported 15% at age 71.) Recent research suggests, however, that lifestyle changes (increased exercise, decreased smoking, improved diet) may be helping to reduce the onset of NCDs in older people.

Not Exclusively a Delirium

An NCD cannot be diagnosed if the symptoms occur only when the patient is delirious. However, these two conditions can (and often do) coexist, as when a patient with NCD due to Alzheimer's is given medication that produces a substance intoxication delirium.

Not Accounted for by Another Mental Disorder

Decline of cognitive ability is sometimes associated with, for example, schizophrenia (which was once called *dementia praecox*—early dementia). The NCD criteria state that such causes of cognitive decline must be ruled out before an NCD can be diagnosed.

Confirmed by Testing

NCD criteria require that testing confirm the patient's decline. Of course, formal tests of the appropriate cognitive domain(s) are preferred, but for many patients, that's simply not going to happen. Then bedside estimates of ability will have to serve as a substitute.

Testing is especially important for patients who present as "the worried well." As people age, they notice little lapses of memory or quirks of behavior that make them wonder, "Am I losing it?" (Trust me on this.) Then the results of objective testing can provide the reassurance they, their relatives, and their health care providers all need to enable them to get on with their lives.

There is at least one instance in which testing alone could lead us astray. That is the case of a really high-functioning person whose formal testing reveals functioning at an average, or even better, level. But for this person, who would formerly have tested off the charts, functioning at a normal level represents a substantial decline. That's why DSM-5 now emphasizes a combination of two requirements—testing and concern on the part of those who know the person.

Impairment

And here's the big difference between a mild NCD and a major one: In the case of a major NCD (dementia), the loss of cognitive ability must be severe enough to have a definite impact on the patient's work or social life. This impact doesn't have to be severe; some patients will be able to function satisfactorily with some help—paying bills or shopping, for example. People with mild NCD, on the other hand, can continue to function *independently* if they put forth more effort. The difference between major and mild NCD, then, is one of degree. Note that for many patients, mild NCD will not progress to major NCD. The trouble is, we might not be able in advance to tell one group from the other.

The onset of NCD is often gradual (though, of course, this depends a lot on the cause). The first indication may be loss of interest in work or leisure activities. Family or friends may note a change in long-standing personality traits. When executive functioning is affected, judgment and impulse control suffer. Loss of the social graces ensues, as shown when the patient makes crude jokes or neglects personal hygiene and appearance. Stripped of the ability to analyze, to understand, to remember, and to apply old knowledge to new situations, the patient may be left to rely upon a skeleton of habit.

Patients with NCDs become increasingly vulnerable to psychosocial stresses: What would have been a minor problem a few years earlier can now assume monumental proportions. Some become apathetic, some irritable; others may ignore the interests or desires of their group. Another might try to compensate for a failing memory by compulsively making lists. The misperceptions (hallucinations or illusions) so common in delirium are often absent, especially early in the process. As major NCD worsens, paranoid ideas and delusions of infidelity can lead to abusive, even assaultive behavior.

Some patients are placid, especially early in the illness as apathy leads to gradually reduced activity. Those who retain some insight may become depressed or anxious. Later, especially, a person who becomes frustrated or frightened may experience outbursts of anger. Restlessness and pacing can lead to wandering from home; patients sometimes remain lost for hours or days. A person in the final stage of major NCD may lose all useful speech and self-care, and end up confined to bed, unaware of attendants or family.

Although most cases of NCD are found in older patients, it can be diagnosed any time after the age of 3 or 4, which is when a person's cognitive functioning becomes reliably measurable. The course depends on the underlying cause. Most often it is one of chronic deterioration; however, some NCDs can become static, or even remit. Remission is especially likely in NCD due to hypothyroidism, subdural hematoma, or normal-pressure hydrocephalus. When one of these causes is diagnosed early and successfully treated, full recovery can occur.

The suspicion of NCD demands medical and neurological evaluation to confirm causation and, whenever possible, to intervene with treatment. In many cases, a biological cause can be identified. These include primary diseases of the central nervous system, such as Huntington's disease, multiple sclerosis, and Parkinson's disease; infectious diseases, such as neurosyphilis and acquired immune deficiency syndrome (AIDS); vitamin deficiencies; tumors; trauma; various diseases of the liver, lungs, and cardiovascular system; and endocrine disorders. (A fuller listing is given in the "Physical Disorders . . ." table in the Appendix.) However, some NCDs must be diagnosed not on the basis of demonstrated pathology, but by inference from clinical features and by ruling out other nonorganic causes. This is often the case with NCD due to Alzheimer's or frontotemporal lobar disease.

Dementia is the term formerly applied to patients with major NCD, which in some situations is preferable to the older term. A good example is a young person whose cognitive problems stem from traumatic brain injury—you want to call attention to a significant problem without using the pejorative term *dementia*. Another might be the people we used to diagnose as having amnestic disorder, whose cognitive problems are generally focused on a single cognitive area. However, the terms *dementia* and *demented* are still understood—and used—by most of the world (even DSM-5 includes the term in parentheses) to denote patients we would formally diagnose as having major NCD. For convenience, not to mention my own sanity, I'll continue to use them occasionally in the rest of this chapter, but only when I want to refer to *major* NCD.

Essential Features of {Major}{Mild} Neurocognitive Disorder

Someone (the patient, a relative, the clinician) suspects that there has been a {marked}{modest} decline in cognitive functioning. On formal testing, the patient scores below accepted norms by {2+}{1–2} standard deviations. Alternatively, a clinical evaluation reaches the same conclusion. The symptoms {materially}{do not materially} impair the patient's ability to function independently. That is, the patient {cannot} {can} negotiate activities of daily life (paying bills, managing medications) by putting forth increased effort or using compensatory strategies such as keeping lists.

The Fine Print

One standard deviation below norms would be at the 16th percentile; 2 would be at the 3rd percentile.

The D's: • Duration (symptoms tend to chronicity) • Differential diagnosis (delirium, normal aging, major depressive disorder [pseudodementia], psychosis)

Coding Notes

Specify if:

> **With behavioral disturbance (*specify type*).** The patient has clinically important behaviors such as apathy, agitation, or responding to hallucinations or mood problems.
> **Without behavioral disturbance.** The patient has no such difficulties.

The wording and actual codes are given in Tables 16.1a and 16.1b.

For major NCD, specify current level of severity:

Mild. The patient requires help with activities of daily living, such as doing housework or managing money.
Moderate. The patient needs help even with such basics as dressing and eating.
Severe. The patient is fully dependent on others.

Recording Major and Mild Neurocognitive Disorders

Using Tables 16.1a and 16.1b, follow the scheme described here when you are recording a diagnosis of a major or mild NCD.

A total of 10 specific (and several nonspecific) disorders are named in DSM-5, though dozens could be classified as etiological in NCD. You assign them different numbers and different descriptions, depending on whether the NCD is major or mild. *Don't worry; this will become clear soon.* The five etiologies in Table 16.1a can be based on a diagnosis due either to probable or possible disease, depending on the criteria that are met. In all other etiologies (Table 16.1b), there should be sufficient certainty about the cause (lab testing, imaging) that a possible diagnosis isn't necessary. *Remember, keep calm.*

For each etiology, the first (upper) code is for the associated (causative) medical condition. The second (lower) code is for major NCD, which occupies two columns—allowing you to make, when necessary, adjustments for the patient's having a behavioral disturbance. Mild NCD offers only a single pair of codes, regardless of etiology. *Easy does it.*

After DSM-5 was published, its editors revised the convention for naming the major NCDs. We are now advised that, wherever applicable, the *possible* and the *probable* labels should come just before the name of the etiological disorder, not before the NCD. After all, the reasoning goes, the fact of the NCD isn't at question—it's the cause that's a bit uncertain. So ignore the formal titles as printed in DSM-5, steady your nerves, and follow these examples:

Major neurocognitive disorder due to {probable}{possible} Alzheimer's disease

Major neurocognitive disorder due to {probable}{possible} frontotemporal lobar degeneration

Major neurocognitive disorder with {probable}{possible} Lewy bodies

Major neurocognitive disorder {probably}{possibly} due to vascular disease

Major neurocognitive disorder {probably}{possibly} due to Parkinson's disease

I'm quoting exactly here from the DSM-5 website. With consistency not the watchword of the day, I'd venture that you can get away with something less than total fidelity to these examples.

TABLE 16.1a. Coding for Major and Mild NCDs: Five Etiologies

| Etiology[a] | Major NCD due to {probable}{possible} [etiology][b] | | Mild NCD {with} {without} behavioral disturbance[c] |
	With behavioral disturbance	Without behavioral disturbance	
Alzheimer's disease	G30.9 [331.0] Alzheimer's disease		(No medical disorder code) — G31.84 [331.83] Mild NCD due to [etiology] State whether {probable} or {possible} and whether the NCD is {with} {without} behavioral disturbance
	F02.81 [294.11]	F02.80 [294.10]	
Frontotemporal lobar degeneration	G31.09 [331.19] Frontotemporal disease		
	F02.81 [294.11]	F02.80 [294.10]	
Lewy body disease	G31.83 [331.82] Lewy body disease		
	F02.81 [294.11]	F02.80 [294.10]	
Parkinson's disease	G20 [332.0] Parkinson's disease		
	F02.81 [294.11]	F02.80 [294.10]	
Vascular disease	—		
	F01.51 [290.40]	F01.50 [290.40]	

[a]Only these five etiologies for NCD (Table 16.1a) include probable and possible levels of certainty.

[b]Under revised rules (not printed in DSM-5), we must state in words whether the major NCD is due to *probable* or *possible* disease—the numbering is the same. The "Recording Major and Mild Neurocognitive Disorders" section of the text gives examples of how names should be listed.

[c]In mild NCD, you don't include the suspected causative factor (for example, Alzheimer's disease). That's because the level of certainty about cause is so much lower in mild than in major NCD. Also, there's no code number for behavioral disturbance, though you should indicate it in the verbiage. Finally, for each Table 16.1a mild NCD, you can add verbiage indicating whether it is probable or possible; however, there is no difference in the code number.

TABLE 16.1b. Coding for Major and Mild NCDs: All Other Etiologies

| Etiology | Major NCD | | Mild NCD[c] |
	With behavioral disturbance	Without behavioral disturbance	
Traumatic brain injury	S06.2X9S [907.0][d]		(No medical disorder code) — G31.84 [331.83] Mild NCD due to [etiology] No statement of {probable}{possible.} You can state {with} {without} behavioral disturbance.
	F02.81 [294.11]	F02.80 [294.10]	
HIV disease	B20 [042] HIV infection		
	F02.81 [294.11]	F02.80 [294.10]	
Huntington's disease	G10 [333.4] Huntington's disease		
	F02.81 [294.11]	F02.80 [294.10]	
Prion disease	A81.9 [046.79] Prion disease		
	F02.81 [294.11]	F02.80 [294.10]	
Other medical condition	## [##] ICD-10 name [ICD-9 name]		
	F02.81 [294.11]	F02.80 [294.10]	
Substance/medication-induced	See Table 15.2 (p. 465)		
Multiple etiologies[e]	(Multiple sets of numbers and names)		
	F02.81 [294.11]	F02.80 [294.10]	

[d]The two code titles for TBI were just too long to squeeze into a table: S06.2X9S = diffuse traumatic brain injury with loss of consciousness of unspecified duration, sequela; 907.0 = late effect of intracranial injury without skull fracture.

[e]If a vascular disorder contributes to the multiple causation, list it along with the multiple-causes bit. Don't ask me why; it's just another rule.

By the way, I've just read over the footnotes to Tables 16.1a and 16.1b, and I apologize for their complexity. You might do better to ignore the explanations and just stare at the tables for a few minutes, or you might prefer to work your way through a couple of vignettes. I've included enough examples throughout this chapter that things should become clear eventually. *Breathe slowly.*

Mild NCD is a new name that comes with a lot of built-in synonyms. They include *age-associated cognitive decline*, *mild cognitive impairment*, *age-associated memory impairment*, and *nondementia cognitive impairment*. These people do not have full-fledged dementia, but they aren't exactly normal, either. Although they have symptoms, their functional abilities are largely intact, but they need increased effort to carry them out. Don't confuse mild NCD with *age-related cognitive decline*, which is more or less normal (where did I put my keys?) for the person's age—and which in ICD-10 no longer has diagnostic status. And don't, please, overinterpret this designation. Although some patients who can be diagnosed with mild NCD will later develop the major form of the disorder, by no means will all do so.

Here's an additional quibbling note about mild NCD. The Good Book tells us that if we make this diagnosis, we are not to write down code for the presumed causative agent. I find myself pushing back against this stricture. Surely, if we know that a person has had, for example, a traumatic brain injury, and that the result is a mild NCD, then we are allowed (heck, I'd say *obligated*) to indicate as much. It is information that could be valuable to the next clinician who sees the patient, and hence it may be of considerable value to the patient. As I understand it, the editors of DSM-5 wanted to be consistent in not writing down causes when the clinician cannot be certain of etiology, which with mild NCD is often the case. But when we have pretty darned strong evidence, our duty is to the patient, not to a book.

Neurocognitive Disorder Due to Alzheimer's Disease

The most common cause of what was once called *senility*, NCD due to Alzheimer's disease, has been recognized since the early 1900s. Alzheimer's accounts for well over half of all dementia cases, which increase steadily with age; the majority of elderly patients in nursing homes have been stricken with this degenerative disorder. It is also common among patients over 40 who have Down syndrome. Indeed, any clinician who treats older patients is bound to encounter it frequently. Patients with early-onset Alzheimer's disease are especially likely to have relatives with the same disorder.

NCD due to Alzheimer's disease is also important because so many other disorders, both cognitive and otherwise, can be mistaken for it. Despite our diagnostic advances, it is *still* a diagnosis of exclusion that should only be made once all other causes (especially those that can be treated) have been ruled out.

Memory loss is the first symptom experienced by about half of patients with

Alzheimer's, but eventually, as in other dementias, all patients will become forgetful. Recent memory (the ability to remember information that was learned within the previous few minutes) is usually the first aspect to be involved; remote memory is affected later on. Patients may forget familiar names or repeatedly ask questions that have just been answered. To compensate, some write themselves notes or compile lists. Although a sense of self is generally preserved until late in the disease, severely demented patients may fail to recognize their relatives or long-time friends, and ultimately may even fail to answer to their own names.

An apparent change in personality can occur early in Alzheimer's. Commonly, existing personality traits are accentuated: A patient may become more obsessional, secretive, or sexually active. Other early indications of dementia can include apathy, emotional lability (sudden weeping or temper outbursts), or the loss of a previously acute sense of humor.

Loss of executive functioning (usually attributed to frontal lobe damage) can be tested directly by asking the patient to identify similarities and differences or to carry out a sequence of steps, as on the Mini-Mental State Exam (MMSE). But executive functioning is often best evaluated from the history or from observation of some of these behaviors: closely trailing the clinician or a companion (imitation behavior); frozen expression until prompted (lack of spontaneity), putting on more than one pair of trousers (perseveration); or repeatedly getting lost on the ward, though oriented at home (environmental dependency). The emerging picture may be that of a person who can navigate and function reasonably well in a fixed, familiar environment, but who has difficulty adapting to changing circumstances. Some patients are referred for evaluation only when they cannot cope with the unfamiliar surroundings of a new residence. As is true of most intellectual tasks, patients with Alzheimer's may do better when they are rested.

Language functions may be manifested at first by trouble finding words (aphasia). The vocabulary contracts as clichés and stereotyped phrases are substituted for real communication, and the patient no longer uses complex sentences. Reading and writing may deteriorate; conversation rambles.

Many patients with Alzheimer's disease will also have perceptual defects such as illusions or hallucinations. They may become inordinately suspicious and develop paranoia. About 20% have depression; even those who are not depressed often experience insomnia or anorexia. Therefore, it is important to consider Alzheimer's (or other causes of dementia) in the differential diagnosis of any older patient who presents with symptoms that suggest a depressive disorder.

The typical patient lives 8 or 10 years after Alzheimer's disease begins (I knew a woman who recently died in her 14th postdiagnosis year). The clinical course, though variable, is typically a steady decline through three stages:

1. From 1 to 3 years of growing forgetfulness.

2. From 2 to 3 years of increasing disorientation, loss of language skills, and

inappropriate behavior. Until they reach advanced stages, most patients look grossly normal, though physical exam may reveal typical "frontal release signs" such as the *palmomental reflex* (pursing of lips when the palm is stroked— though some elderly people develop frontal release signs without having evidence of dementia). Hallucinations and delusions may appear during this stage.

3. A final period of severe dementia, during which there is disorientation for person and complete loss of self-care.

Insight is almost always absent, and sooner or later judgment becomes impaired. At the end, complete muteness and unresponsiveness may ensue. Patients with Alzheimer's tolerate physical illness poorly; infection or reduced nutrition that a person without the disease would shrug off may trigger a superimposed delirium.

Although Alzheimer's disease is depressingly common, the etiological relationship must usually be inferred from the absence of other possible causes. Because some of these are treatable, and because Alzheimer's disease has such a dismal prognosis, it is vitally important to rule out all other possible alternatives. (DSM-5 lists NCD due to Alzheimer's first, as do I; don't let this lead you astray.)

Although nearly every patient with dementia will have problems with memory and learning, it is only one of the six cognitive domains that can be affected by NCD. In DSM-5, however, an early defect of memory is a requirement for the diagnosis of NCD due to Alzheimer's.

Essential Features of **Neurocognitive Disorder Due to Alzheimer's Disease**

The patient has a {major}{mild} neurocognitive disorder (see p. 492) that begins slowly and progresses gradually.

The Fine Print

The D's: • Duration (chronic) • Differential diagnosis (delirium; age-related cognitive decline; intellectual disability; depressive, anxiety, or psychotic disorders; substance intoxication; other causes of NCD, especially vascular, frontotemporal, and Lewy body diseases)

There are two ways to arrive at a diagnosis of probable major NCD due to Alzheimer's dementia, and one way each to a diagnosis of possible major, probable mild, or possible mild NCD due to Alzheimer's disease. See the chart below.

	Major NCD due to Alzheimer's		Mild NCD due to Alzheimer's	
	Probable	Possible	Probable	Possible
	Meets criteria for {major}{mild} NCD			
	Insidious onset, gradual progression of disability			
# domains affected	Two or more		One or more	
Positive genetic evidence (testing or family history) for Alzheimer's disease	Major NCD due to probable Alzheimer's disease	—	Mild NCD due to probable Alzheimer's disease	—
Steady, gradual decline; no extended plateaus	All three factors present: Major NCD due to probable Alzheimer's disease	If any of these 3 is missing: Major NCD due to possible Alzheimer's disease		All three factors present: Mild NCD due to possible Alzheimer's disease
No evidence of mixed causes[a]				
Decline in memory and learning				

[a]Any evidence for mixed causes forces a diagnosis of NCD due to multiple etiologies.

Coding Notes

Record the diagnoses and code numbers from Table 16.1a.

Hank Altig

Two years before Hank Altig moved to Sunny Acres, he took a job as greeter with a "big box" store. He had been retired for several years, and at the age of 66, he wanted more activity. "I just don't feel like sitting around idle any longer," he told the screener at the preemployment physical exam. "I've still got some good years in me." Though he gave his address, Social Security number, and new cell phone number from memory, still he wondered aloud why he occasionally walked into a room and then couldn't remember why he was there. "Don't we all?" was the response.

Hank's former profession (he had worked nearly 40 years as an accountant) required concentration and a high tolerance for boredom; being a greeter required only his presence and a willingness to smile. These he gave in good measure. "Eighty percent of success is just showing up," he quoted.

For months, every time Hank showed up, he'd carefully shaved and paid meticulous attention to his clothes, his shoes—even his hair and nails. "I want to be the greeter's greeter," he had told his daughter, Sandy, who lived just down the street and was the principal informant at his clinical assessment.

But nearly a year into the job, he began to have problems. When first he'd hired on, he had memorized the location of "half the items in the store." But every few days, something would get moved, and now he couldn't seem to keep the new locations in his head. Sandy bought him a tiny Moleskine notebook in which he kept track of the items people asked about most. He also used it for his appointments—mostly they were dinner dates with Sandy—and other important information. Whenever Hank had trouble remembering something, Sandy would smile and say, "Where's Moley?" Often Hank could look up what he wanted to know.

By the time a year and a half had passed, Sandy had really begun to worry. There'd been no dramatic change, just a steady slide. Once or twice when waiting for Hank to get off work, she had noticed that he seemed at first unaware when someone asked for assistance. She knew that he'd been late several times, and sometimes he hadn't bothered to shave. If she pointed it out, he'd just shrug and turn away.

Last week, they were back at the clinician's office. Sandy reported that Hank had stopped cooking. Mostly he ate cold cereal, unless Sandy fixed something for him and brought it over.

"Where do you like to shop for groceries?" asked the interviewer. With no response forthcoming, Sandy prompted, "Where's Moley?" But Hank just looked blank, and the little booklet never left the pocket of his cardigan.

Evaluation of Hank Altig

Even when Hank first sought employment as a greeter, he was concerned about his memory. Concern (on the part of the patient or someone else) is necessary, but not sufficient, for a diagnosis of NCD of any degree. Hank's early concern was based on a common occurrence that had no clinical significance, as his clinician noted at the time. The requirement for a diagnosis is that there be concern about a decline plus objective evidence—the kind that can only be obtained by actual neuropsychological testing or by "bedside" evaluations such as the MMSE. (We're at something of a disadvantage in this discussion because we don't have the results of testing; we'll have to interpolate a bit, as we'll do in discussions of subsequent vignettes.)

In any event, we can be reasonably confident that Hank didn't have any important cognitive deficit at the time he started work. He not only quoted Woody Allen accurately, but his executive abilities were intact: He got himself up, nicely groomed, and to work on time, and he was able to commit to memory the locations of numerous items in the store. However, by the time months had passed, he had begun to falter.

Hank was concerned, as was Sandy (NCD criterion A1), that he was having difficulty learning new material. His memory wasn't quite what it had been: He appeared to have lost his former ability to memorize and recall the new locations of products in his store. However, he compensated for his difficulty with "Moley," the little notebook that Sandy gave him (B), setting us up for a diagnosis of mild NCD. To complete the evaluation, we'd need objective evidence of cognitive decline—formal testing of some sort, whether a cognitive evaluation or just the MMSE done by the clinician in the office (A2). The remaining criteria, that neither a delirium (C) nor some other mental disorder such as depression or schizophrenia (D) was present, are fulfilled in the vignette.

Now we can move on to his subsequent history. By the time a year had passed, Sandy noticed that Hank's attention was wandering while on the job, and that he had begun showing up for work less well groomed than had formerly been the case—presumptive evidence for reduced executive functioning. And he was no longer compensating for his memory problems by using his pocket notebook. The result, as we infer from the fact that he subsequently moved into Sunny Acres, was a decline that was gradual (his entire story spanned nearly 2 years) and in important ways interfered with Hank's independent capacity to pursue the activities of everyday life (B).

Now his clinician would need to complete the evaluation with a formal mental status evaluation, at least a bedside evaluation of cognitive ability such as the MMSE, and a neurological exam and enough laboratory (especially radiological) testing to pinpoint, to the extent possible, the cause of his dementia. In an elderly person, you'd want to rule out a **traumatic brain injury** by the absence of history of blows to the head; a **substance-induced dementia** would feature a prominent history of substance or medication use. Physical exam would reveal no evidence of **Parkinson's disease**, and history and preserved affect would eliminate **pseudodementia due to a depressive disorder.** Skull X-rays and MRI would rule out **brain tumors** and **normal-pressure hydrocephalus**; blood tests would rule out **hypothyroidism** and **vitamin B12 deficiency** as possible causes. The steady rather than stepwise decline renders unlikely a **vascular disease** etiology, which is a common cause of dementia in the elderly. As far as we can tell from the vignette, Hank had none of the core or suggestive features that would suggest a dementia due to **Lewy body disease** or **frontotemporal lobar degeneration.**

All this seems to leave NCD due to Alzheimer's disease as the disorder of exclusion—but would it be probable or possible? The DSM-5 criteria are a little finicky about this, but we can puzzle our way through them. Let's start with the time that Hank first began to have problems with mild NCD.

The criteria for mild NCD due to Alzheimer's disease would allow a probable (the stronger) diagnosis only for patients who have positive evidence from genetic testing or family history; neither condition applies to Hank. So let's examine the other evidence summarized in the Essential Features. His decline would appear to be steady; at least we have no evidence that he had ever reached some sort of plateau. Next, we should look for evidence that he had other possible etiologies for his symptoms: A couple of paragraphs above, we have discarded them all. Finally, his principal symptom was a decline in his memory and his ability to learn. Therefore, at that time he fulfilled the criterion (C) for mild NCD due to *possible* Alzheimer's disease.

Now for the last evaluation, this one to determine the exact type of his major NCD. Once again, there's no genetic or family history to help us out. But, as noted just above, Hank did have a gradually progressive course of declining memory and learning, with no evidence for mixed causes. And this time, we can find evidence of impairment in other cognitive domains—executive functioning and attention—and formal testing might reveal still more. We've therefore at last collected the evidence to support a diagnosis of major NCD due to *probable* Alzheimer's disease (also criterion C). But before we wrap up, what about behavioral disturbance? Hank didn't really respond to Sandy's last question, and he had lost interest in cooking and shaving. I'd interpret this as apathy, which by the liberal DSM-5 definition (along with depression, psychosis, and agitation) constitutes behavioral disturbance.

So, other than giving Hank's GAF score (twice), this is where we'll stop.

First evaluation (GAF = 65):

G31.84 [331.83]   Mild neurocognitive disorder due to possible Alzheimer's
                    disease, without behavioral disturbance

Second evaluation (GAF = 40):

G30.9 [331.0]   Alzheimer's disease
F02.80 [294.10]   Major neurocognitive disorder due to probable Alzheimer's
                   disease, without behavioral disturbance (apathy)

Neurocognitive Disorder with Lewy Bodies

One of the newest NCD diagnoses in the book, NCD with Lewy bodies (I'll call the major form dementia with Lewy bodies, or DLB) was until the mid-1990s only a gleam in the eyes of a few researchers and clinicians. Now DLB is recognized as the second largest cause of dementia—it accounts for about 15% of cases, as against 60–75% for Alzheimer's. There are currently well over a million such patients in the United States alone.

Discovered a full century ago, Lewy bodies are spherical bits of protein (α-synuclein) found in the cytoplasm of brain cells located especially in the brainstem nuclei, substantia nigra, and locus ceruleus. Patients with DLB also frequently have amyloid plaques that are typical of Alzheimer's disease; they have clinical features of both Parkinson's and Alzheimer's diseases as well. Those similarities probably explain why DLB remained so obscure for so long.

- *Fluctuating attention.* Early on, patients with DLB tend to experience less of the early memory loss that is typical for patients with Alzheimer's. Most affected are attention span and alertness, which in fact tend to wax and wane over minutes, hours, or even days in over half of patients with DLB. This fluctuation of symptoms constitutes the first of the principal ("core") features.

- *Hallucinations.* The second core feature is well-formed visual hallucinations, which occur early and tend to persist. Typically, they are of animals or intruders. They can occur with or without insight, and may be accompanied by (sometimes systematized) delusions.

- *Later onset of Parkinson's-type symptoms.* Typical motor features of Parkinson's disease—immobile face, hand tremor, shuffling gait—constitute the third core symptom, but they cannot predate the dementia. If they do, the diagnosis is not DLB at all, but rather Parkinson's disease with dementia. The rule of thumb: DLB symptoms must begin at least a year before motor symptoms appear.

Patients with DLB are also prone to dizziness, falls, and unexplained fainting spells. Depression is common, as is autonomic dysfunction (orthostatic hypotension, incontinence of urine). REM sleep behavior disorder (see p. 343) is sometimes noted. Early diagnosis is especially important in DLB, because these patients can be exquisitely sensitive to neuroleptics: Relatively low doses cause muscle rigidity, fever, and other symptoms of neuroleptic malignant syndrome.

DLB typically begins around age 75; men are affected somewhat more often than are women. After diagnosis, the typical patient lives about 10 years.

It isn't at all clear that Parkinson's dementia and DLB are different entities; some authorities believe that they exist on a continuum. They both involve α-synuclein protein and degeneration of the substantia nigra of the brain. Both feature Parkinson's motor symptoms, though with disparate timing: For a diagnosis of DLB, the movement disorder must show up only after cognitive symptoms have been present for a year or more. Preexisting movement disorder shifts the diagnosis to Parkinson's dementia.

Of course, this creates something of a dilemma for the clinician who needs to make a diagnosis *now*, using as a criterion something that hasn't occurred yet. Actually, not all of these patients do develop the motor symptoms of parkinsonism. And you only need two of the core features to diagnosis the probable form of the disease. Finally, there can be no definitive diagnosis without pathological verification.

Essential Features of **Neurocognitive Disorder with Lewy Bodies**

The patient has a {major}{mild} neurocognitive disorder (p. 492).

Beginning slowly and progressing gradually, the disease has these *core* features: wide fluctuation in attentiveness; elaborate, clear hallucinations; and symptoms of parkinsonism that begin a year or more after the cognitive symptoms.

Some patients have features that *suggest* DLB: REM sleep behavior disorder, marked sensitivity to neuroleptic drugs.

The Fine Print

The D's: • Duration (tends to chronicity) • Differential diagnosis (delirium; substance-related disorders; depressive or psychotic disorders; other causes of NCD—especially Alzheimer's, vascular, and frontotemporal diseases)

See the chart below for guidance in arriving at a diagnosis.

		Probable NCD with Lewy bodies	Possible NCD with Lewy bodies
Core features	Fluctuating alertness and attention	One core feature plus one or more core or suggestive feature yields a diagnosis of {mild} {major} NCD with probable Lewy bodies	One core or suggestive feature is enough for a diagnosis of {mild} {major} NCD with possible Lewy bodies
	Repeated, vivid, detailed hallucinations		
	Parkinsonism that begins only *after* the cognitive decline		
Suggestive features	REM sleep behavior disorder		
	Exquisite sensitivity to neuroleptics		

Coding Notes

Record the diagnoses and code numbers from Table 16.1a.

You can't code *with behavioral disturbance*, but if you note it's there, you should mention it in writing anyway.

Sheila Wilton

"Dr. Brantleigh said she had schizophrenia," Sophia reported. Sophia was Sheila Wilton's grown stepdaughter, and she provided most of the historical information. The shape of her lips said she didn't believe Dr. Brantleigh.

The problems had begun about 3 months earlier, when Sheila had trouble finding her way back from the store. She'd shopped at the Safeway on the corner for many years, but twice now she'd apparently turned left instead of right, and ended up many blocks astray. The first time, a policeman brought her home. The second, a neighbor recognized her and called Sophia, who came and got her. "At first, she seemed fuzzy, confused," Sophia lamented, "but when I asked her later to tell me our address and such, she responded with all the facts."

A few days later, Sophia found Sheila sitting on the edge of the bed in her room, talking to a vivid hallucination of her husband standing beside her. "He was motioning to me to get up and fix breakfast," was what Sheila had finally been able to relate. "And Dad's been dead for 7 years," Sophia finished up.

They'd gone to their local medical provider, who, finding nothing wrong, referred Sheila for psychological evaluation. A tentative diagnosis of schizophrenia and another trip to the doctor had netted a prescription for haloperidol, "and then all hell broke loose."

Sheila's quiet little hallucination turned hostile. Still using mime, her phantom husband now threatened, her sometimes with a closed fist, sometimes with the heavy walking stick he had always carried. She responded first with agitation, then with fury that ultimately dwindled into perplexity that seemed to wax and wane. Within a day or two, she became overly sedated, then rigid—so stiff she could hardly walk. "Now they're saying she's catatonic and needs shock treatments," Sophia said. "I don't understand it. No one in her family has ever had any sort of mental illness."

Off and on during the day, Sheila would be confused, at times not knowing where she was. But in the doctor's office she was fully oriented, missing the correct date by only 2 days. "That's about as well as *I* can do," remarked Sophia. "But it's so typical of the way she's been—first out of it, then back in. The implication was that she was doing it for all the attention I was giving her. Brantleigh used the word *malingering*."

Evaluation of Sheila Wilton

Let's for a moment put aside the hallucinations and focus instead on the domains of Sheila's other cognitive symptoms. These were perceptual–motor (aside from the hallucinations, she couldn't find her way home) and complex attention (she had fluctuating awareness). We'd have to do formal testing to get a number to put on the extent of her decline, but from this and the other information in the vignette, I'd judge her clinically as being moderately impaired, thereby earning a diagnosis of major NCD. Her symptoms interfered with her independence—at least for such important activities of daily living as working around the house and managing money. It would appear that she was able to feed and dress herself, so her current level of severity would be mild. (Note the distinction: She would have mild *major* NCD, not *mild* NCD. *That* semantic nightmare is bound to cause some clinicians heartburn.)

And while we're talking about the basic NCD diagnosis, let's consider the specifiers. Sheila did have rather pronounced hallucinations, which would earn her the qualifier *with behavioral disturbance (hallucinations)*.

Though we could mount a cogent argument for a neurological consultation, there wouldn't appear to be **other medical disorders**, and certainly not **other mental disorders** (the diagnosis of schizophrenia was obviously bogus), that could better explain her symptoms. In short, she would appear to have some sort of a dementia. But which one?

First, a couple of facts—sobering ones for those who would like to achieve certainty while life endures. For many patients with dementia, only the fullness of time (read: a postmortem examination) can deliver a final, accurate diagnosis. And even with imaging and laboratory information, discriminating one form of dementia from another can be devilishly hard. But here goes.

Sheila had had no history of **traumatic brain injury**, so we can pretty well rule out dementia due to that cause. She didn't have early and prominent difficulties with her memory, so we can put **Alzheimer's** aside (though it would not be completely off the radar). There was neither hypertension nor stepwise progression of her symptoms, rendering unlikely a **vascular** cause. History and physical symptoms were inconsistent with **Huntington's**, **Parkinson's**, or **HIV infection.** The criteria for two types of **frontotemporal NCD** are infuriatingly complicated, as I'll discuss later, but neither her behavior nor her language appeared to have deteriorated enough to sustain a diagnosis of either subtype.

Of course, that still leaves many other disorders that can cause dementia, but our diagnostic foray shouldn't be one exclusively of elimination. There are affirmative reasons to consider **NCD with Lewy bodies**—in Sheila or in any patient. The main one is that there is an immediate important implication for treatment. This is the risk that using antipsychotic drugs can lead, as it apparently did in Sheila's case, to worsening of the cognitive symptoms and the physical symptoms of neuroleptic malignant syndrome. (That's one of the suggestive symptoms of DLB.) In addition, she had the wide fluctuations in alertness and attention and the well-formed hallucinations that constitute core features.

For a diagnosis of probable major NCD with Lewy bodies, Sheila would need at least one core symptom plus at least one other (core or suggestive); Sheila had two core and one suggestive, more than enough for her working diagnosis. I'd put her GAF score (at her current level of functioning) as 45, but I wouldn't disagree if you argued for a different value. She'd been all over the map.

The narrative of Sheila Wilton includes two of my differential diagnosis *bêtes noires*—malingering and schizophrenia. It's not that they never happen; of course they do. But they are two "explanations" that clinicians sometimes use to get themselves off the hook for symptoms that are hard to evaluate, hard to understand, hard to treat, and hard to view optimistically. Each of these diagnoses appears late in my evaluative process.

G31.83 [331.82]   Lewy body disease
F02.81 [294.11]   Major neurocognitive disorder with probable Lewy bodies, mild, with behavioral disturbance (hallucinations)

Neurocognitive Disorder Due to Traumatic Brain Injury

Each year in the United States, more than a million people suffer a blow to the head or some other injury that ushers in traumatic brain injury (TBI). Though most cases of TBI are mild, the damage from war and sports injuries can be devastating. And of course, a few percent die as a result of their injuries.

The largest number of patients with TBI are adolescents or young adults (males predominate); the elderly, because they injure themselves in falls, are the next most affected age group. Low socioeconomic status is another risk factor, but the biggest risk of all is use of alcohol and drugs—which contribute to nearly half of TBIs. Motor vehicle accidents (including those that strike pedestrians) are the leading proximate cause; falls (especially in the elderly) are second. Sports injuries are an important source for younger people (women athletes are more likely to be affected than are men).

The symptoms of TBI are caused by a disruption of brain structure or physiology that results from external force exerted upon the head. Immediate loss of consciousness is usual; after awakening, patients may have trouble focusing and maintaining attention. Delirium is common; even after it clears, deficits in attention are commonplace. Many patients complain of trouble with memory (anterograde or retrograde). Language functions affect about a third of patients with severe TBI. These especially include fluent (receptive) aphasias, though nonfluent (expressive) aphasias are also well represented. Executive functioning is commonly affected. Patients with TBI will also complain of problems with sleep, headaches, and irritability.

Though it can take months, most patients eventually recover. But common sequels include depressive disorders (most frequent), anxiety disorders, and substance misuse. Personality change is sometimes noted. A preinjury mental disorder greatly increases the risk for a postinjury disorder. And TBI, especially if repeated, may increase the likelihood of Alzheimer's—perhaps by as much as fourfold.

Some writers note that the differentiation of NCD due to TBI from posttraumatic stress disorder can be challenging.

Chronic traumatic encephalopathy doesn't fit neatly into the TBI paradigm, caused as it is by *repeated* injury to the brain. It's associated with contact sports such as boxing (then, it's sometimes called *dementia pugilistica*), American football, soccer, ice hockey, rugby, and even professional wrestling. Symptoms—which include failing memory, aggression, poor impulse control, parkinsonism, depression, and suicide—have been found, tragically, in athletes as young as 17. At least two professional football players, apparently realizing that their brains had been damaged by repetitive playing injuries, have killed themselves, carefully choosing means that would preserve their brains for postmortem examination. The phenomenon makes for riveting scientific studies, television specials, and lawsuits.

Essential Features of **Neurocognitive Disorder due to Traumatic Brain Injury**

Immediately following head trauma that causes rapid movement of the brain inside the skull, the patient becomes unconscious or may develop amnesia, disorientation and perplexity, or neurological signs such as seizures, blind spots in the visual field, loss of smell, hemiparesis, or an injury demonstrated by imaging (CT, MRI). Subsequently, the patient has symptoms of a {mild}{major} neurocognitive disorder (p. 492).

The Fine Print

The D's: • Duration (starts immediately, lasts a week or more) • Differential diagnosis (delirium, age-related cognitive decline, depression, psychotic disorders, substance intoxication, anxiety disorders, other causes of NCD—especially Alzheimer's disease)

Coding Notes

See Table 16.1b.

Thornton Naguchi

When Thornton Naguchi arrived home, his reception wasn't what he or anyone in his family had imagined. The brass band and confetti (his fantasy) were missing; on the other hand, so was the pine box, which was what his mother had feared all along. "She's a firm believer in Murphy's law—if something can go wrong, it will," he told the interviewer at the VA hospital where he stayed for a few days.

Thornton's grandparents had been interned in Idaho during World War II, leaving his grandfather extremely bitter, often railing against the government. He was something of a tyrant; Thornton's revenge had been to join the military as soon as he was of age. Within a few months, the Army had posted him to "a part of Iraq so remote they'd never heard of tofu."

During Thornton's first week in country, as he was riding in the last non-up-armored Humvee in the unit, they'd hit an improvised explosive device. A shard of metal had sliced right through his helmet strap as he was launched into the air, and he fell back squarely on his head. When he awakened nearly 24 hours later, he remembered starting off on the mission—but nothing of the actual explosion. It was his sergeant who'd reconstructed it for him.

After the accident he'd been grateful to be alive, but he initially had some trouble focusing even on watching TV. Though he had always been bright and personable, he was cross, snapping at a nurse who suggested that he could get up and change the channel for himself.

While he was still awaiting his discharge papers, Thornton got a job selling cell phones at an electronics outlet near his home. He'd grown up with electronic devices and had kept current with the industry while he was in the Army, so he had little trouble demonstrating the basic features of smart phones.

But holding in mind the nuances of the different models was a chore—far more so for him than for the other young people who worked with him. "I needed a crib sheet—on my phone—just to keep up," he remarked. "I mean, we're talking 15 or 20 different models here, not to mention the tablets." If he was talking to a customer and a co-worker asked an incidental question, he found that he'd lose his train of thought completely. "I'd have to ask the customer where we were. I *know* it cost me bonus money."

Thornton lived with Yuki, his girlfriend of 4 years. She reported that he seemed distracted, "forever drifting out of the picture," as she put it. He wasn't really depressed, she thought, but cranky and impulsive, occasionally flinging on his clothes and slamming out the door. When he returned, he'd say that he just walked. "And he just freaks out at loud noises."

That was apparently what happened one afternoon as he was installing curtains in their apartment. Yuki dropped a pan lid in the kitchenette, not 10 feet from where he was standing on a ladder. He jerked, overbalanced, and fell hard on the terrazzo floor.

"Murphy was an optimist," he'd told the paramedics who loaded him up for his second ambulance ride in 6 months.

Evaluation of Thornton Naguchi

The first step in the diagnosis of any NCD, major or mild, is to ascertain that there has been some decline from previous functioning. This appeared to be the case for Thornton, who needed help remembering the different types of cell phone he was supposed to be selling. He managed to avert significant interference with his work by keeping a crib sheet—the extra effort required to compensate for his problems with memory. He had also been irritable, perhaps a sign of a mild decline in the social cognition domain. And there were also some minor problems with his executive functioning, as suggested by the trouble he had picking up on an interrupted conversation.

Formal testing would probably confirm these modest declines in his cognitive abilities (mild NCD criterion A2), but even without it, a diagnosis of mild NCD could be sustained on the basis of a clinical interview. He had continued to support himself (B), wasn't delirious (C), and didn't have another mental disorder (D).

Now for the TBI bit. Of course, the sine qua non of TBI is trauma, which in Thornton's case was well established. After the blow to his head, he had suffered both unconsciousness and amnesia for the event; either of those would complete his diagnostic criteria (criterion B for NCD due to TBI). Long afterwards (certainly well past the immediate postinjury period—criterion C), he remained irritable and unfocused, without definite symptoms of a mood disorder. Still, I don't think that his emotional or behavioral sequelae rise to the level of the *with behavioral disturbance* specifier.

Based on how long he was unconscious, the duration of his amnesia, and his disorientation and bewilderment at initial assessment, DSM-5 permits us to rate the severity of his TBI. Quite frankly, I consider this one too many numbers:* What we really care about is Thornton, not his injury. Prior to his latest fall, his GAF would have been a comparatively robust 71. I hope that he wouldn't now develop chronic traumatic encephalitis (see the sidebar above). Assuming a "no," his diagnosis would be as follows:

---

*Ratings of TBI severity may be helpful in doing research on head injury sequels. If you want to know more, you can see p. 626 of DSM-5. I won't discuss it further here. I have my standards.

S06.2X4S [907.0]	Diffuse traumatic brain injury with loss of consciousness 6-24 hours, sequela
G31.84 [331.83]	Mild neurocognitive disorder due to traumatic brain injury, without behavioral disturbance

Frontotemporal Neurocognitive Disorder

Once called Pick's disease, frontotemporal NCD—for auld lang syne, I'll use the traditional abbreviation for frontotemporal dementia (FTD)—used to be considered rare. Now, it's known to account for up to 5% of all cases of dementia and perhaps one in six younger patients: Its mean age of onset is somewhere in the 50s. FTD appears to respect neither gender nor race, but it is often familial; about half of cases are transmitted as an autosomal dominant trait.

You won't be surprised to hear that FTD affects frontal and temporal lobes of the brain (which lose neurons and accumulate tau protein); in so doing, it can produce diverse clinical pictures. The behavioral variant is characterized either by apathy and social withdrawal or by disinhibition. Apathetic folks basically stay in bed and stop providing their own care, whereas the disinhibited ones do things that are socially inappropriate—make rude sexual comments, for example, or steal items or otherwise subvert social norms. In both types, though, it's the behavior that you notice.

The language variant often begins with patients unable to find the right word (*anomia*) for a particular object or concept—though they can point to the correct object when it is presented to them. Reading aloud and understanding of spoken language are both initially unimpaired, but with time, they may become increasingly unable to produce fluent, meaningful speech. Both the behavioral and the language types begin insidiously and progress slowly, with relative sparing of memory and visuoperceptual skills. Both culminate in compromised activities of daily living. As they progress, the boundaries of the two subtypes become less distinct.

In part because of variability and overlapping features, the syndromes of FTD often go unrecognized. Final diagnosis depends heavily on imaging and neuropsychological testing. Here we'll focus on a couple of vignettes to illustrate what you might expect to confront in patients who haven't yet received the necessary workup.

As Pick's disease, FTD is a venerable diagnosis, dating back to the 1890s. It is remarkable how similar its symptoms are to what was for many years called *simple schizophrenia*, which was retained in the official nomenclature until 1980. Here is the DSM-II description: It is "characterized chiefly by a slow and insidious reduction of external attachments and interests and by apathy and indifference leading to impoverishment of interpersonal relations, mental deterioration, and adjustment on a lower level of functioning." The entry goes on to explain that there is less in the way of dramatic psychosis than in other subtypes of schizophrenia, yet far more progression than with schizoid personality.

Essential Features of **Frontotemporal Neurocognitive Disorder**

The patient has a {mild}{major} neurocognitive disorder (p. 492). The symptoms begin slowly and progress gradually. The patient's symptoms will be mainly of one of these two types:

Behavioral variant. The patient behaves in socially inappropriate ways that may include poor manners, loss of decorum, or rash impulsivity; apathy or inertia; reduced capacity for compassion; compulsive behavior; and hyperorality (binge eating, pica, drinking, smoking) and alterations of diet. Visuomotor skills will be relatively unimpaired, but there tends to be clear evidence of impaired frontal/executive functioning, such as reduced mental flexibility, decreased generation tasks, planning deficits, and reversal learning errors.

Language variant. In the face of relatively unimpaired memory and visuomotor function, there is gradual loss of the ability to produce speech, to find the right word, to attach names to objects, and to use grammar and understand the meaning of words.

The Fine Print

The D's: • Duration (chronic) • Differential diagnosis (mood and psychotic disorders; other causes of NCD—especially Alzheimer's, Lewy bodies) • Definitiveness of diagnosis (see coding notes as regards probable/possible diagnosis)

Coding Notes

Specify if:

Probable frontotemporal NCD. A pathogenic mutation is known to exist (via genetic tests or family history), *or* imaging shows heavy frontotemporal involvement.

Possible frontotemporal NCD. Neither characteristic of a probable diagnosis is present.

Record and code as indicated in Table 16.1a.

Toby Russo

The telephone request came from a man in Chicago, who was worried about his dad. "When I saw him over the holidays, he wasn't himself," the caller began. "For a long time, maybe a year, he's been losing interest in things. He's only 56, but he was recently fired from his job—he worked for a package delivery service. I called his former boss, who told me that customers had complained he had left their packages without ringing, or just dropped them on the steps—not even inside the gate. 'He just didn't seem to give a—to care any longer,' was his exact quote. He said my dad only just shrugged and pocketed his final pay envelope. That was 6 months ago." Since then, he'd apparently had a number of car accidents, but he kept right on driving. The caller ended by asking the clinician to pay a home visit to his dad, who had refused to make an office appointment.

While talking with the clinician, Toby Russo sat in his apartment and stuffed his mouth with Cheetos. He admitted that his weight had shot up in the past couple of years, though he didn't much care. In mute affirmation, about him lay empty Cheetos bags and cereal boxes. His shirt was gray around the neckline and badly frayed; he didn't appear to have showered recently. But both his recent and remote memory appeared intact, and he wasn't depressed; he'd had no delusions or hallucinations. The car accidents? He just ran into a lot of other vehicles; no problem. Maybe he'd get his car fixed, only they'd stopped his insurance. However, on simple testing (the MMSE), he scored 28 out of a possible 30, missing the day of the week and one of the three objects he'd been asked to remember.

Toby had been sleeping in his living room on a mattress tossed onto the floor. Beside it lay a tattered pair of boxer shorts covered in—just what were those spots and blotches, the clinician wanted to know. "I smoke, so I have to cough a lot," Toby explained blandly. "In the night, I don't want to get up, so I just spit it there." He guessed that the same shorts had lain there, night after night, maybe for weeks.

Within days, Toby had slipped rapidly downhill. His son, again visiting in town, had found him alone in his apartment. Apparently, he hadn't stirred from his mattress for a day or two. He was hospitalized, where an MRI revealed marked bilateral atrophy of his frontal and anterior temporal lobes.

Trudy Cantor

At her 60th birthday party, Trudy Cantor's brother had noticed that she hesitated—maybe *stammered* was a better word—a bit when responding to the toast. She'd repeatedly seemed to struggle to find the right word ("Yes, that's it. *Happy*," she'd say at a helpful suggestion; her relief was evident.) Then she'd joke, "My senior moments are growing together."

That was 2 years earlier. Now, though she could read aloud from a printed source, her spontaneous speech was rambling and she never managed to convey any point. "Here's the way it's been. I first wanted to get, um, no that's not right, I thought it was another thing. Most of the time, I've been quite, uh, quite, you know, well . . . that's just the way it is. It's been, I mean."

By this time, she had difficulty identifying a pen by name, yet—it seemed a near miracle—she had continued her part-time employment drafting house plans for a local architect.

Evaluation of Toby Russo and Trudy Cantor

Each of these patients had long-standing cognitive changes that would qualify for a diagnosis of major NCD (frontotemporal NCD criterion A). And each had a personal history of gradually deteriorating (B) cognitive status that, at least initially, was not remarkable for memory impairment.

In Toby's case, there were signs of apathy (criterion C1a-ii), as well as behavioral disinhibition (repeatedly crashing his car and not caring,—C1a-i) and hyperorality (stuffing himself on Cheetos, though other people will smoke or drink to excess, or just put objects into their mouths,—C1a-v). From the results on the MMSE, his memory and perceptual–motor functions were probably relatively spared at the time of his initial evaluation (D, though one wonders what was happening that repeatedly caused him to crash his car). It was only with his deteriorating status that the definitive MRI was forthcoming (probable frontotemporal NCD criterion 2), which allowed us to state that his diagnosis was, um, probable. DSM-5 would allow us to add "with behavioral disturbance" to Toby's diagnosis, but under the circumstance that would seem a little silly, but it lets us state the behavior type. Because his was a probable case, we list first the medical diagnosis. With a GAF score of 10, Toby's diagnosis would be as follows:

| G31.09 [331.19] | Frontotemporal disease |
| F02.81 [294.11] | Major neurocognitive disorder due to probable frontotemporal lobar degeneration, behavioral variant, severe, with behavioral disturbance (apathy and disinhibition) |

Over the years, Trudy had experienced a remarkable loss of her language skills, beginning with problematic word finding and gradually (criterion B) progressing to speech that was normally produced but content-free (C2a). The fact that she was still able to work at drafting indicates sparing of perceptual–motor functioning (D); to evaluate whether her ability to learn was spared would require some testing. However, her problems with language were serious, far past the level of mild NCD. Therefore, on clinical grounds (with a GAF score somewhere in the 50s, I feel her diagnosis should be possible (no testing, no genetic information) major frontotemporal NCD. Though she had terrible problems with communication, she didn't require help with instrumental activities of daily living, so I'd rate her overall severity as mild.

| G31.09 [331.19] | Frontotemporal disease |
| F02.80 [294.10] | Major neurocognitive disorder due to possible frontotemporal lobar degeneration, language variant, without behavioral disturbance, mild |

Wait a minute: There isn't anything in Table 16.1a about stating *language variant* or *behavioral variant*, is there? And the answer is, of course, "No, but there should be." It is additional information that may be of value to the patient and to later clinicians, so I went right ahead and put it in. There's no code number attached, so what's the problem?

Vascular Neurocognitive Disorder

Approximately 10% of dementias have a vascular origin. Vascular dementia has also been called *multi-infarct dementia* because its presumed cause is so often a series of strokes, though some patients are affected by a single event and others may have small vessel disease that doesn't produce infarcts. Whereas patients with Alzheimer's disease deteriorate gradually, many patients with vascular NCD worsen through a series of small steps as the strokes occur. Sometimes, however, progression can appear slow and gradual—probably due to the accumulating involvement of multiple small vessels. Vascular NCD is especially likely to develop in a patient who has diabetes or hypertension.

Besides failing memory, patients experience the loss of executive functioning, which (as noted above) can show up as the inability to deal with novel tasks. Apathy, slowed thinking, and deteriorating hygiene are also often noted. Relatively mild stressors may precipitate pathological laughing or crying. These patients are less likely than patients with Alzheimer's to have aphasia, apraxia, and agnosia, though any aspect of mental functioning can be affected.

The symptoms of vascular NCD depend on the exact location of brain lesion(s), but several characteristics are typical, especially of what's known as *subcortical ischemic vascular disease.* They include early impairment of executive function and attention, slowed motor performance, and slowed processing of information. Episodic memory is less affected than in Alzheimer's, but mood symptoms (depression, lability) and apathy are especially prominent.

In naturalistic studies, the rate of advance of vascular NCD is about the same as for Alzheimer's; illness in treated patients progresses more slowly.

Some authorities advocate a division of dementias into the *cortical* (or degenerative, such as dementia due to Alzheimer's disease) and *sub-cortical* (dementia due to most other causes). The subcortical dementias (some texts also call these *secondary* dementias) are allegedly less likely to produce agnosia, apraxia, and aphasia. Other authorities object, pointing out that the pathology of disease is never that neat and that all dementias have some degree of both cortical and subcortical pathology. Because there is so much overlap in symptoms, DSM-5's seems the safer classification. It categorizes the NCDs much more simply, on the basis of presumed underlying cause.

Essential Features of **Vascular Neurocognitive Disorder**

The patient has a {mild}{major} neurocognitive disorder (p. 492). The symptoms begin after a vascular event and often progress stepwise. There is often prominent decline in complex attention and frontal/executive functioning.

The Fine Print

The D's: • Duration (tends to chronicity) • Differential diagnosis (delirium; other causes of NCD—especially Alzheimer's and frontotemporal; mood and psychotic disorders)

Coding Notes

Specify if:

> **Vascular NCD probably due to vascular disease.** The diagnosis is reinforced by neuroimaging, by proximity (following a cerebrovascular accident), or by both clinical and genetic evidence.
> **Vascular NCD possibly due to vascular disease.** None of the three sorts of evidence cited above obtains.

Specify if: **{With}{Without} behavioral disturbance.**

Minnie Bell Leach

At their family physician's request, her daughter and son-in-law had brought Minnie Bell Leach for consultation. She had lived with them for the past year, since her second stroke. Nearly 5 years earlier, her first stroke had left her with a partly paralyzed left leg, but she had been able to care for herself and even do her marketing until the second stroke a year ago. Since then, she had rarely left her wheelchair. Her daughter provided an increasing share of her personal care.

Over the last few months, Minnie Bell had begun to slip. At first she often forgot to take her medicine for high blood pressure. Despite the fact that she kept them in their container (which had three compartments for each day of the week), she had at first needed reminding to take the pills at breakfast, lunch, and bedtime. After a week or two, this had improved, and for a time she had seemed almost back to her former self.

But when she awakened the previous Sunday morning, it was clear that Minnie Bell had slipped some more. She had neglected to zip her skirt and had gotten the buttons of her blouse into the wrong holes. Neither of these mistakes did she seem to notice. She also had trouble expressing herself—at breakfast she asked for "red stuff" for her toast (it was strawberry jam that she and her daughter had made together last summer). And she had reverted to taking her medicine only when reminded.

Minnie Bell looked a bit older than her 68 years. She sat quietly in her wheelchair, cradling her left wrist in her right hand. Over her cotton house dress she wore a cloth overcoat that had fallen off one shoulder; she did not appear to notice. Although she maintained good eye contact throughout the consultation, she spoke only when spoken to. Her speech was clear and coherent. She denied having hallucinations, delusions, or depression, but she spontaneously complained of a cough, shortness of breath, and numerous aches and pains. She overlooked the fact that she couldn't walk.

On the MMSE, Minnie Bell scored 20 out of 30. She knew the year but missed the month and date by over 2 months; she could name the city and state, a watch, and a pencil. Although she could repeat the names of three objects (ball, chair, telephone) immediately after she heard them, 5 minutes later she could recall only the ball. She became confused when asked to follow the three-part instruction, and she persistently forgot to place the folded paper on the floor. There were no apraxias: She could use a pencil to copy a simple figure.

On neurological exam, Minnie Bell's left hand was weak; there was an abnormal Babinski sign (upgoing great toe when the sole of her foot was scratched) on that side.

Evaluation of Minnie Bell Leach

The evidence for Minnie Bell's having an NCD was as follows: She had had increasing difficulty with her memory, as shown by the history of forgetting to take her medication and by the obvious problem with short-term memory. From the MMSE, she appeared to have no agnosias or apraxias. However, her daughter noted the aphasia of "red stuff" for jam (a language problem). She also had increasing problems with executive functioning, as shown by her neglected appearance and her inability to follow a three-step instruction. These problems represented a major decline from her previous level of functioning, and they did interfere at least moderately with her everyday life.

The prolonged course of her disease would also argue against **delirium.** Minnie Bell denied depression, delusions, or hallucinations, rendering unlikely the diagnosis of a noncognitive disorder such as a **pseudodementia** (vascular NCD criterion D). A vascular etiology for her disease was suggested by her history of hypertension and by the stepwise progression of her disability following several strokes (B1). Her neurological signs (weakness of her hand, upgoing toe) from the start of her decline provided further evidence for a vascular etiology (C). Her clinical course supports a probable vascular etiology (B2).

Because Minnie Bell's principal symptom seemed to be trouble with executive functioning, she would be diagnosed as follows (with a GAF score of 31:

F01.50 [290.40]   Major vascular neurocognitive disorder probably due to vascular disease, without behavioral disturbance, moderate

Neurocognitive Disorder Due to Other Medical Conditions

Also detailed in DSM-5 are several other causes of NCD, most of which are responsible for just a tiny percentage of total cases. Below, I've summarized the features to look for in those accorded specific criteria in DSM-5. A more complete list can be found in the "Physical Disorders . . . " table in the Appendix.

Parkinson's disease. The stooped posture, slow movements, rigidity, back-and-forth ("pill-rolling") tremor, and rapid, shuffling gait characteristic of Parkinson's disease are well known and often obvious. Less well known may be the degree to which NCD occurs—affecting a quarter or more of patients with Parkinson's, with the likelihood of major NCD increasing to as high as 75% with advancing age.

Note that in contrast to dementia with Lewy bodies, the physical aspects of Parkinson's appear before the cognitive features appear. That's one leg of two qualifying factors for a probable or possible diagnosis. The other is that there must be no evidence that another disorder—cerebrovascular disease, Alzheimer's, or any other mental, neurological, or physical disease—is contributing to the development of the NCD. Presence of both factors yields a *probable* diagnosis; presence of only one yields a *possible* diagnosis. See Table 16.1a for details of recording.

Huntington's disease. Age of onset for Huntington's disease averages around 40 years; the first symptoms may be apparently minor changes in personality and executive functioning, followed by deteriorating memory and judgment. A generalized restlessness may precede the characteristic involuntary choreiform movements and slowing of voluntary movements. Prevalence is about 6 per 100,000 in North America and Europe. The cause is an autosomal dominant gene on chromosome 4.

Prion disease. Prion disease is at once miniscule and huge. It accounts for a tiny fraction of all dementias—perhaps 1 case per million population per year—yet its "mad cow disease" form is so dramatic (and unusual) that it makes headlines whenever it occurs. The more common type, Creutzfeldt–Jakob disease, is caused by an infectious protein that contains no nucleic acids (that is, no DNA or RNA). These diseases attack the brain, creating the holes in microscopic sections that account for the collective name *spongiform encephalopathies.* Symptoms include memory loss, hallucinations, personality change, and motor problems. Though the age range is wide, it usually occurs in the elderly; a few cases are familial. Usually fatal within a year, prion disease is essentially untreatable.

HIV infection. Improvements in antiviral therapy have reduced the various threats posed by HIV infection; yet up to half of those infected will have some symptoms of cognitive dysfunction, and up to a third meet criteria for mild or major NCD. It is principally a subcortical type of infection with a variable presentation. Although HIV infection is not one of the more common causes of dementia, it has rapidly become one of the most important, occurring in young people and laying waste otherwise vigorous lives. That's why I've used it below as the exemplar for this NCD category.

Other causes. The symptoms and course of illness depend heavily on the underlying medical cause. Obviously, so do treatment and prognosis. They might include normal-pressure hydrocephalus. hypothyroidism, brain tumor, vitamin B12 deficiency, and many others. See Appendix A for more.

Essential Features of **Neurocognitive Disorder Due to Other Medical Conditions**

The patient fulfills criteria for a {major}{mild} neurocognitive disorder. In addition:

	Huntington's disease	**Parkinson's disease[a]**	**Prion disease**	**HIV infection**	**Other medical condition**
Patient has evidence of:	Huntington's disease (family history or genetic testing)	Motor symptoms of Parkinson's disease	Motor features of prion disease (ataxia, myoclonus, tremor)	Documented HIV infection	History, physical exam, or lab evidence of another non-mental disorder
Symptoms not better explained by:	Another mental or medical disorder			Non-HIV mental, cognitive, medical disorders	Another mental disorder or specific NCD
Onset is:	Insidious, gradually progressive		Insidious; often rapid progression	—	—

[a]Recorded as probable or possible NCD; see text.

Coding Notes

See Tables 16.1a and 16.1b for coding procedures.

Arlen Wing

When he was admitted to the hospital for the third time in 4 months, Arlen Wing had lost 30 pounds, which was nearly 20% of his body weight. With it seemed to have gone much of his will to live: He had often neglected to take the cocktail of antiviral medications prescribed to shore up his failing immune system. This, plus the apathy that was so obvious on admission, prompted the request for mental health consultation. Arlen's physician noted that a CT brain scan showed diffuse cortical atrophy; an EEG had been read as indicating "nonfocal slowing."

Arlen had trained to be a dancer. After he just missed landing a job with the Joffrey Ballet, he had joined his long-time companion, Alex, in the business of buying and selling antique dolls. The two had made a good living traveling around the country to auctions and doll shows, until Alex rather suddenly died of *Pneumocystis* pneumonia. Arlen soon discovered that he was HIV-positive; he promptly began taking prophylactic medications. He had continued to operate his business until the last few months, when his CD4 cell count dropped below 200, triggering his recent series of hospitalizations.

While the consultant explained the purpose of the visit, Arlen made eye contact and listened politely. His speech was slow and labored, but there were no other abnormalities in the flow of his speech. He had no delusions, hallucinations, or other abnormal content of thought. He denied feeling especially sad or anxious—"just tired."

Arlen knew his own name, the name of the hospital, and the month, but he gave the date and year incorrectly. He thought that he had been admitted only the day before, whereas it had actually been a week earlier. He could not recall the name of the physician who had attended him for the past 3 years. He scored only 14 out of 30 on the MMSE. When asked to pick up a sheet of paper, fold it, and put it on the floor, he twice dropped the paper unfolded onto the floor. When asked to tell how an apple and an orange were similar, he could offer no response. Although he acknowledged being seriously ill, he admitted that recently he had often neglected to take his cocktail of pills. "I was feeling terrible," he said, "and I thought they might be making me sick."

Evaluation of Arlen Wing

Arlen's history and obvious intellectual decline (major NCD criterion A) point clearly to the NCDs. He was alert, and he adequately focused his attention on the exam, making a delirium extremely unlikely (C). (However, the trouble he had pursuing a task or shifting attention from one task to another can occur later in the course of NCD due to HIV infection.) His loss of recent memory was obvious; this is especially common in an HIV-related dementia. Also typical were his apathy and slowed speech (slowed-down motor movements in general are characteristic of this disorder). His impairments represented a significant decline from his previous level of functioning (B). There were no obvious agnosias, apraxias, or aphasias, which is what we'd expect from a non-Alzheimer's type of dementia. In all, he clearly conformed to the criteria for an NCD, and his HIV-positive status would provide the necessary information as to etiology. We note that Arlen had the behavioral disturbance of apathy. Because he had given up on self-care, I would score his GAF as only 21, though other clinicians might rate him somewhat higher. The severity rating for his major NCD would be less dire; he wasn't yet fully dependent for all care.

Informants who knew him well would be the most satisfactory source of information about Arlen's executive functioning (had he been having trouble dressing himself, shopping, or taking care of other routine daily tasks?). However, his inability to follow a sequence of events in the MMSE also provided evidence. Discontinuing his medications suggested a lapse in judgment, typical of the later stages of an HIV-related dementia. He denied feeling depressed—evidence (though not definitive) against a mood disorder with pseudodementia.

| B20 [042] | HIV infection |
| F02.81 [294.11] | Major neurocognitive disorder due to HIV infection, moderate, with behavioral disturbance |

Substance/Medication-Induced Neurocognitive Disorder

NCDs can result from prolonged use of alcohol, sedatives, and inhalants, though in the vast majority of instances, alcohol is the chief culprit. Patients will have difficulty with constructional tasks (e.g., drawing), behavioral problems, and memory defects. These patients are often described as having delusional jealousy or hallucinations. Although the onset is typically gradual, nothing may be noted amiss until the patient has dried out for several days or weeks.

One form of this disorder is the type variously known as Korsakoff's psychosis or, as it was called in DSM-IV, substance-induced persisting amnestic disorder. (DSM-5 has swept the entire former class of amnestic disorders into alcohol-induced major NCD, amnestic–confabulatory type.)

Essential Features of **Substance/Medication-Induced Neurocognitive Disorder**

The use of some substance appears to have caused a patient to have a {major}{mild} neurocognitive disorder (p. 492).

The Fine Print

For tips on identifying substance-related causation, see sidebar page 95.

The D's: • Differential diagnosis (numerous other causes of NCD)

Coding Notes

When writing down the diagnosis, use the exact substance in the title—for instance, alcohol-induced major neurocognitive disorder. See Table 15.2 in Chapter 15.

Specify if:

Persistent. Symptoms of the NCD continue long past the time it should take to recover with prolonged abstinence.

Mark Culpepper

Despite drinking nearly a fifth of bourbon every day until he was 56, Mark Culpepper had successfully avoided hospitalization. He had taught developmental biology for 30 years, but 6 months earlier the university had offered him early retirement. Soon afterwards, his daughter, Amarette, had moved in with him as housekeeper and companion. She provided most of the history of his illness.

Amarette never understood how her father had managed to retain his position while drinking as much as he did. Of course, in later years his teaching assignments had always been lower-division, and he had published no research for over a decade. He was "COT," as the students put it—"coasting on tenure." Tenure was a powerful influence at the university; it forgave him the occasional missed class he was too hung over to attend, and the fact that he hardly ever graded a paper at all.

By the time his daughter moved in, Mark was fully retired and devoting all of his time to drinking. Amarette quickly took care of that. She confiscated the contents of his bar and, by combining shame with threats, obtained such control over his finances that he was forced into total abstention. She remained steadfast through a week during which he vomited and had the shakes. At a stroke, she had rid her father of a 30-year habit.

The results were both more and less than Amarette had expected. In the next 4 months Mark didn't touch a drop, but neither did he accomplish much of anything else. Even sober, he neglected his appearance, often going for days without shaving. He spent much of his time "working on a paper" that was, as far as she could tell, recycled material from decades-old notebooks. He had simply copied it out unaltered. "Anything there that made any sense at all, you could read in an old freshman biology text. A very old text," she said while he was being admitted.

An event the day before had precipitated the admission. When she returned from a brief errand, she found him in the living room trying to mop up water from the bathtub that he had turned on and apparently forgotten about. The taps were still running.

Mark was a pleasant enough man whose red nose and cheeks gave him a somewhat boyish appearance. He carried a sheaf of papers in a dog-eared manila folder; the title page read, "Limb Regeneration in the Newt." His speech was normal, and he denied delusions, hallucinations, depression, and suicidal ideas. Although he seemed to pay attention during the MMSE, he scored only 19 out of 30. He was unable to recall two of three objects after 5 minutes. With difficulty, he correctly spelled *world* backward. When asked to follow the three-part instruction (to pick up a piece of paper, fold it, and place it on the floor), he persistently neglected to fold the paper. When asked about this, he brushed it off, saying, "Well, I was thinking about my research."

Evaluation of Mark Culpepper

Central to many cases of NCD is memory impairment. In Mark's case, this was not apparent on casual observation. He was pleasant, carried on a conversation in a natural manner, and even appeared to be working on a scientific paper. However, after 5 minutes he could recall only one of the three objects given to him on the MMSE.

Mark gave no evidence of problems with language, attention, social cognition, or perceptual–motor issues, but Amarette's history suggested that he'd developed real problems in caring for himself (neglecting his appearance, flooding the house with bathwater). This loss of executive functioning was reflected in bedside testing by his inability to follow a three-part instruction. It was enough to count as a major NCD (criterion A), though I'd rate it as mild—so far.

Mark focused attention well, and it did not appear to wander during the interview, suggesting that a **delirium** was not responsible; persistence of his symptoms past the usual time course for withdrawal would fulfill this requirement (B). Heavy, prolonged alcohol use could certainly produce his symptoms (C), the course of which was consistent with the fact that they continued long after Amarette dragged him onto the wagon (D). Other mental pathology was not evident: Mark denied symptoms of **depression** and **psychosis**, which are the two major conditions that might present with neglect and memory loss. Of course, a physical exam, and perhaps some testing, would be needed to rule out **other medical illnesses** (E). Considering his history, however, an **alcohol-induced major NCD** would seem highly probable.

The matter of Mark's **alcohol use disorder** requires some thought. At the time he stopped drinking, when he developed shakiness and vomiting, we'd have said he was in alcohol withdrawal. That, and the fact that alcohol had clearly interfered with both his work and his relationship with Amarette, would have been enough to diagnose alcohol use disorder. Unaddressed in the vignette are many of the remaining criteria for substance use disorder—craving for alcohol and tolerance, to name just two. A full exploration would probably yield enough symptoms to qualify him for the severest level of involvement. At any rate, we couldn't score it as *mild*, which would be misleading and inconsistent with alcohol withdrawal. OK, perhaps it's going a bit beyond the data, but it seems clinically appropriate to rate Mark's alcohol use disorder as severe; I'll select the appropriate codes from Table 15.2 in Chapter 15.

Mark had recently retired and had time on his hands, which could be a problem— or an opportunity. (He might profit from occupational or recreational therapy, or even from referral to day care.) Either way, I'd give him the appropriate Z-code. I can hardly believe that there would be nothing to report as regards his medical condition; we'll have to revisit it later. His GAF score would be 41.

In the coding indicated just below, I've indicated the numbers for both ICD-10 and ICD-9. However, I've given only the terminology for the former (ICD-9 requires separate statements for the alcohol use disorder and NCD).

F10.27 [303.90, 291.2]	Severe alcohol use disorder in early remission, with alcohol-induced major neurocognitive disorder, nonamnestic–confabulatory type, persistent
Z60.0 [V62.89]	Phase of life problem (retirement)

Charles Jackson

A powerfully built 6-footer, Charles Jackson still showed traces of a military bearing. Before he left the Army a year before, he had been busted to buck private; this was the culmination of a string of disciplinary actions for drunkenness. Fortunately, he had served 21 years and did not forfeit his retirement pay.

For over a year, he had had monthly consultations with the current interviewer. On his last MMSE, Charles had scored 17: the full 9 points for language, 3 for spelling *world* backwards as *drolw*, 3 for registration (immediately repeating three items), and 2 for knowing the city and state.

On this occasion, the interviewer asked when they had last met. Charles replied, "Well, I just don't know. What do you think?" To the follow-up question, he said that he guessed he had seen the interviewer before. "Maybe it was last week."

Asking him to remain seated, the interviewer went into the waiting room to ask Mrs. Jackson how she thought her husband was doing. She said, "Oh, he's about the same as before. He sketches some. He can still draw a pretty good caricature of you, as long as you're sitting right in front of him. But mostly he just sits around the house and watches TV. I come home and ask him what he's been watching, but he can't even tell me."

At any rate, Charles was no longer drinking, not since they had moved to the country. It was at least 2 miles to the nearest convenience store, and he didn't walk very well any more. "But he still talks about drinking. Sometimes he seems to think he's still in the Army. He orders me to go buy him a quart of gin."

Charles remembered quite a few things, if they had happened long enough ago—the gin, for example, and getting drunk with his father when he was a boy. But he couldn't remember the name of his daughter, who was 2½ years old. Most of the time, he just called her "the girl."

The interviewer walked back into the inner office. Charles looked up and smiled.

"Have I seen you before?" asked the interviewer.

"Well, I'm pretty sure."

"When was it?"

"It might have been last week."

Evaluation of Charles Jackson

Charles had not only an especially severe anterograde memory loss (he could form no new memories), but also a considerable degree of retrograde amnesia (he couldn't even recall his daughter's name). We hardly need objective testing to conclude that he'd suffered a significant cognitive decline (major NCD criterion A). His wife testified that he just sat around; from that, I'm going to extrapolate that he didn't do any of the bill-paying or household chores (B). We haven't determined, however, the extent to which he was able to provide self-care. Charles showed no evidence of shifting attention or reduced awareness, which would rule out a delirium (C).

Given a little rope, Charles appeared to confabulate a previous meeting with the examiner. Although confabulation is not a criterion for diagnosis, it is one of the classic symptoms, to the extent that it even helps make up the named subtype. In alcohol-induced amnestic–confabulatory syndrome, memory is the principal disturbance.

However, problems with executive functioning (suggested by Charles's performance on the MMSE) can and do occur.

The main items in the differential diagnosis would include **other causes of major NCD** and other complications of alcoholism. Either of these sources of confusion should be clear from the history. Of course, there was little danger that his condition would be mistaken for the memory blackouts associated with **alcohol intoxication.**

Although elements of history are missing from the vignette, Charles should also receive a diagnosis of **alcohol use disorder.** Other than the ongoing desire to drink, he had not met the criteria during the past year, so he would earn the qualifier of *in sustained remission.* (I'm almost tempted to add *in a controlled environment*, because where he lived, he couldn't get anywhere to obtain alcohol. Almost, but not quite.) His GAF score would be only 41. His diagnosis would come from Table 15.2:

F10.26 [303.90, 291.1]   Alcohol use disorder, in sustained remission, with
                           alcohol-induced major neurocognitive disorder,
                           amnestic–confabulatory type, persistent

Neurocognitive Disorder Due to Multiple Etiologies

Whether it has one cause or many, the basic symptoms of NCD remain the same. Many medical and neurological disorders can be at fault, so the combinations are nearly endless. Any patient's symptoms should be consistent with the underlying pathology, but it may be hard to discriminate the contributing factors on purely clinical grounds.

Dementias with more than one cause are especially common in older people, who are prone to falls and multiple illnesses, and in persons whose drinking or drug use puts them at risk for a variety of medical disorders. For example, a patient with alcohol-induced major NCD may also have head trauma, infection, or a degenerative condition such as Marchiafava–Bignami disease (in which the corpus callosum of the brain is affected by chronic alcohol intake).

The symptoms are much the same as with other causes of NCD, so I've given no case example. In fact, I haven't even provided Essential Features; they seem pretty self-evident. Once you've collected the symptoms and made the diagnosis, the only real remaining problem is this: How the heck do you code it? Basically, here's the plan (from Table 16.1b):

First write down the names and codes for each of the contributing medical conditions. Then you add the appropriate code for major NCD {with}{without} behavioral disturbance.

Below is the full diagnosis for a patient with long-established Huntington's disease who has also suffered a blow to the head.

G10 [333.4]   Huntington's disease
S06.2X9S [907.0]   Diffuse traumatic brain injury with loss of consciousness of
                       unspecified duration, sequela
F02.81 [294.11]   Major neurocognitive disorder due to multiple etiologies,
                       with behavioral disturbance

Of course, there's a fly in the ointment. Three flies, in fact.

Fly 1. If your patient has a vascular disorder that contributes to the NCD, you need to mention it separately. Suppose our unfortunate patient has Huntington's *and* a vascular NCD. Here's how the diagnosis would appear:

G10 [333.4]	Huntington's disease
F02.80 [294.10]	Major neurocognitive disorder due to multiple etiologies, without behavioral disturbance
F01.50 [290.40]	Major vascular neurocognitive disorder {probably} {possibly} due to vascular disease, without behavioral disturbance

Fly 2. Suppose, after all that diagnosing, that your patient has "only" a mild NCD. Then you'd list it this way:

G31.84 [331.83]	Mild neurocognitive disorder due to multiple etiologies

Note that you don't code the etiologies. However, you can add in the wording, "{with}{without} behavioral disturbance."

Fly 3. The DSM-5 criteria state that a diagnosis of probable major NCD due to Alzheimer's disease requires that there be no evidence of mixed etiology, and specifically mentions the example of vascular disease. However, NCD due to multiple etiologies specifically states the example of major NCD due to both Alzheimer's disease and vascular disease. If ever you face this irreconcilable contradiction, code as probable major NCD due to Alzheimer's disease *and* as major vascular NCD, but do *not* use the multiple-etiologies code. At least, that's what you should do until DSM-5 comes up with a better solution.

G30.9 [331.0]	Alzheimer's disease
F02.80 [294.10]	Major neurocognitive disorder due to probable Alzheimer's disease, without behavioral disturbance
F01.50 [290.40]	Major vascular neurocognitive disorder probably due to vascular disease, without behavioral disturbance

R41.9 [799.59] Unspecified Neurocognitive Disorder

The unspecified NCD category includes patients whose cognitive deficits do not clearly suggest delirium or NCD (mild or major), yet cause undeniable distress or impaired functioning.

CHAPTER 17

Personality Disorders

Quick Guide to the Personality Disorders

DSM-5 retains the 10 specific personality disorders (PDs) that were listed in DSM-IV. Of these, perhaps 6 have been studied reasonably well and have a lot of support in the research community. The rest (paranoid, schizoid, histrionic, and dependent PDs), while perhaps less well founded in science, retain their positions in the diagnostic firmament because of their practical use and, frankly, tradition.

Speaking of tradition, ever since DSM-III in 1980 the personality disorders have been divided into three groups, called *clusters*. Heavily criticized for a lack of scientific validity, the clusters are perhaps most useful as a device to help us call to mind the full slate of PDs.

Cluster A Personality Disorders

People with Cluster A PDs can be described as withdrawn, cold, suspicious, or irrational. (Here and throughout the Quick Guide, as usual, the page number following each item indicates where a more detailed discussion begins.)

Paranoid. These people are suspicious and quick to take offense. They often have few confidants and may read hidden meaning into innocent remarks (p. 533).

Schizoid. These patients care little for social relationships, have a restricted emotional range, and seem indifferent to criticism or praise. Tending to be solitary, they avoid close (including sexual) relationships (p. 535).

Schizotypal. Interpersonal relationships are so difficult for these people that they appear peculiar or strange to others. They lack close friends and are uncomfortable in social situations. They may show suspiciousness, unusual perceptions or thinking, eccentric speech, and inappropriate affect (p. 538).

Cluster B Personality Disorders

Those with Cluster B PDs tend to be rather theatrical, emotional, and attention-seeking; their moods are labile and often shallow. They often have intense interpersonal conflicts.

Antisocial. The irresponsible, often criminal behavior of these people begins in childhood or early adolescence with truancy, running away, cruelty, fighting, destructiveness, lying, and theft. In addition to criminal behavior, as adults they may default on debts or otherwise behave irresponsibly; act recklessly or impulsively; and show no remorse for their behavior (p. 541).

Borderline. These impulsive people engage in behavior harmful to themselves (sexual adventures, unwise spending, excessive use of substances or food). Affectively unstable, they often show intense, inappropriate anger. They feel empty or bored, and they frantically try to avoid abandonment. They are uncertain about who they are, and they lack the ability to maintain stable interpersonal relationships (p. 545).

Histrionic. Overly emotional, vague, and desperate for attention, these people need constant reassurance about their attractiveness. They may be self-centered and sexually seductive (p. 548).

Narcissistic. These people are self-important and often preoccupied with envy, fantasies of success, or ruminations about the uniqueness of their own problems. Their sense of entitlement and lack of compassion may cause them to take advantage of others. They vigorously reject criticism and need constant attention and admiration (p. 550).

Cluster C Personality Disorders

Someone with a Cluster C PD will tend to be anxious and tense, often overcontrolled.

Avoidant. These timid people are so easily wounded by criticism that they hesitate to become involved with others. They may fear the embarrassment of showing emotion or of saying things that seem foolish. They may have no close friends, and they exaggerate the risks of undertaking pursuits outside their usual routines (p. 553).

Dependent. These people so much need the approval of others that they have trouble making independent decisions or starting projects; they may even agree with others whom they know to be wrong. They fear abandonment, feel helpless when they are alone, and are miserable when relationships end. They are easily hurt by criticism and will even volunteer for unpleasant tasks to gain the favor of others (p. 556).

Obsessive–Compulsive. Perfectionism and rigidity characterize these people. They are often workaholics, and they tend to be indecisive, excessively scrupulous, and preoccupied with detail They insist that others do things their way. They have trouble expressing affection, tend to lack generosity, and may even resist throwing away worthless objects they no longer need (p. 558).

Other Causes of Long-Standing Character Disturbance

Personality change due to another medical condition. A medical condition can affect a patient's personality for the worse. This would not qualify as a PD, because it may be less pervasive and not present from an early age (p. 560).

Other mental disorders. When they persist for a long time (usually years), a variety of other mental conditions can distort the way a person behaves and relates to others. This can give the appearance of a personality disorder. Especially good examples include dysthymia, schizophrenia, social anxiety disorder, and cognitive disorders. Some studies find that patients with mood disorders are more likely to show personality traits or PDs when they are clinically depressed; this may be especially true of Cluster A and Cluster C traits. Personality pathology noted in depressed patients should be reevaluated once the depression has remitted.

Other specified, or unspecified, personality disorder. Use one of these categories for personality disturbances that do not meet the criteria for any of the disorders above, or for PDs that have not achieved official status (p. 563).

Introduction

All humans (and numerous other species as well) have personality traits. These are well-ingrained ways in which individuals experience, interact with, and think about everything that goes on around them. PDs are collections of traits that have become rigid and work to individuals' disadvantage, to the point that they impair functioning or cause distress. These patterns of behavior and thinking have been present since early adult life and have been recognizable in the patient for a long time.

Personality, and therefore PDs, should probably be thought of as dimensional rather than categorical; this means that their components (traits) are present in normal people, but are accentuated in those with the disorders in question. But for good reasons and bad, DSM-5 has retained the traditional categorical structure that has been used for more than 30 years. There are promises that this will change in the coming years; indeed, DSM-5 devotes a long portion of its Section III (material not officially approved for use) to exploring alternative diagnostic structures. However, the experts will first have to agree as to which dimensions to use, then how best to measure and categorize them, and then how to interpret the results. In the meantime, we will continue to muddle along pretty much as before.

As currently defined in DSM-5, all PDs have in common the following characteristics.

Essential Features of **a General Personality Disorder**

There is a lasting pattern of behavior and internal experience (thoughts, feelings, sensations) that is clearly different from the patient's culture. This pattern includes problems with affect (type, intensity, lability, appropriateness); cognition (how the patient sees and interprets self and the environment); control of impulses; and interpersonal relationships. This pattern is fixed and applies broadly across the patient's social and personal life.

The Fine Print

The D's: • Duration (lifelong, with roots in adolescence or childhood) • Diffuse contexts • Distress and disability (work/educational, social, and personal) • Differential diagnosis (substance use, physical illness, other mental disorders, other PDs, personality change due to another medical condition)

The information PDs convey gives the clinician a better understanding of the behavior of patients; it can also augment our understanding of the management of many patients.

As you read these descriptions and the accompanying vignettes, keep in mind the twin hallmarks of the PDs: early onset (usually by late teens) and pervasive nature, such that a disorder's features affect multiple aspects of work, personal, and social life.

Diagnosing Personality Disorders

The diagnosis of PDs presents a variety of problems. On the one hand, they are often overlooked; on the other, however, they are sometimes overdiagnosed (borderline PD is, in my opinion, a notorious example). One (antisocial PD) carries a terrible prognosis; most, if not all, are hard to treat. Their relatively weak validity suggests that no PD should be the sole diagnosis when another mental disorder can explain the signs and symptoms that make up the clinical picture. For all of these reasons, it is a good idea to have in mind an outline for making the diagnosis of a PD.

1. Verify the duration of the symptoms. Make sure that your patient's symptoms have been present at least since early adulthood (before age 15 for antisocial PD). Interviewing informants (family, friends, coworkers) will probably give you the most valid material.

2. Verify that the symptoms affect several areas of the patient's life. Specifically,

are work (or school), home life, personal life, and social life affected? This step can present real problems, in that patients themselves often don't see their behavior as causing problems. ("It's the world that's out of step.")

3. Check that the patient fully qualifies for the particular diagnosis in question. This means checking all the characteristics and consulting all 10 sets of diagnostic criteria. Sometimes you have to make a judgment call. Try to be as objective as possible. As with other mental disorders, with enough motivation you can usually force a patient into a variety of diagnoses.

4. If the patient is under age 18, make sure that the symptoms have been present for at least the past 12 months. (And be really, really sure that they aren't due instead to some other mental or physical disorder.) I personally prefer not making such a diagnosis at such a tender age.

5. Rule out other mental pathology that may be more acute and have greater potential for doing harm. The flip side is that other mental disorders are also often more responsive to treatment than are PDs.

6. This is also a good time to review the generic features for any other requirements you may have missed. Note that each patient must have two or more types of lasting problems with behavior, thoughts, or emotions from a list of four: cognitive, affective, interpersonal, and impulsive. (This helps ensure that the patient's problems truly do affect more than one life area.)

7. Search for other PDs. Evaluate the entire history to learn whether any additional PD is present. Many patients appear to have more than one PD; in such cases, diagnose them all. Perhaps more often, you will find too few symptoms to make any diagnosis. Then you can add to your summary note something to the effect: schizoid and paranoid personality traits.

8. Record all personality and nonpersonality mental diagnoses. Some examples of how this is done are shown in the vignettes that follow.

Although you can learn the rudiments of each PD from the material I present here, it is important to note that these abbreviated descriptions only begin to tap their rich psychopathology. If you want to make a study of these disorders, I strongly recommend that you consult standard texts.

Cluster A Personality Disorders

The PDs included in Cluster A share behaviors generally described as withdrawn, cold, suspicious, or irrational.

F60.0 [301.0] Paranoid Personality Disorder

What you notice most about patients with paranoid PD (PPD) is how little they trust—and how much they suspect—other people. The suspicions they harbor are unjustified, but because they fear exploitation, they will not confide in those whose behavior should have earned their trust. Instead, they read unintended meaning into benign comments and actions, and they will interpret untoward occurrences as the result of deliberate intent. They tend to harbor resentment for a long time, perhaps forever.

These people tend to be rigid and litigious, and may have an especially urgent need to be self-sufficient. To others, they can appear to be cold, calculating, guarded people who avoid both blame and intimacy. They may appear tense and have trouble relaxing during an interview. This disorder is especially likely to create occupational difficulties: Patients with PPD are so aware of rank and power that they frequently have trouble dealing with superiors and coworkers.

Although it is apparently far from rare (it may affect 1% of the general population), PPD rarely comes to clinical attention. When it does, it is usually diagnosed in men. Its relationship (if any) to the development of schizophrenia remains unclear, but if you find that it has preceded the onset of schizophrenia, add the specifier (*premorbid*).

Essential Features of **Paranoid Personality Disorder**

In many situations, these patients demonstrate that they distrust the loyalty or trustworthiness of others. Because they suspect that other people want to deceive, hurt, or exploit them, they hesitate to share personal information. Unjustified suspicions about the faithfulness of spouse or partner, or even the (mis)perception of hidden content in everyday events or speech, can lead to the bearing of grudges or to rapid response with anger or attacks in kind.

The Fine Print

The D's: • Duration (begins in teens or early 20s and endures) • Diffuse contexts • Differential diagnosis (physical and substance use disorders; mood, anxiety, and psychotic disorders; posttraumatic stress disorder; schizotypal and schizoid PDs)

Coding Note

If PPD precedes the onset of schizophrenia, add the specifier **(premorbid)**.

Dr. Schatzky

A professor of dermatology at University Hospital, Dr. Schatzky had never consulted a mental health professional. But he was well known to the staff at the medical center and notorious among his colleagues. One of them, Dr. Cohen, provided most of the information for this vignette.

Dr. Schatzky had been around for several years. He was known as a solid researcher and an excellent clinician. A hard worker, he supervised fellows working on two grants and carried more than his share of the teaching load.

One of the trainees working in his lab was a physician named Masters. He was a bright, capable young man whose career in academic dermatology seemed destined to soar. When Dr. Masters got an offer from Boston of an assistant professorship and his own lab space, he told Dr. Schatzky that he was sorry, but he would leave at the end of the semester. Furthermore, he wanted to use some of their data.

Dr. Schatzky was more than upset. He responded by telling Dr. Masters that "what happened in the lab stayed in the lab." He wouldn't allow anyone to "rip him off," and he told Dr. Masters that he would be blackballed if he tried to publish papers based on their findings. Furthermore, Dr. Schatzky told him to keep away from the students until he left. This outraged the other dermatologists. Dr. Masters was one of the most popular young teachers in the department, and the notion that he shouldn't have any contact with the students seemed punitive to all and little short of an assault on academic freedom.

The other dermatologists discussed the situation in a department meeting when Dr. Schatzky was out of town. One of the older professors had volunteered to try to persuade him to let Dr. Masters teach anyway. Subsequently, Dr. Schatzky refused with the response, "What have I done to you?" He now seemed to think that the other professor had it in for him.

This professor told Dr. Cohen that he wasn't really surprised. He'd known Dr. Schatzky since college, and he'd always been a suspicious type. "He won't confide in anyone without a signed loyalty oath," was how the other professor put it. Dr. Schatzky seemed to think that if he said anything nice, it would somehow be turned against him. The only person he seemed to trust completely was his wife, a rabbity little creature who had probably never disagreed with him in her life.

At the meeting, someone else suggested that the department chairman should talk to him and try to "jolly him along a bit." But Dr. Schatzky had little sense of humor and "the longest memory for a grudge of anyone on the face of the planet."

In the collective memory of all the staff, Dr. Schatzky had never had mood swings or psychosis, and at department dinners, he didn't drink. "Never out of touch with reality, only nasty," said Dr. Cohen.

Evaluation of Dr. Schatzky

I begin with a disclaimer: From the information available in this vignette, it would appear that Dr. Schatzky had never been interviewed by a mental health professional. Any conclusions must therefore be tentative. Clinicians simply have no right to make definitive diagnoses of patients—or just plain people—for whom they haven't gathered adequate information.

That said, Dr. Schatzky's symptoms had apparently been quite constant and present throughout his entire adult life (at least since college). His problems involved both his thinking and his interpersonal functioning, which in turn led to problems with his work and personal life.

What symptoms of PPD did Dr. Schatzky have? Without cause, he suspected young Dr. Masters of planning to "rip off" his data (criterion A1). His colleagues noted his long-standing concerns about the loyalty of associates (A2). He would never confide in others (A3), and he refused to let Dr. Masters teach, which sounds a lot like holding a grudge (A5). (However, he had apparently never questioned the loyalty of his wife, which would be another common symptom of this PD.) So we can find a total of four symptoms, which is what's required for a diagnosis of PPD.

Could a non-PD diagnosis explain Dr. Schatzky's behavior as described? Although the information is incomplete, drug or alcohol use appears unlikely. (It also seems unlikely that anyone of middle age could have been taking a medication long enough to produce character disturbance that had lasted his entire adult life.) The vignette provides no evidence of **another medical condition**. According to the information provided, Dr. Schatzky had never had frank psychosis, such as delusional disorder or schizophrenia, and he had no mood disorder (B).

What about other PDs? Patients with **schizoid PD** are cold and aloof, and as a result may appear distrustful, but they do not have the prominent suspiciousness characteristic of patients with PPD. Patients with **schizotypal PD** may have paranoid ideation, but they also appear peculiar or odd (not the case here). And Dr. Schatzky didn't appear to prefer solitude. Those with **antisocial PD** are often cold and unfeeling, may be suspicious, and have trouble forming interpersonal relationships. However, they rarely have the perseverance to complete professional school, and Dr. Schatzky had no history of criminal behavior or reckless disregard for the safety of others.

With a GAF score of 70, Dr. Schatzky's tentative diagnosis would be as follows:

F60.0 [301.0]   Paranoid personality disorder

F60.1 [301.20] Schizoid Personality Disorder

People with schizoid personality disorder (SzPD) are indifferent to the society of other people, sometimes profoundly so. Typically, they are lifelong loners who show a restricted emotional range; they appear unsociable, cold, and reclusive.

Patients with SzPD may succeed at solitary jobs that others find difficult to tolerate. They may daydream excessively, become attached to animals, and often do not marry or even form long-lasting romantic relationships. They do retain contact with reality, unless they develop schizophrenia. However, their relatives are not at increased risk for that disease.

Although it is uncommonly diagnosed, SzPD is relatively common, affecting perhaps a few percent of the general population. Men may be at greater risk than women. The following patient was the younger brother of Lyonel Childs, whose history has been presented in connection with schizophrenia (p. 67).

Essential Features of **Schizoid Personality Disorder**

In many situations, these patients remain isolated and have a narrow emotional range. Preferring solitude in their activities, they neither want nor enjoy close relationships, including those with family. They may have no close friends, with the possible exception of relatives. Indeed, they enjoy few activities, even showing little interest in sex with other people. Emotionally cold or detached, they seem indifferent to both criticism and praise.

The Fine Print

The D's: • Duration (begins in teens or early 20s and endures) • Diffuse contexts • Differential diagnosis (physical and substance use disorders, mood and psychotic disorders, autism spectrum disorder, schizotypal and paranoid PDs)

Coding Note

If schizoid personality disorder precedes the onset of schizophrenia, add the specifier **(premorbid).**

Lester Childs

"We brought him in because of what happened to Lyonel. They seemed so much alike, and we were worried." Lester's mother sat primly on the office sofa. "After Lyonel was arrested, that's when we decided."

At 20, Lester Childs was in many ways a carbon copy of his older brother. Born several weeks prematurely, he had spent his first few weeks of life in an incubator. But he gained weight rapidly and was soon well within the norms for his age.

He walked, talked, and was toilet-trained at the usual ages. Perhaps because they both worked so hard on the farm, or perhaps because there were no other young children for Lester and his siblings to play with, his parents noticed nothing wrong until Lester entered first grade. Within a few weeks, his teacher had telephoned to set up a conference.

Lester seemed bright enough, they were told; his schoolwork wasn't in question. But his sociability was next to nil. At recess, when the other children played dodge ball or pom-pom-pullaway, he remained in the classroom to color. He seldom participated in group discussions, and he always sat a few inches back from the others in the reading circle. When his turn for show and tell came, he stood silently in front of the class for a few moments, then pulled a length of kite string from his pocket and dropped it onto the floor. Then he sat down.

Most of this behavior was quite a lot like Lyonel's, so the parents hadn't been too worried. Even so, they took him to see their family doctor, who agreed that it was probably normal for their family and that he would "grow out of it." But Lester never did; he only grew up. He never even participated in family activities. At Christmas, he would open a present, take it over to a corner, and play with it by himself. Even Lyonel never did that.

When Lester entered the room, it was clear that he didn't regard the appointment as much of an occasion. He wore jeans with one knee missing, tattered sneakers, and a T-shirt that at one time surely had had sleeves. Through much of the interview, he continued to leaf through a magazine devoted to astronomy and math. After waiting more than a minute for Lester to say something, the interviewer began. "How are you today?"

"I'm OK." Lester kept on reading.

"Your mom and dad asked you to come in to see me today. Can you tell me why?"

"Not really."

"Do you have any ideas about it?"

[Silence.]

Most of the interview went that way. Lester willingly gave information when he was directly asked, but he seemed completely uninterested in volunteering anything. Sitting quietly, nose in his magazine, he showed no other abnormalities or eccentricities of behavior. His flow of speech (what there was of it) was logical and sequential. He was fully oriented, and he scored a perfect 30 on the MMSE. His mood was "OK"—neither too happy nor too sad. He had never used alcohol or drugs of any kind. He calmly but emphatically denied ever hearing voices, seeing visions, or having beliefs that he was being watched, followed, talked about, or otherwise interfered with. "I'm not like my brother," he said in his longest spontaneous speech up to that point.

When asked who he *was* like, Lester said it was Greta Garbo—who famously wanted to be left alone. He claimed he didn't need friends, and he could also do without his family. Neither did he need sex. He had checked out the sex magazines and anatomy books. Females and males were equally boring. His idea of a good way to spend his life was to live alone on an island, like Robinson Crusoe. "But no Friday."

Tucking his magazine under his arm, Lester left the office, never to return.

Evaluation of Lester Childs

Any diagnosis of a PD requires that the difficulties be both pervasive and enduring. Although he was only 20 years old, Lester's problems had certainly been enduring: They were noticeable when he was 6. And as far as we can tell, his rejection of interpersonal contact extended into every facet of his life—family, social, and school.

Lester rejected close relationships, even with his family (criterion A1); he preferred solitary activities (A2); he rejected the notion of having a sexual relationship with anyone (although this could conceivably change with maturity and opportunity—A3); he had always lacked close friends (A5); his affect seemed quite flat and detached (although this could have been an artifact of a first interview with a reluctant interviewee—A7). In any event, Lester met at least four and possibly five diagnostic criteria (four are required) for SzPD. These symptoms would satisfy three of the areas (cognition, affect, and interpersonal functioning) mentioned in the generic criteria for a PD. His interest in mathematics and astronomy would not be unusual in persons with this disorder, who typically thrive on work that others might find too lonely to enjoy.

Could any other disorder better explain Lester's clinical picture? Patients with **depressive disorders** are often withdrawn and unsociable, but these seldom persist life-long. Besides, Lester specifically denied feeling depressed or lonely; any doubts on the point could be settled by asking about vegetative symptoms of depression (changes in appetite or sleep). He also denied having symptoms (delusions and hallucinations) that would suggest **schizophrenia**, and this was supported by collateral information from his mother. There were no stereotypies or symptoms of impaired communication, as we'd expect for **autism spectrum disorder**, or disturbance of consciousness of memory, as would be required for a **cognitive disorder**. From the information we have, he was physically healthy and did not use drugs, alcohol, or medications (B).

What other PDs should we consider? Patients with **schizotypal PD** can have constricted affect and unusual appearance. Lester's clothing was out of keeping for most visits to a professional office but would probably be quite usual for someone 20 years old, and he denied having any beliefs that might seem odd. He did not voice any ideas of deep suspicion or distrust, such as might be encountered in **paranoid PD**. Patients with **avoidant PD** are also isolated from other people; unlike patients with SzPD, however, they don't choose this isolation, and they suffer for it.

If Lester later developed schizophrenia, the qualifier (*premorbid*) would be added at that time to his diagnosis. I find it difficult to place him squarely on the GAF Scale. The score of 65 is to some extent a matter of taste, and arguable.

F60.1 [301.20]   Schizoid personality disorder

F21 [301.22] Schizotypal Personality Disorder

From an early age, patients with schizotypal personality disorder (StPD) have lasting interpersonal deficiencies that severely reduce their capacity for closeness with others. They also have distorted or eccentric thinking, perceptions, and behaviors, which can make them seem odd. They often feel anxious when with strangers, and they have almost no close friends. They may be suspicious and superstitious; their peculiarities of thought include magical thinking and belief in telepathy or other unusual modes of communication. Such patients may talk about sensing a "force" or "presence," or have speech characterized by vagueness, digressions, excessive abstractions, impoverished vocabulary, or unusual use of words.

Patients with StPD may eventually develop schizophrenia. Many of them are depressed when they first come to clinical attention. Their eccentric ideas and style of thinking also place them at risk for becoming involved with cults. They get along poorly with others, and under stress they may become briefly psychotic. Despite their odd behavior, many marry and work. This disorder occurs about as often as schizoid PD.

Essential Features of **Schizotypal Personality Disorder**

In many situations, these patients tend to be isolated and exhibit a narrow emotional range with other people. They will have paranoid or suspicious ideas, even ideas of reference (which, however, are not held to a delusional extent). Their dress or mannerisms may give them an odd appearance, with affect that is inappropriate or constricted; speech can be vague, impoverished, or overly abstract. They may report strange perceptions or physical sensations, and their peculiar behavior may be affected by magical thinking or other odd beliefs (superstitions, a belief in telepathy). With severe social anxiety (which doesn't improve with acquaintance), they tend to have no intimate friends.

The Fine Print

The D's: • Duration (begins in teens or early 20s and endures) • Diffuse contexts • Differential diagnosis (physical and substance use disorders, psychotic disorders, mood disorders with psychotic features, autism spectrum disorder and other neurodevelopmental disorders, paranoid and schizoid PDs)

Coding Note

If StPD precedes the onset of schizophrenia, add the specifier **(premorbid)**.

Timothy Oldham

"But it's my baby! I don't care what he had to do with it!" Hugely pregnant and miserable, Charlotte Grenville sat in the interviewer's office and wept with frustration. She was there at the request of the presiding judge in a battle over visitation rights with her yet-unborn child.

The identity of the father was never in doubt. The week after her second missed period, Charlotte had visited a gynecologist and then called Timothy Oldham with the news. She had considered threatening to sue him for child support, but that hadn't been necessary. He made good money installing carpets and had no dependents. He offered her a generous monthly stipend, beginning immediately. But he wanted to help rear their child. Charlotte had rejected that idea out of hand and then filed suit. With a crowded court docket, the case had dragged on nearly as long as Charlotte's pregnancy.

"I mean, he's really weird!"

"What do you mean, 'weird?' Give me some examples."

"Well, I've known him for the longest time—several years, anyway. He had a sister who died; he talks about her like she's still alive. And he does weird things. Like, when we were making love, right in the middle he started this babble about 'holy love' and dedicating his seed. It put me right off. I told him to stop and get off, but it was too late. I mean, would you want your kid growing up with that for a father?"

"If he's so peculiar, how did you get involved with him?"

She looked abashed. "Well, we only did it once. And I might have been a little bit drunk at the time."

Timothy was not only sedate, but nearly immobile. He sat quietly in the interview chair, a gangly blond whose hair swept across his forehead nearly to his eye brows. He told his story in a dull monotone that didn't reveal the slightest trace of emotion.

Timothy Oldham and his twin sister, Miranda, had been orphaned when they were 4 years old. He had no memory of his parents, other than a vague impression that they might have made their living from a marijuana farm in northern California. The two children had been taken in by an aunt and uncle—Southern Baptists who, he said, made the farm couple in Grant Woods's *American Gothic* look cheerful by comparison. "That painting, it's really them. I have a copy of it in my bedroom. Sometimes I can almost see my uncle moving the pitchfork back and forth to signal me."

"Is it really your uncle, and does the pitchfork really move?" the interviewer wanted to know.

"Well, it's more of a feeling I get . . . not really . . . a sign of my Christian endeavor . . ." Timothy's voice trailed off, but he kept gazing straight ahead.

The "Christian endeavor," he explained, meant that everyone was put on earth for some special purpose. His uncle always used to say that. He thought his own purpose might be to help raise the baby growing inside Charlotte. He knew there had to be more to life than laying carpets all day.

Timothy had only a few friends, none of them close. He and Charlotte had spent no more than a few hours together. In response to a question, he talked about his sister. Miranda and he had been understandably close; she was the only real friend he had ever had. She died of a brain tumor when they were 16, and Timothy was devastated. "We were webbed together when we were born. I swore at her graveside it would never be undone."

With still no inflection in his voice, Timothy explained that being "webbed together" was something you were born with. He and Miranda still were webbed. It was a Christian endeavor, and she was directing him from beyond the grave to have a baby girl. He said that it would be having Miranda back again. He knew that the baby wouldn't actually *be* Miranda, but said he knew it would be a girl. "It's just one of those feelings. But I know I'm right."

Timothy responded in the negative to the usual questions about hallucinations, delusions, abnormal moods, substance use, and medical problems such as head injury and seizure disorders. Then he arose from his seat and left the room without another word.

That evening Charlotte Grenville gave birth—to a healthy boy.

Evaluation of Timothy Oldham

Charlotte's testimony suggested that Timothy's peculiarities had been present for years. Although we don't know much about his school career or work, his symptoms would seem likely to affect most areas of his life. This point should be more fully explored.

Timothy's schizotypal symptoms included odd beliefs (his conviction that the baby would be his sister returned to earth; there is no evidence that he came from a subculture where this sort of thinking was the norm—criterion A2), illusions (the farmer in the picture waving his pitchfork—A3), constricted affect (A6), and absence of close friends (A8). His words ("webbed together," "Christian endeavor") seemed metaphorical and odd (A4). Unexplored by the interviewer were the presence of ideas of reference, paranoid ideas, odd behavior, and excessive social anxiety. Cognitive, affective, and interpersonal symptoms were represented here, however (see the Essential Features for a general PD).

This evaluation turned up no indications of another mental disorder. Timothy specifically denied the actual psychotic symptoms necessary to support a diagnosis of **delusional disorder** or **schizophrenia**. Other conditions that could entail psychotic symptoms include **mood disorders** and **cognitive disorders**, but we've seen evidence against both (B).

Other PDs to consider would include **schizoid** and **paranoid PDs**. Each of these implies some degree of social isolation, but not the eccentric thinking of StPD. Patients with any of these three Cluster A disorders can decompensate into brief psychoses—a trait held in common with **borderline PD**. Some patients may qualify for two diagnoses simultaneously: borderline PD and one of the Cluster A PDs. Patients with **avoidant PD** are socially isolated, but they suffer from it and lack odd behavior and thinking. Of course, a **personality change due to another medical condition** must be considered in those who have a severe or chronic illness; Timothy didn't.

As of this evaluation, Tim would receive a GAF score of 75. He hadn't developed schizophrenia, so we wouldn't use the qualifier *(premorbid)*.

F21 [301.22]	Schizotypal personality disorder
Z65.3 [V62.5]	Litigation regarding child visitation

Cluster B Personality Disorders

People with Cluster B PDs tend to be dramatic, emotional, and attention-seeking, with moods that are labile and often shallow. They often have intense interpersonal conflicts.

F60.2 [301.7] Antisocial Personality Disorder

Those with antisocial PD (ASPD) chronically disregard and violate the rights of other people; they cannot or will not conform to the norms of society. This said, there are a number of ways in which people can exhibit ASPD. Some are engaging con artists; others are, frankly, graceless thugs. Women (and some men) with the disorder may be involved in prostitution. In still other individuals, the more traditional antisocial aspects may be obscured by the heavy use (and often purveyance) of illicit drugs.

Although some of these people seem superficially charming, many are aggressive and irritable. Their irresponsible behavior affects nearly every life area. Besides substance use, there may be fighting, lying, and criminal behavior of every conceivable sort: theft, violence, confidence schemes, and child and spouse abuse. They may claim to have guilt feelings, but they don't appear to feel genuine remorse for their behavior. Although they may complain of multiple somatic problems and will occasionally make suicide attempts, their manipulative interactions with others make it difficult to determine whether their complaints are genuine.

DSM-5 criteria for ASPD specify that, beginning before age 15, the patient must have a history that would support a diagnosis of conduct disorder (p. 381); as an adult, this behavior must have continued and been extended, with at least four ASPD symptoms.

As many as 3% of men, but only about 1% of women, have this disorder; it is found in about three-quarters of penitentiary prisoners. It is more common among lower-socioeconomic-status populations and runs in families; it probably has both a genetic and an environmental basis. Male relatives have ASPD and substance-related disorders; female relatives have somatic symptom disorder and substance-related disorders. Childhood attention-deficit/hyperactivity disorder is a common precursor, and childhood conduct disorder is a requirement (see above).

Although treatment seems to make little difference to patients with ASPD, there is some evidence that the disorder decreases with advancing age, as these people mellow out to become "only" substance users. Death by suicide or homicide is the lot of others.

Generally, the diagnosis of ASPD will not be warranted if antisocial behavior occurs only in the context of substance abuse. Individuals who misuse substances sometimes engage in criminal behavior, but only when in pursuit of drugs. It is crucial to learn whether patients with possible ASPD have engaged in illicit acts when not using substances.

Although these patients often have a childhood marked by incorrigibility, delinquency, and school problems such as truancy, fewer than half the children with such a background eventually develop the full adult syndrome. Therefore, we should never make this diagnosis before age 18.

Finally, ASPD is a serious disorder, with no known effective treatment. It is therefore a diagnosis of last resort. Before making it, redouble efforts to rule out other major mental disorders and PDs.

Essential Features of **Antisocial Personality Disorder**

These patients have a history dating to before age 15 of destroying property, serious rule violation, or aggression against people or animals (that is, they fulfill criteria for conduct disorder, p. 381). Since then, in many situations, they lie, con, or give an alias while engaging in behaviors that merit arrest (whether or not they are actually detained). They tend to fight or assault others, and generally fail to plan their activities, relying instead on the inspiration of the impulse. For none of this behavior do they show remorse, other than feeling sorry if caught. They will refuse to pay their debts or maintain steady employment. They may irresponsibly place themselves or other people in danger.

The Fine Print

The D's: • Duration and demographics (diagnosis cannot be made prior to age 18; behavior patterns are enduring) • Diffuse contexts • Differential diagnosis (physical and substance use disorders, bipolar disorders, schizophrenia, other PDs, ordinary criminality)

Milo Tark

Milo Tark was 23, handsome, and smart. When he worked, he earned good money installing heating and air conditioning. He had broken into that trade when he left high school, which happened somewhere in the middle of his 10th-grade year. Since then, he had had at least 15 different jobs; the longest of them had lasted 6 months.

Milo was referred for evaluation after he was caught trying to con money from elderly patrons at an ATM. The machine was one of two that served the branch bank where his mother worked as assistant manager.

"The little devil!" his father exclaimed during the initial interview. "He was always a difficult one to raise, even when he was a kid. Kinda reminded me of me, sometimes. Only I pulled out of it."

Milo had picked a lot of fights when he was a boy. He had bloodied his first nose when he was only 5, and the world-class spanking administered by his father had taught him nothing about keeping his fists to himself. Later he was suspended from the seventh grade for extorting $3 and change from an 8-year-old. When the suspension was finally lifted, he responded by ditching class for 47 straight days. Then began a string of encounters with the police, beginning with shoplifting (condoms) and progressing through breaking and entering (four counts) to grand theft auto when he was 15. For stealing the Toyota, he was sent for half a year to a camp run by the state youth authority. "It was the only 6 months his mother and I ever knew where he was at night," his father observed.

Milo's time in detention seemed to have done him some good, at least initially. Although he never returned to school, for the next 2 years he avoided arrest and intermittently applied himself to learning his trade. Then he celebrated his 19th birthday by getting drunk and joining the Army. Within a few months he was out on the street again, with a bad-conduct discharge for sharing cocaine in his barracks and assaulting two corporals, his first sergeant, and a second lieutenant. For the next several years, he worked when he needed cash and couldn't get it any other way. Not long before this evaluation, he had gotten a 16-year-old girl pregnant.

"She was just a ditsy broad." Milo lounged back, one leg over the arm of the interview chair. He had managed to grow a scraggly beard, and he rolled a toothpick around in the corner of his mouth. The letters H-A-T-E and L-O-V-E were clumsily tattooed across the knuckles of either hand. "She didn't object when she was gettin' laid."

Milo's mood was good now, and he had never had anything that resembled mania. There had never been symptoms of psychosis, except for the time he was coming off speed. He "felt a little paranoid" then, but it didn't last.

The ATM job was a scam thought up by a friend. The friend had read something like it in the newspaper and decided it would be a good way to obtain fast cash. They had never thought they might be caught, and Milo hadn't considered the effect it would have on his mother.

He yawned and said, "She can always get another job."

Evaluation of Milo Tark

Milo's behavior persistently affected all aspects of his life: school, work, family, and interpersonal relations. By the time he was 15, he easily met criteria for conduct disorder (ASPD criterion C). Afterwards, he moved on to full-blown adult criminality that persisted through his early 20s: repeated illegal acts (A1), assaults (on Army personnel—A4), irresponsible work record (A6), impulsivity (no planning about breaking into the ATM—A3), and lack of remorse (toward his mother and the girl he impregnated—A7). His symptoms touched on the areas of cognition, affect, interpersonal functioning, and impulse control (see the description of a general PD). Of course, he was now old enough (over 18—criterion B) to qualify for a diagnosis of ASPD.

People with a **manic episode** or **schizophrenia** will sometimes engage in criminal activity, but it is episodic and accompanied by other manic or psychotic symptoms. Milo steadfastly denied any behavior suggesting either a mood or a psychotic disorder (D). Patients with **intellectual disability** may break the law, either because they do not realize that it is wrong or because they are so easily influenced by others. Although Milo didn't do especially well in school, there is no indication that he was held back because of low intelligence.

Because many addicted patients will do nearly anything to obtain money, **substance use disorders** are important in the differential diagnosis. Milo had used cocaine and amphetamines, but (according to him) only briefly, and most of his antisocial behaviors were not associated with drug use. Patients with impulse-control disorders will engage in illegal activities, but this is confined to the context of **conduct disorder** in younger people and fighting or property destruction in **intermittent explosive disorder**. Patients with **bulimia nervosa** sometimes shoplift, but Milo had no evidence of bulimic episodes. Of course, many of these conditions (as well as the **anxiety disorders**) can be encountered as associated diagnoses in patients with ASPD.

Career criminals whose antisocial behavior is confined to their "professional lives" may not fulfill all of the criteria for ASPD. They may instead be diagnosed as having **adult antisocial behavior**, which would be recorded as Z72.811 [V71.01]. It constitutes part of the differential diagnosis of the PD.

With a GAF score of 35, Milo's complete diagnosis would be as follows:

| F60.2 [301.7] | Antisocial personality disorder |
| Z65.3 [V62.5] | Arrest for ATM fraud |

F60.3 [301.83] Borderline Personality Disorder

Throughout their adult lives, people with borderline PD (BPD) appear unstable. They're often at the crisis point as regards mood, behavior, or interpersonal relationships. Many feel empty and bored; they attach themselves strongly to others, then become intensely angry or hostile when they believe they are being ignored or mistreated by those they depend on. They may impulsively try to harm or mutilate themselves; these actions are expressions of anger, cries for help, or attempts to numb themselves to their emotional pain. Although patients with BPD may experience brief psychotic episodes, these resolve so quickly that they are seldom confused with psychoses like schizophrenia. Intense and rapid mood swings, impulsivity, and unstable interpersonal relationships make it difficult for these patients to achieve their full potential socially, at work, or in school.

BPD runs in families. These people are truly miserable—so much so that up to 10% complete suicide.

The concept of BPD was devised about the middle of the 20th century. These patients were originally (and sometimes still are) said to hover between neurosis and psychosis—a "borderline" whose existence is disputed by many clinicians. As the concept has evolved into a PD, it has achieved remarkable popularity, perhaps because so many patients can be shoehorned into its capacious definition.

Although 1–2% of the general population may legitimately qualify for a diagnosis of BPD, it is probably applied to a far greater proportion of the patients who seek mental health care. It may still be one of the most overdiagnosed conditions in the diagnostic manuals. Many of these patients have other disorders that are more readily treatable; these include major depressive disorder, somatic symptom disorder, and substance-related disorders.

Essential Features of **Borderline Personality Disorder**

These patients exist in a perpetual crisis of mood or behavior. They often feel empty and bored. Disturbed identity (insecure self-image) can lead them to attach themselves strongly to others and then reject these same people with equal vigor. On the other hand, they may frantically try to avert desertion (it can be actual or fantasied). Pronounced impulsiveness can lead them to harm or mutilate themselves or to engage in other potentially harmful behaviors, such as sexual indiscretions, spending sprees, eating binges, or reckless driving. Although stress can cause brief episodes of dissociation or paranoia, these quickly resolve. Intense, rapid mood swings may yield to anger that is inappropriate and uncontrolled.

The Fine Print

The D's: • Duration (begins in teens or early 20s and endures) • Diffuse contexts • Differential diagnosis (physical and substance use disorders, mood and psychotic disorders, other PDs)

Josephine Armitage

"I'm cutting myself!" The voice on the telephone was high-pitched and quavering. "I'm cutting myself right now! Ow! There, I've started." The voice howled with pain and rage.

Twenty minutes later, the clinician had Josephine's address and her promise that she would come in to the emergency room right away. Two hours later, her left forearm swathed in bandages, Josephine Armitage was sitting in an office in the mental health department. Criss-crossing scars furrowed her right arm from wrist to elbow. She was 33, a bit overweight, and chewing gum.

"I feel a lot better," she said with a smile. "I really think you saved my life."

The clinician glanced at her nonswathed arm. "This isn't the first time, is it?"

"I should think that would be pretty obvious. Are you going to be terminally dense, just like my last shrink?" She scowled and turned 90 degrees to look at the wall. "Sheesh!"

Her previous therapist had seen Josephine for a reduced fee, but had been unable to give her more time when she requested it. She had responded by letting the air out of all four tires of that clinician's new BMW.

Her current trouble was with her boyfriend. One of her girlfriends had been "pretty sure" she'd seen James with another woman two nights ago. Yesterday morning, Josephine had called in sick to work and staked out James's workplace so she could confront him. He hadn't appeared, so last evening she had banged on the door of his apartment until neighbors threatened to call the police. Before leaving, she'd kicked a hole in the wall beside his door. Then she got drunk and drove up and down the main drag, trying to pick up a date.

"Sounds dangerous," observed the clinician.

"I was looking for Mr. Goodbar, but no one turned up. I decided I'd have to cut myself again. It always seems to help." Josephine's anger had once again evaporated, and she had turned away from the wall. "Life's a bitch, and then you die."

"When you cut yourself, do you ever really intend to kill yourself?"

"Well, let's see." She chewed her gum thoughtfully. "I get so angry and depressed, I just don't care what happens. My last shrink said all my life I've felt like a shell of a person, and I guess that's right. It feels like there's no one living inside, so I might just as well pour out the blood and finish the job."

Evaluation of Josephine Armitage

The first thing this clinician should do is to determine whether the behaviors reported (and observed) had been present since Josephine's late teen years. From her report of the comment made by her "last shrink," this would seem to be the case, but it should be verified. These behaviors were pervasive: Her work was affected (calling in sick on a whim), as were her relations with her boyfriend and her previous therapist.

Josephine had an abundance of symptoms. The entire episode of staking out James's apartment could be seen as a frantic effort to avoid abandonment (BPD criterion A1). Even her initial moments with the present clinician revealed some swings between idealization and devaluation (criterion A2). She showed evidence of dangerous impulsivity (driving while under the influence of alcohol, trying to pick up a stranger—A4), and she had made repeated suicide attempts (A5). Her mood, even within the confines of this vignette, would seem markedly unstable and reactive to what she perceived to be the clinician's attitude toward her (A6); her anger was sudden, inappropriate, and intense (A8). She agreed with a description of herself as an "empty shell" (A7). Although patients with BPD are often described as having identity disturbance and occasional, brief psychotic lapses, Josephine's vignette gives no evidence of either of these. Even so, she had six or seven symptoms, whereas only five are required.

A long list of other mental disorders can be confused with BPD; each must be considered before settling on this disorder as a sole (or principal) diagnosis. (This isn't a criterion for BPD, but it is one of the generic PD criteria, as well as one of my personal mantras.) Many patients with BPD also have **major depressive disorder** or **dysthymia**. It's important to establish that suicidal behaviors, anger, and feelings of emptiness are not experienced only during episodes of depression. Similarly, we need to know that affective instability is not due to **cyclothymic disorder**. Note that the official criteria don't mention any of these possibilities, but they are featured in the text.

Patients with BPD can have psychotic episodes, but these tend to be brief and stress-related, and they resolve quickly and spontaneously—all of which makes them unlikely to be confused with **schizophrenia**. The misuse of various **substances** can lead to suicide behavior, instability of mood, and reduced impulse control. Substance-related disorders are also often found as concomitants with BPD, and should always be asked about carefully. Patients with **somatic symptom disorder** are often quite dramatic and may misuse substances and make suicide attempts. Although this vignette contains no evidence for any of these (other than getting drunk—was this an isolated event?), the evaluating clinician would need to consider carefully the list just given.

Patients with BPD can also show features of additional PDs. Josephine's presentation was dramatic, suggesting **histrionic PD**. Patients with **narcissistic PD** are also self-centered, though they don't have Josephine's impulsivity. Patients with **antisocial PD** are impulsive and do not control their anger; although some of Josephine's behaviors were destructive, she did not engage in overtly criminal activity.

Finally, **dissociative identity disorder** is sometimes encountered in patients with BPD. Further interviewing and observation would be needed to rule out this rare condition. Assuming the verification of Josephine's history, her diagnosis would be as given below. I would place her GAF score at 51.

F60.3 [301.83]	Borderline personality disorder
S51.809 [881.00]	Lacerations of forearm

There's no such thing as a late-life PD. By definition, the PDs are conditions present, more or less, from the get-go. If you encounter a patient whose character structure appears to have changed during the adult years, search for the cause until you find it. Usually, you'll turn up a personality change due to another medical condition, a mood or psychotic disorder, something substance-related, a cognitive issue, or a severe adjustment disorder.

F60.4 [301.50] Histrionic Personality Disorder

Patients with histrionic PD (HPD) have a long-standing pattern of extreme attention seeking and emotionalism that seeps into all areas of their lives. These people satisfy their need to be at center stage in two main ways: (1) Their interests and topics of conversation focus on their own desires and activities; and (2) they continually call attention to themselves by their behavior, including speech. They are overly concerned with physical attractiveness (of themselves and of others, as it relates to them), and they will express themselves so extravagantly that it can seem almost a parody of normal emotionality. Their need for approval can cause them to be seductive, often inappropriately (even flamboyantly) so. Many lead normal sex lives, but some will be promiscuous, and still others may be uninterested in sex.

These people are often so insecure that they constantly seek the approval of other people. Dependence on the favor of others may cause their moods to seem shallow or excessively reactive to their surroundings. Low tolerance for frustration can spawn temper tantrums. They usually like to talk with mental health professionals (it is another chance to be the center of attention), but because their speech is often vague and full of exaggerations, they can prove frustrating to interview.

Quick to form new friendships, people with HPD are also quick to become demanding. Because they are trusting and easily influenced, their behavior may appear inconsistent. They don't think very analytically, so they may have difficulty with tasks that require logical thinking, such as doing mental arithmetic. However, they may succeed in jobs that set a premium on creativity and imagination. Their craving for novelty sometimes leads to legal problems as they seek sensation or stimulation. Some have a remarkable tendency to forget affect-laden material.

HPD has not been especially well studied, but it is reportedly quite common. It may run in families. The classic patient is female, though the disorder can occur in men.

Essential Features of **Histrionic Personality Disorder**

These patients not only crave the limelight, but are unhappy when they are not the focus of attention. They actively attempt to draw attention to themselves with their physical appearance and mannerisms. Their manner of speaking may be overly dramatic, but what they say tends to be vague, lacking specificity. They can be gushing or effusive when expressing their emotions, which, however, tend to be superficial and fleeting. Too open to suggestion, too readily influenced, these people may interpret relationships as being intimate when they're not—even to the extent of behaving in ways that are improperly suggestive or seductive.

The Fine Print

The D's: • Duration (begins in teens or early 20s and endures) • Diffuse contexts • Differential diagnosis (physical and substance use disorders, somatic symptom disorder, other personality disorders)

Angela Black

Angela Black and her husband, Donald, had come for marriage counseling; as usual, they were fighting.

"He never listens to me. I might as well be talking to the dog!" Tears and mascara dripped onto the front of Angela's low-cut silk dress.

"What's there to listen to?" Donald retorted. "I know I irritate her, because she complains so much. But when I ask how she'd like me to change, she can never put her finger on it."

Angela and Donald were both 37 years old, and they had been married nearly 10 years. Already they had been separated twice. Donald made excellent money as a corporate lawyer; Angela had been a fashion model. She didn't work often any more, but her husband made enough to keep her well dressed and comfortably shod. "I don't think she's ever worn the same dress twice," Donald grumbled.

"Yes, I have," she snapped back.

"When? Name one time."

"I do it all the time. Especially recently." For several moments Angela defended herself, without ever making a concrete statement of fact.

"Res ipsa loquitur," said Donald with satisfaction.

"Oh, God, Latin!" She nearly howled. "When he puts in his superior, gratuitous Latin, it makes me want to cut my wrists!"

The Blacks agreed on one thing: For them, this was a typical conversation.

He worked late most nights and weekends, which upset her. She spent far too much money on jewelry and clothing. She relished the fact that she could still attract men. "I wouldn't do it if you paid more attention to me," she said, pouting.

"You wouldn't do it if you didn't listen to Marilyn," he retorted.

Marilyn and Angela had been best friends since their cheerleading days in high school. Marilyn was wealthy and independent; she didn't care what people thought, and behaved accordingly. Usually Angela followed right along.

"Like the pool party last summer," put in Donald, "when you took off your suits to 'practice cheers' for the races. Or was that your idea?"

"What would you know about it? You were working late. Besides, it was only the tops."

Evaluation of Angela Black

Angela's personality style had a profound effect on her marriage, though the vignette hints that her other social relationships (for example, men at the party) were affected as well. More information would be needed to establish that she had been this way throughout her adult life. However, it would seem unlikely that her way of doing business with the world had developed recently.

Angela's symptoms included a strong need to be the center of attention (HPD criterion A1) and sexual provocation (inferred from her dancing topless—A2); excessive concern with physical appearance (A4); dramatic emotional expression (A6); suggestibility (following the lead of her friend Marilyn—A7); and vague speech (commented on by her husband—A5). I thought she might have expressed a touch of rapidly shifting emotional expression (A3), too, but maybe that's just me. Conservatively scored, she had at least six symptoms of HPD (five are required by the DSM-5 criteria).

Her clinician should gather information adequate to determine that Angela did not have any of the major mental disorders that commonly accompany HPD. These include **somatic symptom disorder** (had she been in good physical health?) and **substance-related disorders**.

Would Angela qualify for other PD diagnoses? She was centrally focused on herself, and she liked to be admired. However, she lacked the sense of grandiose accomplishment that characterizes patients with **narcissistic PD**. You can often identify histrionic features in people with **borderline PD**. Angela's mood was somewhat labile, but she did not report interpersonal instability, identity disturbance, transient paranoid ideation, or other symptoms that characterize borderline patients. Her easy suggestibility might suggest **dependent PD**, but she was so far from leaning on her husband for support that she actively fought with him. With a GAF score of 65, I'd diagnose her as follows:

F60.4 [301.50]	Histrionic personality disorder
Z63.0 [V61.10]	Relationship distress with spouse

F60.81 [301.81] Narcissistic Personality Disorder

People with narcissistic PD (NPD) have a lifelong pattern of grandiosity (in behavior and in fantasy), a thirst for admiration, and an absence of empathy. These attitudes permeate most aspects of their lives. They regard themselves as unusually special; they are self-important individuals who commonly exaggerate their accomplishments. (From the outset, however, we need to note that these traits constitute a PD only in adults. Children and teenagers are naturally self-centered; in kids, narcissistic traits don't necessarily imply ultimate PD.)

Despite their grandiose attitudes, people with NPD have fragile self-esteem and often feel unworthy; even at times of great personal success, they may feel fraudulent or undeserving. They remain overly sensitive to what others think about them, and feel compelled to extract compliments. When criticized, they may cover their distress with a façade of icy indifference. As sensitive as they are about their own feelings, they have little apparent understanding of the feelings and needs of others and may feign empathy, just as they may lie to cover their own faults.

Patients with NPD often fantasize about wild success and envy those who have achieved it. They may choose friends they think can help them get what they want. Job performance can suffer (due to interpersonal problems), or it can be enhanced (due to their eternal drive for success). Because they tend to be concerned with grooming and value their youthful looks, they may become increasingly depressed as they age.

NPD has been seldom studied. It appears to occur in under 1% of the general population; reportedly, most patients are men. There is no information about family history, environmental antecedents, or other background material that might help us to understand these difficult personalities.

Essential Features of **Narcissistic Personality Disorder**

These people possess grandiosity, together with a craving for admiration. To get it, they typically exaggerate their own abilities and accomplishments. They tend to be preoccupied with fantasies of beauty, brilliance, perfect love, power, or limitless success, and believe that they are so unusual that they should only associate with people or institutions of rarefied status. Often arrogant or haughty, they may believe that others envy them (though the reverse may actually be true). Lack of empathy engages their feelings of privilege in justifying the exploitation of others to achieve their own goals.

The Fine Print

The D's: • Duration (begins in teens or early 20s and endures) • Diffuse contexts • Differential diagnosis (physical and substance use disorders, bipolar disorders, other personality disorders)

Berna Whitlow

"Dr. Whitlow, you're my backup for emergency clinic this afternoon. I've got to have some help from you!" Eleanor Bondurak, a social worker at the mental health clinic, was red-faced with anger and frustration. It wasn't the first time she had had difficulty working with this clinician.

At the age of 50, Berna Whitlow had worked at nearly every mental health clinic in the metropolitan area. She was well trained and highly intelligent, and she read voraciously in her specialty. Those were the qualities that had landed her job after job over the years. The qualities that kept her moving from one job to another were known better to those who worked with her than to those who hired her. She was famous among her colleagues for being pompous and self-centered.

"She said she wasn't going to take orders from me. And her attitude said for her, 'You're nothing but a social worker.'" Eleanor was now reliving the moment in a heated discussion with the clinical director. "She said she'd talk to my boss or to you. I pointed out that neither of you was in the building at the time, and that the patient had brought in a gun in his briefcase. So then she said I should 'write it up and submit it,' and she would 'decide what action to take.' That's when I had you paged."

With the crisis over (the gun had been unloaded, the patient not dangerous), the clinical director had dropped in to chat with Dr. Whitlow. "Look, Berna, it's true that ordinarily the social worker sees the patient and does a write-up before you step in. But this wasn't exactly an ordinary case! Especially in emergencies, the whole team has to act together."

Berna Whitlow was tall, with a straight nose and jutting chin that seemed to radiate authority. Her long hair was thick and blond. She raised her chin a bit higher. "You hardly need to lecture me on the team approach. I've been a leader in nearly every clinic in town. I'm a superb team leader. You can ask anyone." As she spoke, she rubbed the gold rings that encircled nearly every finger.

"But being a team leader involves more than just giving orders. It's also about gathering information, building consensus, caring about the feelings of oth—"

"Listen," she interrupted, "it's her job to work on my team. It's my job to provide the leadership and make the decisions."

Evaluation of Berna Whitlow

From the material we have (which does not include a clinical interview, so our conclusions must be tentative), Dr. Whitlow's personality traits would seem to have caused difficulties for many years. They affected her life broadly, interfering with work (many jobs) and interpersonal relationships. Of course, a full assessment would inquire about her personality as it affected her home and social life.

Symptoms suggestive of NPD included her haughty attitude (NPD criterion A9), exaggerating her own accomplishments ("I'm a superb team leader"—A1), insisting that she receive orders or requests only from persons of high rank (A3), expecting obedience (from a sense of entitlement—A5), and lacking empathy with fellow workers (A7). Five criteria are needed; affective, cognitive, and interpersonal features were present (see the Essential Features of a general PD).

Several other PDs can either accompany or be confused with NPD. Patients with **histrionic PD** are also extremely self-centered, but Dr. Whitlow was not as theatrical (although she did wear a lot of rings). As is the case in **borderline PD** (and most other PDs), patients with NPD have a great deal of trouble relating to other people. But they (including Dr. Whitlow) are not especially prone to unstable moods, suicidal behavior, or brief psychoses under stress. Although there is a hint of the deceitful in narcissistic exaggerations, these people lack the pervasive criminality and disregard for the rights of others that are typical of **antisocial PD**.

Although **dysthymia** and **major depressive disorder** frequently accompany NPD, there is no evidence in the vignette to support either of those diagnoses. Dr. Whitlow's tentative diagnosis (GAF score of 61) would be as follows:

F60.81 [301.81]   Narcissistic personality disorder

Cluster C Personality Disorders

Patients with Cluster C PDs are characteristically anxious, tense, and overcontrolled.

F60.6 [301.82] Avoidant Personality Disorder

People with avoidant PD (APD) feel inadequate, are socially inhibited, and are overly sensitive to criticism. These characteristics are present throughout adult life, and affect most aspects of daily life. (Like narcissistic traits, avoidant traits are common in children and don't necessarily imply eventual PD.)

Their sensitivity to criticism and disapproval makes these people self-effacing and eager to please others, but it can also lead to marked social isolation. They may misinterpret innocent comments as critical; often they refuse to begin a relationship unless they are sure they will be accepted. They will hang back in social situations for fear of saying something foolish, and may avoid occupations that involve social demands. Other than their parents, siblings, or children, they tend to have few close friends. Comfortable with routine, they may go to great lengths to avoid departing from their set ways. In an interview they can appear tense and anxious; they may misinterpret even benign statements as criticism.

Although APD has appeared in the DSMs since 1980, relevant research is *still* sparse. In frequency, it occupies middle ground (about 2% of the general population) as PDs go, roughly equal for men and women. Many such patients marry and work, although they may become depressed or anxious if they lose their support systems. Sometimes this disorder is associated with having a disfiguring illness or condition. APD is not often seen clinically; these patients tend to come to evaluation only when another illness supervenes. There is considerable overlap with social anxiety disorder.

Essential Features of **Avoidant Personality Disorder**

These patients are socially inhibited, are overly sensitive to criticism, and feel inadequate. Feeling themselves inferior, unappealing, or clumsy, they are reluctant to form new relationships. Such people so fear ridicule or shame that they will only become involved with others if they can know in advance they will be accepted. Otherwise, their worry about being rejected or criticized (or embarrassed) on the job or in social situations will lead them to avoid new pursuits.

The Fine Print

The D's: • Duration (begins in teens or early 20s and endures) • Diffuse contexts • Differential diagnosis (physical and substance use disorders, social anxiety disorder, paranoid and schizoid PDs)

Jack Weiblich

Jack Weiblich was feeling worse when he ought to be feeling better. At least, that's what his new acquaintances in Alcoholics Anonymous had told him. One had reminded him that 30 days' sobriety was "time enough to detox every last cell" in his body. Another thought he was having a "dry drunk."

"Whatever a 'dry drunk' is," Jack observed later. "All I know is that after 5 weeks without alcohol, I'm feeling every bit as bad as I did 15 years ago, before I'd ever had a drop. I've enjoyed hangovers more than this!"

At age 32, Jack had a lot of hangovers to choose from. He'd had his first drink when he was only a senior in high school. He had been a strange, lonely sort of kid who'd had a great deal of difficulty meeting other people. While he was still in high school, he had begun to lose his hair; now, with the exception of his eyebrows and eyelashes, he was totally bald. He was also afflicted with a slight, persistent nodding of his head. "Titubation," the neurologist had said; "don't worry about it." The sight of his balding, nodding head in the mirror every morning looked grotesque, even to Jack. As a teenager he found it almost impossible to form relationships; he was positive that no one could like someone as peculiar as he was.

Then one evening Jack found alcohol. "Right from the first drink, I knew I'd discovered something important. With two beers on board, I forgot all about my head. I even asked a girl out. She turned me down, but it didn't seem to matter that much. I had found a life." But the following morning, he found that he still had his old personality. He experimented for months before he learned when and how much he could drink and maintain a glow sufficiently rosy to help him feel well, but not too rosy to function. During a 3-week period in his senior year at law school when he sobered up completely, he discovered that without alcohol, he still had the same old feelings of isolation and rejection.

"When I'm not drinking, I don't feel sad or anxious," Jack observed. "But I'm lonely and uncomfortable with myself, and I feel that other people will feel the same about me. I guess that's why I just don't make friends."

After law school, Jack went to work for a small firm that specialized in corporate law. They called him "The Mole," because he spent nearly all of every work day in the law library doing research. "I just didn't feel comfortable meeting the clients—I never get along well with new people."

The only exception to this lifestyle was Jack's membership in the stamp club. From his grandfather, he had inherited a large collection of commemorative plate blocks. When he took these to the Philatelic Society, he thought they'd welcome him with open arms, and they did. He continued to build upon his grandfather's collection and attended meetings once a month. "I guess I feel OK there because I don't have to worry whether they'll like me. I've got a great stamp collection for them to admire."

Evaluation of Jack Weiblich

Jack's symptoms were pervasive (profoundly affecting his work and social life) and had been present long enough (since he was a teenager) to qualify for a PD. They included the following typical APD features: He avoided interpersonal contact (for example, with clients at the law firm—criterion A1); he felt that he was unappealing (A6); although he joined the stamp club, he was pretty sure that his collection would be accepted (A2); he worried a lot about being rejected (A4). Only four criteria are needed; cognitive, occupational, and interpersonal areas were involved for Jack Weiblich (see the Essential Features for a general PD).

Depression and anxiety are both common in patients with APD. Therefore, it is important to search for evidence of **mood disorders** and **anxiety disorders** (especially **social anxiety disorder**) in patients who avoid contact with others. Jack stated explicitly that he felt neither sad nor anxious, but he admitted that he had severely misused alcohol. The **substance-related disorders** also commonly bring a patient with APD to the attention of mental health care providers.

In both APD and **schizoid PD**, patients spend most of their time alone. The difference, of course, is that patients with APD are unhappy with their condition, whereas people with schizoid PD prefer it that way. A somewhat more difficult differential diagnosis may be that between APD and **dependent PD**. (Dependent patients avoid positions of responsibility, as Jack did.) Note that Jack's avoidant lifestyle may have been bound up in his twin physical peculiarities, his baldness and nodding head.

Although Jack had an alcohol use disorder, his clinician felt that it was causing him little current difficulty and that the PD was the fundamental problem needing treatment (other clinicians might argue with this interpretation). That's why the PD was listed as his principal diagnosis. Of course, he didn't qualify for any course modifiers for alcohol use disorder, because he'd only been on the wagon for 5 weeks (p. 409); I thought his alcoholism was pretty mild, actually (and note that the PD doesn't enter into the coding of the substance use disorder; see Table 15.2 in Chapter 15). I'd put his GAF score at 61.

F60.6 [301.82]	Avoidant personality disorder
F10.10 [305.00]	Alcohol use disorder, mild
L63.1 [704.09]	Alopecia universalis
R25.0 [781.0]	Nodding of head

F60.7 [301.6] Dependent Personality Disorder

Much more so than most, patients with dependent PD (DPD) feel the need for some-one else to take care of them. Because they desperately fear separation, their behavior becomes so submissive and clinging that it may result in others' taking advantage of them or rejecting them. Anxiety blossoms if they are thrust into a position of leadership, and they feel helpless and uncomfortable when they are alone. Because they typically need much reassurance, they may have trouble making decisions. Such patients have trouble starting projects and sticking to a job on their own, though they may do well under the careful direction of someone else. They tend to belittle themselves and to agree with people who they know are wrong. They may also tolerate considerable abuse (even battering).

Though it may occur commonly, this condition has not been well studied. Some writers believe that it is difficult to distinguish it from avoidant PD. It has been found more often among women than men. Bud Stanhope, a patient with the sleep terror type of non-rapid eye movement sleep arousal disorder, also had DPD; his history is given on page 334.

Essential Features of **Dependent Personality Disorder**

The need for supportive relationships draws these people into clinging, submissive behavior and fears of separation. Fear of disapproval makes it hard to disagree with others; to gain support, they will even take extraordinary steps, such as assuming unpleasant tasks. Low self-confidence prevents them from starting or carrying out projects independently; indeed, they want others to take responsibility for their own major life areas. If they do make even everyday decisions, they require lots of advice and reassurance. Exaggerated, unrealistic fears of abandonment and the notion that they cannot care for themselves will cause these people to feel helpless or uncomfortable when alone; they may desperately seek a replacement for a lost close personal relationship.

The Fine Print

The D's: • Duration (begins in teens or early 20s and endures) • Diffuse contexts • Differential diagnosis (physical and substance use disorders, mood and anxiety disorders, other PDs)

Janet Greenspan

A secretary in a large Silicon Valley company, Janet Greenspan was one of the best workers there. She was never sick or absent, and she could do anything—she'd even had some bookkeeping experience. Her supervisor noted that she was polite on the phone, typed like a demon, and would volunteer for anything. When the building maintenance crew went out on strike, Janet came in early every day for a week to clean the toilets and sinks. But still, somehow, she just wasn't working out.

Her supervisor complained that Janet needed too much direction, even for simple things—such as what sort of paper to type form letters on. When she was asked what *she* thought the answer should be, her judgment was good, but she always wanted guidance anyway. Her constant need for reassurance took an inordinate amount of her supervisor's time. That was why she had been referred to the company mental health consultant for an evaluation.

At 28, Janet was slender, attractive, and carefully dressed. Her chestnut hair already showed streaks of gray. She appeared at the doorway of the office and asked, "Where would you like me to sit?" Once she started talking, she spoke readily about her life and her work.

She had always felt timid and unsure of herself. She and her two sisters had grown up with a father who was affectionate but dictatorial; their mouse of a mother seemed to welcome his loving tyranny. At her mother's knee, Janet had learned obedience well.

When Janet was 18, her father suddenly died; within a few months, her mother remarried and moved to another state. Janet felt bereft and panic-stricken. Instead of beginning college, she took a job as a teller in a bank; soon afterward, she married one of her customers. He was a 30-year-old bachelor, set in his ways, and he soon let it be known that he preferred to make all of the couple's decisions himself. For the first time in a year, Janet relaxed.

But even security bred its own anxieties. "Sometimes at night I wake up, wondering what I'd do if I lost him," Janet told the interviewer. "It makes my heart beat so fast I think it might stop from exhaustion. I just don't think I could manage on my own."

Evaluation of Janet Greenspan

Janet had the following symptoms of DPD: She needed considerable advice to make everyday decisions (criterion A1); she wanted her husband to make their decisions (A2); panic-stricken when her father died and her mother left town, she fled into an early marriage (A7); she feared being left to fend for herself, even though she had had no indication that this was likely (A8). She even volunteered to clean the office toilet, probably to secure the favor of the rest of the staff (A5). We have no evidence that she was reluctant to disagree with others, but otherwise the criteria fit like a rubber glove. Five are needed for diagnosis. Janet reported that she had been this way since childhood; from the history, her character traits would seem to have affected both work and social life. Fortunately, she married someone whose need to be in charge matched her dependency. Cognitive, affective, and interpersonal areas were involved (see the criteria for a general PD).

Dependent behavior is found in several mental disorders that Janet did not appear to have, including **somatic symptom disorder** and **agoraphobia**. The person with the secondary psychosis in what used to be called *folie à deux* (or shared psychotic disorder—now it is usually diagnosed as **delusional disorder**) often has a dependent personality. **Major depressive disorder** and **dysthymia** are important in the differential diagnosis; either of these may become prominent when patients lose those upon whom they depend. Even if Janet had all the required physiological symptoms for **generalized anxiety disorder**, she would not be given this diagnosis, because her worries were evidently limited to fears of abandonment.

Patients with DPD must be differentiated from those with **histrionic PD**, who are impressionable and easily influenced by others (but Janet did not seem to be especially attention-seeking). Other PDs usually included in the differential diagnosis are **borderline** and **avoidant**.

With a GAF score of 70, Janet's diagnosis would be simple:

F60.7 [301.6]   Dependent personality disorder

F60.5 [301.4] Obsessive–Compulsive Personality Disorder

People with obsessive–compulsive PD (OCPD) are perfectionistic and preoccupied with orderliness; they need to exert interpersonal and mental control. These traits exist on a lifelong basis, at the expense of efficiency, flexibility, and candor. However, OCPD is not just obsessive–compulsive disorder (OCD) in miniature. Many patients with OCPD have no actual obsessions or compulsions at all, though some do eventually develop OCD.

The rigid perfectionism of these patients often results in indecisiveness, preoccupation with detail, scrupulosity, and insistence that others do things their way. These behaviors can interfere with their effectiveness in work or social situations. Often they seem depressed, and this depression may wax and wane, perhaps to the point that it drives them into treatment. Sometimes these people are stingy; they may be savers, refusing to throw away even worthless objects they no longer need. They may have trouble expressing affection.

Patients with OCPD are list makers who allocate their own time poorly, workaholics who must meticulously plan even their own pleasure. They may plan their own vacations only to postpone them. They resist the authority of others, but insist on their own. They may be perceived as stilted, stiff, or moralistic.

This condition is probably fairly common; prevalence in various studies centers around 5%. It is diagnosed more often in males than in females, and it probably runs in families.

Essential Features of **Obsessive–Compulsive Personality Disorder**

These people are intensely focused on control, orderliness, and perfection. They can become so absorbed with details, organization, and rules of an activity that they lose sight of its purpose. They tend to be rigid and stubborn, perhaps so perfectionistic that it interferes with the completion of tasks. They can be overly conscientious, inflexible, or scrupulous about ethics, morals, and values. Some are workaholics; others won't work unless others agree to do things the patients' way. Some may save worthless items; others are stingy with themselves and with other people.

The Fine Print

The D's: • Duration (begins in teens or early 20s and endures) • Diffuse contexts • Differential diagnosis (physical and substance use disorders, OCD, hoarding disorder, other PDs)

Robin Chatterjee

"I admit it—I'm over the top in neatness." Robin Chatterjee straightened a fold in her sari. Born in Mumbai and educated in London, Robin was a graduate student in biology. Now she spent part of her time as a teaching assistant in biology, and the rest struggling through her own coursework at a major U.S. university. She gazed steadily at the interviewer.

According to her preceptor, a slightly dour Scot named MacLeish who had asked her to come for the interview, the problem wasn't neatness. It was completing the work. Every paper she turned in was wonderful—every fact was there, every conclusion correct, not even a misspelling. He had asked her why she couldn't learn to let go of them a little sooner, "before the rats die of old age?" She had thought it funny at the time, but it made her think.

Robin had always been orderly. Her mother had made her keep neat little lists of her chores, and the habit stuck. Robin admitted that she became so "lost in lists" that sometimes she hardly had time to finish her work. Her students seemed fond of her, but several had said they wished she'd give them more responsibility. One had told Dr. MacLeish that Robin seemed afraid even to let them do their own dissections; their methods weren't as compulsively correct as hers were, so she'd try to do them herself. Finally, she also admitted that nearly every night, her work habits kept her in the lab until late. It had been weeks since she'd had a date—or any social life at all. This realization was what spurred her to follow Dr. MacLeish's advice and come in for a mental health evaluation.

Evaluation of Robin Chatterjee

Although the prototype for OCPD seems a pretty good fit for Robin, she would just barely meet the official criteria. She was workaholic and perfectionistic (OCPD criteria A3 and A2), to the point that these traits interfered with the learning of her students. She had a great deal of difficulty delegating work—even the students' own dissections (A6)! And she concentrated so fiercely on her lists of tasks that she sometimes didn't accomplish the tasks themselves (A1). She had had these tendencies throughout her young adult life.

Depressed mood is common in these people. The common disorders that should be looked for in a patient with OCPD include **OCD** itself, **major depressive disorder**, and **dysthymia**. Robin was not depressed and, unlike so many patients with OCPD, seemed to have no other disorder. Because she barely met the criteria and was functioning well overall, I would place her GAF score at a relatively high 70.

F60.5 [301.4]   Obsessive–compulsive personality disorder

Other Personality Conditions

F07.0 [310.1] Personality Change Due to Another Medical Condition

Some medical conditions can cause a personality change, which is defined as an alteration (usually, a worsening) of a patient's previous personality traits. If the medical condition occurs early enough in childhood, the change can last throughout the person's life. Most instances of personality change are caused by an injury to the brain or by some other central nervous system disorder, such as epilepsy or Huntington's disease; however, systemic diseases that affect the brain (for example, systemic lupus erythematosis) are also sometimes implicated.

Several sorts of personality changes commonly occur. Mood may become unstable, perhaps with outbursts of rage or suspiciousness; other patients may become apathetic and passive. Changes in mood are especially common with damage to the frontal lobes of the brain. Patients with temporal lobe epilepsy may become overly religious, verbose, and lacking in a sense of humor; some may turn markedly aggressive. Paranoid ideas are also common. Belligerence can accompany outbursts of temper, to the extent that the social judgment of some patients becomes markedly impaired. Use the type specifiers in the Coding Notes to categorize the nature of the personality change.

If there is a major alteration in the structure of the brain, these personality changes will probably persist. If the problem stems from a correctable chemical problem, they may resolve. When severe, they can ultimately lead to dementia, as is sometimes the case in patients with multiple sclerosis.

Essential Features of **Personality Change Due to Another Medical Condition**

A physical illness or injury appears to have caused a patient to suffer a lasting personality change.

The Fine Print

From their *expected* developmental pattern, children will experience a personality change that lasts at least 1 year.

The D's: • Duration (enduring) • Distress or disability (work/educational, social, or personal) • Differential diagnosis (delirium, other physical or mental disorders)

Coding Notes

Depending on the main feature, specify type:

> **Aggressive type**
> **Apathetic type**
> **Disinhibited type**
> **Labile type**
> **Paranoid type**
> **Other type**
> **Combined type**
> **Unspecified type**

Use the actual name of the general medical condition when you code this disorder, and also code separately the medical condition.

Eddie Ortway

Eddie Ortway, now age 28, had been born in central Los Angeles, where he was reared by his mother—whenever she was neither hospitalized (for drug and alcohol use) nor jailed (for prostitution). His parents, Eddie always suspected, had been only briefly acquainted.

Eddie avoided school whenever possible, and grew up with no role model in sight. His principal accomplishment was learning to use his fists. By the time he was 15, he and his gang had participated in several turf wars. He was making a name for himself as an aggressive enemy.

But Eddie was not a criminal, and the necessity for earning a living soon set him to work. With little education and no training, he found his opportunities pretty much limited to fast food and hard labor. Sometimes he held several jobs at a time. But, as an old probation report noted, he still had "a raging sense of injustice." Although he gradually stopped associating with his gang, through his middle 20s he continued to deal aggressively with any situation that seemed to require direct action.

His 27th birthday was one of these. Eddie was delivering a pizza to an apartment building in his old neighborhood when he encountered a teenager forcing an old woman into an alley at gunpoint. Eddie stepped forward and for his pains received a bullet that entered his head through the left eye socket and exited at the hairline.

He was admitted to the hospital by way of the operating room, where surgeons debrided his wound. He never even lost consciousness and was released in less than a week. But he didn't return to work. The social worker's report noted that Eddie's physical condition had rebounded within a month, but that he "lacked drive." He appeared for every scheduled job interview, but his prospective employers uniformly reported that he "just didn't seem very interested in working."

"I needed time to recuperate," Eddie told the interviewer. He was a good-looking young man whose hair had begun receding from his forehead. An incisional scar ran up onto his scalp. "I still don't think I'm quite ready."

He had been recuperating for 2 years. Now he was being tested to try to learn why. Other than a slight droop to his left eyelid, his neurological examination was completely normal. An EEG showed some slow waves over the frontal lobes; the MRI revealed a localized absence of brain tissue.

Eddie never failed to cooperate with testing procedures, and all of the clinicians who examined him noted that he was polite and pleasant. However, as one of them put it, "There seems something slightly mechanical about his cooperation. He complies but never anticipates, and he shows little interest in the proceedings."

His affect was about medium and showed almost no lability. His speech was clear, coherent, and relevant. He denied delusions, hallucinations, obsessions, compulsions, or phobias. When asked what he was interested in, he thought for a few seconds and then answered that he guessed he was interested in going back home. He made a perfect score on the MMSE.

In the time since his injury, Eddie admitted, he had lived on workers' compensation and spent most of his time watching television. He didn't argue with anyone any more. When one examiner asked him what he would do if he again saw someone being mugged, he shrugged and said that he thought people should "just live and let live."

Evaluation of Eddie Ortway

Eddie's history and examinations presented an obvious general medical cause for his persistent personality change (criterion A). Note that it was the physiology of trauma to the brain that produced Eddie's personality change. This is the explicit requirement (B) for this diagnosis, which cannot be made when personality change accompanies a nonspecific medical condition such as severe pain.

Eddie's normal attention span and lack of memory deficit would rule out **delirium** (D) and **major neurocognitive disorder** (**dementia**); however, neuropsychological testing should be requested. A PD such as **dependent PD** could not explain Eddie's condition, because his behavior represented a marked change from his premorbid personality (that is, the way he was until his injury). And the features of Eddie's personality change were not better explained by a different physically induced mental disorder. A **mood disorder** due to brain trauma would be one of several possible examples.

Besides head trauma, a variety of neurological conditions can cause personality change. These include multiple sclerosis, cerebrovascular accidents, brain tumors, and temporal lobe epilepsy. Other causes of behavioral change that could resemble a change in personality include **delusional disorder**, **intermittent explosive disorder**, and **schizophrenia**. But Eddie's personality change began abruptly after he was shot, and he had no prior history that was consistent with any of the other disorders mentioned (C). However, many other patients experience apparent personality change associated with mental disorders, including addiction to substances.

The fact that Eddie's condition impaired him both occupationally and socially completed the criteria (E) for this diagnosis. In his clinical picture, apathy (and passivity) clearly stood out as the main feature. This determined the specific subtype. His GAF score would be a heart-breaking 55.

S06.330 [851.31]	Open gunshot wound of cerebral cortex, without loss of consciousness
F07.0 [310.1]	Personality change due to head trauma, apathetic type

F60.89 [301.89] Other Specified Personality Disorder

F60.9 [301.9] Unspecified Personality Disorder

The discussion in DSM-5 suggests that patients who have some traits of certain PDs, but who don't fully meet criteria for any of them, could be listed in one of these two categories. Here's my problem with that strategy: We would be branding someone who may be much less impaired than is the typical patient with a PD. My personal belief is that it would be better just to note in the summary the traits we've identified, and *not* make a firm diagnosis of any sort.

CHAPTER 18

Paraphilic Disorders

Quick Guide to the Paraphilic Disorders

The paraphilias include a variety of sexual behaviors that most people reject as distasteful, unusual, or abnormal: They involve something other than genital sex with a normal, consenting adult. A paraphilic disorder is diagnosed when a person feels distressed or is impaired by such a behavior. Nearly all of them are practiced largely, perhaps exclusively, by males.

Exhibitionistic disorder. The patient has urges for genital exposure to a stranger who does not expect it (p. 567).

Fetishistic disorder. The patient has sexual urges related to the use of inanimate objects (p. 569).

Frotteuristic disorder. The patient has urges related to rubbing his genitals against a person who has not consented to this (p. 571).

Pedophilic disorder. The patient has urges involving sexual activities with children (p. 574).

Sexual masochism disorder. The patient has sexual urges related to being injured, bound, or humiliated (p. 578).

Sexual sadism disorder. The patient has sexual urges related to inflicting suffering or humiliation on someone else (p. 580).

Transvestic disorder. An individual has sexual urges related to cross-dressing (p. 583).

Voyeuristic disorder. The patient has urges related to viewing some unsuspecting person disrobing, naked, or engaging in sexual activity (p. 586).

Other specified, or unspecified, paraphilic disorder. Quite a few paraphilic disorders are not widely practiced or have received too little clinical attention to warrant codes of their own (p. 588).

Introduction

Defining Paraphilias and Paraphilic Disorders

Literally, *paraphilia* means "abnormal or unnatural affection." Paraphilic sexual relationships differ from normal ones with respect to the preferred sexual objects or to how an individual relates to those objects. (Let us take *normal* to mean sex activity that focuses on genital stimulation with a consenting adult partner.) These sexual activities revolve around themes of (1) inanimate objects or nonhuman animals; (2) humiliation or suffering of the patient or partner; or (3) nonconsenting persons, including children. DSM-5 alternatively divides paraphilias into those that involve abnormal target preferences (children, fetishes, cross-dressing) and those involving abnormal activities (exhibitionism, voyeurism, sadism, masochism, frotteurism). There are many additional paraphilias in the world; those listed in DSM-5 are those that are more common and, in some cases, have a greater impact.

We must further differentiate between a *paraphilia* and a *paraphilic disorder*. The latter is a paraphilia that causes distress to the individual or harm to other people. This distinction allows a bit of parsimony in dispensing mental health diagnoses. For example, we don't have to attach a label of *disorder* to the behavior of a cross-dresser who is comfortable with and in no important way inconvenienced by the behavior. (In a 1991 survey of college students, over half admitted they engaged in some sort of paraphilic behavior.) In short, we identify the paraphilia by the urge, but the paraphilic disorder by the distress or impairment the urge provokes.

Mere desire or fantasy about these sexual activities can upset some patients enough to warrant a diagnosis, but it's far more common for patients to act upon their desires. (Indeed, DSM-5 carefully states that a person who claims to have no distress or disability—work/educational, social, personal, or other impairment—can still receive the diagnosis if the ideas have been repeatedly acted upon.) In descending order, the most common paraphilic disorders are pedophilic, exhibitionistic, voyeuristic, and frotteuristic. The rest are encountered much less frequently.

Several of these behaviors involve victims who do not consent. Frotteurs, voyeurs, sadists, and exhibitionists are acutely aware of their precarious legal state and usually take pains to avoid detection or to plan their escape. Pedophiles may delude themselves that what they are doing somehow benefits the children they target ("education," perhaps), but they nonetheless caution their victims not to tell their parents—or anyone else. Patients who seek clinical help because they have run afoul of the law may not reliably describe the motivation for their activities.

Paraphilic behavior may represent a high percentage of sexual episodes for many patients, whereas others may only indulge themselves occasionally, perhaps when under stress. Many patients have multiple paraphilias (the average is three or four). They may move from one paraphilic behavior to another, and may switch between classes of victim identified by gender, age, touching versus nontouching, and intra- versus extrafamilial status.

Although none of the criteria specify gender, apart from pedophiles, almost all patients with paraphilic disorders are male. Most fantasize sexual contact with their victims.

A paraphilic disorder is hardly ever due to another medical condition. However, unusual sexual behavior may be encountered in several other mental disorders: schizophrenia, bipolar I disorder (manic episodes), intellectual disability, and obsessive–compulsive disorder. In addition, personality pathology is frequently a concomitant of paraphilic behavior.

Although none of these criteria sets specify age, most paraphilias begin during adolescence. This is also the time when people begin to discover and explore their sexuality; adolescent boys, in particular, typically experiment with a variety of sexual behaviors. However, any teenager so involved with paraphilic behavior as to meet the diagnostic criteria that appear below should also be considered a candidate for diagnosis.

It should also be noted that the boundaries of what is considered normal in human sexual behavior are not sharply drawn. Although pedophilia is universally condemned, even by imprisoned felons, most other paraphilias have parallel behaviors in the general population. Revealing oneself, watching, and touching constitute part of everyday sexual experience. Even coercion and pain (in moderation) figure in the sexual activities of many people whose sex lives would be considered fairly conventional. Cross-dressing has for centuries been an important part of theater. I admit that I have trouble imagining a "normal" context for fetishism, however.

Specifiers for the Paraphilic Disorders

Note that, for each of the paraphilic disorders, there are two specifiers you can use to indicate that the person is no longer pursuing that particular behavior. Each of these specifiers is more likely to be applied to someone whose behavior can lead to legal difficulties—specifically, patients with exhibitionistic, frotteuristic, pedophilic, voyeuristic, and sometimes sexual sadism disorders.

In a controlled environment is intended for patients who are currently living in places that physically prevent pursuit of their paraphilic interests. These would include prisons, hospitals, nursing homes, and other facilities locked against the unsupervised freedom to roam.

In remission is a less restrictive term you can add to the diagnosis of a person who is *not* living in a controlled environment, yet has had no recurrence of the behavior in question and no distress or impairment from it for at least 5 years.

F65.2 [302.4] Exhibitionistic Disorder

Although no one knows just how many exhibitionists there are in the world, exhibitionism is one of the most commonplace sexual offenses (second only to voyeurism). Despite the fact that some women turn up in general population surveys, people who come to clinical or legal attention are almost invariably male, and their victims are nearly always female. In most cases, the victims are unsuspecting strangers; however, a small percentage of exposures are made to people known to the exhibitionist. Men who expose themselves to children may be quite different from those who expose to adults; for example, their recidivism rate is higher.

An exhibitionist tends to follow the same pattern with each offense. He may fantasize while driving around looking for a victim (often he is careful to leave himself an escape route to use if spotted by someone other than the victim). One individual may expose himself with an erection; another may be flaccid. Some are quite aggressive, savoring the look of shock or terror they produce. An exhibitionist may masturbate when he shows himself to the woman or later when he relives the scene in his imagination. Many will fantasize having sex with their victims, but most exhibitionists don't attempt to act upon such fantasies.

Exhibitionism usually begins before the age of 18, but it may persist until 30 or later. Often the urge to exhibit comes in waves: The patient may yield daily for a week or two, then remain inactive for weeks or months. Exhibitionistic behavior most often occurs when a patient is either under stress or has free time. The use of alcohol is seldom a factor.

Many exhibitionists have spouses or partners and pursue relatively normal sex lives, though their interest in sex may be greater than average. Although the behavior has traditionally been regarded as more a nuisance than an actual danger to others, it can coexist with other paraphilias. Perhaps 15% will have an offense involving contact, such as coercion, pedophilia, or rape. Clearly, a full assessment of paraphilic interests is indicated for any patient involved in exhibitionism.

Essential Features of **Exhibitionistic Disorder**

The person is aroused by genital self-exposure to an unwary stranger and has repeatedly acted on the urge (or feels distress/disability at the idea).

The Fine Print

The D's: • Duration (6+ months) • Distress or disability (work/educational, social, or personal) • Differential diagnosis (physical and substance use disorders, psychotic and bipolar disorders)

Coding Notes

Specify type:

Sexually aroused by exposing genitals to prepubertal children
Sexually aroused by exposing genitals to physically mature individuals
Sexually aroused by exposing genitals to prepubertal children and to physically mature individuals

Specify if:

In full remission (no symptoms for 5+ years)
In a controlled environment

Ronald Spivey

Ronald Spivey was a 39-year-old attorney who occasionally served as a judge *pro tem* in the municipal court of his home city. He referred himself because of the anxiety symptoms he developed after he became concerned that a woman would report him for displaying his erect penis at the swimming pool of the apartment complex where they both lived.

"I thought she had been looking at me in an interested way," he said, smoothing back his toupee. "She was wearing a very skimpy bikini, and I thought she was inviting me to reveal myself. So I sat in such a way that she could look up the leg of my swimming trunks."

Ronald had gone to law school on a scholarship. He had grown up in an inner-city neighborhood that included Hoofer's, a strip-tease joint not far from the Navy recruiting station. When he was in grade school, his friends and he sometimes sneaked in through a side door to watch part of the show. On a dare when he was 15, he pulled down his pants in front of two strippers who were just leaving the building. The women laughed and applauded; later, he masturbated as he fantasized that they were fondling him.

From time to time after that, through college and law school, Ronald would occasionally drive around "trolling," as he called it—looking for a girl or young woman walking by herself in a secluded area. As he drove, he would masturbate. When he found the right combination of circumstances (a woman who took his fancy in a secluded location, with no one else around), he would hop out of his car and confront the woman with his erection. Often the look of surprise on her face would cause him to ejaculate.

With his marriage, which coincided with his graduation from law school, Ronald's exhibitionistic activity subsided for a time. Although sexual intercourse with his wife was fully satisfactory to both of them, he continued to imagine showing himself to a stranger, with whom he would then fantasize having intercourse. As a practicing lawyer, he sometimes had afternoons when a continued court case left him at loose ends. Then he might go trolling again, sometimes several times in a month. At other times he might go months without activity.

About the woman at the swimming pool, Ronald said, "I really think she did want to." Her bikini had been very revealing, and he'd been thinking for several days about having sex with her. He contrived to sit so that she was virtually sure to glance between his thighs. When she noticed what he had intended her to see, her response was "That confirms what I've always thought about lawyers!" Since then he had been in near-panic at the thought that she would notify the state bar association.

Evaluation of Ronald Spivey

Ronald's history of experiencing excitement from exhibiting himself to a nonconsenting person dated to his teenage years and had persisted for at least two decades (criteria A, B). If he were apprehended, he could lose his livelihood, if not his liberty. The fact that he continued this illegal behavior despite its possible consequences indicates the strength of his urge. (Note that whereas "trolling" is typical behavior for an exhibitionist, exposing himself to someone he might expect to meet again is not—though it's hardly unheard of.)

Ronald's assumption that the woman wanted him to "reveal" himself is fairly typical of the cognitive distortion to which these people fall prey. It would be a pretty unusual woman who took any interest at all in a relative stranger who flashed her at a public swimming pool.

Although it is possible that another mental disorder could present together with exhibitionistic disorder, it is unlikely that either **schizophrenia** or **bipolar I disorder** would have been present for over 20 years without detection and thus account for the behavior. Of course, **intellectual disability** would have prevented Ronald from entering, much less completing, law school. The clinician should take pains to fully evaluate Ronald for additional paraphilic disorders, as well as for **substance use**, **mood**, and **anxiety disorders**. I'd also make a note to self: "Search for personality traits at next interview."

Ronald's exclusive interest in adult women would dictate the specifier; he was not currently in remission, so his complete diagnosis (GAF score of 65) would be as follows:

F65.2 [302.4]   Exhibitionistic disorder, sexually aroused by exposing
                       genitals to physically mature women

F65.0 [302.81] Fetishistic Disorder

In its original sense (it is derived from the Portuguese), a *fetish* was an idol or charm that had magical significance. In the context of sexual activity, it refers to something that excites an individual's sexual fantasies or desires. Such objects include underwear, shoes, stockings, and other inanimate objects. Bras and panties are probably the most common objects used as fetishes.

The DSM-5 definition of fetishistic disorder also includes body parts that aren't integral to the reproductive process. A sexual attraction to feet would be an example of *partialism*, as this is known, which sometimes occurs along with other fetishes. (There are reports of men who are attracted to women *missing* body parts, such as a one-legged woman—a sort of fetishistic *jamais vu*.) Cross-dressing that is sexually exciting, as in transvestic disorder, and arousal achieved via objects designed for use during sex, such as dildos or vibrators, are excluded from the definition of fetishistic disorder.

Some people amass collections of their preferred fetishes; some resort to stealing from stores or clotheslines to get them. They may smell, rub, or handle these objects while masturbating, or they may ask sex partners to wear them. Without a fetish, such a person may be unable to get an erection.

Fetishism usually begins in adolescence, though many patients report similar interests even in childhood. Although some women may show a degree of fetishistic behavior, nearly all those with fetishistic disorder are men. It tends to be a chronic condition, to the extent that for some people, a fetish may come to crowd out more traditional love objects.

Essential Features of **Fetishistic Disorder**

The person is aroused by inanimate objects (such as shoes or underwear) or body parts other than genitals (such as feet) and feels distress/disability at the idea.

The Fine Print

The D's: • Duration (6+ months) • Distress or disability (work/educational, social, or personal) • Differential diagnosis (transvestic disorder)

Coding Notes

Specify type:

> **Body parts**
> **Nonliving objects**
> **Other** (perhaps combinations of the first two types)

Specify if:

> **In remission**
> **In a controlled environment**

Corky Brauner

When he was 13, Corky Brauner found a pair of his older sister's panties that his mother had by accident put away with his own underwear. They were embroidered with flowers and the word "Saturday," and he found them peculiarly exciting. He slept with them under his pillow for a couple of nights and masturbated with them twice before sneaking them back into his sister's bureau drawer Friday evening. From time to time throughout the balance of his adolescence, when he was alone in the house, Corky would appropriate items of his sister's underwear.

In college Corky lived alone, so he was able to collect and keep a small wardrobe of lingerie without concern that it would be discovered. Although he had a few bras and slips, he liked panties best. By his senior year, he owned several dozen. Some of these he had purchased, but he preferred those he could persuade a woman to leave behind after a date. He had even stolen one or two pairs from backyard clotheslines, but that was dangerous and he didn't do it often.

Sometimes when Corky wasn't entertaining company, he would take some panties out of the drawer and play with them. He would smell them, rub them on his face, and masturbate with them. During these activities, he would pretend he was making love to the original owner of the panties. If he didn't know her, he would imagine what she might have looked like.

Corky was driven into treatment by the laughter of his most recent girlfriend when he found that he had to put her underwear under his pillow in order to get an erection when they were making love. "I've gotten totally fixated on panties," he said during his initial interview. "I seem to prefer them to women."

Evaluation of Corky Brauner

Corky's excessive interest in panties is a typical example of fetishistic disorder. It had persisted for years—far longer than the 6-month requirement (criterion A). Over the years, he had assembled quite a collection, obtained from a variety of sources. Corky's distress (B) stemmed not from his own perception of his behavior, but from the fact that a girlfriend criticized him for it. In this way, he learned that he preferred panties to people—a not infrequent progression for fetishists.

The differential diagnosis of fetishistic disorder includes **transvestic disorder**, in which men (almost always men) are stimulated by wearing and viewing themselves in women's clothing. Fetishists may put on clothing of the opposite sex, but wearing it is incidental to the sexual gratification they derive from the clothing itself, and they don't fantasize about their own attractiveness when so attired. Corky showed no interest in cross-dressing (C).

Many fetishists have also been involved in **rape, exhibitionism, frotteurism, pedophilia,** or **voyeurism**, but none of these behaviors are mentioned in Corky's vignette (his clinician should ask). Pending the outcome of such an inquiry, Corky's full diagnosis (with a GAF score of 61) would be as follows:

F65.0 [302.81]   Fetishistic disorder, nonliving objects (panties)

F65.81 [302.89] Frotteuristic Disorder

Frottage (the term is derived from the French word *frotter*, meaning "to rub") usually takes place on crowded sidewalks or public transportation. (Ready means of escape is a concern for the frotteur.) The perpetrator (invariably a man) selects a victim (usually a woman) who is accessible and whose allure may be enhanced by tight clothing. The frotteur rubs his genitals against her thighs or buttocks, or he may fondle her breasts or genitalia. The process is efficient; on subways, ejaculation usually occurs within the transit time between stops.

The victim typically does not make an immediate outcry, perhaps because she hopes she is mistaken about what appears to be happening. Note that it is the act of touching or rubbing, not the coercion involved, that is exciting to the frotteur. However, over half have a history of involvement in other paraphilias, especially exhibitionism and voyeurism. A frotteur often fantasizes about an ongoing intimate relationship with the victim.

This condition usually begins in adolescence and is sometimes started off by observing others engaged in frottage. Most acts occur when the frotteur is between the ages of 15 and 25; frequency gradually declines thereafter. No one appears to know how common this condition is, and it may be underreported.

Essential Features of **Frotteuristic Disorder**

Aroused by rubbing against or feeling someone who hasn't consented, the patient has repeatedly acted on the urge (or feels distress/disability at the idea).

The Fine Print

The D's: • Duration (6+ months) • Distress or disability (work/educational, social, or personal) • Differential diagnosis (physical and substance use disorders, psychotic and bipolar disorders)

Coding Notes

Specify if:

In full remission (no symptoms for 5+ years)
In a controlled environment

Henry McWilliams

Henry McWilliams had been born in London. Dressed in his short gray pants, white shirt, and school tie, he rode the Underground every day to his exclusive school. One day, when he was 9, he saw a man rubbing up against a woman.

Henry was small when he was 9, and even in the crowded subway car he had an excellent eye-level view. The woman (she was an adult, though Henry had no idea how old) was a bit overweight and dressed in a tight-fitting miniskirt. She was facing away from the man, who allowed the weight of the crowd surging through the doors to press him up against her. The man tugged at his crotch, and then, as the train began to move, rubbed himself against her.

"I never saw her face, but I could tell she didn't like it," said Henry. "She tried to push him away, she tried to move, but there was no place for either of them to go. Then the train stopped and he ran out the door."

Henry had moved with his parents to the United States when he was 15. Now age 24, he had referred himself for treatment with this story.

Since his graduation from high school, he had worked as a messenger for a large legal firm. Many days he spent several hours on the subway in his official capacity. He guessed that he had rubbed against 200 women in 5 years. He was seeking help at the insistence of one of the partners in his law firm, who the week before had happened to ride the same train and had watched him in action.

When Henry was in need, he would go into the men's room and put on a condom so as not to stain his trousers. Then he would roam up and down the outskirts of a crowd on a subway platform until he found a woman who interested him. This would be someone who was youngish but not young ("They're less likely to scream"), and well-rounded enough to stretch tight the material of her skirt or slacks. He especially liked it if the material was leather. He would board after she did, and if she did not turn around, would rub his erect penis up and down against her buttocks as the train began to roll.

Henry was very sensitive, so it didn't take much pressure. Sometimes the woman didn't even seem to realize what was going on, or maybe she didn't want to acknowledge it, even to herself. He usually climaxed within a minute. Then he would bolt out the door at the next stop. If interrupted prior to climax, he would hang around the platform until he spotted another woman in another crowd.

"It helps if I imagine that we're married or engaged," he explained. "I'll pretend that she's wearing my ring, and I've come home for a quickie."

Evaluation of Henry McWilliams

Henry's method of operation was fairly typical for frotteurs, most of whom tend to follow the same pattern each time. Henry had offended on many occasions (criteria A, B). Like most, he had had many episodes of this behavior over the years and fantasized having a romance with each victim. Henry was not especially upset about his own behavior; he came for treatment because his employers demanded it.

Although patients with **schizophrenia** or **intellectual disability** will sometimes engage in sexual behavior that is inappropriate to the context, Henry bore no evidence whatsoever of either condition. With a GAF score of 70, his diagnosis would simply be this:

F65.81 [302.89]   Frotteuristic disorder

F65.4 [302.2] Pedophilic Disorder

Pedophilia is Greek meaning "love of children." In the context of a paraphilia, of course, it means sex with children. Pedophilic disorder is far and away the most common of the paraphilic disorders that involve actual contact. Estimates vary, but by the age of 18, up to 20% of American children have in some way been interfered with sexually. Most perpetrators are not strangers but relatives, friends, or neighbors. The vast majority of pedophiles are men, but women may account for up to 12% of recorded offenses (though some of these involve allowing children to be abused, rather than committing the act personally).

The type of act preferred varies with the offender. Some pedophiles only view (child pornography or actual children); others want to touch or undress a child. But most acts involve oral sex or touching of the child's genitals—or of the perpetrator's genitals by the child. In cases other than incest, most pedophiles don't require actual penetration. Those who do, however, may use force to achieve it.

Though some pedophiles do not start until midlife, this behavior usually begins in later teenage years. (The definition of pedophilic disorder specifically excludes perpetrators who are adolescents themselves or who aren't at least 5 years older than the victim.) It may be more common among persons who were themselves abused as children. Once pedophilia has begun, it tends to be chronic. Up to 50% use alcohol as a prelude to contact with children. Half or more have other paraphilias.

Many pedophiles limit themselves to children (this type of pedophilia is called *exclusive*); they often further confine themselves to children of a particular sex and age range. However, the majority are also attracted to adults, and their pedophilia is called *nonexclusive*. Like other paraphilic individuals, pedophiles may develop a degree of cognitive distortion about their activities: They persuade themselves that children enjoy the sexual experience or that it is important for their development. Most pedophiles do not force their attentions on children, but depend on friendship, persuasion, and guile. A number of studies suggest that children who are lonely or otherwise uncared for may be especially susceptible to the advances of a pedophile.

Overall, perhaps 15–25% of those convicted reoffend within a few years of their release from prison. Alcohol use and trouble forming intimate relationships with adults increase the chances of recidivism. Men who prefer boys are about twice as likely to reoffend as are those who prefer girls.

Some pedophiles limit their attentions to daughters, stepdaughters, or other victims related to them. Then the specifier *limited to incest* can be used, though it isn't clear what benefit it confers. Some perpetrators of incest may be pedophiles, but many men (most incestuous adults are male) only become interested in daughters or stepdaughters who have reached puberty.

Collateral information is especially important in evaluating pedophiles, who have strong reasons to lie about their behavior. And often there's little motivation to tell the truth: Sentences are long; convicted pedophiles may face harsh treatment in prison; and the prospect of suppressing sex interest through the use of drugs is unappealing to many such people.

One aspect of the criteria that can be confusing is the required 5-year age difference between perpetrator and victim. As the Coding Notes indicate, a 15-year-old having a sexual relationship with someone of any age would not be diagnosed as having pedophilic disorder. Someone who is 20 having an affair with a 14- or 15-year-old, however, would.

And that raises another difficult issue. According to DSM-5 criteria, the child involved must be prepubescent. If we interpret strictly what DSM-5 says, we won't be making the diagnosis in someone whose victim has begun to develop sexually. This has caused a lot of heartburn among clinicians as well as some members of the relevant DSM-5 committee, who worry that by maintaining the current definition DSM-5 depathologizes men who prefer certain children 13 and under who are not prepubertal.

Essential Features of **Pedophilic Disorder**

The patient is sexually aroused by prepubescent children and has acted on the urge (or feels distress/interpersonal impairment at the idea).

The Fine Print

The D's: • Duration (6+ months) • Demographics (the patient must be at least 16 years old and at least 5 years older than the victim) • Differential diagnosis (physical and substance use disorders, psychotic and bipolar disorders, intellectual disability, criminal abuse of children for profit)

Coding Notes

Specify if:

In a controlled environment (see sidebar below)

Specify:

Exclusive type (aroused solely by children)
Nonexclusive type

Specify if:
Sexually attracted to males
Sexually attracted to females
Sexually attracted to both

Specify if:

Limited to incest

There's a bit of an issue here: The criteria for pedophilic disorder are the only ones in this DSM-5 chapter that do not specifically allow the specifier *in a controlled environment*. Of course, it also is the only one that doesn't allow *in full remission*, but that is at least logical: pedophilia has been long established as a lifelong condition. However, who is more likely to do hard time than a pedophile? And just how likely is that person to reoffend while inside? Were I to evaluate such a person again, I'd go right ahead and use the *in a controlled environment* specifier.

Raymond Boggs

At age 58, Raymond Boggs seemed an unlikely convict. His orange prison jumpsuit was stretched tightly over his pear-shaped body; in contrast to the swagger of the younger inmates, he shuffled, head down, along the corridor to the interview room.

Raymond had become interested in sex when he was very young. One of his earliest memories was of sex play with a teenage girl who was babysitting him and his infant sister. As an adult, the sight of little girls' bodies particularly fascinated him. He remembered watching his sister having her bath when he was 7 or 8, hanging around until his mother had to shoo him from the bathroom. When they were teenagers, he had watched outside his sister's window at night, trying to get a glimpse of her as she undressed for bed. When she entered puberty, his evening vigils stopped. "It was the body hair. It seemed so coarse and disgusting. That was when I discovered that I only really liked girls who were, um, smooth."

Despite these tastes, in his mid-20s Raymond married the daughter of the foreman in the printing shop where he worked. During the early years of their marriage, the couple maintained an active sex life. Usually he would try to fantasize that he was having sex with a young girl. Once he persuaded his wife to shave off all her pubic hair, but she complained that it itched as it grew back and refused to do it again. They had three children, all sons, which in retrospect seemed a minor miracle: Little boys didn't tempt him at all.

As the years went by, Raymond acquired a small stack of pornographic magazines that featured children. He kept them hidden under a pile of rags in his tool shed. When his sexual tension became too high, he would masturbate while he imagined himself frolicking with the naked children in these pictures.

By his early 50s, Raymond's life had taken a turn for the worse. His sons had all left home, and a series of pelvic operations caused his wife to reject his sexual advances, sometimes for months at a time. To fill his time, he took up photography. Especially over the long summer months, he found ready subjects in the neighborhood children he befriended. Some of the little girls he could persuade to pose partly or completely disrobed.

He preferred those who were 5 or 6 years old, but on occasion he would photograph a girl as old as 8. (The older children were more independent and harder to persuade.) These sessions occurred principally in a secluded spot behind his tool shed. He used candy and quarters as bait, afterwards reminding each child that her parents wouldn't like it if she told.

"I'm not proud of it," he said as he tried to ease the bulging waistband of his jumpsuit. "It was just something I couldn't resist. The feeling I'd get when she'd slip down her panties—it was anxiety and ecstasy and butterflies in my stomach. Sort of the way you'd feel if you won the lottery. But I never touched one; all I did was look. And I never thought it might hurt them any."

Raymond had been looking and taking pictures for the better part of 10 years when he was discovered by a 12-year-old boy who had ventured behind the tool shed to collect native plant specimens for a science exhibit. The boy told his father, who called the girl's mother, who called the police. The trial—a 3-week media feeding frenzy—featured the corroborative testimony of no fewer than seven neighborhood girls, now in varying stages of adolescence, who had at one time or another been victimized by Raymond Boggs.

Sentenced to 5–10 years in the penitentiary, Raymond still faced millions of dollars in civil lawsuits. The day after he was arrested, his wife filed for divorce and entered therapy. One of his sons broke off contact with him; another moved out of state.

Evaluation of Raymond Boggs

When the facts of the case are clear, there is little to dispute the diagnosis of pedophilic disorder. Someone with **substance intoxication** may perpetrate an isolated incident of fondling a child, but then it is usually evident that this is not a frequent sexual outlet. As an example of their overall defective judgment, patients with **intellectual disability** or **schizophrenia** may sometimes fall into this mode of sexual release. Parents (notoriously celebrities) are sometimes accused of child molestation as a part of a messy divorce; frequently the facts do not bear out these allegations. In the case of Raymond Boggs, the legal facts were indisputable. He freely admitted to his long-standing interests and behavior (criteria A, B). He insisted that the act was never tactile, only visual, which is typical of a large number of such people.

Those with **exhibitionistic disorder** may show themselves to children, but they don't approach the victims for further sexual activity. Some pedophiles may also have **sexual sadism disorder**; if so, both diagnoses should be made.

We are asked to choose several specifiers to help pinpoint the patient's pathology. Raymond was sexually attracted only to females, and young ones at that. His GAF score would be 55. Even though the criteria for pedophilic disorder don't offer the specifier *in a controlled environment*, I've sneaked in a mention of it anyway.

F65.4 [302.2]	Pedophilic disorder, nonexclusive type, sexually attracted to females, in a controlled environment
Z65.1[V62.5]	Imprisonment

F65.51 [302.83] Sexual Masochism Disorder

Sexual masochism comprises three principal features: pain, humiliation, and absence of control. Many people—perhaps 15% of the general population—derive sexual pleasure from some degree of suffering. However, these behaviors/ideas by themselves are usually benign, and are certainly insufficient for the diagnosis of a disorder. Indeed, most people who engage in masochistic behavior function well, both socially and psychologically. Some women even admit that they like being spanked during sex or that they fantasize about being forced to have sex. Sexual masochism is thus the only paraphilic behavior in which any appreciable number of women appear to participate.

On the other hand, sexual masochism *disorder* (SMD) is a paraphilic disorder that usually begins in childhood. The behaviors involved include bondage, blindfolding, spanking, cutting, and humiliation (by defecation, urination, or forcing the submissive partner to imitate an animal). Some form of physical abuse is probably the most commonly used. As time goes on, patients with SMD may require increasing degrees of torture to experience the same degree of sexual satisfaction; in this sense, SMD resembles an addiction.

By choking, pricking, or shocking, some masochists inflict pain upon themselves. Perhaps 30% of them at times also participate in sadistic behavior. A few pursue an especially dangerous behavior called *asphyxiophilia* (or *hypoxyphilia*), in which they induce near-suffocation by means of a noose around the neck, an airtight bag over the head, or the inhalation of amyl nitrite ("poppers"). These people report that the sensation of restricted breathing promotes an especially intense sexual high. Each year, 1 or 2 accidental deaths per 1 million of the general population occur from these practices.

Although masochists derive sexual gratification from feeling pain or degradation, they do not necessarily surrender *complete* control. Many sadomasochistic relationships are carefully planned; the partners may agree upon a secret word by which the masochist can indicate that it really is time to stop.

Essential Features of **Sexual Masochism Disorder**

The patient is sexually aroused by being struck, restrained, or otherwise made to feel humiliated (and feels distress/disability at the idea).

The Fine Print

The D's: • Duration (6+ months) • Distress or disability (work/educational, social, or personal impairment) • Differential diagnosis (physical and substance use disorders)

Coding Notes

Specify if:

With asphyxiophilia

Specify if:

In full remission (no symptoms for 5+ years)
In a controlled environment

Martin Allingham

Martin Allingham came to medical attention the night he almost died. In the apartment he shared with Samuel Brock, the two had devised an elaborate contraption of pulleys, ropes, collars, and shackles that could turn Martin upside down and partly strangle him while Sam applied the whip.

"I get the most beautiful orgasm when I'm about to pass out," Martin reported, much later.

Sam and Martin had been in school together. Sam was a jock; Martin was the class wimp. How perfectly this suited them they didn't realize until one Saturday afternoon when they were 15. The two were fighting on the deserted playground, and Sam began sitting on Martin, twisting his fingers into pretzels. Although Martin cried, the growing urgency of his erection was evident as the pain increased. After they parted, Sam had masturbated while recalling the sensation of absolute control.

Without discussing it much, by common consent Sam and Martin met again 2 weeks later. When they were 19, they moved in together, and they had been living together ever since. Now they were 28.

Martin didn't have to be hurt to enjoy sex, but it greatly enhanced the pleasure. He had tried spanking and bondage, but asphyxia was the best. When he was younger, he had played the field and tried other partners. But most of them had hurt him either too much or not enough; besides, he and Sam were both afraid of AIDS. For the last several years, they had worked at the same department store and had been faithful to one other.

The night of the accident, Martin got himself into the harness while Sam was at work. He apparently cinched the noose a shade too tight and lost consciousness, though he didn't remember that. When Sam found Martin, he had no pulse and wasn't breathing. In the Boy Scouts, Sam had learned CPR, which he vigorously employed after calling 911.

A police report was made, and a pair of officers interviewed them both. "We're perfectly suited," Sam explained. "I like to do it; he likes it done." He admitted that their sex life had recently become increasingly violent, even death-defying. But that hadn't been his idea; it was Martin who had needed more to produce the same effects. Sam admitted that he "got off" on pain, but some pain seemed to serve about as well as a lot.

"I wouldn't want to really harm him," he said. "I love him."

Evaluation of Martin Allingham

Martin's sexual behavior included elements of pain inflicted upon himself (criterion A). Bondage was one of these elements, as was the practice of asphyxiophilia, with which Martin enhanced his own sexual pleasure. Martin had acted on these urges for years; the impairment it had recently caused was nearly terminal (B). He therefore amply fulfilled the criteria for SMD.

Note that some **sex workers** accept pain within limits, because the pay is better than that for standard sex. Such individuals should not be diagnosed as having SMD unless they also both derive pleasure from the practice and are distressed or impaired by it.

Masochists will sometimes cross-dress in response to the demands of a sadistic partner. If the act of wearing clothing of the opposite gender also produces sexual excitement (and not just the humiliation of cross-dressing), then **transvestic disorder** should also be diagnosed. The vignette is silent on the issue, but Martin's clinician should thoroughly explore the possibility of a **personality disorder**—common among patients with SMD—which could significantly affect therapy. Mention it in the summary. Considering the fact that sexual arousal was augmented by the sensation of restricted breathing, Martin's diagnosis (current GAF score of 25) would be as follows:

F65.51 [302.83]   Sexual masochism disorder, with asphyxiophilia

F65.52 [302.84] Sexual Sadism Disorder

Much of the behavior of sadists complements that of masochists; the difference is that sadists are the perpetrators rather than the recipients. Inflicting pain or humiliation sexually stimulates them. The suffering of others arouses them sexually, and they fantasize about dominance and restraint. Some women admit to engaging in this sort of activity.

Although early childhood experiences with punishment may prefigure this chronic condition for some, overt behavior usually begins with fantasies during the individual's teenage years. The physical methods ultimately employed include bondage, blindfolding, spanking, cutting, and humiliation (such as by defecation, urination, or forcing the submissive partner to imitate an animal). Like those with sexual masochism, individuals with sexual sadism may with time need to increase the severity of the torture to produce the same degree of sexual satisfaction.

Most people who engage in sadistic behavior limit themselves to only a few partners, most of whom are willing; by definition, these people would not meet DSM-5 criteria for sexual sadism disorder unless they were distressed or impaired by their urges. Fewer than 10% of sadists commit rape, but those who do can be even more brutal than other rapists, using more force and inflicting greater pain than is necessary to fulfill their needs.

We don't know the frequency of sexual sadism disorder in the general population.

In a study of 240 hospitalized sexual offenders, 52 (21%) could be diagnosed as having sexual sadism disorder. Of these, only 16 (31% of the total) had been correctly diagnosed before the study.

Essential Features of **Sexual Sadism Disorder**

The patient, who is aroused by someone else's suffering, has acted upon the urge with someone who hasn't consented (alternatively, the patient feels distress/disability at the idea).

The Fine Print

The D's: • Duration (6+ months) • Distress or disability (work/educational, social, or personal impairment) • Differential diagnosis (physical and substance use disorders, personality disorders, nonsadistic rape)

Coding Notes

Specify if:

> **In full remission** (no symptoms for 5+ years)
> **In a controlled environment**

Donatien Alphonse François, the Marquis de Sade

If ever one person has been ineluctably associated with a mental disorder, that would be Donatien Alphonse François, the Marquis de Sade—the patron saint of sadism. It is both interesting and instructive to explore the degree to which the personal history of this man, who flourished over two centuries ago in France, reflects the condition that bears his name.

Sade (as his biographers call him) was born into a family that was poor but socially prominent, which may help explain his development into a proud, arrogant autocrat. An absent father left the nurturing during his early formative years to his libertine uncle.

When he was only 16, Sade entered the army and served with distinction in combat. Forced by his family into a loveless (on his part) marriage, soon after the wedding he demonstrated that his sexual interests could be problematic.

As a child he had yearned for his mother's embrace, but as an adult he sought solace in the arms of prostitutes. Several of those he hired filed formal complaints that he had tried to whip them; one also claimed he had made her ill by spiking her bourbon with the notorious (and overhyped) aphrodisiac, Spanish fly. He asked many of the prostitutes he frequented to whip him—not so unusual a request among 18th-century Frenchmen, who were known sometimes to address impotence by employing the lash.

In prison, he later used huge rectal dildos (which he required his wife, Renée, to procure for him) to gain sexual satisfaction.

What assured his ultimate downfall was neither his passion nor his penury, but the antipathy of his mother-in-law. *Cette dame formidable* reacted to his libertine tendencies by persuading the King to issue a private bill of attainder then popular among French petitioners. It allowed the authorities to toss Sade into prison and hold him without trial, without end.

In confinement—he spent nearly 29 years either in prison or in the asylum at Charenton, and he came within 1 day of execution during the Terror of the French Revolution—he wrote some of the most sexually explicit and violent prose ever composed in any language. *Justine* relates the sexual torture of a young woman at the hands of various men, beginning when she was 12 years old. *The 120 Days of Sodom*, written down in little more than a month while he languished in the Bastille, is a nauseating (pardon the editorial queasy stomach) crescendo of sexual horror that culminates in murder. It is on his writings, rather than his own sexual proclivities, that his reputation rests.

That reputation notwithstanding, Sade's character, at least at this remove, remains to a degree confusing. On the one hand, some regard him as an angry loner with a quick and violent temper who had no true friends. Others describe him as a lifelong charmer who could easily manipulate people, sometimes with threats of suicide.

He was later to develop frequent ideas of persecution that involved Renée. He scrutinized her letters for hidden signals, which he thought contained references to his release date. Yet, during one of his infrequent releases from prison, when he could have exacted revenge on his in-laws, he didn't. His reward was rearrest and incarceration for the rest of his life.

Evaluation of Donatien Alphonse François, the Marquis de Sade

From his own writings and from the work of others, it is clear that Sade was intensely interested in sexual pleasures derived from inflicting pain and humiliation on other people (criterion A). Although he did not appear to suffer distress from these desires, he acted upon them repeatedly with nonconsenting individuals when he was quite a young man (B). That qualifies him, even by today's robust standards, for the diagnosis of sexual sadism disorder. (We cannot doubt that the characters described in Sade's *The 120 Days of Sodom* would more than fully qualify for this diagnosis.)

Yet, when we consider the entirety of his life, Sade even better fulfills the definition of sexual masochism disorder: He was much given to receiving the pain of whippings, which contributed to his prolonged incarceration. Yet the power of tradition is such that his name remains firmly attached to behavior that he appears to have pursued personally during a relatively brief chapter in his career.

What other diagnosis might be appropriate? Of course, for anyone with his inclinations we would consider a **personality disorder**, but it would be in addition to, not instead of, the paraphilic disorder diagnosis. Mention of it belongs in a summary.

With only the information given above, the Marquis de Sade's diagnoses (in order of appearance) would read as given below. And I'd give him a GAF score of 71.

F65.51 [302.83]	Sexual masochism disorder
F65.52 [302.84]	Sexual sadism disorder
F52.32 [302.74]	Delayed ejaculation

Leopold von Sacher-Masoch was a 19th-century Austrian writer who enslaved himself to his mistress for 6 months, on the condition that she would wear fur as often as she could and treat him as her servant. He subsequently wrote about the experience in a novel, *Venus in Furs*. This led to the adaptation of his name (along with Sade's) for their respective paraphilias in the 1886 textbook *Psychopathia Sexualis* by Richard von Krafft-Ebing, whose name, sadly, has not been attached to anything.

Sade and Sacher-Masoch are among the diminishing ranks of individuals whose names are retained as eponyms in DSM-5. And they are the only ones we use as adjectives—as is also the case with the terms *Freudian* and *Jungian*. Disorders using other personal names, such as Münchausen's syndrome, have been rebranded with terms that are more descriptive (though perhaps less evocative).

F65.1 [302.3] Transvestic Disorder

Transvestites cross-dress to achieve sexual excitement; they experience frustration when this behavior is thwarted. There is much variability in the amount of cross-dressing. Some will do it occasionally, while alone; others frequently sally forth in public. Some limit it to underwear; others get completely togged out. Some men (once again, men vastly predominate) spend up to several hours a week getting dressed in and wearing women's clothing. Many will masturbate or have intercourse when they cross-dress. They may fantasize about themselves as girls and keep a collection of female clothing, often wearing it under normal male attire. But only a person who is distressed or impaired in some important way by the pursuit of these behaviors earns the diagnosis of transvestic disorder; those who embrace their own behavior are simply cross-dressers.

Transvestic disorder usually begins during adolescence, or even in childhood. However, most male transvestites were not effeminate as boys; under 20% of them are gay as adults. As happens with some other paraphilias, their aberrant behavior may gradually replace more usual modes of sexual gratification. Through videos, magazines, or personal interaction, there may be considerable involvement in the transvestite sub-culture. A small number gradually come to feel increasingly comfortable with their cross-dressing and become transsexual. Such gender dysphoria may provide the final stimulus to seek treatment. With age, the sexual excitement attached to cross-dressing may give way to a general sense of well-being.

Some patients have been previously involved in voyeuristic, exhibitionistic, or masochistic behaviors. You can add specifiers for those who are sexually aroused by clothing (*with fetishism*) or by thoughts of themselves as female (*with autogynephilia*). Too few females with transvestic disorder are reported to justify the term *autoandrophilia*.

In the general male population, the prevalence of cross-dressing to achieve sexual stimulation appears to be just under 3%, though only half of these might qualify for a diagnosis of transvestic disorder.

Essential Features of **Transvestic Disorder**

Arousal by cross-dressing (thoughts or behaviors) has repeatedly caused the patient to feel distressed or impaired.

The Fine Print

The D's: • Duration (6+ months) • Distress or disability (work/educational, social, or personal impairment) • Differential diagnosis (physical and substance use disorders, gender dysphoria, fetishistic disorder)

Coding Notes

Specify if:

> **With fetishism** (sexual arousal by clothing or fabrics])
> **With autogynephilia** (sexual arousal by self-visualization as female)

Specify if:

> **In full remission** (no symptoms for 5+ years)
> **In a controlled environment**

Paul Castro

When Paul Castro was 7, his parents employed a teenage neighbor to babysit. Julie was precocious and imaginative; she would persuade Paul to play dress-up in her clothing, which she would remove for the occasion. At first Paul only tolerated this, but later he would become excited at the sensation of her silky panties as he drew them up over his skinny thighs.

When Julie acquired a steady boyfriend and lost interest in Paul, he would sometimes covertly borrow a bra and panties from his mother to dress up in. By his late teens, he had collected a small wardrobe of women's underwear, which he would put on as often as once or twice a week. Standing in front of a mirror wearing a bra, its cups attractively padded, he might fantasize himself being embraced—sometimes by a man, sometimes a woman. A time or two he tried on lipstick and an old dress his mother hardly ever wore. But those made him look silly and conspicuous, he thought, and he subsequently limited himself to lingerie. However, he never felt any sense of discomfort about being male or any desire to change his gender.

After a year of junior college, Paul got a job as a clerk in a bookstore and moved to his own apartment. Some days he would wear his panties and bra (without the padding) to work under his sport shirt and slacks. Then, during lunch hour, he might masturbate in the men's room as he imagined himself making love to a beautiful woman, both of them dressed in their silk underwear. If he was otherwise occupied during lunch, throughout the afternoon he would enjoy the delicious sensation of silk next to his skin and the anticipation of release while looking at himself in the mirror that evening.

Paul was thus attired one morning when the paramedics picked him up after a passing bus clipped him on his way to work. He awakened to find his right upper arm in a splint, and passers-by agog over his size 40C Maidenform bra. His shame over this episode caused him to rethink his behavior and seek treatment.

Evaluation of Paul Castro

Western society tolerates some cross-dressing and even considers it normal. Transgender impersonation has had a long and honorable history on the stage and in film; Halloween apparel also comes to mind.

In **sexual masochistic disorder**, patients may be forced to cross-dress to excite a sadistic lover; if they do not also experience sexual excitement, transvestic disorder would not be diagnosed. Patients with **gender dysphoria** often dress in clothing appropriate to the opposite sex, but without sexual stimulation. When gay people cross-dress, it is sometimes done to enhance their appeal to other gay individuals; often, however, it is done to be campy or to make fun of society. In any event, sexual stimulation is not the goal.

Obviously, Paul's behavior fit none of these alternative explanations. In fact, other than his interest in lingerie, he had fairly conventional heterosexual interests (judged by his fantasies when masturbating; criterion A). He therefore would not receive the specifier *with autogynephilia*. He appeared to be aroused by the feel of silk, so we could justify giving him the *with fetishism* specifier. His ultimate distress (GAF score of 71) when he was picked up by the paramedics would fulfill criterion B.

F65.1 [302.3]	Transvestic disorder, with fetishism
S42.009 [810.00]	Fractured clavicle

Women can now be diagnosed as having transvestic disorder. This was not the case in DSM-IV-TR or in any of its predecessors, back to DSM-III. The change is egalitarian in the extreme: The only study reporting any women seeking sexual stimulation from cross-dressing found just 5 of 1,171 (0.4%), and we don't know whether those few had been distressed or impaired by their behavior. In practical terms, this club remains "for men only."

F65.3 [302.82] Voyeuristic Disorder

Voyeurs are aroused by watching people engaged in private activities. Of course, many people who do not have a paraphilia also enjoy such viewing—those who patronize pornographic films and websites, for example. The difference is that a voyeur's gratification derives from viewing ordinary people who do not realize they are being watched and would probably not permit it if they did.

In a 2006 Swedish survey, 12% of men (and 4% of women) admitted to at least one incident of voyeuristic behavior. By current standards, the vast majority of these individuals would not be diagnosed with a paraphilic disorder. Other surveys find that many people of both sexes would watch others undressing or having sex if they felt they wouldn't be caught. As with other paraphilic disorders, DSM-5 requires that the behavior be acted upon repeatedly or cause the individual distress or impairment. The bottom lines: Nearly all practitioners are men, and voyeurism is the most commonly reported sexual crime.

Voyeurism usually begins when individuals are in their teens—almost always by age 15. Once voyeuristic disorder develops, it tends to be chronic. The victims of these "peeping Toms" are almost always strangers. Voyeurs will usually masturbate while they are watching. Afterwards, they may fantasize about having sex with the victim, though activity with that victim is rarely sought. Some voyeurs prefer this method of sexual gratification, but most also have normal sex lives. Like exhibitionists, they take precautions to avoid detection.

Essential Features of **Voyeuristic Disorder**

Aroused by watching an unwary person who is undressing or having sex, the patient has repeatedly acted on these urges or has experienced distress or impairment from them.

The Fine Print

The D's: • Duration and demographics (6+ months, age 18+) • Distress or disability (work/educational, social, or personal) • Differential diagnosis (conduct disorder/antisocial personality disorder, substance use disorders, normal sexual interests)

Coding Notes

Specify if:

> **In full remission** (no symptoms for 5+ years)
> **In a controlled environment**

Rex Collingwood

The referral came at the request of a Superior Court judge, who had been displeased to find Rex Collingwood brought before the bench for the second time in less than a year. This time, at age 23, Rex had been caught literally with his pants down, masturbating outside the master bedroom window of a house on a quiet suburban street. He had been so fascinated by the aspect of the woman inside removing her underwear that he failed to notice the approach of her husband, who was walking the dog.

When Rex was growing up, his family had lived near the campus of a small Midwestern college. He had made friends with the caretaker at the student union—a gangly philosophy major named Rollo who, in exchange for minor custodial work, lived rent-free in a room on the second floor. When Rex was 14, Rollo showed him the tiny hole he had discovered in the floorboards immediately above the women's toilet. Intermittently for some weeks, Rex and Rollo had squatted in the dark above the peephole, waiting for women to enter. Because they were looking straight down, they couldn't see much, but the images provided plenty of grist for the mill of Rex's fantasy life.

When he graduated from high school, Rex went to work in an auto body shop. The bookkeeper, Darlene, was a year or two older than he, and they soon began living together. Rex and Darlene made love four or five times a week; they each expressed satisfaction with the arrangement. Rex sometimes wondered whether he was "oversexed" because he still occasionally had the urge to "go looking." He had tried X-rated videos, but it wasn't the same—those people knew they were being watched, and they were also being paid.

So every 2 or 3 months Rex would spend a couple of evenings driving on dark, quiet streets, seeking the right venue. Catching a glimpse of naked flesh was titillating, but watching a woman undressing added the delicious suspense of not knowing how much would be revealed. Whatever he saw, Rex would add to the stock of images to conjure up when he made love with Darlene.

Best of all was watching people have sex. He had carefully memorized the locations of several such encounters, and he returned to them again and again when the urge struck. Summertime was best, for then people were less likely to get under the covers. He had once or twice stood in the bushes for as long as 2 hours, watching while his targets worked up their passion and his. That was what had drawn him back to the house where he was apprehended—less than four blocks from where he'd been arrested a year before.

"I suppose I should feel ashamed," Rex told the interviewer, "but I'm not. I think it's normal to be interested. And if they really cared about their privacy, they'd close their curtains, wouldn't they?"

Evaluation of Rex Collingwood

There isn't much of a differential diagnosis in a history like Rex's; he easily fulfills criteria A and B. If he had spent his time watching paid performers on a stage or the Internet, we wouldn't think a thing about it; neither would the judge. Although Rex had acted repeatedly on his urges, the only distress he felt was at the prospect of being punished.

With a GAF score of 61, Rex's complete diagnosis would be as follows:

F65.3 [302.82]   Voyeuristic disorder
Z65.3 [V62.5]   Arrest and prosecution

F65.89 [302.89] Other Specified Paraphilic Disorder

A variety of other paraphilic disorders have been described. As compared to the foregoing disorders, most of these are less common, less well studied, or both. Coded as other specified paraphilic disorder, they include the following:

Paraphilic coercive disorder. An individual enjoys the idea of forcing sex upon an unwilling partner.

Telephone scatologia. As the name implies, this is a preoccupation with "talking dirty" on the phone. It has been found to be associated with exhibitionism and voyeurism.

Zoophilia. This paraphilia is a preoccupation with having sex with various mammals and other animals. Uncommon in clinical samples, these individuals often report that the attraction is not just sex, but a love for animals.

Necrophilia. Sex with corpses was said to be the only release undertakers had in ancient Egypt. Sex with contemporary cadavers, rarely reported, almost demands another mental or personality diagnosis (perhaps both).

Klismaphilia. In this paraphilia, somewhat allied to sexual masochistic disorder, some people achieve sexual pleasure by giving themselves enemas. In some such individuals, klismaphilia is linked with cross-dressing. Though it may be fairly common, this behavior has been little studied in the professional literature.

Coprophilia. This is masturbating with one's own feces; it has been rarely reported.

Urophilia. Some people become sexually excited by playing or masturbating with urine. This must be distinguished from the form of sexual masochism in which the person desires to be urinated upon ("golden showers"). Collectively, preoccupations with enemas and urine are termed "water sports" by those who enjoy them.

Infantilism. In this paraphilia, the patient derives sexual satisfaction from being treated like a baby—perhaps wearing diapers and drinking from a bottle.

F65.9 [302.9] Unspecified Paraphilic Disorder

Use unspecified paraphilic disorder when a paraphilic disturbance does not meet the criteria for any of the disorders described in this chapter, and you decide not to state the reason.

CHAPTER 19

Other Factors That May Need Clinical Attention

You can use the codes provided in this chapter to report certain environmental or other physical or psychosocial events or conditions that might affect the diagnosis or management of your patient. When stating them, be as specific as possible. (Other problems are possible; these are samples.) Many of these were listed on Axis IV of DSM-IV. DSM-5 requires that we use ICD-10 [or ICD-9] codes for the problems we identify. Following is a reasonably complete list of those available.

But remember, please, that these behaviors, conditions, and relationships are not mental disorders. I emphasize this point in the attempt to reduce our tendency to carve pathology out of behavior that is, after all, the stuff of normal human existence.

Relational and Family Problems

Z62.820 [V61.20] Parent–Child Relational Problem

Use parent–child relational problem when clinically important symptoms or negative effects on functioning are associated with the way a parent and child interact. The problematic interaction patterns may include faulty communication, ineffective discipline, or overprotection. Various emotional and behavioral problems could ensue.

Z63.0 [V61.10] Relationship Distress with Spouse or Intimate Partner

Use relationship distress with spouse or intimate partner when clinically important symptoms or negative effects on functioning are associated with the way a patient and spouse/partner interact. The problematic interaction patterns may include faulty communication or an absence of communication. However, this category explicitly excludes problems related to abuse (which are described below).

Z62.891 [V61.8] Sibling Relational Problem

Use sibling relational problem when clinically important symptoms or negative effects on functioning are associated with the way siblings interact.

Z62.898 [V61.29] Child Affected by Parental Relationship Distress

Z62.29 [V61.8] Upbringing Away from Parents

Upbringing away from parents is for problems that arise because a child is living in foster care or with relatives or friends, but not in residential care or boarding school.

Z59.3 [V60.6] Problems Related to Living in a Residential Institution

This code is for use with kids (or adults) whose problems arise from living away from home in some sort of institution. It does not include emotional responses to the experience to institutional living.

Z59.2 [V60.89] Discord with Neighbor, Lodger, or Landlord

Res ipsa loquitur.

Z63.5 [V61.03] Disruption of Family by Separation or Divorce

Z63.8 [V61.8] High Expressed Emotion Level within Family

Lots of yelling and screaming in the family unit has been linked with relapse in schizophrenia, but it could affect just about anyone.

Z63.4 [V62.82] Uncomplicated Bereavement

When a relative or close friend dies, it is natural to grieve. When the symptoms of the grieving process are a reason for receiving clinical attention, DSM-5 allows us to code these as uncomplicated bereavement—provided that the symptoms don't last too long and aren't too severe. The problem is that the sadness of grief can resemble the sadness associated with a major depressive episode.

Certain symptoms can help you decide whether, in addition to being bereaved, the patient is suffering from a major depressive episode:

- Guilt feelings (other than about actions that might have prevented the death)
- Death wishes (other than the survivor's wishing to have died with the loved one)
- Slowed-down psychomotor activity

- Severe preoccupation with worthlessness

- Severely impaired functioning for an unusually long time

- Hallucinations (other than of seeing or hearing the deceased)

In addition, people who are "only" bereaved typically regard their moods as normal. Traditionally, a diagnosis of depressive illness has been withheld in these cases until after the symptoms have lasted longer than 2 months. Now we are encouraged to diagnose major depressive disorder regardless of bereavement, should the symptoms warrant. Table 19.1 compares the symptoms of major depression with those of uncomplicated bereavement.

Academic and Occupational Problems

Z55.9 [V62.3] Academic or Educational Problem

Use academic or educational problem for a patient whose problem is related to scholastic endeavors and who does not have a specific learning disorder or other mental disorder that accounts for the problem. Examples include illiteracy, unavailable school, poor academic performance, underachievement, or discord with teacher or other students. Even if another disorder can account for the problem, the academic problem itself may be so severe that it independently justifies clinical attention. For example, see the vignette of Colin Rodebaugh (p. 311).

TABLE 19.1. Comparing Symptoms of Major Depression and Uncomplicated Bereavement

	Major depression	Grief
Expression of mood	Despair and hopelessness	Loss or emptiness
Time course	Steady or waxing	Decrease with time (weeks)
Stability of mood	Persistent	Surges and retreats
Response to humor, distraction	Little or none	May bring relief
Content of thought	Largely unrelieved thoughts of own misery	Memories/thoughts of departed, but some positive thoughts regarding others
Self-esteem	Guilt, blame, worthlessness	"I've done my best"
Passing of time	Time crawls	Time passes as before
Death, dying	Wish for own death; suicidal plans	Life is still worth living
Clinical impairment	Yes	No

Z56.82 [V62.21] Problem Related to Current Military Deployment Status

Don't include psychological reactions here. Rather, use this category when deployment itself is the focus.

Z91.82 [V62.22] Personal History of Military Deployment

Z56.9 [V62.29] Other Problem Related to Employment

Other occupational problems could include issues in choosing a career, job change, troubles getting along with supervisor or coworkers, threat of dismissal, general dissatisfaction with one's job, stressful or hostile work environment, sexual harassment on the job, or unemployment.

Problems Related to Income and Dwelling

Z59.0 [V60.0] Homelessness

A patient has no fixed abode.

Z59.1 [V60.1] Inadequate Housing

Examples: No utilities, overcrowding, vermin, excessive noise.

Z59.4 [V60.2] Lack of Adequate Food or Safe Drinking Water

Z59.5 [V60.2] Extreme Poverty

Z59.6 [V60.2] Low Income

Z59.7 [V60.2] Insufficient Social Insurance or Welfare Support

Z59.9 [V60.9] Unspecified Housing or Economic Problem

Z60.2 [V60.3] Problem Related to Living Alone

Legal/Behavioral Problems

Z65.0 [V62.5] Conviction in Civil or Criminal Proceedings without Imprisonment

Z65.1 [V62.5] Imprisonment or Other Incarceration

Z65.2 [V62.5] Problems Related to Release from Prison

Z65.3 [V62.5] Problems Related to Other Legal Circumstances

Examples include being arrested, suing, or being sued.

Z65.4 [V62.89] Victim of Crime

Z72.811 [V71.01] Adult Antisocial Behavior

If the reason for clinical attention is antisocial behavior that is not part of a pattern (and hence not attributable to antisocial personality disorder, conduct disorder, or a disorder of impulse control), adult antisocial behavior can be coded. Examples would include the activities of career criminals who do not have any of the disorders just mentioned.

Z72.810 [V71.02] Child or Adolescent Antisocial Behavior

Child or adolescent antisocial behavior is the juvenile equivalent of the adult code described above.

Problems Related to Health Care Issues

The labels for many of the codes in the health care category explain themselves.

E66.9 [278.00] Overweight or Obesity

Z64.0 [V61.7] Problems Related to Unwanted Pregnancy

Z64.1 [V61.5] Problems Related to Multiparity

Z64.4 [V62.89] Discord with Social Service Provider, Including Probation Officer, Case Manager, or Social Services Worker

Z71.9 [V65.40] Other Counseling or Consultation

Other counseling or consultation covers matters such as counseling for weight loss or smoking cessation.

Z75.3 [V63.9] Unavailability or Inaccessibility of Health Care Facilities

Z75.4 [V63.8] Unavailability or Inaccessibility of Other Helping Agencies

Problems in these two areas could be due to insufficient health insurance or unavailability of transportation to health care services.

Z91.19 [V15.81] Nonadherence to Medical Treatment

Use nonadherence to medical treatment for a patient who requires attention because the patient has ignored or controverted attempts at treatment for a mental disorder or another medical condition. An example would be a patient with schizophrenia who requires repeated hospitalization for refusal to take medication.

Z91.83 [V40.31] Wandering Associated with a Mental Disorder

The wandering . . . code applies especially to patients with major neurocognitive disorders, who are particularly prone to leaving their dwellings and striking off on their own; the negative consequences sometimes make national headlines. Code first the mental disorder, then the Z-code/V-code.

Z91.5 [V15.59] Personal History of Self-Harm

Problems Related to Abuse or Neglect

The titles of the Z-codes [with V-codes] for various types of abuse or neglect are pretty much self-explanatory. Rather than write out every one of them, I've put them into a table (see Table 19.2). Also, each of the ICD-10 codes in Table 19.2 should have XA (for initial encounter) or XD (for subsequent encounter) appended. Note that some of the code numbers are the same, though the wording is different. This isn't a mistake—or, at least, it isn't my mistake.

Here are three helpful definitions:

Sexual abuse. Any sex act (including those that do not involve contact, such as photography) intended to gratify the perpetrator or others.

Neglect. An act (or omission) that so deprives an individual of basic needs that it could result in physical or psychological harm.

Psychological abuse. Intentional verbal or symbolic acts by a caregiver that could

TABLE 19.2. Codes for Neglect and Abuse

	Abuse confirmed	Abuse suspected
Child physical abuse	T74.12 [995.54]	T76.12 [995.54]
Child sexual abuse	T74.22 [995.53]	T76.22 [995.53]
Child neglect	T74.02 [995.52]	T76.02 [995.52]
Child psychological abuse	T74.32 [995.51]	T76.32 [995.51]
Spouse or partner violence, physical	T74.11 [995.81]	T76.11 [995.81]
Spouse or partner violence, sexual	T74.21 [995.83]	T76.21 [995.83]
Spouse or partner neglect	T74.01 [995.85]	T76.01 [995.85]
Spouse or partner abuse, psychological	T74.31 [995.82]	T76.31 [995.82]
Adult physical abuse by nonspouse or nonpartner	T74.11 [995.81]	T76.11 [995.81]
Adult sexual abuse by nonspouse or nonpartner	T74.21 [995.83]	T76.21 [995.83]
Adult psychological abuse by nonspouse or nonpartner	T74.31 [995.82]	T76.31 [995.82]

result in psychological harm. Examples include berating, scapegoating, threatening, coercion, and physical confinement.

By the way, there are other codes you can use if the focus of the interview is on the encounter for mental health services for the victim or the perpetrator—different codes if the perpetrator is a parent or not (see Table 19.3). And if the patient has a personal history of abuse or neglect, there are some codes for that, too (see Table 19.4).

TABLE 19.3. Codes for Neglect and Abuse When the Emphasis Is on the Encounter for Mental Health Services

Encounter for mental health services for:	Victim	Perpetrator
Child neglect or physical/sexual/psychological abuse by parent	Z69.010 [V61.21]	Z69.011 [V61.22]
Child neglect or physical/sexual/psychological abuse by nonparent	Z69.020 [V61.21]	Z69.021 [V62.83]
Adult spouse/partner neglect, physical/sexual violence, or psychological abuse	Z69.11 [V61.11]	Z69.12 [V61.12]
Adult nonspousal or nonpartner abuse	Z69.81 [V65.49]	Z69.82 [V62.83]

TABLE 19.4. Codes for Use When a Patient Has a Previous Personal History of Neglect or Abuse

Physical or sexual abuse in childhood	Z62.810 [V15.41]
Neglect in childhood	Z62.812 [V15.42]
Psychological abuse in childhood	Z62.811 [V15.42]
Spouse or partner physical or sexual violence	Z91.410 [V15.41]
Spouse or partner neglect	Z91.412 [V15.42]
Spouse or partner psychological abuse	Z91.411 [V15.42]

Medication-Induced Movement Disorders

Medication-induced movement disorders are important in mental health care for two reasons:

- They may be mistaken for mental disorders (such as tic disorders, schizophrenia, or anxiety disorders).

- They can affect the management of patients who are receiving psychotropic medications.

G21.0 [333.92] Neuroleptic Malignant Syndrome

The use of a neuroleptic medication can lead within 3 days to muscle rigidity, fever, and other problems, such as sweating, trouble swallowing, incontinence, and delirium.

G21.11 [332.1] Neuroleptic-Induced Parkinsonism

G21.19 [332.1] Other Medication-Induced Parkinsonism

Many of the antipsychotic agents that have been developed and used over the past 60 years (and a few other medications, too) can induce a frozen face, shuffling gait, and pill-rolling tremor that much resemble naturally occurring Parkinson's disease.

G24.01 [333.85] Tardive Dyskinesia

After a patient has taken a neuroleptic medication for a few months or more, involuntary movements of the face, jaw, tongue, or limbs may become noticeable. Once begun, these movements can become permanent, even if the neuroleptic medication responsible is discontinued.

G24.02 [333.72] Medication-Induced Acute Dystonia

Abrupt contracting in muscles of the head, neck, or other portions of the body can produce painful, often frightening spasms. These are due to the use of neuroleptic medications (and others) and occur quite commonly.

G25.1 [333.1] Medication-Induced Postural Tremor

The use of medications such as antidepressants, lithium, or valproate may cause a fine tremor when the person tries to maintain a position (for example, an outstretched hand).

G25.71 [333.99] Medication-Induced Acute Akathisia

Shortly after beginning or increasing the dose of a neuroleptic (or other) drug, some patients become acutely restless and unable to remain seated.

G25.79 [333.99] Other Medication-Induced Movement Disorder

DSM-5 suggests that other medication-induced movement disorder may be useful for patients who have symptoms resembling neuroleptic malignant syndrome, but who have used drugs other than neuroleptics.

T43.205 [995.29] Antidepressant Discontinuation Syndrome

Within a few days of stopping an antidepressant, a patient may develop nonspecific symptoms that can include dizziness, sleeplessness, a peculiar sensation sometimes described as "electric shocks to the brain," nausea, sweating, and many other symptoms. Its incidence is probably proportional to the dose of the antidepressant.

T50.905 [995.20] Other Adverse Effects of Medication

Other adverse effects of medication can be used for unwanted effects besides movement disorders that become an important focus for clinical attention. Examples include severe hypotension caused by neuroleptics and priapism caused by trazodone.

Miscellaneous Issues

Z65.4 [V62.89] Victim of Terrorism or Torture

Z65.8 [V62.89] Other Problem Related to Psychosocial Circumstances

Z65.9 [V62.9] Unspecified Problem Related to Unspecified Psychosocial Circumstances

Other Conditions That May Be a Focus of Clinical Attention . . .

. . . but are not mental disorders.

R41.83 [V62.89] Borderline Intellectual Functioning

Use borderline intellectual functioning for a patient whose IQ and level of functioning fall within the range of approximately 71–84. In the face of other mental diagnoses (psychotic or cognitive disorders, for example), the differential diagnosis between borderline intellectual functioning and mild intellectual disability can be quite difficult—especially now that DSM-5 has stopped defining intellectual disability by IQ score.

Z60.0 [V62.89] Phase of Life Problem

Use phase of life problem for a patient whose problem is not due to a mental disorder but to a life change, such as marriage, divorce, a new job, an empty nest, or retirement. It must be discriminated from adjustment disorder.

Z60.3 [V62.4] Acculturation Problem

Acculturation problem may be useful for patients whose problems center on a move from one culture to another (e.g., migrants and immigrants).

Z60.4 [V62.4] Social Exclusion or Rejection

Being a victim of bullying would fit in here.

Z60.5 [V62.4] Target of (Perceived) Adverse Discrimination or Persecution

Examples could include racial or sexual discrimination.

Z65.8 [V62.89] Religious or Spiritual Problem

Patients who require evaluation or treatment for issues pertaining to religious faith (or its lack) may be given the religious or spiritual problem code.

Z65.8 [V62.89] Other Problem Related to Psychosocial Circumstances

This catch-all category could include death or illness of a relative, or remarriage of a parent. I realize that it has the same code numbers as religious or spiritual problem; life's imperfect.

Z65.5 [V62.22] Exposure to Disaster, War, or Other Hostilities

Z72.9 [V69.9] Problem Related to Lifestyle

Examples include poor sleep hygiene, high-risk sexual behavior.

Z76.5 [V65.2] Malingering

Malingering is defined as the intentional production of the signs or symptoms of a physical or mental disorder. The purpose is some sort of gain: obtaining something desirable (money, drugs, insurance settlement) or avoiding something unpleasant (punishment, work, military service, jury duty). Malingering is often confused with factitious disorder (in which the motive is not external gain, but a wish to occupy the sick role) and other somatic symptom and related disorders (in which the symptoms are not intentionally produced at all).

Malingering should be suspected in any of these situations:

- The patient has legal problems or the prospect of financial gain.
- The patient has antisocial personality disorder.
- The patient tells a story that does not accord with informants' accounts or with other known facts.
- The patient does not cooperate with the evaluation.

Malingering is easy to suspect and difficult to prove. In the absence of definitive observation (you watch as someone places sand into a urine specimen or holds a thermometer over a glowing light bulb), a resolute and clever malingerer can be almost impossible to detect. When malingering involves symptoms that are strictly mental or emotional, detection may be impossible. Moreover, the consequences of this diagnosis are dire: It provides closure in such a way as to totally alienate the clinician from the patient. I therefore recommend that you make this diagnosis only in the most obvious and imperative of circumstances.

Z91.49 [V15.49] Other Personal History of Psychological Trauma

Z91.89 [V15.89] Other Personal Risk Factors

Additional Codes

Finally, here are a few additional codes useful for administrative purposes. These are not included in DSM-5, but they are a part of ICD-10. I provide them here anyway.

Z03.89 [V71.09] Encounter for Observation for Other Suspected Diseases and Conditions Ruled Out

This rather clumsy and way too long designation (ICD-9 has it as a slightly smaller mouthful—*observation of other suspected mental condition*) means that the patient does not have a major mental disorder or personality disorder. Of course, that won't often be the case, but every mental health practitioner at some time or other is likely to encounter patients who have no mental disorder. If (when) I use it, I'll write down one of the numbers given above but just call it "No mental disorder."

F48.9 [300.9] Unspecified Nonpsychotic Mental Disorder

There are one or two situations in which a diagnosis of unspecified nonpsychotic mental disorder may be appropriate:

- The diagnosis you want to give is not contained in DSM-5.

- You know that a patient has a mental disorder, but you have insufficient information to state what it is, and no other unspecified category seems appropriate. Once you have obtained more information, you should be able to change this to a more specific diagnosis. If you cannot even be sure that the patient has no psychotic symptoms, you'd have to use the next code.

F99 [799.9] Mental Illness, Unspecified (Diagnosis Deferred)

Here is a designation you should hardly ever use—as a final diagnosis—but one that I frequently deploy at first evaluation. It means that you don't have even enough information to be sure what chapter of DSM-5 your patient belongs in (if you did, you could use, for example, unspecified depressive disorder). I most often use this category to describe a patient in an admitting note (where, of course, I don't have to include any code numbers at all). This patient could be psychotic.

R69 [799.9] Unspecified Illness

This one is the least specific of all, but wouldn't you think you'd at least have enough information to know that it's *mental*?

CHAPTER 20

Patients and Diagnoses

Clinicians use rules to decide what diagnoses to give their patients. They don't always realize that they are using rules, but they're there, all right.

Throughout my professional life, I've spent a lot of time thinking, talking, and writing about these rules (OK, I usually call them "principles") and how they should be deployed. Here I'm just going to list them, so we can then use them in diagnosing the mental health patients in this chapter. I hope you'll want to know more about how to understand and apply this important part of mental health practice.

Diagnostic Health Care Principles

As you read the patient vignettes that follow, try not to confuse the principles, which are designated with capital letters, with the DSM-5 criteria, which also have letters. Lots of luck—I've gotten turned around a time or two myself. By the way, I've filched these from one of my own books: *Diagnosis Made Easier*, second edition (The Guilford Press, 2014, pp. 305–306). Highly recommended.

Create a Differential Diagnosis

A. Arrange your differential diagnosis according to a safety hierarchy.

B. Family history can guide diagnosis, but because you often can't trust reports, clinicians should attempt to rediagnose each family member.

C. Physical disorders and their treatment can produce or worsen mental symptoms.

D. Consider somatic symptom (somatization) disorder whenever symptoms don't jibe or treatments don't work.

E. Substance use can cause a variety of mental disorders.

F. Because of their ubiquity, potential for harm, and ready response to treatment, *always* consider mood disorders.

When Information Sources Conflict

G. History beats current appearance.

H. Recent history beats ancient history.

I. Collateral information sometimes beats the patient's own.

J. Signs beat symptoms.

K. Be wary when evaluating crisis-generated data.

L. Objective findings beat subjective judgment.

M. Use Occam's razor: Choose the simplest explanation.

N. Horses are more common than zebras; prefer the more frequently encountered diagnosis.

O. Watch for contradictory information.

Resolve Uncertainty

P. The best predictor of future behavior is past behavior.

Q. More symptoms of a disorder increase its likelihood as your diagnosis.

R. Typical features of a disorder increase its likelihood as your diagnosis; in the presence of nontypical features, look for alternatives.

S. Previous typical response to treatment for a disorder increases its likelihood as your diagnosis.

T. Use the word *undiagnosed* whenever you cannot be sure of your diagnosis.

U. Consider the possibility that this patient should be given no mental diagnosis at all.

Multiple Diagnoses

V. When symptoms cannot be adequately explained by a single disorder, consider multiple diagnoses.

W. Avoid personality disorder diagnoses when your patient is acutely ill with a major mental disorder.

X. Arrange multiple diagnoses to list first the one that is most urgent, treatable, or specific. Whenever possible, also list diagnoses chronologically.

Case Histories

With experience, sorting through the information from a patient's history and mental status exam becomes gradually easier. After you have evaluated 200 patients or so, you will find that the process has become virtually second nature. In the remainder of this chapter, you'll have an opportunity to try your own diagnostic skills on a variety of patients. Some of them have multiple mental disorders, which may be the norm rather than the exception. A national survey of adults in the general population found that of those who had a lifetime history of at least one disorder, over 60% had more than one. About 14% of all Americans have three or more lifetime diagnoses.

Due to space requirements, these case histories have been somewhat abridged. Other clinicians might disagree with some of my conclusions; my main purpose in presenting them is to demonstrate how a clinician reasons through the facts to arrive at a diagnosis.

Here's one additional suggestion. People learn more rapidly when they are actively involved. So rather than just reading the vignettes and my discussions, I suggest that you try to figure out the diagnoses yourself, using the diagnostic principles and my DSM-5 Essential Features. Then compare your answers to mine.

Laura Freitas

Laura Freitas, a 32-year-old divorced woman, was admitted to a mental health unit with this chief complaint: "I'm God." She was referred from an outpatient clinic and served as her own chief informant.

Laura had had her first episode of mental illness at age 19, after her second baby was born. She could remember little about this period, except that it was called a "postpartum psychosis" and she had spent some time in isolation for dancing nude in the hospital day room. She had recovered and remained well until 3 years ago, when, for reasons she could not remember, she was placed on lithium carbonate. She had taken this medication from then until 7 or 8 days ago, when she stopped because "I felt so well, so powerful that I knew I didn't need it." Over the next several days she became increasingly agitated, slept little, and talked a great deal, until friends finally brought her for treatment.

Laura had been born in Illinois, where her father was an automobile mechanic. She was an only child who often felt that her parents "would have been happier with no children at all." She described them both as "alcoholics" and noted that she had run away from them overnight on at least one occasion when she was 13. She had twice experimented with marijuana when she was a teenager, but she denied using other drugs, including alcohol.

At 18 Laura had been briefly married to a bread salesman, with whom she had had two children. The daughter, 13, lived with her father. The son, 14, was hyperactive and had at one time been treated with Ritalin. Laura was a fallen-away Catholic who for the past 2 years had worked at a travel agency. She stated that her health had been "above perfect," meaning that she had had no allergies or medical problems, other than a tonsillectomy when she was 6 and a tubal ligation after the birth of her daughter. Family history was positive for alcoholism in both parents and both grandfathers. A paternal aunt would intermittently "go to pieces," becoming excessively religious and imagining various sins for which she felt excessive guilt.

Laura was a somewhat overweight woman who looked about her stated age. She was quite agitated, jumping out of her chair every few moments to pace to the door and back. Given breakfast during a part of this interview, she intentionally smeared grape jelly onto the trousers of a passing nurse. Subsequently, she lay down on the floor and kicked her legs in the air, apparently in ecstasy.

Laura seemed to be struggling to control her speech; even so, she skipped from one subject to another. However, the rate at which she spoke was approximately normal. Her affect was clearly elevated, and she declared that she had never felt better in her life. She admitted that she might hear voices singing (the interviewer could hear no music); she enjoyed singing along with what she heard. She stated that she was "the All-Powerful One" and that she now realized that she had no need for medication.

Laura was oriented to person, place, and time. She named five recent presidents, and correctly (and extremely rapidly) subtracted serial sevens into the negative numbers. When she finished, she apologized for taking so long to complete a task working with numbers. "After all," she remarked, "I created them."

Evaluation of Laura Freitas

Two diagnostic areas stand out in Laura's case—psychosis and mood disturbance. Psychosis can be dealt with summarily: Her delusions were too brief for any of the psychotic diagnoses except **brief psychotic disorder** or **substance-induced psychotic disorder**. However, each of these requires that a mood disorder not better explain the symptoms, and that, as we will note, was not the case: Laura's previous manic episodes would disqualify her for any psychotic disorder.

Laura's current symptoms strongly suggest a **manic episode**. It appears that a previous clinician also had thought so: She was successfully treated with lithium (specific for the bipolar disorders) until shortly before this admission. Let us work through the steps necessary to diagnose manic episode (see p. 116):

1. *Quality of mood.* Elevated mood was shown in the expansive way Laura expressed herself and in her statement that she had never felt better.

2. *Duration.* Her current symptoms had lasted at least 1 week. Information from informants (principle I) would probably establish that the onset of her present episode was even longer ago, perhaps at the point that she began to feel increasingly "well."

3. *Symptoms.* Laura had at least four symptoms (three are required) for manic

episode. She was grandiose (she was calling herself God and claiming that her physical health was "above perfect"). She also had agitation, excessive speech, and decreased need for sleep. I might point out, too, that she had a *lot* of typical symptoms of mania (principle R).

4. *Impairment.* This was clearly demonstrated by Laura's admission to the hospital, where she smeared jelly on a nurse.

5. *Exclusions.* None were noted, including substance use (she had used marijuana only when she was a teenager) and general medical conditions. However, hyperthyroidism and other endocrine disorders should be ruled out by routine laboratory testing upon admission.

Laura would therefore fulfill the basic criteria for manic episode. No general medical condition or cognitive disorder would seem more likely (diagnostic principle C). If any further confirmation was needed, she had an aunt who might have had a recurrent psychosis. This sort of family history (principle B) would better support a remitting condition such as bipolar I disorder than a chronic psychosis such as schizophrenia. Furthermore, the safety principle (A) demands that we consider more treatable disorders first. And, just to rub it in, reread principle F.

The vignette does not indicate whether Laura had ever had an episode of depression; for coding purposes, it doesn't matter. Her most recent (current) episode was manic, and she had had at least two prior episodes (one 13 years ago, one 3 years ago when she started lithium). Psychosis would qualify her for a severity level of severe, with psychotic features. Her delusion that she was God would be mood-congruent for mania.

By the way, in rereading this discussion, I note that I haven't indicated any differential diagnosis. The symptoms of mania just overwhelmed me, and I didn't think it would add anything to our understanding of this patient with classic bipolar I disorder.

Laura would not qualify for any episode specifiers (see Table 3.3 in Chapter 3). The vignette gives no information suggesting that she also had a personality disorder. Her physical health was good. There is no evidence that her divorced status or the treatment of her son for hyperactivity would have any effect on the treatment of her mania, so I didn't list any Z-codes for her. I placed her GAF score at 25 on the basis that she was currently quite ill, with behavior influenced by delusions, though she did not seem to be in danger of hurting herself or others. Her full diagnosis would read:

F31.2 [296.44]   Bipolar I disorder, current episode manic, severe with mood-congruent psychotic features

Adrian Branscom

Adrian Branscom was a 49-year-old executive who referred himself to his company's mental health clinician. "I never thought I'd be talking to a shrink," was his first comment upon entering the office.

After serving 2 years as a junior officer in the Army Ordnance Corps, Adrian had been recruited by a subsidiary of one of the large petroleum companies that specialized in oil field development. Bright and energetic, he had climbed rapidly through the ranks of middle management and was in line for a vice-presidency when the recession hit. Although his share of the restructuring turned out to be no vice-presidency and a 10% pay cut, Adrian felt lucky that he still had a job. His wife's view was less sanguine.

Yoshiko was a Japanese service bride. They had married during a whirlwind 2-week leave he had spent in Tokyo during Adrian's tour of duty in Asia. For the past 20 years, since the births of their daughter and son, she had stayed home with the children.

"She wishes she had stayed home in Japan," Adrian commented wryly. Almost since their wedding, Yoshiko had accused him of taking her away from her people so he could "dump her." In all the years they had lived together, she had never made friends. She spent most of her free time acquiring a collection of Japanese porcelain artifacts. Now she deeply resented her husband's demotion and their loss of income.

"We hadn't been getting along well for years," said Adrian, "but for the last several years we've hit one new low after another. She says if I were a real man, I'd provide better for her."

On many occasions, Adrian had told Yoshiko he thought they should discuss their problems. Her usual response was "So go ahead and discuss it!" When he tried to state his viewpoint, she would listen for half a sentence; then "She always begins to talk over me. After starting six or eight sentences, I usually give up." Every suggestion Adrian made that they seek marital counseling provoked a torrent of invective from Yoshiko and the demand for a divorce. When he tried to discuss divorce, she cried and said that he was trying to get rid of her and that they'd all be better off if she committed suicide. These tirades made him feel guilty, and they had worsened in the past month or so.

Although Adrian was usually a "happy-go-lucky sort of fellow," for most of the past 6 weeks he had been depressed and anxious. His appetite and energy had been unchanged, but he had had trouble sleeping most nights; he had often awakened with a pounding heart and the feeling that he was about to smother. His concentration at work and his self-confidence had both plummeted. Increasingly over the past week, he had been thinking about death and the shotgun he still had somewhere up in his attic. Frightened, he had finally decided to seek help.

Adrian had been born in west central Texas, where his father taught school and did a little farming. He was the youngest of three children, all of whom managed to go to college and succeed in business or a profession. "It wasn't until I was out of college that I realized just how dirt-poor my parents were," he said. "I guess we seemed well off because we were all happy."

The family history was negative for substance use or for any other mental disorder. Adrian had never used drugs or alcohol, and had never had moods that were excessively elevated or irritable. He spent most of his time at work and had very few friends; he had never strayed from the marital bed ("twin beds," as he put it). At home, he enjoyed collecting rocks and hiking with his son.

Adrian was a conservatively dressed, somewhat overweight man who looked his stated age. He sat quietly in the office chair during the interview. Once or twice he reached for a fresh tissue to wipe his eyes. His speech was clear, coherent, relevant, and spontaneous. His mood was appropriate to the content of thought and showed normal lability. He denied having any hallucinations or delusions. He stated that he had always been "a fixer"—that he felt it was his job to make things work for everyone. He earned a perfect score on the MMSE. His insight and judgment seemed unimpaired. "I think we'd all be better off if we lived apart," he concluded. "This is one thing I don't think I can fix."

Evaluation of Adrian Branscom

A rapid reading of Adrian's history suggests three possible diagnostic areas: mood disorder, anxiety disorder, and problems of adjustment. To consider adjustment disorder first, it would be easy to suppose that Adrian's difficulties could be laid completely at the doorstep of his marital difficulties. After all, he had no past history of mental disorder, and he did have an extremely troubled marriage. But he had enough symptoms to qualify for a mood disorder (see below), and the criteria for adjustment disorder with depressed mood quite clearly require that the criteria for no other mental disorder be fulfilled.

From the information we have, his character structure, though perhaps a bit naïve, revealed none of the sorts of interpersonal difficulties we would expect for a personality disorder. However, in a later interview, the clinician should obtain information from informants (principle I); the vignette gives only Adrian's interpretation of his marital strife.

As for the anxiety disorders, Adrian had episodes of awakening from sleep with pounding heart and shortness of breath, and he had felt anxious for much of the previous few weeks. These symptoms weren't enough to qualify for a panic attack (which can occur during sleep); naturally, we won't diagnose **panic disorder**. None of his symptoms would suggest **specific phobia**, **social anxiety disorder**, **agoraphobia**, or **obsessive– compulsive disorder**. Although he was a war veteran, he was evidently not exposed to extremely traumatic events (as would be the case in **posttraumatic stress disorder**). **Generalized anxiety disorder** requires a 6-month duration and more symptoms. Although Adrian was overweight, obesity does not have any known relationship to anxiety symptoms; it should be mentioned in his diagnostic summary, however.

Finally, Adrian did have some clear-cut mood symptoms, and when you hear hoofbeats in the street, think of horses, not zebras (principle N). His symptoms included feeling depressed most of the time, insomnia, problems with concentration, feelings of guilt, and an increasing preoccupation with suicide. (DSM-5 does not credit low self-confidence and weeping as qualifying depressive symptoms.) His symptoms had been constantly present for over a month and were causing him trouble with his job. None of the exclusions would apply (general medical condition or substance use), so he would fulfill criteria for a major depressive episode and for a single episode of **major depressive disorder**. None of the course or episode specifiers would apply (see Chapter

3, Table 3.3). He fulfilled only the minimum number of symptoms, but one of these (suicidal ideas) was serious, so his clinician thought this deserved a severity rating of at least moderate. His moderate symptoms would earn him a GAF score of 60. Although Adrian had had some thoughts about suicide, he had no plans and did not appear to be at serious immediate risk. His complete diagnosis would be as follows:

F32.1 [296.22]	Major depressive disorder, single episode, moderate
E66.9 [278.00]	Obesity
Z63.0 [V61.10]	Marital discord

Wait a minute! What about Yoshiko? Surely she deserves some sort of diagnosis. A personality disorder, you might think.

Of course, Yoshiko's personal characteristics sound pretty alarming, very possibly enough to earn some sort of mental disorder diagnosis. There are just two problems: We haven't nearly enough information, and she isn't our patient. We haven't even interviewed her. All we have to go on is information from Adrian, who may well be an acute observer; however, he isn't exactly a disinterested one, and we really must have her side of the story before making any diagnosis for her. That isn't one of my diagnostic principles, but it's one that every clinician should follow, nonetheless.

Reggie Ansnes

When he was 35, Reggie Ansnes was admitted to a mental hospital 3,000 miles from home. The admitting note reported that he was agitated, was somewhat grandiose, and didn't even know what city he was in. Although he talked a lot, nothing he said made much sense. "I have schizophrenia," was one of his few unambiguous statements.

"It must be his schizophrenia," Faye, his wife, said on the telephone to the clinician who admitted him. "He told me he had it once before. We've only been married 3 years."

Five years earlier, Reggie had been admitted with psychosis to a mental hospital in Boston. Faye thought that he had then believed he was the son of Jesus, but she didn't know anything else about his symptoms. A doctor had told him he had paranoid schizophrenia. He had been treated with chlorpromazine; Faye knew that because he was still taking it when they began dating.

For about 2 years after that hospitalization, Reggie had been depressed. He used to complain of trouble concentrating at work, and Faye thought that not long after the hospital released him, he had had suicidal ideas. However, the depression had gradually remitted, leaving him with relatively mild problems with appetite and sleep. Even these had resolved by the time they got married, and he had been well ever since. It had now been several years since he had taken any medication at all.

For several days before Reggie's recent business trip, he had been unusually cheerful. He talked a lot, seemed to have increased energy, and arose early to complete the work he would miss while he was gone.

Faye stated that her husband was in good physical health except for a "slight thyroid condition," for which he took a small dose of a thyroid medication. She thought it had been checked the last time he visited his doctor, 3 months earlier. To her knowledge, he neither drank nor used drugs.

During his first 24 hours in the hospital, Reggie was extremely hyperactive and did not sleep at all. His mood was markedly elevated, and he spoke so fast that he was often unintelligible. His statements that could be understood included "I am the son of God," and he shared some ideas for improving the operation of the hospital. He paid little attention to whatever task was at hand, so the MMSE could not be completed.

Evaluation of Reggie Ansnes

Thyroid disease is a general medical condition that can cause mood symptoms; however, Reggie's physician had recently evaluated his thyroid condition, and it had never before produced symptoms that resembled his current condition. Reevaluation of thyroid function tests would be a reasonable course to follow, in any event. (You're right, I *am* getting tired of typing "principle C.")

As for substance use, Faye's information would militate against **substance-induced psychotic disorder**, with onset during withdrawal. However, the blood toxicity screen should rule out any possibility of such a psychosis with onset during intoxication (such as phencyclidine intoxication). With the other history available, this would seem highly unlikely. It is much more usual for patients to use alcohol to attenuate the uncomfortable, driven feeling caused by mania or other psychosis.

A **mood disorder** would seem a much stronger candidate. Five years earlier, Reggie had had grandiose delusions; afterward, he had been depressed for months or years. After a 2-year period of apparent complete normality, he had once again become psychotic, with elevated mood, hyperactivity, insomnia (a decreased need for sleep), and distractibility. Assuming that the tests for thyroid function and toxicity screen came back normal, he would completely fulfill the Essential Features of a manic episode (p. 116), and thus for **bipolar I disorder**, current episode manic (p. 129). If you like, you can check out these criteria in DSM-5—it's tedious, but great exercise.

The previous history of **schizophrenia** might appear to provide a readymade diagnosis for this obviously psychotic patient. If Reggie's earlier illness really had been schizophrenia, it would have been in full remission until the current episode. This would be highly unusual, and with mood symptoms as prominent then as they were now, his new history would demand a serious rethink (principle H). Furthermore, no matter how psychotic Reggie might appear on cross-sectional appearance, his history of episodic illness with complete recovery virtually compels (principle G) us to diagnose bipolar I disorder. An apparent mood disorder now and schizophrenia years ago would also violate the parsimony rule (principle M), not to mention the basic criteria for schizophrenia.

Reggie's current manic symptoms were markedly disabling; severe would be the only appropriate level for him. His psychotic features were completely congruent with manic themes—he thought he was the son of God—which dictates the code numbers listed below. The other possible specifiers (Chapter 3, Table 3.3) do not apply. His previous schizophrenia diagnosis was simply wrong, and should be expunged (as far as possible) from his records. On admission, his GAF score was a low 30; by discharge, his GAF had rebounded to 90.

F31.2 [296.44]	Bipolar I disorder, current episode manic, severe with mood-congruent psychotic features
E03.9 [244.9]	Acquired hypothyroidism

James Chatterton

When James Chatterton was 18, he cut his wrist on the glass of a window he had just broken; this earned him his first admission to a mental hospital. James's aunt was the chief informant on this occasion. "He always seemed a little cold. Kind of like his cousin, my Betty," she said.

James had been pretty unconventional, even when he was little. He cared so little what other people thought that in fourth grade, when he called the teacher "Gristle Butt," he didn't even acknowledge the suppressed laughter of the other children. "I don't think he had a single friend in school," said his aunt. "He never cracked a smile, never got angry—not even when he said he thought the other kids were talking about him. He said that quite a lot, as I recall." Even when he was older, he had never showed the slightest interest in girls or curiosity about sex.

When James was 14, his mother died suddenly. His father, working in another state, had no time for child care, so he was sent to live with his aunt. With no friends to speak of, he had plenty of time to study, and he did well during his first 2 or 3 years in high school. He was fond of science. Well past the time when most boys give up that sort of thing, he continued to play with the chemistry set he had received for Christmas the year he was 9. One day toward spring of his senior year, when his cousin Betty was home with her "monthlies," she lifted her skirt and offered to let James touch her. "He came and told me about it immediately," said his aunt. "He said it made him feel nauseated." On the following day, the entire family was relieved when Betty was rehospitalized for schizophrenia.

For the next several months, James seemed to go into a decline. When his grades fell and his aunt asked why, he only shrugged. He showed no interest either in going to college or in getting a job. He spent most of his free time reading chemistry texts and making notes in the margins. Sometimes when his aunt awakened in the early hours of the morning, she thought she heard him walking around in his room. Several times he seemed to be laughing to himself. He took to sleeping late, often past noon; gradually he stopped going to school at all.

That summer Betty returned from the hospital, vastly improved on neuroleptic medication. Within a week she confided to her mother that James had warned her not to take the medication. It was part of a plot by Mormons, he had told her, to make her sterile. Several times during the next 2 months, he lectured her about extraterrestrials.

James had stopped eating much of anything and lost at least 20 pounds. Weight loss and sleep disturbance made him look gaunt and older. Just before Thanksgiving he broke the window and cut himself, and was finally admitted to the same hospital where Betty had been a patient.

Apart from his lack of friends and his separation from his parents, James's early life had not been remarkable. He had experimented with marijuana a few times, but had never used other street drugs or alcohol. He smoked about a pack of cigarettes a day. His only medical problem had been an operation for an umbilical hernia when he was 5. Besides his cousin, the family history was positive for alcoholism in his paternal grandfather and hyperthyroidism in both his father and an uncle. His mother had been "nervous."

James was thin and sallow, and looked several years older than his age. He was dressed in tattered, cut-off blue jean shorts and a T-shirt. His tennis shoes had no laces, so he scuffed slowly into the interview room, head down, gazing at the ground. Though his facial expression was almost always blank, he would occasionally laugh and turn his head to the side as if he had heard something. He initially denied that he was hearing voices, but later in the day admitted to a second interviewer that a woman's voice kept telling him to "jack off." He denied having any delusions, including grandeur or persecution. Asked directly about a Mormon conspiracy to sterilize his cousin, he said that he wasn't at liberty to discuss it.

James claimed not to be depressed or suicidal; he said he had broken the window and lacerated his arm because he was "upset." He scored 28 out of 30 on the MMSE (he did not know the date within 2 days or the name of the hospital). Although he agreed that he needed medical attention for his arm, he had no insight about his mental disorder.

Evaluation of James Chatterton

James had symptoms in three areas of clinical interest: psychotic thinking, somatic symptoms, and social and personality problems. The somatic symptoms (which included loss of appetite and weight loss), and a family history of hyperthyroidism, should cause his clinician to consider a general medical condition as a possible cause of his psychosis (principle C). Upon admission he would receive a complete physical exam and relevant laboratory testing, which would include thyroid tests. For the purposes of this discussion, let us assume the absence of thyroid disease.

The discussion of James's psychotic thinking follows the outline of the section in Chapter 2 called "Distinguishing Schizophrenia from Other Psychotic Disorders" (p. 60). First, the extent of symptoms must be considered: Did James have enough to meet criterion A for **schizophrenia**? His active psychotic symptoms included persecutory delusions (the Mormon plot, extraterrestrials) and the hallucinated woman's voice giving him commands. These two symptoms by themselves would be enough to fulfill criterion A, but he also had the negative symptom of loss of volition (his grades declined and he showed no interest in work or college). Although his behavior suggested otherwise, James at first denied hearing voices. This demonstrates the value of principle J (signs beat symptoms), which was confirmed later when he admitted to another interviewer that he was in fact having auditory hallucinations. Laughing to himself (possibly responding to something funny his hallucinated voices said) and having a relative with schizophrenia (principle B) also point strongly to a diagnosis of schizophrenia.

The course of a psychotic disorder is extremely important in determining diagnosis. James's disorder began gradually, without precipitating factors, and progressed without remission or recovery. That doesn't constitute a criterion, but it sure sounds like schizophrenia. Here's the criterion (DSM-5 schizophrenia criterion C, actually): Including the prodromal period when he began to withdraw and show lack of volition, he had been ill longer than 6 months (from about April to November). Premorbid personality is discussed below. The consequences were also severe enough for a diagnosis of schizophrenia: They severely interfered with James's social life and his ability to attend school (principle B). With this many typical symptoms of schizophrenia, we become increasingly persuaded that that should be the diagnosis (principle Q).

The rest of our job vis-à-vis the schizophrenia criteria is just to rule out other diagnoses. The possibility of **another medical condition** causing psychotic symptoms has already been discussed and, for the sake of argument, dismissed (DSM-5 criterion E for schizophrenia). James had tried marijuana a few times, but had not used **substances** enough to account for his remarkable deterioration (also criterion E). He scored 2 points short of perfect on the MMSE, well above the range for a **cognitive disorder**. Although James had lost weight, slept poorly, and cut his wrist on glass, when he was admitted to the hospital he could not explain why he had cut his wrist. Moreover, he not only denied feeling depressed; his affect was at times inappropriate. Ergo, I'd dismiss **mood disorders**, even though, for safety reasons, they almost always appear toward the top of my differential diagnoses (principle A).

Finally, we must consider **social** and **personality problems**. According to his aunt, from the time he was a little boy, James had been identified by others as "different." He was emotionally distant (schizoid personality disorder criterion A1), didn't care what others thought (A6), had no close friends (A5), showed few expressions of emotion (A7), and preferred solitary activities (A2). We have only his aunt's perspective on his lack of interest in sex, but still he has one symptom more than the required four for **schizoid personality disorder**. He also had some ideas of reference (the other children might be talking about him)—a symptom of **schizotypal personality disorder**—but his aunt did not report other odd beliefs or peculiar speech or behaviors; James was generally more aloof than peculiar. The absence of any other symptoms of suspiciousness would also rule out **paranoid personality disorder**.

In *DSM-IV Made Easy*, I discussed James's schizophrenia subtype. With delusions, hallucinations, and an affect that was both flat and at times inappropriate (giggling), the only conclusion I could reach was that his was schizophrenia of the undifferentiated type. With the DSM-5 criteria, however, that exercise has been rendered moot, though it's still interesting—to clinicians of a certain age. He had not yet been ill with active-phase symptoms for a year, so he would receive no course specifier. I have already noted his personality disorder, to which the qualifier *(premorbid)* would be added because it was present long before his schizophrenia began.

James also had a notable problem with sleep, but should it receive an independent diagnosis? He would meet most of the criteria for insomnia related to schizophrenia, but it was neither the predominant complaint nor a major focus for treatment. Persistent insomnia of this sort usually normalizes once the underlying psychosis has been successfully treated, so we cannot say it deserves independent evaluation. With a GAF score of 20, James's full diagnosis would be as follows:

F20.9 [295.90]	Schizophrenia
F60.1 [301.20]	Schizoid personality disorder (premorbid)
S61.519A [881.02]	Laceration of wrist

You may have noticed that at the start of my evaluation of James, I mentioned "areas of clinical interest." Well, what are those?

Many years ago, I thought it would aid explanation to divide all the symptoms you might encounter in patients into groups. I ended up with seven groups, three of which were *psychotic thinking*, *somatic symptoms*, and *social and personality problems*. Here are the rest: *mood symptoms*, *anxiety symptoms*, *cognitive problems*, and *substance use*. I've written much, much more about them in my book *The First Interview*, now in its fourth edition (The Guilford Press, 2014).

Gail Downey

"Go ahead, cut!" Gail Downey lay flat on her hospital bed, staring at the ceiling. Her hair was carefully washed and combed, but her expression was stiff. "I want a lobotomy. I'll sign the papers. I can't take this anymore."

Gail was an attractive 34-year-old divorcee with three children. For 5 years she had had depressions but no manias or hypomanias. Her treatment had been marked by frequent suicide attempts and hospitalizations. In her current episode, which had lasted nearly 5 weeks, she had felt severely depressed throughout nearly every day. She complained that she lay awake each night until the early hours; she had no pep, interest, or appetite. She cried frequently, and she was so distracted by her emotional turmoil that her boss had reluctantly let her go.

Gail had been prescribed at least six antidepressants, often in combination. Most of these seemed to help the depression initially, raising her mood enough that she could at least return home. She also had responded positively to each of several courses of ECT. Within a few months of each new treatment she would relapse and return to the hospital, often with a fresh set of stitches in her wrist. While on a brief pass from the present hospitalization, she had swallowed a nearly fatal overdose of chloral hydrate.

After Gail's parents had divorced when she was 9, she had been reared by her mother. Since the age of 13, Gail had been arrested three or four times for taking small items such as pantyhose or a tube of lipstick from department stores. Each of these incidents had occurred while she was under particular stress, usually because a job or personal relationship was going sour. She always noted increasing tension before taking these items, and felt nearly explosive joy each time she left the store with her trophy in the pocket of her overcoat. As a juvenile, whenever she was caught she had been remanded to the custody of her mother; once she had paid a fine. The most recent episode had occurred just before this hospitalization. This time, the charges had been dropped because of her repeated suicide attempts.

Gail's medical history was a catalog of symptoms. It included urinary retention, a lump in her throat that seemed about to strangle her, chest pains, severe menstrual cramps, vomiting spells, chronic diarrhea, heart palpitations, migraine headaches (a neurologist said they were "not typical"), and even a brief episode of blindness (from which she had recovered without treatment). At the time of the divorce, Gail's husband had confided that she had been "frigid" and often complained of pain during intercourse. Starting in her teens, she had taken medicine or consulted a physician for more than 30 such symptoms. The doctors had never found much wrong with her physically; they had either given her tranquilizers or referred her to a succession of psychiatrists.

After several years Gail had been evicted from her apartment, and her husband had obtained custody of their three children. The only nonmedical person she ever talked to was her mother. Now she was demanding an operation that would permanently sever some of the connections within her brain.

Evaluation of Gail Downey

Gail had more than enough mood symptoms (low mood, loss of pleasure, insomnia, anorexia, suicide ideas, loss of energy, trouble thinking) to qualify her current episode as a major depressive episode (you can review the features on p. 112). Any patient who presents with severe depression should be evaluated for **major depressive disorder** (principle F), which can be potentially life-threatening and often responds quickly to the appropriate therapy.

Gail had had numerous episodes of depression, but no manias or hypomanias and no psychotic symptoms; she had also apparently recovered for at least 2 months between episodes. She would therefore qualify for a diagnosis of major depressive disorder, recurrent. The persistent suicide attempts would mark it as severe without psychotic features. The vignette does not give enough information to support other specifiers. But the fact that Gail's depression had been treated so often and so unsuccessfully is a problem. Response to typical treatment for a disorder points in favor of it (principle S), but can we say the inverse? There's no diagnostic principle to that effect, but perhaps there should be: "Repeated failure to respond to typical treatment should prompt consideration of some other condition."

However, since her teens Gail had also had a variety of somatic symptoms, at least some of which (like the migraines) were atypical, so we need to consider **somatic symptom disorder** (principle D). We're going to evaluate her somatic symptoms twice; first with the official DSM-5 description (p. 251), then with the old DSM-IV guidelines for somatization disorder (sidebar, p. 256). She would adequately fulfill the former: at least one somatic symptom that caused marked distress and disrupted her life in some important ways. She had been symptomatic far longer than the 6 months required, and she had experienced a high degree of anxiety relevant to her symptoms.

Of course, she would also meet the DSM-IV somatization disorder criteria, which I believe are far more valuable for identifying actual pathology. These symptoms were distributed appropriately for that diagnosis. Among the **medical** and **neurological disorders** to consider would be multiple sclerosis, spinal cord tumors, and diseases of the heart and lungs. The fact that she had been unsuccessfully treated by so many physicians would reduce the likelihood that she instead had a series of other medical conditions (principle C). The vignette provides no evidence that Gail consciously feigned her symptoms for gain (**malingering**) or for less concrete motives (**factitious disorder**).

No additional diagnosis is needed for Gail's anorexia (principle M); any problem with maintaining body weight was not due to refusal of food, but to her lack of appetite. Her insomnia could be given a separate diagnosis (**insomnia disorder with non-sleep disorder mental comorbidity**) had it been serious enough to warrant independent clinical evaluation; it wasn't. Similarly, her **sexual dysfunction** would not be independently coded (even if the vignette gave enough specifics as to its exact nature), because it is easily explained as a symptom of somatic symptom disorder. Oh, and she didn't abuse **substances**, so that's one more item to cross off our list.

Finally, Gail's history revealed a pattern of repeated shoplifting (see **kleptomania**, p. 390) characterized by tension and release. These features cannot be explained on the basis of anger or revenge or indeed on the basis of some other mental disorder. Hence we must also give her a diagnosis of kleptomania (principle V).

Gail thus had three codable mental diagnoses. How should they be listed? Her major depressive disorder was serious enough that it had been the focus of treatment for at least 5 years; at the beginning of her treatment, that approach was probably sound (principle X). Now, however, that same principle X suggests something quite different: If we make somatization disorder (OK, we can call it somatic symptom disorder for the sake of DSM-5) the focus of her care, it will suggest a common approach to several of her problems. Although the somatic symptom disorder criteria don't specify severity, Gail's clinician, who wanted to indicate how seriously ill she had been, used "clinician's prerogative" and rated her as severely ill.

The vignette gives little information about her personality; we need to add a note to her diagnostic summary that indicates the need for further exploration. Besides, it's best to avoid diagnosing a personality disorder while depression and other matters are so acute (principle W). Considering all of her recent history, she would earn a low GAF score of 40.

F45.1 [300.82]	Somatic symptom disorder, severe
F33.2 [296.33]	Major depressive disorder, recurrent, severe without psychotic features
F63.2 [312.32]	Kleptomania
Z56.9 [V62.29]	Unemployed
Z65.3 [V62.5]	Loss of child custody
Z59.0 [V60.0]	Eviction

Reena Walters

Reena Walters was more than happy to tell her story to the handful of students. In the 4 days she'd been hospitalized (this time), she'd mainly sat around awaiting many tests to be run.

"It's an aneurysm, I'm afraid," she told the class with a wry smile. "I had a seizure on Christmas Day, right as we were about to carve the turkey, and instead I ended up here. As a pediatrician, I've got lots better things to do."

"But how did you come to be here, on the locked unit?" the student interviewer wanted to know.

Reena settled comfortably into her chair. "It's the only ward in the hospital that has no TVs in the rooms." The student looked perplexed. "They're afraid my seizures will be exacerbated by the flicker of the televisions," she explained patiently. "You're familiar with the phenomenon of induced seizures, right? Good. Over the years, I had a couple of kid patients with the same problem. Never dreamed I'd someday be the one affected." She was controlled pretty well now, on medication—the name of which she couldn't recall right now.

Reena continued her story. She had grown up near Modesto, the daughter of itinerant farm workers who made their living picking fruit and hoeing tomatoes. The family had moved around a good deal, so by age 18 she'd attended "literally dozens of different schools." But a scholarship committee at her last high school had plucked her from the fields and sent her off to college. From there, her intelligence and her determination to escape her parents' lifestyle carried her through medical school in southern California and into a career caring for children. She had been instrumental, she remarked with pride, in developing one of the definitive tests for cystic fibrosis in neonates. "I believe it was my finest hour," she almost whispered.

Now 59, her chief regret was that a botched D&C and subsequent hysterectomy when she was in her early 30s meant she'd never been able to have children of her own.

By now, the student interviewer had bogged down, unsure what to ask next. "Maybe you'd like to hear about my family," Reena prompted with a kind smile. She told about her father (a quiet, gentle man who had never spoken a cross word) and her mother (still living at 97, a saint among women, who still drove her own car). Reena had married twice, first to a fellow medical student, who had years ago died as a medical missionary in Uganda. About 10 years later she had married again, this time to a psychiatrist who was still practicing in the town where they lived. Because of his workload, he hadn't yet been able to visit her.

"Could you tell us how you got to the hospital—I mean, what led up to it?"

Reena explained that when she had one of her seizures, she would often behave automatically. "It's called a complex partial seizure, you know? Good. I'll lose track of where I am, but my body plugs right ahead. I can walk and walk, sometimes miles. This time, they found me outside the home of an actor I used to know. The police said I was 'lurking.'" She laughed with infectious humor, and the class joined in.

A few minutes later, Reena had departed, and the instructor asked the students how they'd evaluate her. Her calm and pleasant demeanor and logical presentation seemed highly persuasive to several in the class. "Perhaps, then, we should just take her story at face value," suggested the instructor. That would make hers one of the rare (on mental health wards) cases of no mental diagnosis (principle U).

On the other hand, one student pointed out, there was the niggling matter of her medication, the name of which she couldn't recall despite her own status as a medical practitioner. Of course, it could have been just a senior moment, but was it instead the sort of contradictory evidence (principle O) that encourages us to rethink her whole story? Now that they considered it further, wouldn't it be possible just to turn off the television in a room on any medical ward in the hospital? Until they had more data, the class agreed to consider her as undiagnosed (principle T).

That's when the student who, during the discussion, had been smiling quietly to herself offered some context. She had been involved in discussions with the team that cared for Reena, and she shared the following additional information.

About the only wholly accurate statement Reena had made was her name. She'd never been to medical school, never even graduated from college. None of her *three* husbands had been a physician—she was now once again divorced—and her parents had both been dead for years. Reena herself had once worked as a medical receptionist; there she had picked up the jargon that she deployed with such precision.

Reena's belief that she had a seizure disorder seemed genuine (time after time, she'd been closely quizzed on this issue). She could describe the early sensation of a smell of tomatoes ("from the fields of my childhood, I suppose"), followed by the sense of *déjà vu* that almost always preceded the prolonged periods of unconsciousness, during which she would often wander through strange neighborhoods. Over the years, she'd been worked up several times for a seizure disorder, but all of her MRIs and EEGs (some with pharyngeal leads) had been normal. No one had ever seen her actually having a seizure. (Did she then have **factitious disorder**, someone asked? But she'd only ever been treated in one town, and at one hospital, and she hadn't been observed to manufacture symptoms. Was she **malingering**? If so, where was the gain?)

On the other hand, she did have a rather long rap sheet with local police. Each contact had been related to her fascination (if that was the appropriate word) with a local actor who had had occasional success in television. For years she had followed his career, the actor himself, and her inclination to be near him, leading to repeated arrests for stalking and half a dozen restraining orders. The student ended with, "And if you ask her, she'll be happy to tell you that she's pregnant. Never mind her age, and the hysterectomy."

Evaluation of Reena Walters

The presence of multiple delusions for many years (delusional disorder criterion A) without ever fulfilling criterion A for schizophrenia (delusional disorder criterion B) launches this rare condition to the forefront of our differential diagnosis. (OK, Reena did mention the olfactory hallucination of tomatoes, but this was closely associated with her delusional seizures; this sort of hallucination doesn't really count toward fulfilling criterion A for schizophrenia and is often encountered in delusional disorder.) Outside the context of her specific delusions, her behavior and affect seemed rather ordinary (C), and there was no evidence of associated mood episodes (D).

Of course, her personal history presents any number of possible confounds that we have to eliminate before making a definitive diagnosis. We'd need to learn whether she used **substances** (F)—and, considering the mendacity of her other statements, that information should come from some more reliable source. There was no information to support a different mental condition, specifically **body dysmorphic disorder** or **obsessive–compulsive disorder** (D). As to the type of delusions, I'd say they were largely somatic (she believed she had temporal lobe epilepsy). Only hinted at were her possibly grandiose ideas of having a relationship with the actor. If you prefer a more comprehensive (but vague) classification, call the delusions mixed type. I'd rate her GAF as about 35, though I'd be happy to entertain arguments. And I'd certainly support something in her summary that points the way to a full evaluation of her personality structure—but later.

F22 [297.1]	Delusional disorder, somatic type
Z65.3 [V62.5]	Restraining orders

Sara Winkler

Before she sat down, Sara Winkler crossed herself three times. She and her husband were each 25, and they had been married 4 years. "I've known her since we were 16," Loren Winkler said, "and she's always been pretty careful. You know, checking the stove to see that it's turned off, or the doors to make sure that they're really locked before we go out. It's only been the last couple of years that it's been so much worse."

Sara was a college graduate who had worked briefly as a paralegal assistant before taking time out to have a family. She was healthy and had no history of alcohol or drug use. When their son, Jonathan, was only 6 months old, she had had a terrifying dream in which she plunged a paring knife into the chest of a doll as it lay on the kitchen table. She recognized the doll as one she had owned as a child. But as the knife entered the plastic body, its arms and legs began to move, and she saw that it was a real child. On the kitchen wall, the word *KILL* seemed to scroll upward before her eyes, and she awakened screaming. It had taken her several hours to get back to sleep.

The following evening, while slicing carrots for a salad, she suddenly had this thought: "Would I ever harm Jonathan?" Although the idea seemed absurd, it was accompanied by some of the same anxieties she had felt the night before. She took the baby in to Loren while she finished preparing dinner.

After that, thoughts of knives and of stabbing someone smaller and weaker had increasingly wormed their way into Sara's consciousness. Even if her mind was fixed on reading or watching television, she might suddenly visualize the giant block letters *KILL* arising before her eyes.

The idea that she would actually harm Jonathan seemed irrational to her, but the nagging doubts and anxiety tormented her daily. She no longer trusted herself in the kitchen with him. Sometimes she could almost feel the muscles of her forearm begin to contract in the act of reaching for a knife. Although she had never followed through on one of these impulses, the thought that she might do so terrified her. Now she refused even to open the knife drawer; any cutting had to involve scissors, the food processor, or her husband.

Not long after her dream, Sara began trying to ward off her troubling thoughts and impulses. A fallen-away Catholic, she reverted to some of the practices she had known as a child. When she had one of her frightening thoughts, she initially felt comforted if she crossed herself. If she was carrying packages or Jonathan, she muttered a Hail Mary.

With time, the power of these simple measures seemed to weaken. Then Sara found that if she crossed herself three times or said three Hail Marys (or any combination, in threes), she felt better. Eventually, however, she needed nine of these behaviors before she felt she had adequately protected her son and herself. When she was in public, she could cross herself once and complete the ritual by murmuring Hail Marys under her breath.

Now Jonathan was nearly a year old, and several hours a day were being consumed by Sara's repetitive thoughts and activities. Jonathan was fretful, and Loren was cooking virtually all of their meals. For several weeks she had felt increasingly depressed; she admitted that her mood was bad nearly all the time, though she had not had suicidal ideas or death wishes. Nothing interested her much, and she was always tired. She had lost over 10 pounds and had insomnia; she frequently awakened screaming at night. When her husband found her doing penance 27 times in a row, he insisted they come for help.

"I know it seems crazy," Sara said tearfully, "but I just can't seem to get these stupid ideas out of my head."

Evaluation of Sara Winkler

For longer than 2 weeks, Sara had been depressed most of the time. Her symptoms also included insomnia, fatigue, and loss of interest and weight, all symptoms consistent with a **major depressive episode**. She was physically healthy (principle C) and had no history of substance use (principle E). It is hard to be sure whether she was being impaired by the depression or the symptoms of **obsessive–compulsive disorder (OCD)**; it seems reasonable that she would be having problems from both. With no prior major depressive, manic, or hypomanic episodes, her diagnosis would be **major depressive disorder, single episode**. I'd rate the severity specifier as moderate (relatively few symptoms, no suicidal ideas, but considerable distress). There was very little risk that she would actually harm her son.

As for Sara's anxiety, she had neither **panic attacks** nor **generalized anxiety disorder**. Rather, she had obsessions and compulsions, both of which fulfilled the criteria for OCD (p. 200). (Although she had another mental disorder, her obsessions were not confined to guilty ruminations related to her major depressive disorder.) Her OCD symptoms occupied more than an hour a day, and she was severely distressed. Clearly, Sara's concern was not just an exaggeration of a **real-life problem**, so her focus of concern was pathological. She herself recognized that she was being unreasonable; we'd grade her insight as pretty good.

In recording of Sara's diagnoses, the depression was listed first to indicate that her clinician regarded it as the aspect that most required clinical attention. (Others might well disagree.) Her GAF score of 45 would be justified by the severity of her rituals.

F32.1 [296.22]	Major depressive disorder, single episode, moderate
F42 [300.3]	Obsessive–compulsive disorder, with good insight

Gemma Livingstone

"I eat, then I throw up." That was how Gemma Livingstone described her problem during her first interview. Beginning when she was 23, this behavior had been almost continual in the intervening 4 years.

Even as a teenager, Gemma was concerned about the way she looked. Along with classmates, she had crash-dieted from time to time during high school. But her weight had seldom varied by more than a few pounds from 116. At 5 feet, 6 inches tall, she had been svelte but not too thin. Throughout her adolescence and early adulthood, she had the feeling that if she did not tightly control her eating habits, she would rapidly gain weight—"puff up like a toad," as she put it.

Dealing with the aftermath of an unwanted pregnancy and a subsequent abortion, Gemma had had the opportunity to test her theory. Eating what she wanted, she had ballooned from a size 8 to a size 14 in less than half a year. Once she finally regained control, she vowed she would never lose it again. For 3 years, she had bought nothing larger than a size 4.

Back when Gemma was a teenager, she and her friends simply didn't eat. Whenever dining in a restaurant or with friends, she would still push her food around on her plate to disguise how little she was actually taking in. But when she was at home she would often eat a full meal, then retire to the bathroom and throw up. At first, this had required touching the back of her throat with the handle of a teaspoon she kept in the bathroom for that purpose. With practice, she had learned to regurgitate just by willing it. "It's as easy as blowing your nose," she reported later.

Gemma's fear of obesity had become the organizing principle of her life. On her refrigerator door, she kept a picture of herself when she was in her "toad" phase. She said that every time she looked at it, she lost her appetite. Whereas she previously relied on laxatives only for constipation, recently she had begun to use them as another means of purging her system: "If I don't have a bowel movement every day, I feel as if I'll burst. Even my eyes get all puffy." She had also taken some diuretics, but had stopped doing so when her periods stopped. She didn't really believe there was a connection, but recently she had begun to menstruate again. If there was one thing she feared more than getting fat, it was getting pregnant. She had never been very active sexually, but now she and her husband seldom had intercourse more than once a month. Even then, she insisted on using both a diaphragm and a condom.

Other than her weight, which had fallen under 90 pounds, Gemma appeared to be in good health. A review of systems was positive only for abdominal bloating. Although she occasionally had a day or two of low mood and feeling sorry for herself, she laughed it off as "PMS" and added that it certainly wasn't bothering her now. She had never had manic episodes, hallucinations, obsessions, compulsions, phobias, panic attacks, or thoughts about suicide.

Gemma had been born in Virginia Beach, where her father was stationed with the Navy. Subsequently he owned his own heating and air conditioning company, and the family was reasonably well off. Gemma was an only child. She'd had no history of any kind of difficulties with learning or conduct while she was in school. She and her husband were married when she was 21, after she had worked 3 years as a bank teller. They had two children, a son who was 7 and a daughter age 5.

Gemma's only brush with the law had occurred 2 years earlier, when she'd forged some prescriptions to obtain amphetamines for dieting. She had copped a plea and been placed on probation for a year; she'd scrupulously avoided amphetamines since then. She had tried marijuana once or twice when she was first out of high school, but had never used alcohol or tobacco. Her only surgical procedure had been bilateral breast augmentation, which had been done with autologous fat rather than silicone.

In a separate interview, Gemma's husband stated that he thought his wife felt inadequate and insecure. He said that she usually dressed in revealing, even alluring clothing, which looked less enticing now that she had lost so much weight. When she was denied her way, she would sometimes pout for hours, though he didn't think there was much real feeling behind this expression of her emotion. "She loves to be the center of attention," he said, "but a lot of people don't buy into her act any more. I think it frustrates her."

Gemma was a dark-haired, slightly built woman who had probably been quite pretty before she'd lost so much weight. She smiled readily and somewhat self-consciously, as if she were trying to make her cheeks dimple. She wore a V-necked blouse and a very short skirt that she did not attempt to pull down when she crossed her legs. She spoke with a good deal of rolling of eyes and varying inflections of her voice, but her answers to the examiner's questions were themselves vague and often discursive. She denied feeling depressed or wishing she were dead; she had never had delusions or hallucinations, but she claimed that she was still "fat as a pig." To illustrate, she pinched between thumb and forefinger a fold of skin that hung loosely from her arm. She scored a perfect 30 on the MMSE.

Evaluation of Gemma Livingstone

Gemma had a history of disordered eating that dated back to her high school years. She bore the following features of **anorexia nervosa**: She was gaunt and fearful of gaining weight, and she perceived herself as being fat. Her current subtype would be binge-eating/purging type; as a teenager, she had been of the restricting type. Just how severe do we rate her anorexia? The DSM-5 criteria grade solely on the basis of body mass index (BMI), which is an error, in my opinion; surely the type of behavior should count for something. Gemma's weight is under 90 (let's say 89), so for a height of 66 inches, her BMI works out to 14.4, putting her in the *extreme* category of severity.

Based only on the information she herself provided, Gemma could not have been diagnosed with a **personality disorder**—that's our usual clinical experience derived solely from a patient's own reports. But from her husband's information (principle I) and from that of the mental status evaluation (principle L), the following criteria for **histrionic personality disorder** were established: needing to be the center of attention, shifting and shallow emotions, drawing attention to herself (wearing revealing clothing and crossing her legs), speaking vaguely, and expressing herself dramatically. Histrionic personality disorder is often associated with **somatization/somatic symptom disorder**, but a review of systems revealed minimal symptoms, and she didn't express the disproportionate health concerns normally attached to a somatic symptom diagnosis.

Forging prescriptions and using drugs are of course illegal, but Gemma hadn't pursued either behavior after her probation; I certainly wouldn't regard them as evidence of diagnosable pathology. With a GAF score of 45, her complete diagnosis would read as follows:

F50.02 [307.1]	Anorexia nervosa, binge-eating/purging type, extreme
F60.4 [301.50]	Histrionic personality disorder

Edith Roman

Seventy-six year-old Edith Roman entered the hospital on the complaint of Sylvia, her daughter: "She's been depressed since her stroke." Beginning about a year earlier, Edith had become forgetful. This first became apparent when for 3 weeks out of 4 she neglected to place her Friday night telephone call to Sylvia, who at that time lived several hundred miles away. Each time her daughter called instead, and Edith seemed surprised to get the call.

When she finally took a week off work for a visit, Sylvia discovered that Edith had also been neglecting the marketing and housecleaning: The sink was full and the refrigerator was nearly empty, and dust blanketed everything. Although Edith's speech and physical appearance hadn't changed, something was clearly wrong. By the end of the week, Sylvia had the answer from a neurologist: early Alzheimer's disease. She took an extra week off work to move her mother across the state and into her own home. A companion was hired to stay with Edith during the day, when Sylvia was absent.

This arrangement worked well for several months. Edith's deterioration was gradual and minimal, until the stroke left her limping and unable to remember words. Now her memory was worse than ever, and this was when the depression began. When Edith talked at all, she complained to the companion about how useless and lonely she felt. She slept poorly, ate very little, cried often, and said she was a burden.

Edith had been born in St. Louis, where until she was 12, her parents had run a small dry-cleaning business. Then her father died and her mother soon married Edith's paternal uncle, who came equipped with two teenagers of his own. They all got along quite well, and Edith graduated from high school, got married, and had her only child.

Throughout life, she had been pleasant and spunky, interested in crafts and many other aspects of homemaking. After her husband died, she continued to be active in her social and bridge clubs. Until a year ago, her physical health had been good; she had never used alcohol or tobacco.

An elderly woman dressed in a cotton nightgown and a quilted wrap, Edith sat upright on the edge of her bed, her useless left hand lying in her lap. She made good eye contact with the examiner; although she did not speak spontaneously, she did respond to all questions. Her speech was clear, but she sometimes had difficulty finding the words she wanted. Asked to identify a magazine, she thought for a moment and called it "this papers." She admitted feeling depressed, said that she saw no future for herself, and hoped she could die soon. She denied ever experiencing hallucinations or delusions. On the MMSE, she scored only 16 out of a possible 30.

Evaluation of Edith Roman

The symptoms of Edith's **major neurocognitive disorder** included failing memory and deteriorating ability to care for herself (p. 492). These symptoms, consistent with **Alzheimer's disease** (p. 498), had begun gradually and were gradually worsening when she had her stroke. At that point, her memory abruptly worsened further, and she developed aphasia (she couldn't think of certain words she wanted to use). She maintained eye contact and appeared to focus her attention on the examiner—evidence against **delirium**. A neurological exam earlier had not found evidence of other **medical conditions** that might better explain her symptoms.

For far longer than 2 weeks, Edith had also had symptoms of depression. These included constantly depressed mood, loss of appetite and sleep, death wishes, and the feeling of being a burden (more or less equivalent to a sense of worthlessness). Her symptoms would seem to qualify for **major depressive episode**, which we should diagnose whenever relevant, despite the presence of other disorders (principles F, V). However, because of the presumed etiology (that is, her Alzheimer's disease), we will list her disorder as **depressive disorder due to another medical condition**. The exact wording for this diagnosis appears below, to which we add verbiage indicating that her symptoms are those of a major depressive episode.

Edith's dementia had two causes, each of which had created difficulties with communication and with everyday functioning for her and her daughter. This would fulfill the criteria for **major neurocognitive disorder due to multiple etiologies**, which is not really a diagnosis. Instead, it is a reminder that we can record a single set of codes for the dementia, but a separate code for each cause of dementia (p. 526). (An exception exists for vascular disease, which requires its own code.) Her depressive symptoms rate the specifier *with behavioral disturbance*. Her GAF score would be 31.

A funny thing happened on the way to Edith Roman's diagnosis: It got tangled in a DSM-5 contradiction. The criteria for probable Alzheimer's dementia (see DSM-5, p. 611) state that there must be no evidence of mixed etiology; they give the example of cerebrovascular disease. The criteria for major or mild neurocognitive disorder due to multiple etiologies (see DSM-5, p. 642) give as an example Alzheimer's plus cerebrovascular disease. Not to worry; we'll do what's best for the patient and give both diagnoses anyway. Anyone want to complain? See me after class.

G30.9 [331.0]	Alzheimer's disease
F02.81 [294.11]	Major neurocognitive disorder due to multiple etiologies, with behavioral disturbance
F01.51 [290.40]	Major vascular neurocognitive disorder, with behavioral disturbance
F06.32 [293.83]	Depressive disorder due to major neurocognitive disorder, with major depressive-like episode

Clara Widdicombe

Clara Widdicombe had been overweight for a long time, but now, age 14, she was round-faced and puffy. For all that, she seemed to have been progressing normally through both school and puberty, until one evening when she suddenly began talking, according to her mother, "a blue streak." She insisted that her parents stay up with her to talk about "my agenda." At first, her mood seemed high, but she became angry when her father said he wanted to go to bed. Within hours, Clara became so agitated that she required hospitalization on a closed ward for adults.

Clara stood 5 feet, 3 inches tall and weighed 211 pounds, which gave her a BMI of 37—well exceeding the level considered obese. Her blood pressure was consistently above 230/110. When she undressed, the hospital staff could see that the skin of her abdomen bore reddened stretch marks (called *striae*) caused by her weight gain.

For the next several days, Clara's mood was elevated, and she needed little sleep. Even when interrupted, she wouldn't stop talking longer than a few moments. Over and over, she claimed to be the mother of Jesus; she'd divined the solution to many problems—AIDS, sin, and global warming. She had flight of ideas, and she even admitted that her thoughts were racing. It was impossible to interrupt her longer than a moment, and hard to get her attention at all. At one point, she undressed right in front of her several visitors—immodest behavior that was completely out of character for her.

Clara had no previous personal history of depression or mania, and her family history was negative for mood disorder. What she did have was an abnormal serum cortisol level. An endocrinologist recommended an MRI, which revealed a pituitary adenoma. After it was surgically removed, she no longer required psychotropic medications. She became euthymic and returned to school.

Evaluation of Clara Widdicombe

Of course, after a successful operation that yields the desired outcome, it's pretty easy to attribute mood symptoms to a tumor. The trick is to make the connection before too many months or years have elapsed. Clara's age at onset (young for bipolar disorder), her appearance (typical "moon" face, marked overweight, classical abdominal striations) were diagnostic giveaways. Other patients have been less fortunate.

For a week Clara was ill. She was in turns euphoric and irritable, *and* she had increased activity (both required for manic episode criterion A). (Note that although she had several other symptoms of mania—she spoke rapidly, needed little sleep, was grandiose, and was even delusional in that she thought she was Jesus's mother—a full symptom list isn't required for the diagnosis of an induced bipolar condition.) Although we might infer from her inability to connect with other people that she was distractible, there isn't enough detail here to diagnose delirium (D). As far as the severity of her symptoms, she suffered from all three consequences mentioned in criterion E: psychosis, hospitalization, and impaired functioning.

Finally, I don't see evidence of another mental disorder (C)—do you? High on the list of her differential diagnoses would be **bipolar I disorder**, but that would require that other **medical conditions** and **substance-induced mood disorders** be ruled out first. And this brings us back to her pituitary tumor and Cushing's syndrome, which are well known to produce manic symptoms (B). On admission, I'd give her a GAF score of 25.

Once the final diagnosis was made, her clinicians would have to determine which (if any) of the possible specifiers she had. A handful of other medical conditions can produce symptoms of mania (see the chart in Appendix A).

D35.2 [227.3]	Pituitary adenoma
E24.9 [255.0]	Cushing's syndrome
F06.33 [293.83]	Bipolar disorder due to Cushing's syndrome, with manic-like episode

> Clara's is a somewhat unusual case, in that it fully meets the DSM-5 symptomatic requirements for manic episode. That's unusual? Probably, in that most patients in my experience have the euphoria (irritability) and overactivity, but may come up short when you look for the other qualifying symptoms—grandiosity, decreased need for sleep, pressure of speech, flight of ideas, distractibility, and frenetic rushing from one activity to the next. Using ICD-10, we can now differentiate a Clara-type episode from those that don't fully meet manic episode criteria—and depressions that do meet full symptomatic criteria for major depressive episode from those that don't. Another benefit courtesy of the international community.

Jeremy Dowling

"I feel miserable," was the chief complaint of Jeremy Dowling, a 24-year-old graduate student. For a lifelong perfectionist, a thesis deadline a fortnight off wasn't improving matters. He was weeks behind schedule, partly because he needed to perfect every paragraph before he began to write the next.

Most of the time since his teen years, he had felt "not good enough" and somewhat depressed. He had never had a manic episode. He was socially withdrawn and claimed never to take much pleasure in things. "I'm a pessimist, more or less," he said.

Jeremy described his appetite as being fine, and he had never had suicidal ideas. His sleep, however, was another matter. With the approaching thesis deadline, he felt that he had to stay up most nights in order to do his work. Therefore, he drank lots of coffee. "If I have to sleep less than 8 hours a night, I drink a cup every 2 or 3 hours. When I'm up all night, it's four or five cups. Strong coffee." Other than coffee, Jeremy denied ever misusing substances such as alcohol or street drugs. Lately, Jeremy had stayed up all night three nights a week; he always felt tired. He also admitted to chronic feelings of guilt and irritability. He had never had crying spells, but his concentration was "a lifelong major problem." For example, while he was working at the computer, other thoughts and worries intruded upon his consciousness, to the point that he had difficulty getting his work done.

Jeremy also complained of anxiety. Toward the end of supper, for example, he would begin to worry about the amount of work he had to do. A knot would tighten in his stomach, and the world would seem to be closing in. Time of day made little difference to how he felt, but he would usually improve briefly once he turned in a term paper or other major assignment. He denied ever having problems with shortness of breath, muscle twitching, or palpitations of his heart, unless he had had an extraordinarily large amount of coffee. At those times, he also would notice that he felt nervous and often had an upset stomach, sometimes to the point that he had to stay home from class. He denied feelings of impending doom or disaster.

Though Jeremy had always been a list maker, he didn't describe any obsessional thinking or compulsive behavior. ("I do sometimes straighten out my sock drawer," he was careful to point out.) He described himself as a person who had always had difficulty making decisions, even to the point that he couldn't discard worthless things that he no longer needed—an Easter basket from when he was 10 was one example.

Jeremy had been born in Brazil, where his father had been studying insects of the rain forests. The family returned to live in southern California when Jeremy was 4. His mother was a professional harpist; she had been in therapy with one counselor or another for 25 years. She had always been somewhat dour and had never gotten much pleasure out of life. When Jeremy was 16, she had obtained a divorce, because she had never felt that her husband was committed to their relationship. After the divorce, she had changed to such an extent that she had finally consented to take an antidepressant medication. It had "turned her life around," and now she was happy for the first time in her life. It was partly at her urging that Jeremy was now seeking treatment.

Several maternal relatives had had depression, including a cousin who'd killed himself by drinking antifreeze. Another relative had also committed suicide, but Jeremy didn't know the details.

When Jeremy was in high school, he had been "born again"; since then he had attended a fundamentalist church. He so strongly condemned his father for living with another woman without marrying her that for over 2 years, father and son hadn't spoken. Jeremy's only physical problem was that he bit his nails. He had never had any legal difficulties. He had a serious girlfriend, and they were "trying very hard" to refrain from overcommitting themselves sexually until they got married.

Jeremy was a tall, rather gangling man whose haggard face and baggy eyes made him look almost aged. Although he moved normally and smiled readily, prominent worry lines were emerging on his forehead. His speech was clear, coherent, relevant, and spontaneous. When he talked spontaneously, it was largely to discuss his concerns about getting his thesis done; he denied any death wishes or suicidal ideas. He was fully oriented, had an excellent fund of information, and could do calculations quickly. His recent and remote memory were unimpaired; his insight and judgment seemed excellent: "Life is too meaningful, and I'm wasting it."

Evaluation of Jeremy Dowling

In evaluating any mood disorder, the first business at hand is to determine whether either a **major depressive episode** or a **manic episode** has been present. Jeremy came close to satisfying criteria for the former: He had been "somewhat depressed" for a long time, perhaps most of his adult life. The depression was present most of the time, and he never took much pleasure in things; He felt chronically guilty and had poor concentration and low self-esteem. However, from history and direct observation he had had no problems with appetite or weight, suicidal ideas, or level of psychomotor activity. Although he did complain of fatigue, this symptom appeared related to his coffee drinking. His family history was strongly positive for a mood disorder (his mother had been depressed, and two relatives had committed suicide).

Jeremy had four symptoms (five required) of major depressive episode, and two symptoms (two required) of **persistent depressive disorder**, or **dysthymia** for short. So we have to ask: Is it reasonable to insist that a patient exactly fulfill the criteria? After all, Jeremy nearly met criteria for major depressive episode, and his family history was strongly positive. A diagnosis of **major depressive disorder** would point the way to treatment and alert clinicians to possible worsening symptoms (such as suicidal ideas) later on. But this clinician felt that it was more important to emphasize the prolonged course of Jeremy's symptoms, which seemed almost to shade into his **personality disorder** (see below). Dysthymia often sets the stage for later major depressive disorder, and the DSM-5 criteria have blended them anyway, by explicitly stating that even a full major depressive disorder can be diagnosed as a specifier to dysthymia.

I wouldn't waste a lot of time in argument about this area—where two excellent diagnosticians may disagree forever, and where you can see the benefits of judging a patient not on the basis of (obsessively) counting symptoms but matching to a prototype of an idealized patient. Let's go ahead and give him a diagnosis that will promote possibly effective treatment.

There's also the matter of Jeremy's anxiety symptoms. He had never had actual anxiety attacks, phobias, obsessions, or compulsions. But he'd certainly been anxious, however. He worried about a variety of things—school, his personality, the intensity of his relationship with his girlfriend. He complained of fatigue, troubles with his sleep, and concentration, which would seem (barely) enough to qualify for a diagnosis of **generalized anxiety disorder**. However, these symptoms occurred during the course of a mood disorder, so his clinician felt that no concurrent anxiety diagnosis was needed. (He even failed to meet the criteria for the mood specifier *with anxious distress*; see p. 159). Besides, his anxiety symptoms could be all bound up with his caffeinism, so I'd not add this extra dollop of diagnostic verbiage.

As for substance use, although Jeremy had never used alcohol or street drugs, his coffee use had on many occasions produced nervousness, upset stomach, palpitations, muscle twitching, and insomnia. These were sometimes serious enough that he couldn't go to school; the symptoms would qualify for a diagnosis of **caffeine intoxication**. You might wonder about a diagnosis of **caffeine use disorder**, but this is one that isn't sanctioned by DSM-5. His usage does make one wonder, though.

Finally, self-described as a perfectionistic pessimist who chronically felt he was not good enough, Jeremy was also a maker of lists and a straightener of drawers who had trouble making decisions and couldn't discard things. These features, plus his moralistic condemnation of his father, would be diagnostic of **obsessive–compulsive personality disorder**.

Jeremy's dysthymia appeared to have begun years ago, probably when he was still a teenager. His hypersomnia and increased appetite would qualify him for the specifier *with atypical features* (p. 160), were it not for the fact that I couldn't find any evidence of mood reactivity in the vignette. Maybe we just needed to interview some more. A psychosocial/environmental problem was noted with a Z-code because it could affect management, at least for the next couple of weeks. His GAF score of 65 was assigned on the basis of his combined disorders.

F34.1 [300.4]	Persistent depressive disorder, early onset
F15.929 [305.90]	Caffeine intoxication
F60.5 [301.4]	Obsessive–compulsive personality disorder
Z55.9 [V62.3]	Academic problem (thesis deadline)

Cookie Coates

Cookie Coates was a 23-year-old single woman who was admitted to a mental health unit with the chief complaint of "seeing spiders."

According to the records, the doctor had arrived late for Cookie's birth, which a nurse had tried to hold back by pressure on her head. "I don't know if it would have made any difference, anyway," her mother reportedly told a social worker at the time. "I had measles during my pregnancy."

Whatever the cause, Cookie was slow to develop. She walked at 18 months, spoke words at 2 years, and formed sentences at 3. She was a withdrawn, frightened child who had clung so tightly to her mother that she could not even be left with a babysitter. She didn't begin school until she was nearly 7. With an IQ that hovered in the low 70s, she attended special classes for her first 2 years and was then mainstreamed.

In her early school years, Cookie developed a reputation for biting and kicking other children. When she was 11, she was repeatedly disciplined for stealing (and eating) lunches belonging to other children. At about the same time, she began to pull out her hair. She would usually pull only a few strands at a time from the front of her head, but worked away at it assiduously throughout the day. By the end of the school day, there would be little accumulations of hair all around her desk.

However, it was Cookie's persistent tendency to hurt and mutilate herself that first brought her into mental health care. At 9, she bit her lip until it bled. The following year, she gradually fell into the habit of repeatedly banging her forearms on the edge of a table; this produced chronic swelling and bruising, and eventually a constantly running sore. When she was 13, she cut long troughs in her face with a razor and then rubbed dirt into the wounds, producing permanent, hypertrophic scars.

Several of these episodes prompted admission to mental health facilities. Most of them were for short stays, but once, when she was 16 and had set fire to her pantyhose, she was kept for 4 months. During this admission it was learned that from the age of 7, Cookie had been sexually molested almost weekly by her father and two older brothers. She was subsequently admitted to the first in a series of group homes for persons with developmental disabilities.

Cookie's pattern in each of these facilities was to form an immediate, strong relationship with one or more staff members, especially males. Typically, she would call one of them "Daddy." When a staff member disappointed her (as each inevitably did), she would say that she hated that staffer. Her animosity could last for weeks, during which she would sometimes sulk and say she was depressed, and sometimes lose her temper and throw things in her room. At still other times she would accuse her counselors of conspiring to drive her crazy, so they could return her to the hospital. As she became more familiar with a facility, she would request special privileges (extra food at supper, staying up late) and injure herself in some dramatic way when these were not forthcoming.

Gradually, Cookie began to act out sexually. During parties or other activities with patients from the men's group home, she would lie with her head in the lap of nearly any male patient or run her hand between his thighs. Repeated cautioning and counseling from her own staff counselors did nothing to eliminate this sort of behavior; she only became more cautious about where and when she did it. Also in the various group homes, she was found to eat in binges. Habitually a big eater, now she also ate from the plates of others when they were finished; often she volunteered to clear away the table, even when it was not her turn. None of the staffers who provided information to the admitting clinician was aware of any self-induced vomiting or use of laxatives. And they described her usual activity level as "couch potato."

On admission to the unit, Cookie was an obese woman who wore no makeup and was dressed in a sweatshirt and sweatpants. She fiddled with strands of her hair; although she did not pull any out during the interview, her scalp bore half-dollar-sized patches of near-baldness. She denied feeling a sense of either tension or relief in regard to her hair pulling, and she didn't show any evidence of distress about it. She sat quietly, showing no evidence of abnormal movements, and cooperated with the examiner. She said that she felt "hopeless"; her somewhat flattened mood was generally appropriate to these thoughts. She spoke slowly and did not volunteer information, but she always responded to questions. Her thinking was sequential and goal-oriented, with no evidence of loose associations.

Cookie reported occasionally seeing "showers of spiders" falling from the ventilator in the ceiling of her bedroom. For several years she had intermittently heard voices directing her to harm herself. She usually noticed them when she was unhappy. They were quite clearly audible, were not the voices of anyone she knew, and were located within her own head. Upon close questioning, she agreed that they could be her own thoughts. She did not think anyone else could hear them. She talked freely about the sexual abuse she had suffered from her father and brothers, and described it in graphic (and seemingly accurate) detail. However, she offered no evidence of either reliving or repressing these experiences.

Cookie scored 28 out of 30 on the MMSE (she could remember only two of three objects at 5 minutes, and she missed the correct date by several days). Although she maintained good attention, she could only perform very simple calculations. She recognized that there was something wrong with her, but attributed it to others: her parents and a worker at her previous residence who had "dissed" (disrespected) her by laughing when she said she heard voices. She did not feel that she needed to be in the hospital, and said that she would like to get her own apartment and a job as a waitress.

Evaluation of Cookie Coates

Cookie presented with a wide variety of clinical problems and symptoms, potentially encompassing psychotic, mood, anxiety, impulse-control, eating, and personality disorders, as well as low intellectual functioning.

Let's consider the last factor first. Slow to develop, Cookie consistently had IQ scores that were in the low 70s. She performed well on the MMSE and had no problems with attention, so she would not seem to qualify for **delirium** or a **major or minor neurocognitive disorder**. Her clinician felt that the extent of her deficits (problems with self-care, home living, social/interpersonal skills, self-direction, and safety) warranted a diagnosis of **mild intellectual disability**.

Cookie also reported feeling hopeless and depressed, but these symptoms appeared to be transitory, reactive to her circumstances, and to some extent manipulative. Symptoms of psychosis (seeing spiders, hearing voices) did not carry the conviction of true hallucinations: They often occurred when she was unhappy (principle K), and she noted that the voices could be her own thoughts. She had no loose associations, catatonic behavior, or negative symptoms typical of schizophrenia. In fact, no diagnosis of **psychosis** seemed justified. Although she had **abnormal eating behavior**, she didn't appear distressed about it, and she had no history of vomiting or use of laxatives or diuretics; her self-evaluation did not overemphasize her weight or body shape. One clinician who reviewed the case felt that her history had some of the features of **posttraumatic stress disorder**, but she had no history of reliving the sexual abuse she had endured as a child.

Cookie's acting out included biting, kicking, hair pulling, and stealing, which began when she was about 11. These behaviors did not appear to be part of a larger problem with violating societal norms or the rights of others, ruling out **conduct disorder**. The hair pulling was not associated with stress, and there was no information that she'd tried to stop it, so we wouldn't diagnose **trichotillomania**. Self-injury can be encountered in **stereotypic movement disorder**, but Cookie's behavior did not appear to be repetitive and stereotypical. As a small child, she might have qualified for a diagnosis of **disinhibited social engagement disorder** (because of the excessive readiness to approach strangers), but we don't have information enough for the diagnosis even in retrospect, and it wouldn't appear to be a problem now.

And so, having ruled out major mental disorders as the cause of these behaviors, we can now consider a **personality disorder** (principle W). Indeed, most of her self-destructive behaviors seemed well explained by **borderline personality disorder**. Beginning in her teens and affecting many life areas, the relevant symptoms included self-harm, intense interpersonal relations (those with various staff members), impulsivity (eating, sexual acting out), reactive mood (temper tantrums), and paranoid ideation.

Although Cookie by no means had every symptom of borderline personality disorder, those she did report I'd call severe. Her GAF score of 30 would reflect a composite of all her difficulties.

F70 [317]	Intellectual disability, mild
F60.3 [301.83]	Borderline personality disorder, severe
E66.9 [278.00]	Obesity

Dean Wannamaker

"I keep hearing voices that I can't turn off," said Dean Wannamaker. They bothered him every day, and he wasn't sure how much longer he could stand it. Dean was 54, but he had first heard voices when he was only in his early 40s. In fact, he had been hospitalized on three separate occasions; each time he had been successfully treated with medication. It had now been over 6 years since he was last hospitalized.

"They're in my head, but they sound just as loud and clear as a radio," Dean said. The voices were mostly men, but there were a few women as well; none of them were at all familiar. They spoke only phrases, not sentences, but they tried to order him around. They'd tell him it was time to go home or that it would be OK to have another drink. "Mostly they seemed to be looking out for me." He thought they'd been talking for about 3 weeks this time.

Dean admitted that he was a drinker. He had begun drinking sweet wine when he was only 12. In the military he had had a few fights and was even threatened with court-martial once, but he'd managed to "escape with an honorable discharge." Over the years, he'd been arrested several times for driving while under the influence of alcohol; the most recent time was only 2 weeks ago.

Dean's usual pattern was to drink heavily for several months, then stop suddenly and stay dry for years. His three previous benders had occurred 3, 5, and 11 years earlier. It was during the bender of 11 years ago that his wife walked out on him for good; she was tired of paying his traffic tickets and supporting him when he got fired for missing work. But he had a girlfriend then, Annie—the same woman he was with now—so he didn't mind so much about his wife. What he remembered most vividly was the time he'd heard voices for nearly 3 months. "It was enough to drive a man to drink," he commented, without a trace of irony.

On the present occasion, it was the IRS that had supplied the drive. He made good money at his trade (he was a meat cutter), and, apparently while he was in the coils of his last bender 3 years earlier, he had neglected to report some of it. Now he was being dunned for back taxes, interest, and penalties, and he didn't even have any records.

"I didn't intend to start drinking," he said. "I only meant to take a drink." Now he had been drinking over a quart of bourbon a day for 2 months. Annie added that he "never seemed drunk," and she confirmed that he only had these hallucinations after he'd been drinking for a while.

The middle of three children, Dean had been born in Chicago, where his father worked as a meat salesman. His parents had divorced when he was 9; his mother had remarried twice. In the course of a depression 4 years earlier, his older brother had shot and killed himself. His sister was a nurse who had once been hospitalized for abusing barbiturates.

After the military, Dean had attended 2 years of junior college, but he didn't think it ever did him much good. "I've never been anything more than a big, dumb city slicker who cuts up dead animals for a living," he said.

Annie reported that Dean had been depressed most of the time for the last month and a half—not quite as long as he'd been drinking. He had cried some and slept poorly, often awakening early in the morning, unable to get back to sleep. His appetite had diminished, and he'd lost about 20 pounds. He seemed chronically tired, and his sex interest was diminished except when he was drunk, which was most of the time.

Dean looked closer to 60 than to 54. He had clearly lost weight. He was over 6 feet tall, but his outsized clothes seemed to diminish his size. He slumped quietly in his chair and only spoke when spoken to. His voice was a low monotone, but his speech was relevant and coherent. He was fully alert, and he paid close attention to the conversation. There was very little variation in his mood, which he admitted was depressed. He was fully oriented to time, place, and person; he scored 29 out of 30 on the MMSE, failing only to recall a street address after 5 minutes. He had never had delusions, but neither did he seem to have any insight into the fact that what he heard was not real.

Dean had had some thoughts about dying. They had begun with the depression, and now the voices had jumped on the idea. "They aren't ordering me to do it or anything like that," he said. "They just think I might be a lot better off."

Evaluation of Dean Wannamaker

Here's how I'd analyze this complex history.

To begin with, what were Dean's diagnosable drinking behaviors? Of course, he had a variety of the criteria for **alcohol use disorder** (p. 397): There were social symptoms (divorce, arrests). During the current episode of drinking, he demonstrated tolerance (he didn't appear drunk on a quart per day of hard liquor), continued to drink despite having hallucinations, and used more alcohol than he intended ("I only meant to take a drink"). Even if withdrawal symptoms were not taken into account, he would qualify for a diagnosis of alcohol use disorder. He had been actively drinking within the past month, so he could have no course specifier.

Dean's somatic complaints included appetite and weight loss, reduced libido, and insomnia. These represent three separate DSM-5 categories (eating, sleep–wake, and sexual disorders), and a differential diagnosis could be constructed for each. However, the resulting burden of independent major mental diagnoses would be highly unlikely, from either a statistical or a logical viewpoint (principle M—keep it simple). These somatic complaints can all be found in patients who have depression, psychosis, or alcohol-related disorders. A **mood disorder due to another medical condition** must always be considered, especially in a patient who has been ignoring health needs (principle B). Although we'd need a physical examination and laboratory tests to be certain, no information given in the vignette suggests that Dean had any such medical disorder.

Throughout his later adult life, Dean had intermittently heard voices. A principal concern for any psychotic patient is whether schizophrenia is a possibility. But Dean lacked the A portion of the basic criteria—he heard voices, but that was the only psychotic symptom he had—knocking out **schizophrenia**, as well as **schizophreniform** and **schizoaffective disorders**. He had hallucinations but no other symptoms (OK, his affect was constricted, but I'd chalk that up to the depression). Annie pointed out that he only developed hallucinations subsequent to drinking. The results of his MMSE would rule out **delirium** and a **major or mild neurocognitive disorder**; the history would exclude **psychotic disorder due to another medical condition**. Of course, all other psychotic disorders require that the symptoms not be directly related to the use of a substance. Furthermore, neither **delusional disorder** nor **brief psychotic disorder** can be diagnosed if a mood disorder is a more likely etiology.

Look at the criteria for **substance/medication-induced psychotic disorder** in Chapter 2 (p. 93). These require prominent hallucinations or delusions (or disorganized speech). Inasmuch as Dean always drank before the hallucinations appeared, and they never lasted longer than a few weeks after the drinking stopped, he would seem to fulfill the criteria for alcohol-induced psychotic disorder, with hallucinations. If this became the working diagnosis, we'd add the qualifier *with onset during withdrawal*.

As for mood disorder, Dean fulfilled the inclusion criteria for **major depressive episode**: He had had more than 2 weeks of persistent low mood, fatigue, weight loss, insomnia, and thoughts of suicide. His symptoms weren't due to a medical condition, represented a change from his usual self, and certainly distressed him. However, they did occur subsequent to the time he began drinking, and therefore could be alcohol-related; if so, this would rule out **major depressive disorder**.

The criteria for **substance-induced mood disorder** are simple, and Dean would appear to fulfill them: He was persistently depressed, meeting full criteria for a major depressive disorder; he had also been drinking for several months, and we know that alcohol is fully capable of inducing severe depression. DSM-5 mentions several bits of evidence that would support a non-substance-related depression. Although his brother had shot himself during a depression, we do not know whether he was also a drinker; a sister had used drugs. OK, genetic information isn't a criterion, but it is a useful principle (B).

Major depressive disorder is treatable, and it can be lethal. It should be given a high priority for investigation and possible treatment (principle F). However, it should not be diagnosed automatically in a substance-using patient; many instances of mood disorder will improve when the patient stops using the substance.

Therefore, symptoms of substance use, mood disorder, and psychosis must be accounted for in Dean's final diagnosis. It would not appear that cognitive or general medical conditions can explain these symptoms (principle C). It would be elegant to explain all of them simply, on the basis of one underlying disease mechanism (principle M). Because substance use was surely the first of these symptom groups to appear (principle X)—Dean began drinking at age 12 and had some behavioral problems resulting from it when he was a young man in the military—it is reasonable to consider it first.

Now we have two ways of looking at Dean's symptoms: (1) Alcohol usage induced a psychosis, and he had an independent major depressive disorder; or (2) alcohol usage induced both a psychosis and a mood disorder. The simplicity of the second formulation, plus the desire not to rush in with possibly unnecessary treatment before it is needed, would lead a conservative clinician initially to regard the mood disorder as substance-induced—at least until Dean could be withdrawn completely from alcohol. Under ICD-9, the clinician's perception that the alcoholism was the underlying problem, and thus the one that should be addressed first, would determine the order in which we list the diagnoses. Under ICD-10, where we code the use disorder at the same time as the psychosis or depression, I'd list the psychosis first; it seems to require treatment more urgently. But I'd be happy to entertain arguments. Dean's GAF score would be about 40.

F10.259 [303.90, 291.9]	Severe alcohol use disorder, with alcohol-induced psychotic disorder, with onset during withdrawal
F10.24 [303.90, 291.89]	Alcohol-induced depressive disorder, with onset during intoxication

Essential Tables

Global Assessment of Functioning (GAF)

As you will note, you have to get fairly far down the list (around 50–70) to arrive at a point at which most patients described in this book were awarded a diagnosis. Although we can interpolate between these numbers, trying to interpolate at a finer degree than 5-unit intervals (65, 25, etc.) is probably futile. As you will notice, that hasn't stopped me from trying on some occasions, however.

Global Assessment of Functioning (GAF) Scale

Consider psychological, social, and occupational functioning on a hypothetical continuum of mental health-illness. Do not include impairment in functioning due to physical (or environmental) limitations.

Code (Note: Use intermediate codes when appropriate, e.g., 45, 68, 72.)

100 | 91	**Superior functioning in a wide range of activities, life's problems never seem to get out of hand, is sought out by others because of his or her many positive qualities. No symptoms.**
90 | 81	**Absent or minimal symptoms** (e.g., mild anxiety before an exam**), good functioning in all areas, interested and involved in a wide range of activities. socially effective, generally satisfied with life, no more than everyday problems or concerns** (e.g. an occasional argument with family members).
80 | 71	**If symptoms are present, they are transient and expectable reactions to psychosocial stressors** (e.g., difficulty concentrating after family argument); **no more than slight impairment in social, occupational or school functioning** (e.g., temporarily falling behind in schoolwork).
70 | 61	**Some mild symptoms** (e.g., depressed mood and mild insomnia) **OR some difficulty in social, occupational, or school functioning** (e.g., occasional truancy, or theft within the household), **but generally functioning pretty well, has some meaningful interpersonal relationships.**
60 | 51	**Moderate symptoms** (e.g., flat affect and circumstantial speech, occasional panic attacks) **OR moderate difficulty in social, occupational, or school functioning** (e.g., few friends, conflicts with peers or co-workers).
50 | 41	**Serious symptoms** (e.g., suicidal ideation, severe obsessional rituals, frequent shoplifting) **OR any serious impairment in social, occupational, or school functioning** (e.g., no friends, unable to keep a job).
40 | 31	**Some impairment in reality testing or communication** (e.g., speech is at times illogical, obscure, or irrelevant) **OR major impairment in several areas, such as work or school, family relations, judgment, thinking, or mood** (e.g., depressed man avoids friends, neglects family, and is unable to work; child frequently beats up younger children, is defiant at home, and is failing at school).
30 | 21	**Behavior is considerably influenced by delusions or hallucinations OR serious impairment in communication or judgment** (e.g., sometimes incoherent, acts grossly inappropriately, suicidal preoccupation) **OR inability to function in almost all areas** (e.g., stays in bed all day; no job, home, or friends).
20 | 11	**Some danger of hurting self or others** (e.g., suicide attempts without clear expectation of death; frequently violent; manic excitement) **OR occasionally fails to maintain minimal personal hygiene** (e.g., smears feces) **OR gross impairment in communication** (e.g., largely incoherent or mute).
10 | 1	**Persistent danger of severely hurting self or others** (e.g., recurrent violence) **OR persistent inability to maintain minimal personal hygiene OR serious suicidal act with clear expectation of death.**
0	Inadequate information.

Note. Reprinted by permission from the *Diagnostic and Statistical Manual of Mental Disorders,* 4th ed., text rev. (p. 34), by the American Psychiatric Association, 2000, Washington, DC: Author. Copyright 2000 by the American Psychiatric Association.

Physical Disorders That Affect Mental Diagnosis

Medical disorder	Anx	Depr	Mania	Psych	Delir	Dem	Cata	Pers chg	Erect	Ejac	Sex Pain	Anorg
Cardiovascular												
Anemia	×											
Angina	×											
Aortic aneurysm									×			
Arrhythmia	×				×							
A-V malformation							×					
Congestive heart failure	×				×				×			
Hyperthyroidism	×				×							
Myocardial infarction	×											
Mitral valve prolapse	×											
Paroxysmal atrial tachycardia	×											
Shock	×				×							
Endocrine												
Addison's (adrenal insufficiency)	×	×			×							
Carcinoid tumor	×											
Cushing's disease	×	×	×		×				×			
Diabetes	×								×			×
Hyperparathyroidism							×					
Hyperthyroidism	×	×	×		×				×			
Hypoglycemia	×	×			×	×						
Hypoparathyroidism	×	×										
Hypothyroidism	×	×		×		×		×	×			×
Inappropriate ADH secretion					×							
Klinefelter's syndrome									×			
Menopause	×										×	
Pancreatic tumor		×										
Pheochromocytoma	×											
Premenstrual syndrome	×											
Hyperprolactinemia												×

(cont.)

Note. Key to column heads: Anx, anxiety; Depr, depression; Psych, psychosis; Delir, delirium; Dem, dementia (major neurocognitive disorder); Cata, catatonia symptoms; Pers chng, personality change; Erect, erectile dysfunction; Ejac, ejaculatory dysfunction; Sex pain, sexual pain syndromes (male or female); anorg, anorgasmia.

Physical Disorders That Affect Mental Diagnosis (*cont.*)

Medical disorder	Anx	Depr	Mania	Psych	Delir	Dem	Cata	Pers chg	Erect	Ejac	Sex Pain	Anorg
Infections												
AIDS	×	×	×		×			×				
Brain abscess					×							
Subacute bacterial endocarditis	×											
Systemic infection	×				×							
Urinary tract infection					×							
Vaginitis											×	
Viral infections		×										
Toxicity												
Aminophylline					×							
Antidepressants	×			×	×				×	×		×
Aspirin intolerance	×											
Bromide				×								
Cimetidine					×							
Digitalis					×							
Disulfiram				×	×							
Estrogens									×			
Fluorides							×					
Heavy metals	×	×										
Herbicides									×			
L-dopa					×							
Steroids	×			×								
Theophylline	×											
Metabolic												
Electrolyte imbalance	×				×							
Hepatic disease		×			×	×			×			
Hypercarbia					×							
Hyperventilation	×											
Hypocalcemia	×											
Hypokalemia	×	×										
Hypoxia					×							
Malnutrition		×			×				×			
Porphyria	×							×				
Renal disease	×			×	×				×			

Medical disorder	Anx	Depr	Mania	Psych	Delir	Dem	Cata	Pers chg	Erect	Ejac	Sex Pain	Anorg
Neurological												
Alzheimer's/frontotemporal						×						
Amyotrophic lateral sclerosis						×			×			
Brain tumor	×			×	×	×	×	×				
Cerebellar degeneration						×						
Cerebrovascular accident	×					×			×			
Creutzfeldt-Jakob						×						
Encephalitis	×				×	×	×					
Epilepsy, seizures	×	×			×	×			×			
Extradural hematoma					×							
Head trauma	×				×	×	×	×				
Huntington's	×	×				×			×			
Intracerebral hematoma					×							
Ménière's	×											
Meningitis					×							
Migraine	×											
Multiple sclerosis	×	×	×			×			×	×		
Multi-infarct						×						
Neurosyphilis			×		×	×			×	×		
Normal-pressure hydrocephalus						×						
Parkinson's						×			×			×
Post-anoxia						×						
Progressive supranuclear palsy						×						
Spinal cord disease									×			
Subarachnoid hemorrhage					×		×					
Subdural hematoma					×	×	×					
Transient ischemic attack	×				×							
Wilson's disease	×								×			

(cont.)

Physical Disorders That Affect Mental Diagnosis (*cont.*)

Medical disorder	Anx	Depr	Mania	Psych	Delir	Dem	Cata	Pers chg	Erect	Ejac	Sex Pain	Anorg
Pulmonary												
Asthma	×											
Chronic obstructive lung disease	×				×				×			
Hyperventilation	×											
Pulmonary embolus	×											
Other												
Collagen	×											
Endometriosis											×	
Pelvic disease									×		×	×
Peyronie's disease									×			
Postoperative states					×							
Systemic lupus erythematosus	×	×		×	×			×				
Temporal arteritis	×											
Vitamin deficiency												
B^{12} (pernicious anemia)	×	×				×						
Folic acid						×						
Niacin (pellagra)					×	×						
Thiamin (B^1) (Wernicke's)					×	×						

Classes (or Names) of Medications That Can Cause Mental Disorders

	Anxiety	Mood	Psychosis	Delirium
Analgesics	×	×	×	×
Anesthetics	×	×	×	×
Antianxiety agents		×		
Anticholinergics	×	×	×	
Anticonvulsants	×	×	×	×
Antidepressants	×	×	×	×
Antihistamines	×		×	×
Antihypertensives/ cardiovascular drugs	×	×	×	×
Antimicrobials		×	×	×
Antiparkinsonian agents	×	×	×	×
Antipsychotics	×	×		×
Antiulcer agents		×		
Bronchodilators	×			×
Chemotherapeutic agents			×	
Corticosteroids	×	×	×	×
Disulfiram (Antabuse)		×	×	
Gastrointestinal agents			×	×
Histamine agonists				×
Immunosuppressants				×
Insulin	×			
Interferon	×	×	×	
Lithium	×			
Muscle relaxants		×	×	×
NSAIDs			×	
Oral contraceptives	×	×		
Thyroid replacements	×			

Note. Adapted from Morrison J: *Diagnosis Made Easier* (2nd ed.). New York: Guilford Press, 2014. Copyright 2014 by The Guilford Press. Adapted by permission.

Index

In this index, **boldfaced** numbers denote Essential Features diagnostic material.
Italicized page numbers indicate a definition. The letter *t* after a page number denotes a table.